Ancient and Traditional Foods, Plants, Herbs and Spices used in Diabetes

The use of different foods, herbs and spices to treat or prevent disease has been recorded for thousands of years. Egyptian papyrus, hieroglyphics and ancient texts from the Middle East have described the cultivation and preparations of herbs and botanicals to "cure the sick." There are even older records from China and India. Some ancient scripts describe the use of medicinal plants that have never been seen within European cultures. Indeed, all ancient civilizations have pictorial records of different foods, herbs and spices being used for medical purposes. However, there are fundamental questions pertaining to the scientific evidence for the use of these agents or their extracts in modern medicine.

There have been considerable advances in scientific techniques over the last few decades. These have been used to examine the composition and applications of traditional cures. Modern science has also seen the investigation of herbs, spices and botanicals beyond their traditional usage. For example, plants that have been used for "digestion" or "medical ills" since time immemorial are now being investigated for anticancer properties or their toxicity, using high throughput screening. Techniques also include molecular biology, cellular biochemistry, physiology, endocrinology and even medical imaging. However, much of the material relating to the scientific basis or applications of traditional foods, herbs, spices and botanicals is scattered among various sources. The widespread applicability of foods or botanicals is rarely described and cautionary notes on toxicity are often ignored. This is addressed in *Ancient and Traditional Foods, Plants, Herbs and Spices used in Diabetes*.

Ancient and Traditional Foods, Plants, Herbs and Spices in Human Health

Series Editors

Vinood B. Patel *University of Westminster, London*
Victor R. Preedy *King's College, London*
Rajkumar Rajendram *King Abdulaziz Medical City, Riyadh*

Each volume in the series provides an evidence-based ethos describing the usage and applications of traditional foods and botanicals in human health. The content provides a platform upon which other scientific studies can be based. These may include the extraction or synthesis of active agents, *in vitro* studies, pre-clinical investigations in animals, and clinical trials.

The key benefits of each volume:

- Chapters provide a historical background on the usage of food and plant-based therapies.
- Chapters are based on the results of studies using scientific techniques and methods.
- Presents wide references to other foods, herbs, and botanicals reported to have curative properties.
- Chapters are self-contained, focused toward specific conditions.

Ancient and Traditional Foods, Plants, Herbs and Spices used in Cardiovascular Health and Disease
Edited by Rajkumar Rajendram, Victor R. Preedy, and Vinood B. Patel

Ancient and Traditional Foods, Plants, Herbs and Spices used in Diabetes
Edited by Rajkumar Rajendram, Victor R. Preedy, and Vinood B. Patel

For more information about this series, please visit www.routledge.com/Ancient-and-Traditional-Foods-Plants-Herbs-and-Spices-in-Human-Health/book-series/ATFHSH

Ancient and Traditional Foods, Plants, Herbs and Spices used in Diabetes

Edited by
Rajkumar Rajendram, Victor R. Preedy
and Vinood B. Patel

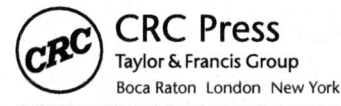

CRC Press
Taylor & Francis Group
Boca Raton London New York

CRC Press is an imprint of the
Taylor & Francis Group, an **informa** business

First edition published 2024
by CRC Press
6000 Broken Sound Parkway NW, Suite 300, Boca Raton, FL 33487-2742

and by CRC Press
4 Park Square, Milton Park, Abingdon, Oxon, OX14 4RN

CRC Press is an imprint of Taylor & Francis Group, LLC

ISBN: 978-1-032-10859-9 (hbk)
ISBN: 978-1-032-11658-7 (pbk)
ISBN: 978-1-003-22093-0 (ebk)

DOI: 10.1201/9781003220930

Typeset in Times
by Apex CoVantage, LLC

Contents

SECTION I Overviews and Dietary Components

SECTION II Specific Agents, Items and Extracts

SECTION III Resources

Editors

Rajkumar Rajendram, AKC, BSc (Hons), MBBS (Dist), MRCP (UK), FRCA, EDIC, FFICM, is a clinician scientist with a focus on internal medicine, anesthesia, intensive care and peri-operative medicine. His interest in traditional medicines began at medical school when he attended the Society of Apothecaries' history of medicine course. He subsequently graduated with distinctions from Guy's, King's and St. Thomas Medical School, King's College London in 2001. As an undergraduate he was awarded several prizes, merits and distinctions in preclinical and clinical subjects. He completed his specialist training in acute and general medicine in Oxford in 2010 and then practiced as a consultant in acute general medicine at the John Radcliffe Hospital, Oxford. He also trained in anesthesia and intensive care in London and was awarded fellowships of the Royal College of Anaesthetists (FRCA) in 2009 and the Faculty of Intensive Care Medicine (FFICM) in 2013. He then moved to the Royal Free London Hospitals as a consultant in intensive care, anesthesia and peri-operative medicine. He has been a fellow of the Royal College of Physicians of Edinburgh (FRCP Edin) since 2017 and the Royal College of Physicians of London (FRCP Lond) since 2019. He is currently a Consultant in Internal Medicine at King Abdulaziz Medical City, National Guard Health Affairs, Riyadh, Saudi Arabia. He recognizes that integration of traditional medicines into modern paradigms for healthcare can significantly benefit patients. As a clinician scientist, he has therefore devoted significant time and effort to nutritional science research and education. He is an affiliated member of the Nutritional Sciences Research Division of King's College London and has published over 300 textbook chapters, review articles, peer-reviewed papers and abstracts.

Victor R. Preedy, BSc, PhD, DSc, FRSB, FRSPH, FRCPath, FRSC, is a staff member of the Faculty of Life Sciences and Medicine within King's College London. He is also a member of the Department of Nutrition and Dietetics (teaching), Director of the Genomics Centre of King's College London and Professor of Clinical Biochemistry (Hon) at Kings College Hospital. He graduated in 1974 with an Honours Degree in biology and physiology with pharmacology. He gained his University of London PhD in 1981. In 1992, he received his Membership of the Royal College of Pathologists and in 1993 he attained his second doctorate (DSc) for his outstanding contribution to protein metabolism in health and disease. He was elected as a Fellow to the Institute of Biology in 1995 and to the Royal College of Pathologists in 2000. Since then he has been elected as a Fellow to the Royal Society for the Promotion of Health (2004) and The Royal Institute of Public Health (2004). In 2009, Professor Preedy became a Fellow of the Royal Society for Public Health and in 2012 a Fellow of the Royal Society of Chemistry. He has carried out research when attached to Imperial College London, The School of Pharmacy (now part of University College London) and the MRC Centre at Northwick Park Hospital. He has collaborated with research groups in Finland, Japan, Australia, the United States and Germany. Professor Preedy is a leading expert on the science of health and has a long-standing interest in dietary and plant-based components. He has lectured nationally and internationally. He has published over 700 articles that include peer-reviewed manuscripts based on original research, abstracts and symposium presentations, reviews, and numerous books and volumes.

Vinood B. Patel, BSc, PhD, FRSC, is currently Reader in Clinical Biochemistry at the University of Westminster and honorary fellow at King's College London. He directs studies on metabolic pathways involved in liver disease, particularly related to mitochondrial energy regulation and cell death. Research is being undertaken to study the role of nutrients, antioxidants, phytochemicals, iron, alcohol and fatty acids in the pathophysiology of liver disease. Other areas of interest are identifying new biomarkers that can be used for the diagnosis and prognosis of liver disease and understanding mitochondrial oxidative stress in Alzheimer disease and gastrointestinal dysfunction in autism. He graduated from the University of Portsmouth with a degree in pharmacology and completed his PhD in protein metabolism from King's College London in 1997. His postdoctoral work was carried out at Wake Forest University Baptist Medical School studying structural-functional alterations to mitochondrial ribosomes, where he developed novel techniques to characterize their biophysical properties. He is a nationally and internationally recognized researcher and has several edited biomedical books related to the use or investigation of active agents or components. These books include *The Handbook of Nutrition, Diet, and Epigenetics; Branched Chain Amino Acids in Clinical Nutrition; Cancer: Oxidative Stress and Dietary Antioxidants; Diet Quality: An Evidence-Based Approach; Toxicology: Oxidative Stress and Dietary Antioxidants;* and *Molecular Nutrition: Vitamins.* In 2014, he was elected as a Fellow to The Royal Society of Chemistry.

Contributors

Sarah M. Abdel Aziz
Beni-Suef University
Beni-Suef, Egypt

Mohammed Abdel-Gabbar
Beni-Suef University
Beni-Suef, Egypt

Reem Fawaz Abutayeh
Applied Science Private University
Amman, Jordan

Snezana Agatonovic-Kustrin
La Trobe University
Bendigo, Australia
I.M. Sechenov First Moscow State Medical
    University
Moscow, Russia

Osama Mohamed Ahmed
Beni-Suef University
Beni-Suef, Egypt

Shaza H. Aly
Badr University in Cairo
Cairo, Egypt

Ehsan Amiri Ardakani
Shiraz University of Medical Sciences
Shiraz, Iran

Vahid Reza Askari
Mashhad University of Medical Sciences
Mashhad, Iran

Anoja Priyadarshani Attanayake
University of Ruhuna
Galle, Sri Lanka

Ana Barabash
Hospital Clínico Universitario San Carlos
    and Instituto de Investigación Sanitaria del
    Hospital Clínico San Carlos (IdISSC)
Centro de Investigación Biomédica en Red
    de Diabetes y Enfermedades Metabólicas
    Asociadas (CIBERDEM)
Universidad Complutense de Madrid
Madrid, Spain

Manjusha Borde
YMT Dental College and Hospital
Navi Mumbai, India

Lynda Bourebaba
Wrocław University of Environmental and Life
    Sciences
Wrocław, Poland

Nabila Bourebaba
Wrocław University of Environmental and Life
    Sciences
Wrocław, Poland

Alfonso L. Calle-Pascual
Hospital Clínico Universitario San Carlos
    and Instituto de Investigación Sanitaria del
    Hospital Clínico San Carlos (IdISSC)
Centro de Investigación Biomédica en Red
    de Diabetes y Enfermedades Metabólicas
    Asociadas (CIBERDEM)
Universidad Complutense de Madrid
Madrid, Spain

Sze Wa Chan
Caritas Institute of Higher Education
Hong Kong SAR, China

Raushan Kumar Chaudhary
NGSM Institute of Pharmaceutical
    Sciences
Mangaluru, India

Matthew James Cheesman
Griffith University
Gold Coast, Australia

Bula Choudhury
IIT Guwahati
Guwahati, India

Ian Edwin Cock
Griffith University
Nathan, Australia

Patricia Daliu
Albanian University
Tirane, Albania

Safa Daoud
Applied Science Private University
Amman, Jordan

Shivsharan Dhadde
Shree Santkrupa College of Pharmacy
Ghogaon, India

Sharanbasappa Durg
Independent Researcher
Bidar, India

Heba A.S. El-Nashar
Ain Shams University
Cairo, Egypt

Omayma A. Eldahshan
Ain Shams University
Cairo, Egypt

Sanaa M. Abd El-Twab
Beni-Suef University
Beni-Suef, Egypt

Ochuko L. Erukainure
University of the Free State
Bloemfontein, South Africa

Madiwalayya S. Ganachari
KLE Academy of Higher Education & Research
Belagavi, India

Daniel Gyamfi
The Doctors Laboratory Ltd
London, UK

Debarupa Hajra
University of Calcutta
Kolkata, India

Lucian Hritcu
Alexandru Ioan Cuza University of Iasi
Iasi, Romania

Md. Shahidul Islam
University of KwaZulu-Natal
Durban, South Africa

Pavithra L. Jayatilake
University of Sri Jayewardenepura
Nugegoda, Sri Lanka

Inés Jiménez
Hospital Clínico Universitario San Carlos
and Instituto de Investigación Sanitaria del
Hospital Clínico San Carlos (IdISSC)
Madrid, Spain

Felipe Jiménez-Aspee
University of Hohenheim
Stuttgart, Germany

B. Jyotirmayee
Centurion University of Technology and
Management
Odisha, India

Pukar Khanal
NGSM Institute of Pharmaceutical Sciences
Mangaluru, India

Selvaa Kumar C
D Y Patil Deemed to be University
Navi Mumbai, India

Abinash Kumar
Karunya Institute of Technology and
Sciences
Coimbatore, India

Pema Lhamo
Karunya Institute of Technology and
Sciences
Coimbatore, India

Hui-Kang Liu
National Research Institute of Chinese
Medicine (NRICM), Ministry of Health and
Welfare
Taipei, Taiwan, Republic of China

Gyanranjan Mahalik
Centurion University of Technology and
Management
Odisha, India

Biswanath Mahanty
Karunya Institute of Technology and Sciences
Coimbatore, India

Asma Ismail Mahmod
Applied Science Private University
Amman, Jordan

Ushashee Mandal
Centurion University of Technology and
  Management
Odisha, India

Krzysztof Marycz
Wrocław University of Environmental and Life
  Sciences
Wrocław, Poland

Verónica Melero
Hospital Clínico Universitario San Carlos
  and Instituto de Investigación Sanitaria del
  Hospital Clínico San Carlos (IdISSC)
Madrid, Spain

Almahi I. Mohamed
University of KwaZulu-Natal
Durban, South Africa

Ipseeta Ray Mohanty
MGM Medical College
Navi Mumbai, India

David W. Morton
La Trobe University
Bendigo, Australia

Helani Munasinghe
University of Sri Jayewardenepura
Nugegoda, Sri Lanka

Leena Omer
Applied Science Private University
Amman, Jordan

Davoud Babazadeh Ortakand
La Trobe University
Bendigo, Australia

Vinood B. Patel
University of Westminster
London, UK

Santanu Paul
University of Calcutta
Kolkata, India

Victor R. Preedy
King's College London
London, UK

Vafa Baradaran Rahimi
Mashhad University of Medical
  Sciences
Mashhad, Iran

Pouria Rahmanian-Devin
Mashhad University of Medical
  Sciences
Mashhad, Iran

Rajkumar Rajendram
King Abdullah International Medical Research
  Center
Riyadh, Saudi Arabia

Antonello Santini
University of Napoli Federico II
Napoli, Italy

Neelima Satrasala
Vasavi Institute of Pharmaceutical Sciences
Kadapa, India

Wamidh H. Talib
Applied Science Private University
Amman, Jordan

Samar Thiab
Applied Science Private University
Amman, Jordan

Brian Tomlinson
Macau University of Science and
  Technology
Macau, China

Nuria García de la Torre
Hospital Clínico Universitario San Carlos
  and Instituto de Investigación Sanitaria del
  Hospital Clínico San Carlos (IdISSC)
Centro de Investigación Biomédica en Red
  de Diabetes y Enfermedades Metabólicas
  Asociadas (CIBERDEM)
Madrid, Spain

Keng-Chang Tsai
National Research Institute of Chinese
  Medicine (NRICM), Ministry of Health and
  Welfare
Taipei, Taiwan, Republic of China

Johanna J. Valerio
Hospital Clínico Universitario San Carlos
    and Instituto de Investigación Sanitaria del
    Hospital Clínico San Carlos (IdISSC)
Madrid, Spain

Laura del Valle
Hospital Clínico Universitario San Carlos
    and Instituto de Investigación Sanitaria del
    Hospital Clínico San Carlos (IdISSC)
Madrid, Spain

Keddagoda Gamage Piyumi Wasana
University of Ruhuna
Galle, Sri Lanka

Asmaa S. Zaky
Beni-Suef University
Beni-Suef, Egypt

Section I

Overviews and Dietary Components

1 Gestational Diabetes Mellitus and Mediterranean Diet

Nuria García de la Torre, Ana Barabash, Johanna Valerio, Laura del Valle, Verónica Melero, Inés Jiménez and Alfonso Calle-Pascual

CONTENTS

ABBREVIATIONS

ADA	American Diabetes Association
BMI	body mass index
CMFO	composite of maternofetal outcomes
CXCR	CX chemokine receptor
ENA78	epithelial neutrophil activating peptide-78
EVOO	extra virgin olive oil
FFQ	food frequency questionnaire
GDM	gestational diabetes mellitus
GW	gestational week
GWG	gestational weight gain
HOMA-IR	homeostatic model assessment insulin resistance
hs-CRP	high-sensitivity C-reactive protein
IADPSG	International Association of Diabetes and Pregnancy Study Groups
IFN-γ	interferon-γ
IL-1β, IL-6, IL-8	interleukin-1β, interleukin-6, interleukin-8
LGA	large for gestational age
MCP-1	monocyte chemoattractant protein-1
MDS	Mediterranean Diet Score
MedDiet	Mediterranean diet
MIP-1β	macrophage inflammatory protein-1
MiRNAs	micro-RNAs

DOI: 10.1201/9781003220930-2

MNT	medical nutritional therapy
RCT	randomized controlled trial
SGA	small for gestational age
SNPs	single nucleotide polymorphisms
TCF7L2	transcription factor 7 like 2
TNF-α	tumor necrosis factor-α
T2DM	type 2 diabetes mellitus

1.1   BACKGROUND

Gestational diabetes mellitus (GDM) is defined as "diabetes diagnosed in the second or third trimester of pregnancy that is not clearly overt diabetes." GDM is associated with important risks to both the mother and the baby in the short and long term. For the mother, these include an increased risk of undergoing a cesarean section, preeclampsia, prematurity, and the development of type 2 diabetes mellitus (T2DM) later in life (Metzger et al. 2008; Bellamy et al. 2009); for the offspring, macrosomia, shoulder dystocia, hyperbilirubinemia, neonatal hypoglycemia, respiratory distress syndrome, large and small for gestational age (LGA and SGA, respectively), intrauterine growth retardation, and obesity with insulin resistance in young adulthood (Metzger et al. 2008; Scholtens et al. 2019; Lowe et al. 2019). In light of this health and economic burden and the increasing incidence reflecting the rising prevalence of obesity and delaying age of maternity, measures that prevent or reduce the risk of developing GDM need to be identified.

In this chapter we review the evidence supporting adherence to the Mediterranean diet (MedDiet) for GDM prevention and treatment and the potential mechanisms involved in its beneficial effects.

1.2   GESTATIONAL DIABETES MELLITUS PREVENTION WITH NUTRITIONAL INTERVENTION

The relationship between maternal body mass index (BMI) and risk of GDM is well described, but randomized controlled trials (RCTs) including overweight and obese women at high risk of GDM have not been able to consistently demonstrate that nutritional interventions are able to reduce GDM risk.

In a study in the United States aimed to detect gestational weight gain as the primary outcome, 257 pregnant women with obesity were randomly assigned to receive either conventional management or an active nutritional and behavioral intervention from 12 weeks of gestation (Thornton et al. 2009). Those in the intervention arm gained significantly less weight (5.0 ± 6.8 kg vs. 14.1 ± 7.3 kg; $p < 0.001$) and there was a significant decrease in the incidence of GDM in the subgroup of women with high adherence to the program within the intervention arm (4% vs. 19%, $p < 0.01$). In a trial led in Australia with a reduction in GDM incidence as the primary outcome, 132 pregnant women who were overweight or obese were randomly assigned to either a multidisciplinary antenatal care approach (obstetrician, food technician, and a clinical psychologist) or to routine antenatal care (Quinlivan et al. 2011). The intervention was associated with significant reductions in mean gestational weight gain (GWG) (7.0 ± 0.65 kg vs. 13.8 ± 0.67 kg, $p < 0.001$) and an 83% reduction in GDM incidence (95% CI [0.03, 0.95]). The RADIEL study conducted in Finland included 293 high-risk women with a history of GDM and/or obesity that were randomly allocated to the intervention group or the control group before the 20th gestational week (GW) (Koivusalo et al. 2016). Subjects in the intervention group received individualized counseling on diet, physical activity, and weight control from trained nurses and had one group meeting with a dietician. The control group received standard antenatal care. The incidence of GDM was 13.9% in the intervention group and 21.6% in the control group (95% CI [0.40, 0.98]) and GWG was lower in the intervention group (20.58 kg, 95% CI [21.12, 20.04]). In the DALI study, 150 pregnant women with a BMI ≥ 29 kg/m^2 from nine European countries were allocated to healthy eating, physical activity, or both (Simmons et al. 2015). Women received face-to-face and telephone coaching sessions. Healthy eating was associated with less GWG (−2.6 kg, 95% CI [−4.9, −0.2], $p = 0.03$) and lower fasting glucose (−0.3 mmol/L, 95% CI [−0.4, −0.1], $p = 0.01$) than those in the physical activity group at 24–28 weeks, with no difference in GDM incidence. Nevertheless, intervention started late in pregnancy (women were included before 20 GWs).

More recently, this protective effect of lifestyle intervention on GDM risk has been shown also in non-obese women. A Chinese study including 281 women allocated in the first trimester of gestation to the intervention arm who received individually modified education on diet and physical activity or to the control group demonstrated that intervention was associated with a lower risk of GDM (OR 0.45, 95% CI [0.22, 0.86], $p < 0.01$) (Lin et al. 2020). In this study all women had at least one risk factor of GDM, but pre-pregnancy BMI were 25.4 ± 3.4 kg/m^2 and 25.9 ± 3.7 kg/m^2.

However, the UPBEAT trial conducted in the UK yielded conflicting results (Poston et al. 2015). This trial assessed the effect of an intense behavior change intervention in 1555 obese pregnant on adverse pregnancy and perinatal outcomes. The intervention was effective in reducing dietary intake of total energy, total fat, saturated fat, and carbohydrates, as well as achieving a diet with a lower glycemic load and index, and increasing protein and fiber intake, but it did not have an effect on the primary outcomes of GDM or LGA neonates. But again, participants in the intervention arm attended the sessions from approximately 19 GWs. The LIMIT trial, performed in women with a BMI ≥ 25kg/m^2 (Dodd et al. 2014), and the NELLY study (Luoto et al. 2011), including women with at least one GDM risk factor (BMI ≥ 25 kg/m^2, glucose intolerance or newborn macrosomia [≥ 4,500 g] in any earlier pregnancy, family history of diabetes, age ≥ 40 years) did not find a reduction in GDM incidence. This heterogeneity could be explained by differences in the characteristics of the study sample, duration, and type of nutritional intervention and when it was initiated. Negative studies based their recommendations on restriction of saturated fats and consumption of carbohydrates with a low glycemic index. However, none of the dietary recommendations provided in these interventions was founded in MedDiet principles rich in extra virgin olive oil (EVOO) and nuts.

1.3 GESTATIONAL DIABETES MELLITUS PREVENTION WITH MEDITERRANEAN DIET

Most studies assessing the effect of a MedDiet on GDM incidence consist of cohort and case-control studies (Table 1.1). To the best of our knowledge, only two RCTs have analyzed the effect of an intervention based on a MedDiet on prevention of GDM to date: the St. Carlos GDM Prevention Study and the ESTEEM study.

In the St. Carlos GDM Prevention Study, 1000 women were randomized in the first trimester of gestation to an intervention group with MedDiet supplemented with EVOO and nuts, or to a control group that followed the standard guidelines in pregnancy (restricted consumption of dietary fat, including EVOO and nuts) (Assaf-Balut et al. 2017). A total of 874 women reached the final analysis. GDM was diagnosed in 23.4% women in the control group and in 17.1% in the intervention group ($p = 0.012$). The crude relative risk for GDM was 0.73 (95% CI [0.56 ± 0.95], $p = 0.020$) and persisted after adjusted multivariable analysis (RR 0.75, 95% CI [0.57 ± 0.98], $p = 0.039$). In addition, an improvement on several maternal and neonatal outcomes was observed: significant reduction in rates of insulin-treated GDM, prematurity, GWG at 24 ± 28 and 36 ± 38 GWs, emergency cesarean section, perineal trauma, and SGA and LGA newborns (all $p < 0.05$). Next, in order to assess its translational effects in the real world our group also evaluated the effect of the MedDiet from the first gestational visit in GDM rate compared with the control and intervention groups from the previous referred study (García de la Torre et al. 2019). In this trial 932 women received a motivational lifestyle interview with emphasis on daily consumption of EVOO and nuts, but without providing any of them, and followed the standard care in the usual clinical setting. GDM rate was significantly lower than the previous control group (RR 0.81, 95% CI [0.73, 0.93], $p < 0.001$) and no different from the intervention group (RR 0.96, 95% CI [0.85, 1.07], $p = 0.468$).

TABLE 1.1

Epidemiological Studies Assessing the Effect of a Mediterranean Diet on GDM Incidence

Authors	Study Design	Participants	Gestational Age at Dietary Assessment	Dietary Assessment	Results
Tobias et al. 2012	Prospective cohort study	15254	Pre-pregnancy	Validated FFQ to calculate an MDS (score range 0–8)	Participants in the fourth quartile of MDS had a 24% lower risk (RR 0.76, 95% CI [0.60, 0.95], p-trend = 0.004) of GDM than women in the first quartile.
Karamanos et al. 2014	Prospective cohort study	1076	24–32 GWs	78-item validated FFQ to calculate a MDS	Incidence of GDM was lower in subjects with better adherence to the MedDiet (higher tertile compared with lowest tertile); 8.0% vs. 12.3%, OR 0.618, p = 0.030 by ADA 2010; 24.3% vs. 32.8%, OR 0.655, p = 0.004 by IADPSG 2012 criteria.
Schoenaker et al. 2015	Prospective cohort study	3853	Pre-pregnancy	101-item validated FFQ	Women in the highest tertile had a 44% lower risk for GDM (95% CI [0.41, 0.77], p for trend = 0.0001) when compared with women in the lowest tertile.
Izadi et al. 2016	Case-control study	460 (200 cases, 260 controls)	5–28 GWs	Average of three 24-hour dietary records to calculate a MDS based on 10-point Trichopoulou score	Women in the highest tertile of the MedDiet had 80% lower risk for GDM compared with those in the lowest tertile (p-trend = 0.006).
Schoenaker et al. 2016	Prospective cohort study	3378	Pre-pregnancy	Validated FFQ to calculate a MDS based on 10-point Trichopoulou score	Low adherence to the MedDiet was associated with higher risk of GDM (OR 1.35, 95% CI [1.02, 1.60]).
Olmedo-Requena et al. 2019	Case-control study	1466 (291 cases, 1175 controls)	Pre-pregnancy	Validated FFQ to calculate a MDS (score range 0–9: low, ≤2; middle, 3–4; high, 5–6; very high, ≥7)	Compared to low adherence, high adherence was associated with GDM reduction (aOR 0.61, 95% CI [0.39, 0.94], p = 0.028), and very high adherence was more strongly associated (aOR 0.33, 95% CI [0.15, 0.72], p = 0.005).

Abbreviations: ADA, American Diabetes Association; FFQ, food frequency questionnaire; GDM, gestational diabetes mellitus; GWs, gestational week; IADPSG, International Association of Diabetes and Pregnancy Study Groups; MDS, Mediterranean Diet Score; MedDiet, Mediterranean diet.

In the ESTEEM study 1252 pregnant women with metabolic risk factors (obesity, chronic hypertension, or hypertriglyceridemia) were randomized to a Mediterranean diet with high intake of nuts and EVOO versus usual care (Al Wattar et al. 2019). The primary endpoints were composite maternal (GDM or preeclampsia) and composite offspring (stillbirth, SGA, or admission to neonatal care unit) outcomes prioritized by a Delphi survey. A total of 1138 reached the final follow-up. There was no significant reduction in the composite maternal (22.8% vs. 28.6%; aOR 0.76, 95% CI [0.56, 1.03], $p = 0.08$) or composite offspring (17.3% vs. 20.9%; aOR 0.79, 95% CI [0.58, 1.08], $p = 0.14$) outcomes. There was an apparent reduction in the odds of GDM by 35% (aOR 0.65, 95% CI [0.47, 0.91], $p = 0.01$) but not in other individual components of the composite outcomes. In addition, the authors performed a pooled effect estimate of the two RCTs (St. Carlos and ESTEEM; 2012 women) showing a consistent reduction in GDM (OR 0.67, 95% CI [0.53, 0.84], $I^2 = 0\%$). The intervention did not reduce the rates of other individual components of the primary composite outcomes such as preeclampsia, SGA, or admission to the neonatal care unit.

In the ESTEEM study, two-thirds of participants were from ethnic minority groups (mainly Black and Asian), and all the patients had metabolic risk factors. In the St. Carlos studies (RCT and the real-world trial) the intervention was applied in unselected pregnant women with a mean BMI < 25 kg/m^2 in both studies, considered as low risk for GDM, and one-third belonged to ethnic minority groups (mainly Latin American). Therefore, we recommend an easy, universal nutritional intervention in pregnant women based on a Mediterranean diet rich in EVOO and nuts applied in the usual clinical setting as early as possible to reduce the burden of GDM.

1.4 MEDITERRANEAN DIET AS MEDICAL NUTRITIONAL THERAPY (MNT) FOR GDM

The first-line therapy for GDM is lifestyle advice, which includes medical nutrition therapy, weight management, and physical activity. Nevertheless, there is no consensus regarding what is the ideal MNT for GDM treatment. This is due to limited data regarding the optimal diet for achieving maternal euglycemia and reducing excessive fetal growth and adiposity.

Different dietary strategies have been reported including low glycemic index, the Dietary Approaches to Stop Hypertension (DASH) diet, low carbohydrates, soy protein-enrichment, fiber, and fat modification diets. All these approaches have been reviewed in a meta-analysis (Yamamoto et al. 2018) that pooled results from 18 RCTs including 1151 women with a variety of modified dietary interventions. Despite the heterogeneity between studies, the authors found a moderate effect of dietary interventions on maternal glycemic outcomes, including changes reduced postbreakfast and postprandial glucose levels, and a lowering of neonatal birth weight.

The MedDiet has a low carbohydrate/higher fat macronutrient distribution with low glycemic index and is rich in fiber, antioxidants, and anti-inflammatory components, and therefore might be a good option for MNT in diabetes, especially knowing that adherence to this dietary pattern has been associated with a 30% reduction in the incidence of GDM, as well as a reduction in adverse perinatal outcomes (Assaf-Balut et al. 2017). To our knowledge there are no published RCTs evaluating the effect of a MedDiet-based MNT on GDM complications (glycemic control and pregnancy outcomes) or comparing these women with those without GDM. Hence, we performed a secondary analysis of the St. Carlos GDM Prevention Study (Assaf-Balut et al. 2018). Women from both the control and intervention groups who were diagnosed with GDM were referred to the Diabetes and Pregnancy Unit and treated according to local guidelines. Regardless of having been previously allocated to the control or intervention group, all women who developed GDM received the same treatment. Using a MedDiet-based MNT as part of GDM management was associated with achievement of near normoglycemia at 36–38 GWs, subsequently making most pregnancy outcomes similar to those women with normoglycemia. Specifically, women with GDM as compared with normoglycemic women had higher HbA$_{1c}$ levels at 24–28 GWs (5.1% ± 0.3% vs. 4.9% ± 0.3%,

$p = 0.001$). Nonetheless, after at least 12 weeks of MNT, 36- to 38-week values were similar between the groups. Similarly, fasting serum insulin and homeostatic model assessment insulin resistance (HOMA-IR) were higher in women with GDM at 24–28 GWs ($p = 0.001$) but became similar at 36–38 weeks. Women with GDM had higher rates of insufficient weight gain (39.5% vs. 22.0%, $p = 0.001$), SGA (6.8% vs. 2.6%, $p = 0.009$), and neonatal intensive care unit admission (5.6% vs. 1.7%, $p = 0.006$) compared with normoglycemic women. The rates of macrosomia, LGA, pregnancy-induced hypertensive disorders, prematurity, and cesarean sections were comparable between the groups. These preliminary results show the potential benefit of using this type of diet as MNT in women with GDM. However, strategies are needed to reduce the rates of SGA newborns and insufficient weight gain and thus avoid potential deleterious consequences.

1.5 BEYOND GDM: OTHER PERINATAL AND POSTPARTUM BENEFITS

Both RCT assessing the effect of a MedDiet on the risk of GDM incidence have shown additional beneficial effects to different extent. In the St. Carlos GDM Prevention Study (Assaf-Balut et al. 2017) the GWG was significantly lower at 24 ± 28 GW and at 36 ± 38 GW in the control group ($p = 0.022$ and $p = 0.037$, respectively). In addition, compared to the control group, fewer women diagnosed with GDM in the intervention group required insulin therapy (14/74 [19%] vs. 33/103 [32%], $p = 0.002$). There was also a significant decrease in the episodes of urinary tract infections, emergency C-sections, and perineal trauma; and lower rates of prematurity and LGA and SGA newborns in the intervention group. In the ESTEEM trial (H Al Wattar et al. 2019), a lower GWG was observed ($M = 6.8$ vs. 8.3 kg, adjusted difference −1.2 kg, 95% CI [−2.2, −0.2, $p = 0.03$) in the intervention versus control group, but with no differences in other perinatal outcomes.

But benefits from adopting a Mediterranean nutritional pattern early in gestation might extend further after pregnancy, since the MedDiet has been associated with the prevention of T2DM and metabolic syndrome (Salas-Salvadó et al. 2015). In order to address this issue, our group conducted a cohort study that clustered 1675 women into two groups: the standard-care group (679) and the early-intervention (<12 GWs) group (999) with a MedDiet rich in EVOO and nuts (Assaf-Balut et al. 2019a). When subjects were evaluated at 12–14 weeks postpartum, significantly less women (%) in the intervention group had fasting glucose ≥ 100 mg/dL and HbA_{1c} ≥ 5.7%. Rates of systolic and diastolic blood pressure ≥ 130 and ≥ 85 mm Hg respectively, HDL cholesterol < 50 mg/dL and triglycerides ≥ 150 mg/dL were lower in the intervention group. In addition, women in the intervention group had lower BMI postpartum, and a higher percentage had a weight retention < 0 kg. Metabolic syndrome was less frequent in the intervention group (11.3 vs. 19.3, $p < 0.005$) and the RR of having metabolic syndrome was 0.74 (95% CI [0.60, 0.90]). In this study, women in the intervention group kept better nutritional scores in pregnancy and postpartum than the standard-care group. This behavior has been reported in previous trials such as the RADIEL (Koivusalo et al. 2016) and the LIMIT (Dodd et al. 2014) studies, where authors also found that an intervention during pregnancy was associated with persistence of improved postpartum dietary habits, while the standard-care group experienced a decline in their nutritional habits. These results show the importance of a nutritional intervention and adoption of healthy dietary habits during pregnancy when women have such a high motivation.

Even though this chapter reviews evidence supporting adherence to MedDiet for GDM prevention and treatment, we would like to highlight its potential benefits also in normoglycemic women. Nutritional recommendations provided in clinical practice limit the intake of fats to avoid excessive gestational weight gain; however, data on effective dietary interventions are inconclusive. Limitation of fats includes trans and saturated fats, but by default it also includes monounsaturated and polyunsaturated fats. These are present in EVOO and nuts, which are indispensable components of MedDiet. This diet is not associated with weight gain during pregnancy; in fact, it is just the opposite (Assaf-Balut et al. 2017; H Al Wattar 2019). Therefore, we performed a secondary analysis of the normoglycemic women participating in the St. Carlos GDM Prevention Study comparing maternal and neonatal outcomes as well as clinical and biochemical parameters of women who followed nutritional guidelines based on a MedDiet supplemented with EVOO and pistachios versus women who followed guidelines provided in regular clinical practice that limit total fat consumption (Assaf-Balut et al. 2019b). The primary outcome was a composite of maternofetal outcomes (CMFO): at least having one event of emergency C-section, perineal trauma, pregnancy-induced hypertension, preeclampsia, prematurity, and LGA or SGA newborns. Surprisingly, the intervention was associated with a significant reduction in the risk of CMFOs (RR 0.48, 95% CI [0.37, 0.63], $p = 0.0001$), with a number needed to treat = 5. Risks of urinary tract infections, emergency C-sections, perineal trauma, and LGA and SGA newborns were also significantly reduced. Therefore, even though current guidelines for pregnancy highlight the importance of reducing total fat intake, with the concern that the opposite will lead to an excessive weight gain, our experience does not support this recommendation, and we advise universal nutritional intervention in all pregnant women based on a MedDiet rich in EVOO and nuts as early as possible.

Moreover, adherence to a MedDiet during pregnancy might provide benefits also in offspring health. The adverse intrauterine environment linked to GDM leads to epigenetic changes that predispose children to develop metabolic disease later in life (Scholtens et al. 2019; Lowe et al. 2019) and worsens respiratory health in infants (Azad et al. 2017). A secondary analysis of the UPBEAT trial has shown that the epigenetic impact of a dysglycemic prenatal maternal environment, assessed by DNA methylation in cord blood from neonates, appeared to be modified by a lifestyle intervention in pregnancy (Antoun et al. 2020).

While the current evidence suggests a possible association between diet in pregnancy and the development of diseases in children, very few have evaluated in an RCT the effect of an intervention based on a MedDiet in the development of metabolic and immune diseases in the offspring. Our group led a prospective analysis of the St. Carlos GDM prevention study including the infants of women who attended the 2-year postpartum follow-up (Melero et al. 2020). From the 874 women who were analyzed in the St. Carlos GDM prevention study, a total of 703 (80.5%) children, 365 from the control group and 338 from the intervention group were assessed. The primary outcome was to assess the incidence of bronchiolitis/asthma, atopic dermatitis, and food allergies as well as the number and duration of all-cause hospital admissions in children at 2 years of age. The secondary outcome was to evaluate the rates of hospital admissions due to severe episodes of bronchiolitis/asthma and other diseases requiring pharmacological treatment with antibiotics, corticosteroids, or both. Even if we did not find differences between intervention and control groups in relation to rates of bronchiolitis/asthma, diseases of autoimmune origin (food allergies and dermatitis eczema), and infectious illness that did not require hospital admission, the study showed that the adherence to the MedDiet seemed to be associated with a lower risk of hospitalization in children requiring antibiotic and corticosteroid treatment, and admissions related to asthma/bronchiolitis. This was especially observed in women who had a pre-gestational BMI < 25 kg/m^2 and in those with normoglycemia. Breastfeeding (followed by more than 90% of women in both groups in the first 5 months) and compliance with the vaccination program (completed by more than 99% of children in both groups) are relevant factors within the first 2 years of life that could have influenced the results. Whether these results are sustained over time remains to be known. Therefore, we will re-evaluate these children's health at 5 to 6 years of age.

1.6 MECHANISMS INVOLVED

When we try to assess the mechanisms involved, we are not dealing with a single exposition but rather a complex set of foods, nutrients, and phytochemicals, each of which may act on the metagenomic, genomic, epigenomic, transcriptomic, and proteomic levels. Apart from their separate effects, all these individual components can have synergetic effects at all levels, making this analysis extremely complex (Corella et al. 2018). Among all foods included in the MedDiet, virgin olive oil is the most representative. Virgin olive oil is obtained from the fruit of the olive tree solely by mechanical means. Its composition consists of major compounds (>98%), with a high content of monounsaturated fatty acids (MUFAs), and minor compounds (~2%), among which are antioxidants. The main antioxidants of virgin olive oil are carotenes and unique bioactive phenolic compounds such as hydroxytyrosol, tyrosol, and oleuropein (Reboredo-Rodríguez et al. 2017). Non-virgin (refined) olive oil has practically no polyphenols or any other of the favorable compounds. This is extremely important because the effects on health are different depending on whether extra virgin olive oil or virgin olive oil is used in the interventions or habitual diet. Olive oil is used for dressing and cooking, improving the texture and taste of vegetables, but also increasing the bioavailability of some nutrients. For example, cooking with olive oil increases the bioavailability of the polar phenolic compounds in tomatoes (Vallverdú-Queralt et al. 2014) and also reduces the formation of toxic compounds in high-temperature frying compared with other fats (Rangel-Zuñiga et al. 2017).

1.6.1 Proteomics

We do not know the specific mechanisms through which the MedDiet exercises its protective effects, but evidence suggests that it may do so through its modulation of chronic inflammation. In an RCT including 285 patients from the PREDIMED study, participants were randomly assigned into three intervention groups: MedDiet supplemented with EVOO or MedDiet supplemented with nuts, and a low-fat diet (Urpi-Sarda et al. 2021). After 3 years of intervention, both MedDiet groups showed a significant reduction in the plasma levels of plasma inflammatory biomarkers IL-1β, IL-6, IL-8, TNF-α, IFN-γ, hs-CRP, MCP-1, MIP-1β, and ENA78 compared to baseline, while no significant changes were observed in these biomarkers in the low-fat diet group. The decreased levels of IL-1β, IL-6, IL-8, and TNF-α after the MedDiet significantly differed from those in the low-fat diet.

Our group is also interested in elucidating the mechanisms involved in GDM development and the protective effects of a MedDiet. Some inflammatory cytokines such as IL-6 and TNF-α and adipokines such as leptin are produced by the placenta, contributing to insulin resistance in GDM (Briana and Malamitsi-Puchner 2009; Fasshauer et al. 2014) and have been even proposed as predictive markers for GDM (Xu et al. 2014; Abell et al. 2015). Another adipokine, adiponectin, decreases progressively throughout pregnancy and is significantly lower in women with GDM compared to controls (Xu et al. 2014). In addition, in a subset of the HAPO study, adiponectin correlated inversely with maternal glucose levels, C-peptide levels, and BMI (Lowe et al. 2010). Therefore, we are currently analyzing these inflammatory cytokines (IL-6 and TNF-α) and adipokines (leptin and adiponectin) in a subgroup of participants from the St. Carlos GDM Prevention Study (172 from the intervention group and 141 from the control group) at baseline, at 24–28 GWs after at least 12 weeks of intervention when GDM was diagnosed, and 2 to 3 years' postpartum when maternal cardiovascular risk profile was also assessed.

1.6.2 Transcriptomics

Transcriptomics allow us to assess the effect of a specific food or diet on gene expression. There is growing evidence analyzing the effects of the MedDiet or its most representative components on the transcriptome. In the RCT from the PREDIMED study assessing inflammatory biomarkers (Urpi-Sarda et al. 2021), an additional pilot study of gene expression was performed. In a subpopulation of 35 participants (12 in the MedDiet supplemented with EVOO group, 12 in the MedDiet supplemented with nuts group, and 11 in the low-fat diet group), a gene expression analysis was carried out at baseline and after 3 years of intervention. The expression of ten genes related to inflammatory stages of atherosclerosis was measured. The mRNA expression of all the studied genes did not change significantly after the MedDiet and the low-fat diet. Nevertheless, the mRNA expression of CXCR2 and CXCR3 (chemokine receptors mediating chemotaxis of leukocytes) showed a slight trend of increase only in the low-fat control group ($p = 0.09$). Although this was a very small sample study, the results suggest that one of the mechanisms by which the MedDiet might exert beneficial effects is through its anti-inflammatory properties. In a previous study by the same group, a sample of 34 patients was studied using the whole-transcriptome approach versus the selected gene expression (Castañer et al. 2013). Participants were distributed randomly in the same three dietary groups and followed the intervention over 3 months. They examined changes in cardiovascular system traditional pathways. Nine pathways were modified by the MedDiet with EVOO and four pathways were modulated by the MedDiet + nuts. Essential pathways in the physiopathology of cardiovascular risk, such as atherosclerosis, renin-angiotensin, nitric oxide and angiopoietin signaling, hypoxia, and endothelial nitric oxide synthase signaling pathways, were modulated by MedDiet. The atherosclerosis signaling pathway was significantly downregulated after the MedDiet with EVOO intervention. Several other studies suggest that the MedDiet and EVOO are capable of producing changes in gene expression related to inflammation and oxidative stress (reviewed by Herrera-Marcos et al. 2017).

1.6.3 EPIGENOMICS

Epigenetics involves the changes in the heritable phenotype that do not involve alterations in the DNA sequence but affect gene activity and expression. The three main mechanisms that produce such changes are DNA methylation, histone modification, and non-coding RNAs (microRNAs). These effects may result from environmental factors such as dietary exposure or maternal hyperglycemia during pregnancy.

DNA methylation has been proposed as a mediating mechanism for maternal hyperglycemia to lead to adverse offspring outcomes. In a subgroup of 557 women from the UPBEAT study (Antoun et al. 2020), cord blood DNA samples from infants were analyzed for genome-wide DNA methylation levels. Maternal dysglycemia at 24 to 28 weeks' gestation was associated with significant changes in the epigenome of the infants. In addition, the epigenetic impact of a dysglycemic prenatal-maternal environment appeared to be modified by a lifestyle intervention in pregnancy.

These epigenomic changes can lead to poorer health outcomes for the offspring later in life. In an analysis of epigenome-wide methylation patterns using umbilical cord blood DNA from 470 participants in the UK, the authors identified differential methylation patterns associated with systolic blood pressure, pulse pressure, arterial distensibility, and descending aorta pulse wave velocity measured by magnetic resonance imaging at 8 to 9 years of age (Murray et al. 2021). Maternal smoking, pre-pregnancy BMI, weight gain during pregnancy, and decreased intake of oily fish in early and late pregnancy, were associated with methylation patterns linked to raised aortic pulse wave velocity, the most widely used measure of increased arterial stiffness. These findings suggest a link between maternal polyunsaturated fatty acid intake and maternal body composition both before and during pregnancy, altered epigenetic regulation of cardiovascular development in the fetus, and childhood measures of cardiovascular disease risk.

On the other hand, it has been shown that specific components of the MedDiet, particularly nuts and EVOO, were able to induce methylation changes in several peripheral white blood cell genes related to inflammation and immune functions in a small group of 36 participants who followed a MedDiet over 5 years (Arpón et al. 2016).

MicroRNAs (miRNAs) are small, single-stranded, non-coding RNA molecules that function in RNA silencing and posttranscriptional regulation of gene expression. Data about miRNA expression in GDM are scarce and controversial. Therefore, our group aims to evaluate whether the circulating miRNAs hsa-miR-29a-3p, hsa-miR-103-3p, and hsa-miR-222-3p are part of the epigenetic mechanisms involved in GDM development and the protective effect of the MedDiet during pregnancy and in the metabolic profile at 2 to 3 years postpartum. So far we have analyzed samples from 284 participants in the St. Carlos GDM Prevention Study: 102 from the control group and 182 from the intervention group. We have observed a hsa-miR-222-3p overexpression in women with GDM and lower adherence to the MedDiet compared to normoglycemic women in the 24–28 GWs that

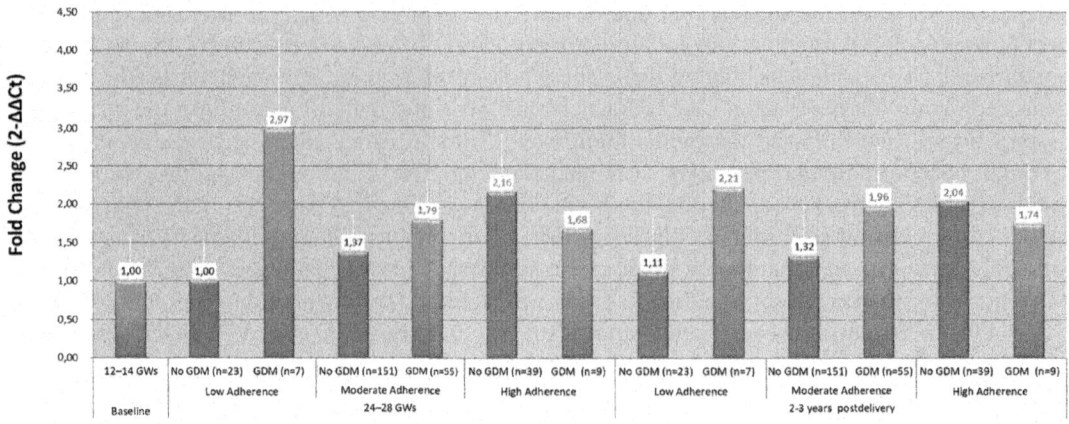

FIGURE 1.1 hsa-miR-222-3p expression at 12–14 gestational weeks (GWs), 24–28 GWs, and 2–3 years postpartum in pregnant women according to MedDiet adherence. GDM, gestational diabetes mellitus; GWs: gestational weeks.

remains 2–3 years postpartum (data not published), suggesting that this miRNA might be a molecular biomarker of GDM risk (Figure 1.1).

1.6.4 GENOMICS

The single nucleotide polymorphism (SNP), a germline substitution of a single nucleotide at a specific position in the genome, leads to differences in human susceptibility to a wide range of diseases. Several SNPs influence the risk of GDM development (Ding et al. 2018). In recent years, nutrigenetic studies have gathered growing evidence that genetic variants confer individual differences in response to nutritional interventions. This research into gene-diet interactions provides us with a better understanding of the heterogeneity of responses to the same dietary intervention. Nonetheless, very a few studies of gene–lifestyle interactions and their influence on GDM development have been published, and to our knowledge only one assessing MedDiet.

There is strong evidence that SNPs within the transcription factor 7 like 2 (TCF7L2 gene influence GDM risk (Ding et al. 2018). The TCF7L2 gene encodes T cell transcription factor 4 (TCF4), which plays a key role in the Wnt signaling pathway. It is crucial in the β cell genesis and function and is considered a main regulator of glucose homeostasis. The T allele has been associated with impaired β cell function and insulin secretion and lower insulin levels (Jin 2016). A post hoc analysis of the St. Carlos GDM Prevention Study (Assaf-Balut et al. 2017) evaluating whether the TCF7L2 rs7903146 polymorphism could modulate the association between late first trimester adherence to the MedDiet and the risk of GDM revealed that the risk of developing GDM in those with high adherence versus low adherence was significantly reduced only in carriers of the T allele (CT + TT), with an aOR of 0.15 (95% CI [0.05, 0.48]). Nevertheless, this effect was not observed in CC carriers (Barabash et al. 2020). Therefore, an unfavorable genetic predisposition may be counteracted by an adequate nutritional pattern. This reinforces the relevance of identifying patients at risk of GDM based on genetic characteristics that are especially sensitive to specific types of diets and the importance of a nutritional education to pregnant women.

1.6.5 METAGENOMICS

Gut microbiota is emerging as a pivotal player in the relationship between dietary habits and health.

Research analyzing whether modification in gastrointestinal microbial diversity is one of the mechanisms involved in GDM reduction in patients following a MedDiet are lacking. Nevertheless, some data back up the etiopathogenic role of microbiota in T2DM (Palacios et al. 2020) and how the MedDiet is able to modify microbiota in pregnant women (Miller et al. 2021). Adherence to the MedDiet pattern is associated with increased maternal gastrointestinal microbial diversity and promotes the abundance of bacteria that produce short chain fatty acids (Miller et al. 2021). Therefore, further studies are needed to determine whether adherence to a MedDiet translates not only into microbial health but also into reduced risk of GDM.

1.7 SUMMARY POINTS

- Several nutritional interventions have been proposed to reduce GDM risk.
- In multiple epidemiological studies and in two RCTs, the MedDiet has shown a consistent reduction in GDM incidence.
- Additional benefits such as lower GWG, a decrease in insulin requirements when GDM was diagnosed; a reduction in episodes of urinary tract infections, emergency C-sections, perineal trauma, prematurity, and LGA and SGA; and lower incidence of postpartum metabolic syndrome have been observed.
- Even more, adherence to a MedDiet during pregnancy is likely to provide benefits also in offspring health later in life.
- Mechanisms involved for this benefit include reduction in the plasma levels of inflammatory biomarkers, modulation of gene expression related to inflammation and oxidative stress, epigenomic changes in DNA methylation and circulating miRNAs, gene-diet interaction, and possibly changes in gut microbiota.

REFERENCES

Abell, S. K., De Courten, B., Boyle, J. A., and Teede, H. J. 2015. Inflammatory and other biomarkers: Role in pathophysiology and prediction of gestational diabetes mellitus. *International Journal of Molecular Sciences*, *16*(6): 13442–13473. https://doi.org/10.3390/ijms160613442.

Al Wattar, B. H., Dodds, J., Placzek, A., Beresford, L., Spyreli, E., Moore, A., Gonzalez Carreras, F. J., et al. 2019. Mediterranean-style diet in pregnant women with metabolic risk factors (ESTEEM): A pragmatic multicentre randomised trial. *PLoS Medicine*, *16*(7): e1002857. https://doi.org/10.1371/journal. pmed.1002857.

Antoun, E., Kitaba, N. T., Titcombe, P., Dalrymple, K. V., Garratt, E. S., Barton, S. J., Murray, R., and UPBEAT Consortium. 2020. Maternal dysglycaemia, changes in the infant's epigenome modified with a diet and physical activity intervention in pregnancy: Secondary analysis of a randomised control trial. *PLoS Medicine*, *17*(11): e1003229. https://doi.org/10.1371/journal.pmed.1003229.

Arpón, A., Riezu-Boj, J. I., Milagro, F. I., Marti, A., Razquin, C., Martínez-González, M. A., Corella, D., et al. 2016. Adherence to Mediterranean diet is associated with methylation changes in inflammation-related genes in peripheral blood cells. *Journal of Physiology and Biochemistry*, *73*(3): 445–455. https://doi. org/10.1007/s13105-017-0552-6.

Assaf-Balut, C., García de la Torre, N., Durán, A., Bordiú, E., Del Valle, L., Familiar, C., Valerio, J., et al. 2019a. An early, universal Mediterranean diet-based intervention in pregnancy reduces cardiovascular risk factors in the "fourth trimester." *Journal of Clinical Medicine*, *8*(9): 1499. https://doi.org/10.3390/ jcm8091499.

Assaf-Balut, C., García de la Torre, N., Durán, A., Fuentes, M., Bordiú, E., Del Valle, L., Familiar, C., et al. 2017. A Mediterranean diet with additional extra virgin olive oil and pistachios reduces the incidence of gestational diabetes mellitus (GDM): A randomized controlled trial: The St. Carlos GDM prevention study. *PLoS ONE*, *12*(10): e0185873. https://doi.org/10.1371/journal.pone.0185873.

Assaf-Balut, C., García de la Torre, N., Durán, A., Fuentes, M., Bordiú, E., Del Valle, L., Familiar, C., et al. 2019b. A Mediterranean diet with an enhanced consumption of extra virgin olive oil and pistachios improves pregnancy outcomes in women without gestational diabetes mellitus: A sub-analysis of the St. Carlos gestational diabetes mellitus prevention study. *Annals of Nutrition & Metabolism*, *74*(1): 69–79. https://doi.org/10.1159/000495793.

Assaf-Balut, C., Garcia de la Torre, N., Durán, A., Fuentes, M., Bordiú, E., Del Valle, L., Valerio, J., et al. 2018. Medical nutrition therapy for gestational diabetes mellitus based on Mediterranean diet principles: A sub-analysis of the St. Carlos GDM prevention study. *BMJ Open Diabetes Research & Care*, 6(1): e000550. https://doi.org/10.1136/bmjdrc-2018-000550.

Azad, M. B., Moyce, B. L., Guillemette, L., Pascoe, C. D., Wicklow, B., McGavock, J. M., Halayko, A. J., and Dolinsky, V. W. 2017. Diabetes in pregnancy and lung health in offspring: Developmental origins of respiratory disease. *Paediatric Respiratory Reviews*, 21: 19–26. https://doi.org/10.1016/j.prrv.2016.08.007.

Barabash, A., Valerio, J. D., Garcia de la Torre, N., Jimenez, I., Del Valle, L., Melero, V., Assaf-Balut, C., et al. 2020. TCF7L2 rs7903146 polymorphism modulates the association between adherence to a Mediterranean diet and the risk of gestational diabetes mellitus. *Metabolism Open*, 8, 100069. https://doi.org/10.1016/j.metop.2020.100069.

Bellamy, L., Casas, J. P., Hingorani, A. D., and Williams, D. 2009. Type 2 diabetes mellitus after gestational diabetes: A systematic review and meta-analysis. *Lancet (London, England)*, 373(9677): 1773–1779. https://doi.org/10.1016/S0140-6736(09)60731-5.

Briana, D. D., and Malamitsi-Puchner, A. 2009. Reviews: Adipocytokines in normal and complicated pregnancies. *Reproductive Sciences (Thousand Oaks, Calif.)*, 16(10): 921–937. https://doi.org/10.1177/1933719109336614.

Castañer, O., Corella, D., Covas, M. I., Sorlí, J. V., Subirana, I., Flores-Mateo, G., Nonell, L., and PREDIMED Study Investigators. 2013. In vivo transcriptomic profile after a Mediterranean diet in high-cardiovascular risk patients: A randomized controlled trial. *The American Journal of Clinical Nutrition*, 98(3): 845–853. https://doi.org/10.3945/ajcn.113.060582.

Corella, D., Coltell, O., Macian, F., and Ordovás, J. M. 2018. Advances in understanding the molecular basis of the Mediterranean diet effect. *Annual Review of Food Science and Technology*, 9: 227–249. https://doi.org/10.1146/annurev-food-032217-020802.

Ding, M., Chavarro, J., Olsen, S., Lin, Y., Ley, S. H., Bao, W., Rawal, S., et al. 2018. Genetic variants of gestational diabetes mellitus: A study of 112 SNPs among 8722 women in two independent populations. *Diabetologia*, 61: 1758e68. https://doi.org/10.1007/s00125-018-4637-8.

Dodd, J. M., Turnbull, D., McPhee, A. J., Deussem, A. R., Grivell, R. M., Yelland, L. N., Crowther, C. A., et al. 2014. Antenatal lifestyle advice for women who are overweight or obese: LIMIT randomised trial. *British Medical Journal*, 348: g1285. https://doi.org/10.1136/bmj.g1285.

Fasshauer, M., Blüher, M., and Stumvoll, M. 2014 Adipokines in gestational diabetes. The Lancet. *Diabetes & Endocrinology*, 2(6): 488–499. https://doi.org/10.1016/s2213-8587(13)70176-1.

García de la Torre, N., Assaf-Balut, C., Jiménez Varas, I., Del Valle, L., Durán, A., Fuentes, M., Del Prado, N., et al. 2019. Effectiveness of following Mediterranean diet recommendations in the real world in the incidence of gestational diabetes mellitus (GDM) and adverse maternal-foetal outcomes: A prospective, universal, interventional study with a single group. The St. Carlos study. *Nutrients*, 11(6): 1210. https://doi.org/10.3390/nu11061210.

Herrera-Marcos, L. V., Lou-Bonafonte, J. M., Arnal, C., Navarro, M. A., and Osada, J. 2017. Transcriptomics and the Mediterranean diet: A systematic review. *Nutrients*, 9(5): 472. https://doi.org/10.3390/nu9050472.

Izadi, V., Tehrani, H., Haghighatdoost, F., Dehghan, A., Surkan, P. J., and Azadbakht, L. 2016. Adherence to the DASH and Mediterranean diets is associated with decreased risk for gestational diabetes mellitus. *Nutrition (Burbank, Los Angeles County, Calif.)*, 32(10): 1092–1096. https://doi.org/10.1016/j.nut.2016.03.006.

Jin, T. 2016. Current understanding on role of the WNT signaling pathway effector TCF7L2 in glucose homeostasis. *Endocrine reviews*, 37(3): 254–277. https://doi.org/10.1210/er.2015-1146.

Karamanos, B., Thanopoulou, A., Anastasiou, E., Assaad-Khalil, S., Albache, N., Bachaoui, M., Slama, C. B., et al. 2014. Relation of the Mediterranean diet with the incidence of gestational diabetes. *European Journal of Clinical Nutrition*, 68(1): 8–13. https://doi.org/10.1038/ejcn.2013.177.

Koivusalo, S. B., Rönö, K., Klemetti, M. M., Roine, R. P., Lindström, J., Erkkola, M., Kaaja, R. J., et al. 2016. Gestational diabetes mellitus can be prevented by lifestyle intervention: The Finnish gestational diabetes prevention study (RADIEL): A randomized controlled trial. *Diabetes Care*, 39(1): 24–30. https://doi.org/10.2337/dc15-0511.

Lin, X., Yang, T., Zhang, X., and Wei, W. 2020. Lifestyle intervention to prevent gestational diabetes mellitus and adverse maternal outcomes among pregnant women at high risk for gestational diabetes mellitus. *The Journal of International Medical Research*, 48(12): 300060520979130. https://doi.org/10.1177/0300060520979130.

Lowe, L. P., and HAPO Study Cooperative Research Group. 2010. Inflammatory mediators and glucose in pregnancy: Results from a subset of the hyperglycemia and adverse pregnancy outcome (HAPO) study. *Journal of Clinical Endocrinology and Metabolism*, 95(12): 5427–5434. https://doi.org/10.1210/jc.2010-1662.

Lowe, W. L. Jr., and HAPO Follow-up Study Cooperative Research Group. 2019. Maternal glucose levels during pregnancy and childhood adiposity in the hyperglycemia and adverse pregnancy outcome follow-up study. *Diabetologia*, 62(4): 598–610. https://doi.org/10.1007/s00125-018-4809-6.

Luoto, R., Kinnunen, T. I., Aittasalo, M., Kolu, P., Raitanen, J., Ojala, K., Mansikkamäki, K., et al. 2011. Primary prevention of gestational diabetes mellitus and large-for-gestational-age newborns by lifestyle counseling: A cluster-randomized controlled trial. *PLoS Medicine*, 8(5): e1001036. https://doi.org/10.1371/journal.pmed.1001036.

Melero, V., Assaf-Balut, C., Torre, N. G., Jiménez, I., Bordiú, E., Valle, L. D., Valerio, J., et al. 2020. Benefits of adhering to a Mediterranean diet supplemented with extra virgin olive oil and pistachios in pregnancy on the health of offspring at 2 years of age. Results of the San Carlos Gestational diabetes mellitus prevention study. *Journal of Clinical Medicine*, 9(5): 1454. https://doi.org/10.3390/jcm9051454.

Metzger, B. E., and HAPO Study Cooperative Research Group. 2008. Hyperglycemia and adverse pregnancy outcomes. *New England Journal of Medicine*, 358: 1991–2002. https://doi.org/10.1056/NEJMoa0707943.

Miller, C. B., Benny, P., Riel, J., Boushey, C., Perez, R., Khadka, V., Qin, Y., Maunakea, A. K., and Lee, M. J. 2021. Adherence to Mediterranean diet impacts gastrointestinal microbial diversity throughout pregnancy. *BMC Pregnancy and Childbirth*, 21(1): 558. https://doi.org/10.1186/s12884-021-04033-8.

Murray, R., Kitaba, N., Antoun, E., Titcombe, P., Barton, S., Cooper, C., Inskip, H. M., and EpiGen Consortium. 2021. Influence of maternal lifestyle and diet on perinatal DNA methylation signatures associated with childhood arterial stiffness at 8 to 9 years. *Hypertension (Dallas)*, 78(3): 787–800. https://doi.org/10.1161/HYPERTENSIONAHA.121.17396.

Olmedo-Requena, R., Gómez-Fernández, J., Amezcua-Prieto, C., Mozas-Moreno, J., Khan, K. S., and Jiménez-Moleón, J. J. 2019. Pre-pregnancy adherence to the Mediterranean diet and gestational diabetes mellitus: A case-control study. *Nutrients*, 11(5): 1003. https://doi.org/10.3390/nu11051003.

Palacios, T., Vitetta, L., Coulson, S., Madigan, C. D., Lam, Y. Y., Manuel, R., Briskey, D., et al. 2020. Targeting the intestinal microbiota to prevent type 2 diabetes and enhance the effect of metformin on glycaemia: A randomised controlled pilot study. *Nutrients*, 12(7): 2041. https://doi.org/10.3390/nu12072041.

Poston, L., Bell, R., Croker, H., Flynn, A. C., Godfrey, K. M., Goff, L., Hayes, L., and UPBEAT Trial Consortium. 2015. Effect of a behavioural intervention in obese pregnant women (the UPBEAT study): A multicentre, randomised controlled trial. *The Lancet. Diabetes & Endocrinology*, 3(10): 767–777. https://doi.org/10.1016/S2213-8587(15)00227-2.

Quinlivan, J. A., Lam, L. T., and Fisher, J. 2011. A randomised trial of a four-step multidisciplinary approach to the antenatal care of obese pregnant women. *The Australian & New Zealand Journal of Obstetrics & Gynaecology*, 51(2): 141–146. https://doi.org/10.1111/j.1479-828X.2010.01268.x.

Rangel-Zuñiga, O. A., Haro, C., Tormos, C., Perez-Martinez, P., Delgado-Lista, J., Marin, C., Quintana-Navarro, G. M., et al. 2017. Frying oils with high natural or added antioxidants content, which protect against postprandial oxidative stress, also protect against DNA oxidation damage. *European Journal of Nutrition*, 56(4): 1597–1607. https://doi.org/10.1007/s00394-016-1205-1.

Reboredo-Rodríguez, P., Figueiredo-González, M., González-Barreiro, C., Simal-Gándara, J., Salvador, M. D., Cancho-Grande, B., and Fregapane, G. 2017. State of the art on functional virgin olive oils enriched with bioactive compounds and their properties. *International Journal of Molecular Sciences*, 18(3): 668. https://doi.org/10.3390/ijms18030668.

Salas-Salvadó, J., Guasch-Ferré, M., Lee, C. H., Estruch, R., Clish, C. B., and Ros, E. 2015. Protective effects of the Mediterranean diet on type 2 diabetes and metabolic syndrome. *The Journal of Nutrition*, 146(4): 920S–927S. https://doi.org/10.3945/jn.115.218487.

Schoenaker, D. A., Soedamah-Muthu, S. S., Callaway, L. K., and Mishra, G. D. 2015. Pre-pregnancy dietary patterns and risk of gestational diabetes mellitus: Results from an Australian population-based prospective cohort study. *Diabetologia*, 58(12): 2726–2735. https://doi.org/10.1007/s00125-015-3742-1.

Schoenaker, D. A., Soedamah-Muthu, S. S., and Mishra, G. D. 2016. Quantifying the mediating effect of body mass index on the relation between a Mediterranean diet and development of maternal pregnancy complications: The Australian longitudinal study on women's health. *The American Journal of Clinical Nutrition*, 104(3): 638–645. https://doi.org/10.3945/ajcn.116.133884.

Scholtens, D. M., and HAPO Follow-up Study Cooperative Research Group. 2019. Hyperglycemia and adverse pregnancy outcome follow-up study (HAPO FUS): Maternal glycemia and childhood glucose metabolism. *Diabetes Care*, *42*(3): 381–392. https://doi.org/10.2337/dc18-2021.

Simmons, D., Jelsma, J. G., Galjaard, S., Devlieger, R., van Assche, A., Jans, G., Corcoy, R., et al. 2015. Results from a European multicenter randomized trial of physical activity and/or healthy eating to reduce the risk of gestational diabetes mellitus: The DALI lifestyle pilot. *Diabetes Care*, *38*(9): 1650–1656. https://doi.org/10.2337/dc15-0360.

Thornton, Y. S., Smarkola, C., Kopacz, S. M., and Ishoof, S. B. 2009. Perinatal outcomes in nutritionally monitored obese pregnant women: A randomized clinical trial. *Journal of the National Medical Association*, *101*(6): 569–577. https://doi.org/10.1016/s0027-9684(15)30942-1.

Tobias, D. K., Zhang, C., Chavarro, J., Bowers, K., Rich-Edwards, J., Rosner, B., Mozaffarian, D., and Hu, F. B. 2012. Prepregnancy adherence to dietary patterns and lower risk of gestational diabetes mellitus. *The American Journal of Clinical Nutrition*, *96*(2): 289–295. https://doi.org/10.3945/ajcn.111.028266.

Urpi-Sarda, M., Casas, R., Sacanella, E., Corella, D., Andrés-Lacueva, C., Llorach, R., Garrabou, G., et al. 2021. The 3-year effect of the Mediterranean diet intervention on inflammatory biomarkers related to cardiovascular disease. *Biomedicines*, *9*(8): 862. https://doi.org/10.3390/biomedicines90808.

Vallverdú-Queralt, A., Regueiro, J., Rinaldi de Alvarenga, J. F., Torrado, X., and Lamuela-Raventos, R. M. 2014. Home cooking and phenolics: Effect of thermal treatment and addition of extra virgin olive oil on the phenolic profile of tomato sauces. *Journal of Agricultural and Food Chemistry*, *62*(14): 3314–3320. https://doi.org/10.1021/jf500416n.

Xu, J., Zhao, Y. H., Chen, Y. P., Yuan, X. L., Wang, J., Zhu, H., and Lu, C. M. 2014. Maternal circulating concentrations of tumor necrosis factor-alpha, leptin, and adiponectin in gestational diabetes mellitus: A systematic review and meta-analysis. *The Scientific World Journal*, 926932. https://doi.org/10.1155/2014/926932.

Yamamoto, J. M., Kellett, J. E., Balsells, M., García-Patterson, A., Hadar, E., Solà, I., Gich, I., et al. 2018. Gestational diabetes mellitus and diet: A systematic review and meta-analysis of randomized controlled trials examining the impact of modified dietary interventions on maternal glucose control and neonatal birth weight. *Diabetes Care*, *41*(7): 1346–1361. https://doi.org/10.2337/dc18-0102.

2 The Use of *Acacia* spp. for the Control of Blood Sugar in Type 2 Diabetes Mellitus

Ian Edwin Cock and Matthew James Cheesman

CONTENTS

ABBREVIATIONS

DM	diabetes mellitus
FBG	fasting blood glucose
GLP-1	glucagon-like peptide 1
GLUT-4	glucose transporter-4
G6Pase	glucose-6-phosphatase
HbA1c	glycosylated hemoglobin
HDL	high-density lipoprotein
LDL	low-density lipoprotein
NF-κB	nuclear factor κB
ROS	reactive oxygen species
STZ	streptozotocin
T2-DM	type 2 diabetes mellitus
VLDL	very-low-density lipoprotein
WHO	World Health Organization

2.1 INTRODUCTION

Although type 2 diabetes mellitus (T2-DM) has been extensively documented historically, there has been a dramatic increase in its incidence in recent years due to the global adoption of energy-intensive diets and decreased exercise levels. Indeed, the World Health Organization (WHO) estimates that the number of people with T2-DM worldwide increased from 108 million in 1980 to 425 million in 2017 (WHO 2019). This figure represents approximately 9% of the adult population over

DOI: 10.1201/9781003220930-3

18 years of age. Both females and males are equally represented in these figures. The incidence of T2-DM increases markedly with age, with substantially more than 25% of the population over 65 years estimated to have T2-DM (WHO 2019). However, it is likely that these figures substantially underestimate the incidence of T2-DM as a large percentage of cases remain unreported, especially in the early phases of the disease. Furthermore, the number of people with T2-DM is expected to continue to rise at the same rate in future years to more than 642 million people by 2040 (International Diabetes Federation 2015).

T2-DM manifests as hyperglycemia, which is maintained over prolonged periods, resulting in a myriad of symptoms including frequent urination, as well as increased thirst and hunger. If T2-DM is not effectively treated to return the blood glucose to manageable levels, ketoacidosis occurs and may result in a myriad of serious comorbidities. These may include blindness, coronary disease, renal disease, and an increased incidence of strokes. The metabolic and physiological conditions established by prolonged hyperglycemia can also create conditions conducive to gas gangrene, which may necessitate limb amputation. Furthermore, as well as increasing an individual's incidence of serious and debilitating comorbidities, T2-DM more than doubles the risk of early death (WHO 2019). Indeed, estimates of the number of deaths globally attributed to T2-DM in 2017 range from 3.2 to 5.0 million (International Diabetes Federation 2017). Additionally, a further 2.12 million deaths that resulted from hyperglycemia but were not directly attributed to T2-DM were also reported in 2012 (WHO 2019). If the current trends continue unabated, T2-DM is expected to become a leading cause of death and disability in the future (Malviya et al. 2010). Of further concern, the increasing incidence of T2-DM morbidity and mortality increases the health care burden and was estimated to cost US$727 billion globally in 2017 (International Diabetes Federation 2017).

Although lifestyle modification (changing to lower energy diets, increasing exercise) is considered the most effective treatment option, pharmacotherapy is also effective. In particular, metformin (a low-affinity sodium-glucose cotransport inhibitor) is effective in lowering plasma glucose levels and improving glucose tolerance (Mudaliar and Henry 2001; Klein et al. 2004; Chao and Henry 2010). Metformin also inhibits gluconeogenesis, lowers intestinal glucose absorption, improves insulin sensitivity, and increases glucose excretion in the urine (Bailey and Turner 1996). However, none of the current T2-DM treatments is completely effective, and new chemotherapies are urgently needed.

2.2   BACKGROUND ON MEDICINAL PLANTS USED TO TREAT DIABETES MELLITUS

A re-examination of traditional and herbal medicines for the development of new therapies to treat T2-DM is an attractive option as plant-based medicines have been used for centuries to regulate glucose homeostasis (Handa et al. 1989; Alarcon-Aguilar and Roman-Ramos 2005). More than 1000 plants are used globally to regulate blood glucose levels in the treatment of T2-DM (Marles and Farnsworth 1995). However, relatively few plant species have been investigated scientifically for antihyperglycemic effects, and even fewer mechanistic studies have been published. This is perhaps surprising, as plant-based therapies have already provided several pharmacological options to treat T2-DM. Indeed, several current anti-diabetes drugs, including metformin, phenformin, and buformin, were initially isolated from *Galega officinalis* L. (commonly known as French lilac, goat's rue) (Maruthur et al. 2016; Cock et al. 2021). There is scope to develop more therapies from other traditional medicines, and substantially more work is required in this field.

A number of studies have identified and itemized plant species used traditionally to lower blood glucose, and the reader is referred to those studies for a comprehensive listing (Cock et al. 2021; El Haouari et al. 2019; Yusuf et al. 2012; Baskaran et al. 1990). Many of the species identified are widely cultivated globally. Examples of traditional treatments for T2-DM include *Allium sativum* L. (garlic), *Annona squamosa* L. (commonly known as custard apple or sweetsop), *Berberis vulgaris* L. (commonly known as sugar beet, beetroot, chard, spinach beet), *Lantana camara* L. (lantana), and *Momordica charantia* L. (bitter melon; Cock et al. 2021; El Haouari and Rosado 2019; Yusuf et al. 2012; Baskaran et al. 1990). The anti-diabetes properties of several of these species have been verified, and some of the bioactive constituents have already been identified (Apaya et al. 2020; Rasouli et al. 2020; Rao et al. 2010). However, few of these studies have evaluated the antihyperglycemic mechanisms of the plants, or of the isolated compounds. Additionally, many plants used traditionally to treat T2-DM have not yet been evaluated to verify their antihyperglycemic activity.

2.3   THE MEDICINAL PROPERTIES OF *ACACIA* SPP.

Reports of the therapeutic potential of *Acacia* spp. are extensive, particularly for *Acacia nilotica* (Lam.) Willd., which has anticancer, antihypertensive, antimicrobial, anti-asthmatic, antiplatelet, and antipyretic properties (Ali et al. 2012). The Taiwanese species *A. confusa* Merr. also possesses powerful antioxidant properties (Lin et al. 2018), whereas *A. catechu* (L.) Willd. is known for its anti-inflammatory effects (Stohs and Bagchi 2015). *A. caesia* (L.) Willd. is rich in antioxidants (Thambiraj and Paulsamy 2012), and the fresh plant segments of *A. arabica* possess astringent, demulcent, aphrodisiac, anthelmintic, antimicrobial, and antidiarrheal properties (Rajvaidhya et al. 2012). Numerous other species have been noted for their biological activities, including (but not limited to) *A. dealbata* L., *A. tortilis* (Forsk.) Hayne, *A. seyal* Delile, and *A. laeta* R.Br. ex Benth. (Paula et al. 2022).

2.4   TRADITIONAL USE OF *ACACIA* SPP. TO CONTROL BLOOD GLUCOSE

The ethnomedicinal value of various *Acacia* spp. to treat diabetes is well established, although less is known about the use by the First Australians for this purpose. However, the Australian *Acacia* spp. have similar phytochemical compositions to species from other regions of the world, and it is likely that they have similar properties. Due to the paucity of information documenting the uses of Australian species, this chapter focuses on species from other regions, and phytochemical similarities are highlighted where relevant. Several traditional Indian healing systems use *Acacia arabica* (Lam.) Willd. and *A. farnesiana* (L.) Willd. for their anti-diabetic effects (Rajvaidhya et al. 2012; Kingsley et al. 2013). Similarly, *A. pennata* (L.) Willd. is also widely used in Thai traditional medicine to treat diabetes (Andrade et al. 2020), and dried decoctions prepared from *A. catechu* wood have traditionally been used in Bangladesh to maintain normal blood sugar levels (Rahmatullah et al. 2013).

2.5   STUDIES ON ANTI-DIABETIC PROPERTIES OF *ACACIA* SPP. AND ISOLATED COMPOUNDS

The blood-lowering properties of multiple *Acacia* spp. have been well investigated. Extracts from *Acacia arabica* pod extracts and powdered seeds of that species exert hypoglycemic effects in experimental animals, presumably by stimulating insulin release from pancreatic β cells (Singh et al. 1976; Wadood et al. 1989; Asad et al. 2011; Abd El-Aziz et al. 2013; Auwal et al. 2013; Hegazy et al. 2013). The flavonoid components quercetin and kaempferol, which were isolated from *A. arabica* bark, are believed to induce increases in insulin secretion *in vivo* (Ansari et al. 2021). *A. catechu* ethyl acetate extracts elicit significant reductions in blood glucose levels in both diabetic and non-diabetic rats (Ray et al. 2006), and 70% ethanol extracts of *A. auriculiformis* A.Cunn. ex Benth. bark and leaf restore blood glucose to normal levels in diabetic animals (Sathya and Siddhuraju 2013). Polysaccharides isolated from *A. tortilis* also have substantial anti-diabetic activity in diabetic rats (Kumar Bhateja et al. 2014), which is mediated via inhibition of α-glucosidase inhibition, and the resultant modulation of glucagon-like peptide 1 (GLP-1) plasma levels (Bhateja et al. 2020). Less is known about the uses of Australian *Acacia* spp. to treat diabetes, although the Australian species *A. kampeana* F.Muell., *A. tetragonophylla* F.Muell., and *A. ligulata* A.Cunn. ex Benth. each possess potent antioxidant and glycemic enzyme inhibitory activities, which indicate that they may be promising species for the management of hyperglycemia, although further investigation is required to confirm their potential (Gulati et al. 2012). There is also evidence that *A. mearnsii* De Wild. bark extracts can lower blood glucose levels in mice due to the abundance of proanthocyanidins, which suppress gluconeogenesis while enhancing the action of insulin (Kashiwada et al. 2021).

2.6 PHYTOCHEMISTRY OF *ACACIA* SPP.

The phytochemistry of *Acacia* spp. is relatively well reported, although a few species have been most extensively studied. The phytochemistry of *Acacia nilotica* (L.) has been well documented and a number of noteworthy constituents have been identified (Rather et al. 2015). Indeed, the phytochemical profile of *A. nilotica* is often used to search for similar compounds in other *Acacia* spp., and as a comparison. The previous studies have identified flavonoids, tannins, fatty acids, and essential oils, as well as polysaccharides as the major classes of compounds in *Acacia* spp. (Rather et al. 2015). Of these, the flavonoids and tannins are particularly interesting due to their physiochemical properties and known bioactivities. Flavonoids have been linked with multiple therapeutic properties including the induction of cellular mechanisms that inhibit carcinogenesis and block cancer cell proliferation, inhibit inflammation, as well as inhibiting and treating other diseases including diabetes (Cock 2013). Furthermore, many of the beneficial properties of flavonoids are mediated through their high antioxidant capacities. Therefore, some flavonoids may be useful in the treatment of diabetes by directly decreasing reactive oxygen species (ROS), as well as by modulating transcription factors and inhibiting the release of inflammatory mediators, which may have downstream effects on glucose homeostasis.

The presence of high levels of tannins is also interesting as they also have high antioxidant capacities and may act via pathways similar to flavonoids. However, it is also likely that the *Acacia* spp. tannins may function by simpler mechanisms. Tannins are well known to bind to proteins and inactivate enzymes, and several plants with high tannin contents have been reported to be effective antihyperglycemic treatments (Cock 2015; Buzzini et al. 2008; Machado et al. 2003). It is therefore likely that the tannin constituents of *Acacia* spp. may directly inactivate polysaccharide catabolic enzymes, thereby decreasing blood glucose levels, as well as functioning via several of the antioxidant mediated pathways much like those used by flavonoids.

2.7 FLAVONOIDS

An abundance and diversity of flavonoids have been identified in multiple *Acacia* spp. This is noteworthy as multiple flavonoids have been reported to decrease hyperglycemia, protein glycation, and insulin resistance *in vivo* (Hussain et al. 2020; Zhou et al. 2020; Mahmoud et al. 2019; Ghorbani 2017; Sarian et al. 2017; Chen et al. 2015) and numerous antihyperglycemic mechanisms have been identified (summarized in Figure 2.1). Many of these mechanisms rely either directly or indirectly on the antioxidant activity of the flavonoids. In particular, flavonoids exert their anti-diabetic effects via:

- Directly scavenging free radicals or decreasing ROS via regulation of cellular antioxidant systems (Hussain et al. 2020; Mahmoud et al. 2019; Sarian et al. 2017; Cock 2013).
- Direct inhibition of enzymes involved in sugar metabolism (Ghorbani 2017; Jadhav and Puchchakayala 2012; Ahmed et al. 2010; Li et al. 2009; Jo et al. 2009; Prince et al. 2006).
- Inhibition of transcription factors (Ghorbani 2017).
- Inhibition of pro-inflammatory cytokines (Ghorbani 2017). This may subsequently upregulate insulin release and stimulate glycogen synthesis.
- Increasing insulin and insulin-like activity. This may occur via both a direct modulation of insulin release (Cai and Lin 2009) and the insulin mimetic effects of some flavonoids (Ahmed et al. 2010).
- Inhibition of insulin resistance (Hussain et al. 2020; Zhou et al. 2020; Mahmoud et al. 2019).

TABLE 2.1

Important Phytoconstituents Identified in *Acacia* spp. and Their Anti-Diabetic Mechanisms (Where Known)

Compound Class	Compound	Known Anti-Diabetic Activities	References

Flavonoids	Acacetin
	Apigenin
	Apigenin-6,8-bis-C-β-D-glucopyranoside
	Catechin
	Catechin-5-gallate
	Catechin-5,7-digallate
	Catechin-3,5-digallate
	Catechin-4,5-digallate
	Catechin-7-O-gallate
	Chalconaringenin-4'-O-β-
	  glucopyranoside
	Chrysoeriol
	Epicatechin
	Flavone
	Isoquercetin
	Kaempferol
	Kaempferol-7-glucoside
	Leucocyanidin
	Luteolin
	Melacacidin
	Mollisacacidin
	Myricetin
	Naringenin
	Naringenin-7-O-β-D-glucopyranoside
	Naringenin-7-O-β-D-(6'-O-galloyl)
	  glucopyranoside
	Rutin
	Quercetin
	Quercetin-3-galactosyl
	Vitexin
		Protection of β cells, stimulation of glycogen synthesis, inhibition of α-glucosidase, sucrase, maltase and α-amylase activities, activation of glucose sport and stimulation of glucose uptake, stimulation of insulin secretion, insulin receptor signaling, inhibition of G-6-Pase, inhibition of glycogen breakdown	Ngaffo et al. 2020; Chen et al. 2015; Rather et al. 2015; El-Toumy et al. 2011; Hsieh and Chang 2010; Leela et al. 2010; Singh et al. 2009

Tannins	Dicatechin Digallic acid Ellagic acid Epigallocatechin-7-gallate Epigallocatechin-5,7-digallate Gallocatechin-5-O-gallate Gallic acid 1-O-galloyl-β-D-glucose 1,6-di-O-galloyl-β-D-glucose Ethyl gallate Methyl gallate Polygalloyltannin	Stimulates β cell regeneration, stimulates insulin release and insulin signaling pathways, decreases serum lipid levels, alleviates oxidative stress, stimulates glucose uptake via activation of GLUT-4 glucose transporter, suppresses cytokine release, modulates levels of TNF-α, IL-6, and C reactive protein and MAD protein, stimulates glucose uptake and glycogen synthesis, inhibits polysaccharide catabolic enzymes, decreases plasma HbA1c, modulates NF-κB release	Vinayagam et al. 2016; Rather et al. 2015; Sharma et al. 2014; Leela et al. 2010; Salem et al. 2011; El-Toumy et al. 2011; Kalaivani et al. 2011; Singh et al. 2009

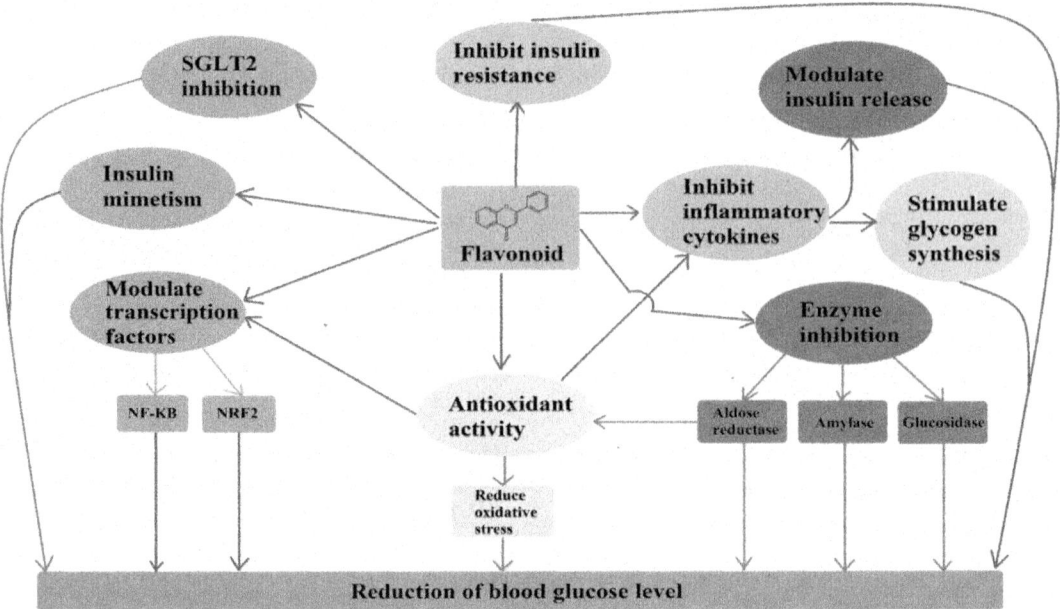

FIGURE 2.1   An overview of the mechanisms through which flavonoids exert antihyperglycemic effects.

The flavonoid rutin has been identified in relative abundance in multiple *Acacia* spp. (Grace et al. 2009; Dongmo et al. 2007; Muhaisen et al. 2002). Interestingly, rutin treatment can decrease blood and serum lipid levels in several ways. Indeed, oral administration of rutin (50 mg/kg body weight) in streptozotocin (STZ)-induced diabetic rats significantly decreases fasting blood glucose (FBG) and glycosylated hemoglobin (HbA$_{1c}$) levels (Niture et al. 2014; Prince et al. 2006). Those studies reported that the effects of rutin on FBG and were comparable to that of pioglitazone (a peroxisome proliferator-activated receptor agonist). Another study reported that rutin had comparable hyperglycemic activity in diabetic rats as the anti-diabetes drug glibenclamide (Jadhav and Puchchakayala 2012). Furthermore, rutin also reduces the development of hyperglycemia (and therefore diabetes) in STZ-induced diabetic rats (Srinivasan et al. 2005). Additionally, rutin treatment has numerous beneficial effects in diabetic patients, including reducing serum triglyceride, very-low-density (VLDL), low-density (LDL), and high-density lipoproteins (HDL) (Dake and Sora 2016; Sattanathan et al. 2011). Rutin also inhibits intestinal cholesterol absorption, thereby reducing serum cholesterol levels in *in vivo* preclinical studies (Ahmed et al. 2010), although these results are not reproducible in human clinical studies (Sattanathan et al. 2011).

Rutin directly inhibits α-glucosidase, α-amylase, maltase, and glucoamylase enzyme activity, thereby reducing intestinal digestion of carbohydrates and subsequent increases in blood glucose levels (Ghorbani 2017; Jadhav and Puchchakayala 2012; Ahmed et al. 2010; Li et al. 2009; Jo et al. 2009). Notably, rutin also stimulates an increase in insulin secretion from pancreatic β cells (Cai and Lin 2009), as well as having an insulin-mimetic role in isolated rat tissue (Ahmed et al. 2010). Rutin also stimulates glucose transport into muscle cells via activation of the GLUT-4 transporter and therefore stimulates glycogen synthesis and storage. Furthermore, it inhibits endogenous glucose synthesis via gluconeogenesis by inhibiting the expression of genes encoding for glucose-6-phosphatase (G6Pase), fructose-1,6-bisphosphatase, and phosphoenolpyruvate carboxykinase (Ahmed et al. 2010; Prince et al. 2006).

Other flavonoids identified in *Acacia* spp. exert antihyperglycemic effects via similar mechanisms to rutin. Apigenin, catechin, chrysoeriol, kaempferol, luteolin, myricetin, vitexin, quercetin, and their glycosides have all been identified in *Acacia* spp. extracts, and anti-diabetes activities have been attributed to all of these molecules (Muhaisen 2020; Ngaffo et al. 2020; Gabr et al. 2018). Many of the flavonoids and their glycosides identified in *Acacia* spp. have been reported to protect pancreatic β cells from damage, inhibit α-glucosidase and α-amylase (as well as several other polysaccharide catabolism enzymes), increase insulin secretion and function, stimulate glucose uptake into muscle and liver cells, and inhibit glycogenolysis (as reviewed in Chen et al. 2015).

2.8 TANNINS

Another notable aspect of *Acacia* spp. phytochemistry is the relative abundance and diversity of tannins that have been identified (Rather et al. 2015; Leela et al. 2010; Salem et al. 2011; El-Toumy et al. 2011; Kalaivani et al. 2011; Singh et al. 2009). Interestingly, several of these tannins have been reported to function via multiple antihyperglycemic mechanisms (Figure 2.2). Generally, the anti-diabetes mechanisms of tannins are substantially more simplistic that those of the flavonoids and can be categorized as affecting blood glucose levels in two main ways:

- Enzyme inhibition via direct interaction (Zhu et al. 2020; Alam et al. 2019; Vinayagam et al. 2016).
- Suppression of pro-inflammatory molecules and pathways, which subsequently stimulates glucose uptake into liver and muscle cells and storage as glycogen (Shanmuganathan and Angayarkanni 2018; Vinayagam et al. 2016).

Gallic acid has considerable antihyperglycemic activity in both insulin deficient and insulin resistant in *in vivo* model systems, inducing significant decreases in blood glucose, cholesterol, and triglyceride levels (Gandhi et al. 2014), while stimulating increases in plasma insulin, C-reactive

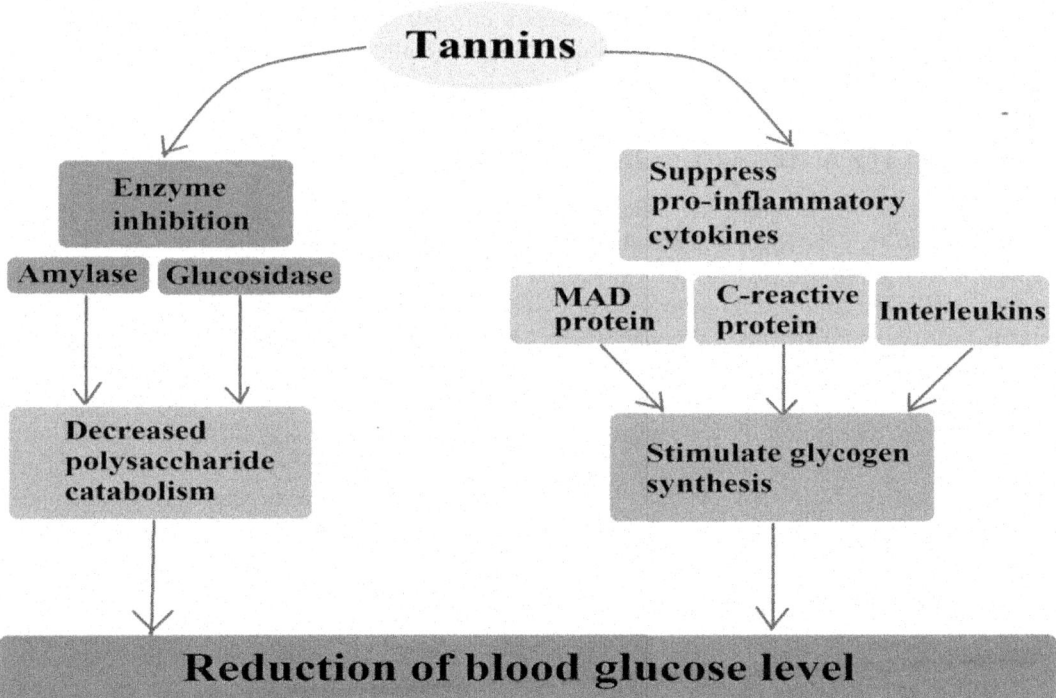

FIGURE 2.2 An overview of the mechanisms through which tannins exert antihyperglycemic effects.

peptide, and glucose tolerance levels. Furthermore, gallic acid treatment has been reported to stimulate insulin secretion in STZ-treated diabetic rats (Punithavathi et al. 2011). Additionally, gallic acid significantly improves β cell regeneration in STZ-induced diabetic rats and stimulates insulin secretion (Vinayagam et al. 2016; Latha and Daisy 2011). It has also been shown to increase glucose uptake into liver and muscle cells by activation of the GLUT-4 glucose transported (Gandhi et al. 2014). Another study also demonstrated that gallic acid suppresses NF-κB activation and inhibits cytokine release (Lee et al. 2015). Therefore, gallic acid alleviates hyperglycemia via a multifaceted approach. Notably, other hydrolysable and condensed gallotannins, including chebulagic acid and chebulinic acid, have been reported to reported to function by many of the same mechanisms (Shanmuganathan and Angayarkanni 2018).

Ellagic acid also has substantial anti-diabetic effects and protects β cells from ROS damage (Vinayagam et al. 2016; Jang et al. 2010). Although the anti-diabetic mechanisms of ellagic acid have not been as extensively studied as for gallic acid, it is known to function via multiple mechanisms. An *in vivo* study demonstrated that ellagic acid decreased hyperglycemia and inflammation, while increasing plasma insulin levels (Ahad et al. 2014). Ellagic acid stimulates insulin-signaling pathways and increases GLUT-4 translocation, thereby stimulating glucose uptake into adipocytes (Scazzocchio et al. 2015). Additionally, ellagic acid inhibits the NF-κB pathway and attenuates the inflammatory pathways.

2.9 FUTURE DIRECTIONS

T2-DM is a chronic illness that reduces patient quality of life. Elevated blood glucose levels may be treated with the few drugs that are currently available on the market, but new modalities of treatment are required. The traditional use of *Acacia* spp. to treat the condition is substantiated by the many studies which provide evidence indicating that the extracts, or compounds isolated from extracts, can reduce plasma glucose levels *in vivo*, and via various pharmacological mechanisms of action that have been discussed in this review. The abundance and variety of phytochemicals in *Acacia* spp. offer new and exciting opportunities for novel drug discovery and development, which may ultimately produce more effective treatment options to alleviate this chronic disease and offer hope for those who have the condition.

2.10 TOXICITY AND CAUTIONARY NOTES

Few studies have yet evaluated the safety of *Acacia* spp. extracts and substantially more work is required before they (or their isolated components) can be adopted for clinical use. Several studies have screened African *Acacia* spp. extracts for toxicity and have generally classified them to be nontoxic within the parameters of those studies (as reviewed in Cock et al. 2021). Fewer studies have screened Australian *Acacia* spp., although where Australian *Acacia* spp. have been evaluated for toxicity, they have also generally been classified as nontoxic across the concentration ranges tested (Cock 2017; Cock 2012). However, the majority of those studies used *Artemia* nauplii toxicity assays or have screened the extracts against limited panels of human cell lines. Substantially further study is required to test against expanded cell libraries to fully evaluate toxicity. Furthermore, there is a paucity of preclinical *in vivo* or clinical studies to date. Until such studies are undertaken, caution is recommended with the use of *Acacia* spp. extracts to treat diabetes, or indeed, for any other therapeutic use.

2.11 SUMMARY POINTS

- Multiple *Acacia* spp. are used in traditional medicine systems to treat various medical conditions, including diabetes.
- Several noteworthy phytochemicals including flavonoids and tannins have been identified in *Acacia* spp. extracts.

- *Acacia* spp. flavonoids and tannins have substantial antioxidant activity, which is associated with the anti-diabetes effects.
- Several flavonoids and tannins directly inhibit glycosidic enzymes, thereby decreasing blood glucose levels.
- Some *Acacia* spp. compounds stimulate insulin release, whereas others are insulin mimetics.
- Other *Acacia* spp. phytoconstituents modulate transcription factors and stimulate glycogen synthesis.
- This chapter reviews the current phytochemical knowledge and the previous studies into the anti-diabetic properties of *Acacia* spp.

REFERENCES

Abd El-Aziz, Ahmed M., Nagwa E. Awad, Ahmed A. Seida, and Zakaria El-khayat. 2013. Biological and chemical evaluation of the use of *Acacia nilotica* (L.) in the Egyptian traditional medicine. *International Bulletin of Drug Research* 3:1–19.

Ahad A., A.A. Ganai, M. Mujeeb, and W.A. Siddiqui. 2014. Ellagic acid, an NF-κB inhibitor, ameliorates renal function in experimental diabetic nephropathy. *Chemico-Biological Interactions* 219:64–75.

Ahmed, Osama Mohamed, Adel Abdel Moneim, Ibrahim Abul Yazid, and Ayman Moawad Mahmoud. 2010. Antihyperglycemic, antihyperlipidemic and antioxidant effects and the probable mechanisms of action of *Ruta graveolens* infusion and rutin in nicotinamide-streptozotocin-induced diabetic rats. *Diabetologia Croatica* 39:15–35.

Alam, Fiaz, Zainab Shafique, Sayyeda Tayyeba Amjad, and Mohammad Hassham Hassan Bin Asad. 2019. Enzymes inhibitors from natural sources with antidiabetic activity: A review. *Phytotherapy Research* 33:41–54.

Alarcon-Aguilar, Francisco Javier, and Ruben Roman-Ramos. 2005. *Antidiabetic Plants in Mexico and Central America*. Boca Raton, FL: CRC Press, Taylor & Francis.

Ali, Atif, Naveed Akhtar, Barkat Ali Khan, Muhammad Shoaib Khan, Akhtar Rasul, Nayab Khalid, Khalid Waseem, Tariq Mahmood, and Liaqat Ali. 2012. *Acacia nilotica*: A plant of multipurpose medicinal uses. *Journal of Medicinal Plants Research* 6:1492–1496.

Andrade, Catarina, Nelson G.M. Gomes, Sutsawat Duangsrisai, Paula B. Andrade, David M. Pereira, and Patricia Valentao. 2020. Medicinal plants utilized in Thai Traditional Medicine for diabetes treatment: Ethnobotanical surveys, scientific evidence and phytochemicals. *Journal of Ethnopharmacology* 263:113177.

Ansari, Prawej, Peter R. Flatt, Patrick Harriott, J.M.A. Hannan, and Yasser H.A. Abdel-Wahab. 2021. Identification of multiple pancreatic and extra-pancreatic pathways underlying the glucose-lowering actions of *Acacia arabica* bark in Type-2 diabetes and isolation of active phytoconstituents. *Plants* 10:1190.

Apaya, Maria Karmella, Tien-Fen Kuo, Meng-Ting Yang, Greta Yang, Chiao-Ling Hsiao, Song-Bin Chang, Yenshou Lin, and Wen-Chin Yang. 2020. Phytochemicals as modulators of β-cells and immunity for the therapy of type 1 diabetes: Recent discoveries in pharmacological mechanisms and clinical potential. *Pharmacological Research* 156:104754.

Asad, Munazza, Muhammad Aslam, Tahir Ahmad Munir, and Amina Nadeem. 2011. Effect of *Acacia nilotica* leaves extract on hyperglycaemia, lipid profile and platelet aggregation in streptozotocin induced diabetic rats. *Journal of Ayub Medical College Abbottabad* 23:3–7.

Auwal, Mohammed Shaibu, Sanni Saka, Abdullahi Shuaibu, Ismail Alhaji Mairiga, Kyari Abba Sanda, Amina Ibrahim, Fatima Abba Lawan, Ahmad Bello Thaluvwa, and Abdulhamid Baba Njobdi. 2013. Phytochemical properties and hypoglycemic activity of the aqueous and fractionated portions of *Acacia nilotica* (Fabaceae) pod extracts on blood glucose level in normoglycemic Wistar albino rats. *Journal of Medical Sciences* 13:111.

Bailey, Clifford J., and Robert C. Turner. 1996. Metformin. *New England Journal of Medicine* 334:574–579.

Baskaran, Kizar, B. Kizar Ahamath, K. Radha Shanmugasundaram, and E.R.B. Shanmugasundaram. 1990. Antidiabetic effect of a leaf extract from *Gymnema sylvestre* in non-insulin-dependent diabetes mellitus patients. *Journal of Ethnopharmacology* 30:295–305.

Bhateja, Pradeep Kumar, Anu Kajal, and Randhir Singh. 2020. Amelioration of diabetes mellitus by modulation of GLP-1 via targeting alpha-glucosidase using *Acacia tortilis* polysaccharide in Streptozotocin-Nicotinamide induced diabetes in rats. *Journal of Ayurveda and Integrative Medicine* 11:405–413.

Buzzini, Pietro, Panagiotis Arapitsas, Marta Goretti, Eva Branda, Benedetta Turchetti, Patrizia Pinelli, F. Ieri, and Annalisa Romani. 2008. Antimicrobial and antiviral activity of hydrolysable tannins. *Mini-Reviews in Medicinal Chemistry* 8:1179–1187.

Cai, Erica P., and Jen-Kun Lin. 2009. Epigallocatechin gallate (EGCG) and rutin suppress the glucotoxicity through activating IRS2 and AMPK signaling in rat pancreatic β cells. *Journal of Agricultural and Food Chemistry* 57:9817–9827.

Chao, Edward C., and Robert R. Henry. 2010. SGLT2 inhibition – a novel strategy for diabetes treatment. *Nature Reviews Drug Discovery* 9:551–559.

Chen, Jian, Sven Mangelinckx, An Adams, Zheng-tao Wang, Wei-lin Li, and Norbert De Kimpe. 2015. Natural flavonoids as potential herbal medication for the treatment of diabetes mellitus and its complications. *Natural Product Communications* 10:187–200.

Cock, I.E. 2012. Antimicrobial activity of *Acacia aulacocarpa* and *Acacia complanta* leaf methanolic extracts. *Pharmacognosy Communications* 1:66–73.

Cock, I.E. 2013. The phytochemistry and chemotherapeutic potential of *Tasmannia lanceolata* (Tasmanian pepper): A review. *Pharmacognosy Communications* 3:13–25.

Cock, I.E. 2015. The medicinal properties and phytochemistry of plants of the genus Terminalia (Combretaceae). *Inflammopharmacology* 23:203–229.

Cock, I.E. 2017. Australian *Acacia* spp. extracts as natural food preservatives: Growth inhibition of food spoilage and food poisoning bacteria. *Pharmacognosy Communications* 7:4–15.

Cock, I.E., N. Ndlovu, and S.F. Van Vuuren. 2021. The use of South African botanical species for the control of blood sugar. *Journal of Ethnopharmacology* 264:113234.

Dake, Andrew W., and Nicoleta D. Sora. 2016. Diabetic dyslipidemia review: An update on current concepts and management guidelines of diabetic dyslipidemia. *The American Journal of the Medical Sciences* 351:361–365.

Dongmo, Alain B., Tomofumi Miyamoto, Kazuko Yoshikawa, Shigenobu Arihara, and Marie-Aleth Lacaille-Dubois. 2007. Flavonoids from *Acacia pennata* and their cyclooxygenase (COX-1 and COX-2) inhibitory activities. *Planta Medica* 73:1202–1207.

El Haouari, Mohammed, and Juan A. Rosado. 2019. Phytochemical, anti-diabetic and cardiovascular properties of *Urtica dioica* L. (Urticaceae): A review. *Mini Reviews in Medicinal Chemistry* 19:63–71.

El-Toumy, Sayed A., Samy M. Mohamed, Emad M. Hassan, and Abdel-Tawab H. Mossa. 2011. Phenolic metabolites from *Acacia nilotica* flowers and evaluation of its free radical scavenging activity. *Journal of American Science* 7:287–295.

Gabr, Sara, Stefanie Nikles, Eva Maria Pferschy Wenzig, Karin Ardjomand-Woelkart, Rania M. Hathout, Sherweit El-Ahmady, Amira Abdel Motaal, Abdelnasser Singab, and Rudolf Bauer. 2018. Characterization and optimization of phenolics extracts from *Acacia* species in relevance to their anti-inflammatory activity. *Biochemical Systematics and Ecology* 78:21–30.

Gandhi, Gopalsamy Rajiv, Gnanasekaran Jothi, Poovathumkal James Antony, Kedike Balakrishna, Michael Gabriel Paulraj, Savarimuthu Ignacimuthu, Antony Stalin, and Naif Abdullah Al-Dhabi. 2014. Gallic acid attenuates high-fat diet fed-streptozotocin-induced insulin resistance via partial agonism of PPARγ in experimental type 2 diabetic rats and enhances glucose uptake through translocation and activation of GLUT4 in PI3K/p-Akt signaling pathway. *European Journal of Pharmacology* 745:201–216.

Ghorbani, Ahmad. 2017. Mechanisms of antidiabetic effects of flavonoid rutin. *Biomedicine & Pharmacotherapy* 96:305–312.

Grace, Mary H., George R. Wilson, Fayez E. Kandil, Eugene Dimitriadis, and Robert M. Coates. 2009. Characteristic flavonoids from *Acacia burkittii* and *A. acuminata* heartwoods and their differential cytotoxicity to normal and leukemia cells. *Natural Product Communications* 4:69–76.

Gulati, Vandana, Ian H. Harding, and Enzo A. Palombo. 2012. Enzyme inhibitory and antioxidant activities of traditional medicinal plants: Potential application in the management of hyperglycemia. *BMC Complementary and Alternative Medicine* 12:1–9.

Handa, S.S., A.S. Chawla, and A. Maninder. 1989. Hypoglycaemic plants – a review. *Fitoterapia* 60:195–202.

Hegazy, Gehan A., Amina M. Alnoury, and Hoda G. Gad. 2013. The role of *Acacia Arabica* extract as an antidiabetic, antihyperlipidemic, and antioxidant in streptozotocin-induced diabetic rats. *Saudi Medical Journal* 34:727–733.

Hsieh, Ching-Yu, and Shang-Tzen Chang. 2010. Antioxidant activities and xanthine oxidase inhibitory effects of phenolic phytochemicals from *Acacia confusa* twigs and branches. *Journal of Agricultural and Food Chemistry* 58:1578–1583.

Hussain, Tarique, Bie Tan, Ghulam Murtaza, Gang Liu, Najma Rahu, Muhammad Saleem Kalhoro, Dildar Hussain Kalhoro, et al. 2020. Flavonoids and type 2 diabetes: Evidence of efficacy in clinical and animal studies and delivery strategies to enhance their therapeutic efficacy. *Pharmacological Research* 152:104629.

International Diabetes Federation. 2015. *IDF Diabetes Atlas*. 7th ed., Brussels, Belgium, International Diabetes Federation. Available from www.diabetesatlas.org. Accessed 3 September 2021.

International Diabetes Federation. 2017. *IDF Diabetes Atlas*. 8th ed., Brussels, Belgium, International Diabetes Federation. Available from www.diabetesatlas.org. Accessed 3 September 2021.

Jadhav, Ramulu, and Goverdhan Puchchakayala. 2012. Hypoglycemic and antidiabetic activity of flavonoids: Boswellic acid, ellagic acid, quercetin, rutin on streptozotocin-nicotinamide induced type 2 diabetic rats. *International Journal of Pharmacy and Pharmaceutical Sciences* 4:251–256.

Jang, Jae Soon, Jong Seok Lee, Jung Hyun Lee, Duck Soo Kwon, Keun Eok Lee, Shin Young Lee, and Eock Kee Hong. 2010. Hispidin produced from *Phellinus linteus* protects pancreatic β-cells from damage by hydrogen peroxide. *Archives of Pharmacal Research* 33:853–861.

Jo, S.H., E.H. Ka, and H.S. Lee. 2009. Comparison of antioxidant potential and rat intestinal α-glucosidases inhibitory activities of quercetin, rutin, and isoquercetin. *International Journal of Applied Research in Natural Products* 2:52–60.

Kalaivani, T., C. Rajasekaran, and Lazar Mathew. 2011. Free radical scavenging, cytotoxic, and hemolytic activities of an active antioxidant compound ethyl gallate from leaves of *Acacia nilotica* (L.) Wild. Ex. Delile subsp. *indica* (Benth.) Brenan. *Journal of Food Science* 76:T144–T149.

Kashiwada, Mayumi, Saho Nakaishi, Ayumi Usuda, Yumi Miyahara, Kenta Katsumoto, Kyoko Katsura, Izumi Terakado, et al. 2021. Analysis of anti-obesity and anti-diabetic effects of acacia bark-derived proanthocyanidins in type 2 diabetes model KKAy mice. *Journal of Natural Medicines* 75:893–906.

Kingsley, R. Bino, S. Aravinth Vijay Jesuraj, P. Brindha, A. Subramoniam, and M. Atif. 2013. Anti-diabetes activity of *Acacia farnesiana* (L.) Willd in alloxan diabetic rats. *International Journal of PharmTech Research* 5:112–118.

Klein, Samuel, Nancy F. Sheard, Xavier Pi-Sunyer, Anne Daly, Judith Wylie-Rosett, Karmeen Kulkarni, and Nathaniel G. Clark. 2004. Weight management through lifestyle modification for the prevention and management of type 2 diabetes: Rationale and strategies. A statement of the American Diabetes Association, the North American Association for the Study of Obesity, and the American Society for Clinical Nutrition. *The American Journal of Clinical Nutrition* 80:257–263.

Kumar Bhateja, Pradeep, and Randhir Singh. 2014. Antidiabetic activity of *Acacia tortilis* (Forsk.) Hayne ssp. raddiana polysaccharide on streptozotocin-nicotinamide induced diabetic rats. *BioMed Research International* 2014:572013.

Latha, R. Cecily Rosemary, and P. Daisy. 2011. Insulin-secretagogue, antihyperlipidemic and other protective effects of gallic acid isolated from *Terminalia bellirica* Roxb. in streptozotocin-induced diabetic rats. *Chemico-Biological Interactions* 189:112–118.

Lee, Wooje, Sang Yeol Lee, Young-Jin Son, and Jung-Mi Yun. 2015. Gallic acid decreases inflammatory cytokine secretion through histone acetyltransferase/histone deacetylase regulation in high glucose-induced human monocytes. *Journal of Medicinal Food* 18:793–801.

Leela, V., L. Kokila, R. Lavanya, A. Saraswathy, and P. Brindha. 2010. Determination of gallic acid in *Acacia nilotica* Linn. by HPTLC. *International Journal of Pharmacy and Technology* 2:285–292.

Li, Yan Qin, Feng Chao Zhou, Fei Gao, Jun Sheng Bian, and Fang Shan. 2009. Comparative evaluation of quercetin, isoquercetin and rutin as inhibitors of α-glucosidase. *Journal of Agricultural and Food Chemistry* 57:11463–11468.

Lin, Huan-You, Tzu-Cheng Chang, and Shang-Tzen Chang. 2018. A review of antioxidant and pharmacological properties of phenolic compounds in *Acacia confusa*. *Journal of Traditional and Complementary Medicine* 8:443–450.

Machado, T.B., A.V. Pinto, M.C.F.R. Pinto, I.C.R. Leal, M.G. Silva, A.C.F. Amaral, R.M. Kuster, and K.R. Netto-dosSantos. 2003. In vitro activity of Brazilian medicinal plants, naturally occurring naphthoquinones and their analogues, against methicillin-resistant *Staphylococcus aureus*. *International Journal of Antimicrobial Agents* 21:279–284.

Mahmoud, Ayman M., Rene J. Hernandez Bautista, Mansur A. Sandhu, and Omnia E. Hussein. 2019. Beneficial effects of citrus flavonoids on cardiovascular and metabolic health. *Oxidative Medicine and Cellular Longevity* 2019:5484138.

Malviya, Neelesh, Sanjay Jain, and S.A.P.N.A. Malviya. 2010. Antidiabetic potential of medicinal plants. *Acta Poloniae Pharmaceutica* 67:113–118.

Marles, Robin J., and Norman R. Farnsworth. 1995. Antidiabetic plants and their active constituents. *Phytomedicine* 2:137–189.

Maruthur, Nisa M., Eva Tseng, Susan Hutfless, Lisa M. Wilson, Catalina Suarez-Cuervo, Zackary Berger, Yue Chu, Emmanuel Iyoha, Jodi B. Segal, and Shari Bolen. 2016. Diabetes medications as monotherapy or metformin-based combination therapy for type 2 diabetes: A systematic review and meta-analysis. *Annals of Internal Medicine* 164:740–751.

Mudaliar, Sunder, and Robert R. Henry. 2001. New oral therapies for type 2 diabetes mellitus: The glitazones or insulin sensitizers. *Annual Review of Medicine* 52:239–257.

Muhaisen, Hasan M.H. 2020. Flavonoid glycosides from *Acacia tortilis*. *Merit Research Journal of Medicine and Medical Sciences* 8:575–580.

Muhaisen, Hasan M.H., M. Ilyas, M. Mushfiq, Mehtab Parveen, and Omer A. Basudan. 2002. Flavonoids from *Acacia tortilis*. *Journal of Chemical Research* 2002:276–278.

Ngaffo, Carine M.N., Rodrigue S.V. Tchangna, Armelle T. Mbaveng, Justin Kamga, Freya M. Harvey, Bonaventure T. Ngadjui, Christian G. Bochet, and Victor Kuete. 2020. Botanicals from the leaves of *Acacia sieberiana* had better cytotoxic effects than isolated phytochemicals towards MDR cancer cells lines. *Heliyon* 6:e05412.

Niture, Netaji T., Ansar A. Ansari, and Suresh R. Naik. 2014. Anti-hyperglycemic activity of rutin in streptozotocin-induced diabetic rats: An effect mediated through cytokines, antioxidants and lipid biomarkers. *Indian Journal of Experimental Biology* 52:720–727.

Paula, Vanessa, Soraia I. Pedro, Maria G. Campos, Teresa Delgado, Letícia M. Estevinho, and Ofélia Anjos. 2022. Special bioactivities of phenolics from *Acacia dealbata* L. with potential for dementia, diabetes and antimicrobial treatments. *Applied Sciences* 12:1022.

Prince, P. Stanley Mainzen, and N. Kamalakkannan. 2006. Rutin improves glucose homeostasis in streptozotocin diabetic tissues by altering glycolytic and gluconeogenic enzymes. *Journal of Biochemical and Molecular Toxicology* 20:96–102.

Punithavathi, Vilapakkam Ranganathan, Ponnian Stanely Mainzen Prince, Ramesh Kumar, and Jemmi Selvakumari. 2011. Antihyperglycaemic, antilipid peroxidative and antioxidant effects of gallic acid on streptozotocin induced diabetic Wistar rats. *European Journal of Pharmacology* 650:465–471.

Rahmatullah, Mohammed, Maraz Hossain, Arefin Mahmud, Nahida Sultana, S. Mizanur, R. Mohammad, R. Islam, M.S. Khatoon, S. Jahan, and F. Islam. 2013. Antihyperglycemic and antinociceptive activity evaluation of "khoyer" prepared from boiling the wood of *Acacia catechu* in water. *African Journal of Traditional, Complementary and Alternative Medicines* 10:1–5.

Rajvaidhya, Saurabh, B.P. Nagori, G.K. Singh, B.K. Dubey, Prashant Desai, and Sanjay Jain. 2012. A review on *Acacia Arabica* – an Indian medicinal plant. *International Journal of Pharmaceutical Sciences and Research* 3:1995–2005.

Rao, M. Upendra, M. Sreenivasulu, B. Chengaiah, K. Jaganmohan Reddy, and C. Madhusudhana Chetty. 2010. Herbal medicines for diabetes mellitus: A review. *International Journal of PharmTech Research* 2:1883–1892.

Rasouli, Hassan, Reza Yarani, Flemming Pociot, and Jelena Popović-Djordjević. 2020. Anti-diabetic potential of plant alkaloids: Revisiting current findings and future perspectives. *Pharmacological Research* 155:104723.

Rather, Luqman Jameel, and Faqeer Mohammad. 2015. *Acacia nilotica* (L.): A review of its traditional uses, phytochemistry, and pharmacology. *Sustainable Chemistry and Pharmacy* 2:12–30.

Ray, D., K.H. Sharatchandra, and I.S. Thokchom. 2006. Antipyretic, antidiarrhoeal, hypoglycaemic and hepatoprotective activities of ethyl acetate extract of *Acacia catechu* Willd. in albino rats. *Indian Journal of Pharmacology* 38:408–413.

Salem, Manar M., Frederick H. Davidorf, and Mohamed H. Abdel-Rahman. 2011. In vitro anti-uveal melanoma activity of phenolic compounds from the Egyptian medicinal plant *Acacia nilotica*. *Fitoterapia* 82:1279–1284.

Sarian, Murni Nazira, Qamar Uddin Ahmed, Siti Zaiton Mat So'ad, Alhassan Muhammad Alhassan, Suganya Murugesu, Vikneswari Perumal, Sharifah Nurul Akilah Syed Mohamad, Alfi Khatib, and Jalifah Latip. 2017. Antioxidant and antidiabetic effects of flavonoids: A structure-activity relationship based study. *BioMed Research International* 2017:8386065.

Sathya, Arumugam, and Perumal Siddhuraju. 2013. Protective effect of bark and empty pod extracts from *Acacia auriculiformis* against paracetamol intoxicated liver injury and alloxan induced type II diabetes. *Food and Chemical Toxicology* 56:162–170.

Sattanathan, K., C.K. Dhanapal, R. Umarani, and R. Manavalan. 2011. Beneficial health effects of rutin supplementation in patients with diabetes mellitus. *Journal of Applied Pharmaceutical Science* 1:227.

Scazzocchio, Beatrice, Rosaria Varì, Carmelina Filesi, Ilaria Del Gaudio, Massimo D'Archivio, Carmela Santangelo, Annunziata Iacovelli, et al. 2015. Protocatechuic acid activates key components of insulin signaling pathway mimicking insulin activity. *Molecular Nutrition & Food Research* 59:1472–1481.

Shanmuganathan, Sivasankar, and Narayanasamy Angayarkanni. 2018. Chebulagic acid Chebulinic acid and Gallic acid, the active principles of Triphala, inhibit TNFα induced pro-angiogenic and pro-inflammatory activities in retinal capillary endothelial cells by inhibiting p 38, ERK and NFkB phosphorylation. *Vascular Pharmacology* 108:23–35.

Sharma, Manisha, A.K. Gupta, and Alok Mukherji. 2014. Invasive *Acacia nilotica* a problematic weed is a source of potent methyl gallate. *International Journal of Scientific Research* 10:1193–1195.

Singh, Brahma N., B.R. Singh, R.L. Singh, D. Prakash, B.K. Sarma, and H.B. Singh. 2009. Antioxidant and anti-quorum sensing activities of green pod of *Acacia nilotica* L. *Food and Chemical Toxicology* 47:778–786.

Singh, K.N., R.K. Mittal, and K.C. Barthwal. 1976. Hypoglycaemic activity of *Acacia catechu*, *Acacia suma*, and *Albizzia odoratissima* seed diets in normal albino rats. *The Indian Journal of Medical Research* 64:754–757.

Srinivasan, K., C.L. Kaul, and P. Ramarao. 2005. Partial protective effect of rutin on multiple low dose streptozotocin-induced diabetes in mice. *Indian Journal of Pharmacology* 37:327–328.

Stohs, Sidney J., and Debasis Bagchi. 2015. Antioxidant, anti-inflammatory, and chemoprotective properties of *Acacia catechu* heartwood extracts. *Phytotherapy Research* 29:818–824.

Thambiraj, J., and S. Paulsamy. 2012. In vitro antioxidant potential of methanol extract of the medicinal plant, *Acacia caesia* (L.) Willd. *Asian Pacific Journal of Tropical Biomedicine* 2:S732–S736.

Vinayagam, Ramachandran, Muthukumaran Jayachandran, and Baojun Xu. 2016. Antidiabetic effects of simple phenolic acids: A comprehensive review. *Phytotherapy Research* 30:184–199.

Wadood, Abdul, Noreen Wadood, and S.A. Shah. 1989. Effects of *Acacia arabica* and *Caralluma edulis* on blood glucose levels of normal and alloxan diabetic rabbits. *The Journal of Pakistan Medical Association* 39:208–212.

World Health Organization. 2019. *Diabetes. Factsheet on Diabetes*. Available from www.who.int/news-room/fact-sheets/detail/diabetes. Accessed 3 September 2021.

Yusuf, Uthman A., Olusola A. Adeeyo, Emmanuel O. Salawu, Bernard U. Enaibe, and Olusegun D. Omotoso. 2012. *Allium cepa* protects renal functions in diabetic rabbit. *World Journal of Life Sciences and Medical Research* 2:86–90.

Zhou, Qian, Ka-Wing Cheng, Jianbo Xiao, and Mingfu Wang. 2020. The multifunctional roles of flavonoids against the formation of advanced glycation end products (AGEs) and AGEs-induced harmful effects. *Trends in Food Science & Technology* 103:333–347.

Zhu, Wei, Ibrahim Khalifa, Ruifeng Wang, and Chunmei Li. 2020. Persimmon highly galloylated-tannins in vitro mitigated α-amylase and α-glucosidase via statically binding with their catalytic-closed sides and altering their secondary structure elements. *Journal of Food Biochemistry* 44:e13234.

3 A Review of the Plants Used for the Management of Diabetes

B. Jyotirmayee, Ushashee Mandal, Ehsan Amiri Ardakani and Gyanranjan Mahalik

CONTENTS

3.1   INTRODUCTION

Diabetes mellitus can be defined as a chronic disease in which a person's body has poor sugar regulation in the blood. As a result, the blood glucose level is abnormally elevated (Nam et al., 2011). It has been found that there are three types of diabetes: type 1 diabetes, type 2 diabetes, and gestational diabetes. In the case of type 1 diabetes, the pancreas cannot secrete the hormone insulin or makes significantly less insulin. Insulin promotes sugar uptake in cells, which can be further used as energy. However, when insulin is not secreted, blood sugar cannot enter the cell and thus accumulates in the bloodstream. Type 1 diabetes (known as insulin-dependent or juvenile diabetes) is generally detected in children, teenagers, and young people but can initiate at any stage of life. Roughly 5%–10% of people have type 1 diabetes. It is unknown how type 1 diabetes can be prevented. Still, it is manageable if one follows the healthcare professionals' advice to maintain a healthy lifestyle, blood sugar control, and have regular health check-ups. Type 1 diabetes is thought to arise from an autoimmune response (in which the body attacks itself), damaging pancreatic β cells that form insulin. This activity can continue for several months before any symptoms comes to light (DiMeglio et al., 2018).

Some specific genes are related to type 1 diabetes and environmental factors, such as exposure to a virus. In the case of type 2 diabetes, the cells usually do not respond to insulin secretion, which is known as insulin resistance, causing further insulin release. The pancreas can't sustain insulin release, and the blood sugar levels increases, leading to type 2 diabetes. This type of diabetes can keep developing in the body yearly without showing any traits. In the case of gestational diabetes, this appears in pregnant women in the absence of diabetic symptoms. About 2%–10% of pregnant women in America are prone to gestational diabetes each year. Insulin resistance results from the cells' reduced ability to utilize insulin. The body's need for insulin is heightened in this condition. Insulin resistance develops in the third trimester in almost all pregnant women (DiMeglio et al., 2018).

DOI: 10.1201/9781003220930-4

In some cases, women experience resistance to insulin before getting pregnant. As a result, their pregnancy begins with a high demand for insulin and they have maximum probability of developing gestational diabetes. This type does not have any particular indications. A person's medical records and any other consequences provide information to a patients risk of developing this type of diabetes (Powers et al., 2020).

It has been shown that medicinal herbs might be a powerful source of α-amylase inhibition in both the *in vitro* and *in vivo* experimental models. As a result, they might serve as prospective candidates for future drug development efforts to treat diabetes with low or no adverse effects. Potential candidate plants with more excellent anti-diabetic characteristics are selected to support the pre-existing ethnobotanical usage of medicinal plants (Khadayat et al., 2020). Several plant species inhibit the enzymes α-amylase and α-glucosidase to lower blood sugar levels. Additionally, several other anti-diabetic herbs may repair pancreatic cells, enhance insulin production, and reduce metabolic syndrome in individuals with type 2 diabetes. Elements such as magnesium (Mg), potassium (K), phosphorus (P), calcium (Ca), zinc (Zn), copper (Cu), and nickel (Ni) all play a role in the mechanism of action. These plant components and elements might be included in new and more effective herbal drugs and nutraceuticals to reduce the global impact of diabetes (Chinsembu, 2019). Research has demonstrated the hypoglycemic effects of medicinal plants, including the ability to increase insulin secretion, inhibit amylase or glucosidase, prevent reactive oxygen species (ROS) and antioxidant activity, increase the translocation of glucose transporter type 4 (GLUT-4), and prevent insulin resistance, to name just a few. Medicinal herbs help with diabetes mellitus and provide several other health benefits, including preventing diabetes complications. Anti-diabetic drugs already on the market may benefit from using these plants as an alternative or supplement (Nazarian-Samani et al., 2018).

3.2   PLANTS USED IN THE MANAGEMENT OF DIABETES

Conventional medicine isn't only about treating diabetes; numerous therapeutic plant-based recipes should be studied and rationalized. Diabetes mellitus may be prevented from 800 reported medicinal plants. However, anti-diabetic characteristics of just 450 medicinal plants have been clinically confirmed, with 109 medicinal plants possessing a comprehensive mechanism of action (Verma et al., 2018). Stem barks were the most common, followed by leaves, and the rest included roots, fibers, fruit, bulbs, flowers, rhizomes, skin, and stems (Tjeck et al., 2017). Plants historically used to treat and control diabetes are included in this list (Tables 3.1–3.3):

> *Allium cepa* (garlic): Clinical trials showed that garlic lowered fructosamine and glycosylated hemoglobin and improved rats' blood glucose and retinal morphological abnormalities (Salleh et al., 2021). Garlic has been reported stimulating nitric oxide (NO) synthesis in various cells. AEG (aqueous extract of garlic) and a purified NO-generating protein from garlic (NGPG) can control hyperglycemia through the stimulation of NO by glucose-activated NO synthase that would play an essential role in the synthesis of insulin/GLUT-4 in liver cells (Bhattacharya et al., 2019).
>
> *Curcuma longa* (turmeric): The β cell activity of diabetic and prediabetic individuals was improved by curcumin, decreasing the course of the disease. However, the pancreas and kidneys of diabetic rats were protected by oral treatment of turmeric extract and curcumin (Essa et al., 2019). In addition, a three-month randomized-controlled experiment using *Curcuma longa* found a substantial reduction in arterial stiffness compared to placebo in individuals with type 2 diabetes (Srinivasan et al., 2019).
>
> *Momordica charantia* (bitter gourd): Recently, it was shown that rats fed either non-fermented or lactic acid fermented *M. charantia* juice reduced fasting and postprandial blood glucose levels when given the latter (Hartajanie et al., 2020). The use of mcIRBP-19, a bitter melon peptide, in diabetic blood glucose management seems promising since it may

provide patients with a more concentrated dosage of anti-diabetic bioactive chemicals (Amiri-Ardekani et al., 2021).

Allium cepa (onion): Organosulfur compounds, phenolic compounds, polysaccharides, and saponins are all onions. Onion's primary bioactive ingredients include phenolic and sulfur-containing compounds, such as onionin A (quercetin, quercetin glucosides, cysteine sulf-oxides). Onion and its bioactive components have been shown to provide several health benefits, including antioxidant, anti-diabetic, anticancer, antibacterial, anti-inflammatory, and anti-obesity properties. Onion bulbs include crude oil, vitamin E, sodium, potassium, zinc, and other nutrients (Zhao et al., 2021). Because of its hypolipidemic action, the juice of the *A. cepa* plant has been shown to reduce total cholesterol, triglyceride levels, low-density lipoprotein cholesterol (LDL-C), and high-density lipoprotein cholesterol (HDL-C) levels. Alloxan-induced diabetic rats treated with *A. cepa* bulb showed hypolipidemic and anti-diabetic effects (Airaodion et al., 2020; Mahmood et al., 2021).

Aloe vera: Anthraquinones, nutrients, lignin, saponins, minerals, sugars, catalysts, unsaturated fats, and amino acids are all found in *A. vera*. Bioactive compounds such as catalysts, regular sugars, unsaturated fats, amino acids, and other bioactive combinations are located in the leaves. The plant has immense healing potential because of its anti-aging, anti-diabetic, antioxidant, anticancer, anti-inflammatory, antibacterial, analgesic, and several other properties. One of the potential candidates for alleviating diabetes is *A. vera* extract, which has a synergistic impact on the pathways implicated in the advancement of diabetes because of its contents (Riaz et al., 2021). Reduced development of age-glycated end products (AGE) and decreased postprandial glucose levels may indicate that aloe vera methanol extract (AVM) might help avoid diabetic problems linked with AGE, as shown by this study. The oxidative breakdown of fructosamine in AVM successfully suppressed the glycation response of proteins in the BSA/glucose system (Babu et al., 2021; Muñiz-Ramirez et al., 2020).

Andrographis paniculata (green chiretta): For generations, *A. paniculata*, also known as green chiretta, has been utilized in Ayurvedic herbal treatment. This plant's biological action is due to its bioactive components, including andrographolide, dehydroandrographolide, neoandrographolide, and deoxyandrographolide in the diterpene lactone group. Andrographolide is in *A. paniculata* in higher concentrations than the other diterpene lactones. This species has also been shown to contain the antioxidants andrographidine, apigenin, and luteolin (Chen et al., 2014; Rafi et al., 2020). Modern medications benefit significantly from the hydroethanolic extract of *A. paniculata*. The study's findings also discovered the extract's potential anti-diabetic properties. Anti-diabetic properties may be inferred from the hypoglycemic action mediated by a decrease in glucose diffusion rate (Dsouza et al., 2020).

Azadirachta indica (neem): The anti-diabetic effects of neem plant components such as leaves, bark, flowers, seeds, oil, and roots are noteworthy since they all reduce blood glucose levels in the body. To treat diabetes, seed and leaf extracts may be combined into a dosage form and administered orally (Gautam et al., 2021). The presence of specific phytochemicals responsible for the experimental animals' increased antioxidant enzyme activity may explain the ability of the aqueous extract of *A. indica* at various dosages to reduce fasting blood glucose levels in streptozotocin-induced diabetic rats. To treat and control diabetes, the aqueous extract of *A. indica* leaves may be utilized as an alternate anti-diabetic therapy (Christian et al., 2019).

Emblica officinalis (amla): Gallotannin, gallic acid, ellagic acid, and corilagin have been found in the *E. officinalis* or *Phyllanthus emblica* Linn. fruits. Antioxidant and free radical scavenging characteristics provide it anti-diabetic benefits. Preventing/reducing hyperglycemia, diabetic nephropathy, and other consequences of diabetic nephropathy have also been possible using amla (D'Souza et al., 2014). Methanolic extracts of *P. emblica* fruit contain a significant amount of quercetin. Quercetin may have anti-diabetic and antihyperglycemic effects because of its ability to alter glucose, cholesterol, and triglyceride levels in the body. This has been shown in both vitro and *in vivo* investigations (Srinivasan et al., 2018).

Moringa oleifera (moringa): The research shows that diverse *M. oleifera* plant components might be ideal candidates for antibacterial, antioxidant, and anti-diabetic supplements, especially since it is currently extensively used in animal and human diets. The leaf extracts had the total phenolics, whereas the lateral roots contained the most condensed tannins and flavonoids. Therefore, using the roots as an antioxidant source is preferable to using the leaves. Compared to root extracts, all leaf extracts demonstrated much better anti-diabetic and antibacterial activities (Alamgir, 2018). This plant's therapeutic properties can be found in every part of it. Vitamin C, vitamin A, and milk protein are abundant in this product. Quinine, saponins, flavonoids, alkaloids, proteins, steroids, glycosides, fixed oil, tannin, and lipids are only some of the active phytoconstituents in this plant (Tshabalala et al., 2020).

Additionally, niazinin A and B and niazimicin A and B make up the rest of the ingredients. Only diabetic rats responded well to *M. oleifera* leaf extract's antihyperglycemic properties. Cryptochlorogenic acid, quercetin 3-D-glucoside, and kaempferol 3-O-glucoside were likely responsible for this action (Irfan et al., 2017; Paikra & Gidwani, 2017).

Ocimum sanctum (tulsi): Glucose-fed rats treated orally with *O. sanctum* extract resulted in a substantial reduction in blood sugar levels. In laboratory mice, *O. sanctum* leaves have hypoglycemic effects. According to results from animal studies, *O. sanctum* leaf extracts may stimulate insulin production by interacting with physiological mechanisms (Gulhane et al., 2021). The anti-diabetic activities of *O. sanctum* have been widely recognized. In both acute and long-term feeding experiments, *O. sanctum* ethanol extract has been demonstrated to lower hyperglycemia in alloxan diabetic rats (Shival et al., 2020).

Trigonella foenum-graecum (fenugreek): *T. foenum-graecum* seed powder solution reduced TC, TG, and LDL-C levels and raised HDL-C levels in newly diagnosed type 2 diabetes individuals. Researchers found that the powdered seed of *T. foenum-graecum* is a powerful dietary supplement for controlling dyslipidemia (Geberemeskel et al., 2019). Fenugreek's anti-diabetic effect is remarkable because it increases insulin secretion while sensitizing insulin. Similarly, the alkaloid found in fenugreek seeds, trigonelline, has been shown to have potent anti-diabetic and analgesic properties. An anti-diabetic herbal drug, SugaHeal, a standardized fenugreek seed extract high in 4-hydroxy isoleucine and trigonelline, is on the market. Fenfuro, a standardized fenugreek extract with high concentrations of furostan saponins, is also beneficial in treating type 2 diabetes. Galactomannan-rich water-soluble fiber possesses anti-diabetic and lipid-lowering properties (Kilambi & Shah, 2021).

Zingiber officinale (ginger): Patients with type 2 diabetes had reduced blood sugar, hemoglobin A_{1C}, and LDL/HDL ratio after oral ginger supplementation. Patients with type 2 diabetes may benefit from ginger's ability to lower fasting blood glucose and hemoglobin A_{1C} levels (Arzati et al., 2017). It was shown that 6-shogaol and 6-paradol could significantly increase the adipocytes and myotubes' glucose consumption. 6-Paradol reduced the levels of blood sugar, cholesterol, and weight. The antihyperglycemic properties of ginger might be attributed to 6-paradol (Wei et al., 2017).

3.3 ETHNOBOTANICAL USES OF PLANTS FOR THE TREATMENT OF DIABETES

Medicinal herbs are used by Santhal tribes in Mayurbhanj, Odisha, to treat diabetes (Aradhna et al., 2021)

- The whole plant of green chiretta is boiled, especially the leaves, and consumed in the morning.

- Jamun ripe fruit and dried seed are used for the treatment. The ripened fruits are consumed orally, and seed powder is mixed with honey or gur (*jaggery*) to cure diabetes.
- Aqueous extract of neem leaves is taken on an empty stomach. Then young leaves are prescribed to the patient, and the seed is also beneficial.
- *Centella asiatica* leaves are taken orally.
- *Moringa oleifera* fruit and the leaves show anti-diabetic properties. Therefore, patients are advised to take leaves, fruits, and flowers as vegetables.
- *Catharanthus roseus* young leaves and flowers are taken daily on an empty stomach.
- *Gymnema sylvestre*, also known as *gurmar*, means "sugar destroyer." Leaf juice, powdered leaves, or young leaves are orally administered once in the morning.
- *Momordica charantia* fruit juice is given to the patient in the morning on an empty stomach, and it is also advised to take the fruit as a vegetable in the daily diet to treat diabetes.

An ethnobotanical study of traditional medicinal plants of Javadhu hill of Tiruvannamalai district used for the treatment of diabetes. Locals utilized plant components such as seeds, rhizomes, leaves, and roots. Diabetes patients were treated using plant materials made as decoctions, infusions, or aqueous extracts in milk or honey (Thirumalai et al., 2012).

- *Aegle marmelos*: The dried and powdered leaves are used.
- *Allium sativum*: Leaf juice is taken.
- *Aloe vera*: Oral ingestion of leaf gel.
- *Andrographis paniculate*: Leaf juice is taken orally.
- *Aristolochia bracteolate*: Leaf juice is ingested orally.
- *Azadirachta indica*: Powdered leaves are used.
- *Brassica juncea*: Every day, the seed decoction is taken.
- *Cajanus cajan*: Boiling and eating the seeds as part of a meal.
- *Cassia auriculata*: Every day, three or four flowers are consumed.
- *Colocasia esculenta*: Diabetic patients might benefit from the usage of powdered leaves.
- *Costus igneus*: Use of the juice obtained from the leaves.
- *Eugenia jambolana*: Taken orally first thing in the morning, seeds powered.
- *Mangifera indica*: The powdered leaves are combined with cow's milk orally.
- *Momordica charantia*: The powdered seed is taken orally after being diluted with water.
- *Moringa oleifera*: Oral ingestion of early-morning leaf juice is recommended.
- *Ocimum sanctum*: A tiny amount of leaf is taken in the morning.
- *Solanum nigrum*: Leaf juice is ingested orally.
- *Spermacoce hispida*: Powered leaves are ingested two times a day.

3.4 FUTURE CHALLENGES

In this review, published studies on human clinical trials for medicinal plants' intervention in diabetes are criticized for their inadequacies. The inconsistency of data findings might be due to various extraction processes and procedures employed on medicinal plants in different regions. Medicinal plants have drawn interest in the past because they had fewer adverse effects than chemically manufactured medications. To obtain more information on the biology and pharmacology of medicinal plants, further research into their impact on diabetes is required. More research is needed to determine if curcumin is safe and effective to consume among plants. New natural inhibitors will need to be developed to understand better how AVM interacts with enzymes such as α-amylase, α-glucosidase, and pancreatic lipase. A thorough evaluation of *Azadirachta indica* for developing plant-based medications and nutraceuticals and assessing their clinical efficacy and safety against diabetes mellitus has been recommended due to research limitations. Several studies have looked into the anti-diabetic properties of *Ocimum*, but its exact action method is still a mystery. Sacred basil should be the focus of future research in the fight against various ailments. To fully understand the mechanism of action of a particular bioactive component found in *Trigonella foenum-graecum* seed powder, additional research is required, including detailed chemical and pharmacological evaluation. In addition, more extensive research is needed to evaluate the long-term effects of *T. foenum-graecum* seed powder solution on a bigger scale. There are several active compounds in fenugreek and the chemical constituents that make up the herb. This spice might become therapeutically potent if the scientific and medical research community and pharmaceutical entrepreneurs take a more targeted approach and work together more closely. It is safe to propose these herbs as vital medicinal plants for the benefit of humanity after thorough evaluation.

3.5   TOXICITY AND CAUTIONARY NOTES

Toxicology investigations use a test preparation to determine whether a material hurts a biological system and to gather typical dose-response data. Using the data, it is possible to assess how dangerous the test preparation is to humans to estimate the dosage for human safety. Human biochemical, physiological, and pathological reactions to a test preparation can be observed utilizing a toxicity test conducted on animals as a model. The results of toxicology tests cannot show human safety. Still, they can provide evidence of relative toxicity and aid in determining the harmful consequences that might be experienced by humans if exposed to a substance or preparation. New, effective therapies and protections against dangerous pharmaceutical items are sought for the market, which is why drug toxicological rules exist. Toxicity can be assessed in three ways: (1) by accidental exposure, (2) through cells/cell lines, and (3) through effects on experimental animals – *in vivo* in all three cases. The recommended dosage level for the therapy of the condition was first tested in animal models for toxicity. The toxicity evaluation is an essential part of pharmaceutical research and the supervision of the quality of health products derived from plants. Acute toxicity is the most widely reported toxicity test. Leaves proved to be the most challenging component to work with. Several plants produce compounds that are hepatotoxic. Whole plant extracts or fractions containing various substances can have multiple biological impacts on the body, some of which may be severe poisonous effects. Certain portions of the plant may have more hazardous effects than others. Healthcare practitioners are reluctant to integrate herbal products because of the potential for toxicity, which is a significant reason. Accurate awareness of the traditional uses of these medicinal herbs is essential because this often helps to prevent their intake.

3.6   CONCLUSION

Diabetes is a dangerous metabolic illness that affects millions of people worldwide. Unfortunately, allopathic drugs are ineffective in treating the disease, resulting in various side effects. As a result, treating diabetes mellitus with plant-derived chemicals that are readily available and do not necessitate time-consuming pharmaceutical production appears to be a compelling option. Therefore, it is concluded that some common plants like *Momordica charantia, Gymnema sylvestre, Catharanthus roseus, Ocimum sanctum*, and *Azadirachta indica* have the potential to reduce the problems of diabetes. Furthermore, if medicinal plants with concurrent effects may be used to treat or prevent diabetes mellitus and its consequences, they might be considered alternative or adjunctive medicine.

3.7   SUMMARY POINTS

- Glucose-focused diabetes is a metabolic and endocrine disorder marked by hyperglycemia and insulin resistance. Diabetic cases are on the rise across the globe. According to the World Health Organization, India is the diabetes capital of the world.
- For drug development, herbal products are a hotspot because of their enormous range and common side effects. Structure diversity and drug-like characteristics are lacking in

synthetic substances. The need to keep looking at natural products as potential sources of new medications is essential.

- This review examines plant-derived chemicals that may be used to combat obesity or be antagonistic to diabetic treatments. Oral hypoglycemic medications and insulin therapy are the most common treatments for type 2 diabetes.
- An alternative to synthetic anti-diabetic drugs is available in the form of medicinal plants. Edible plants are emphasized in this chapter's discussion on anti-diabetic plants. The chapter's focus continues on the use of edible anti-diabetic herbs or products.
- Herbal medicine, a centuries-old practice in areas of India, was found highly effective by the researchers. This old idea should be thoroughly examined in light of modern medical science and may be used in part if proven appropriate. Using this study's application is predicted to speed up the identification and development of drugs from natural resources for treating diabetes. The goal is that medicinal plants can be used to treat diabetes safely and effectively.
- This review provides a comprehensive look at medicinal plants' potential anti-diabetic properties. More research on these plants is needed to support their usage as anti-diabetic medications. To explore the anti-diabetic activity of various untreated plant species, bioactive substances responsible for anti-diabetic qualities must be examined in additional studies.

TABLE 3.1
Plant and Plant Parts Used in Diabetic Treatment

Scientific Name	Common Name	Parts Used	Family
Aegle marmelos	Wood apple	Leaves, fruit	Rutaceae
Aloe barbadensis	Aloe vera	Leaves	Asphodelaceae
Allium sativum	Garlic	Root crop bulbs, stems, tops	Liliaceae
Allium cepa	Onion	Root crop bulbs, stems, tops	Liliaceae
Andrographis paniculate	Green chiretta	Stems, leaves, roots	Acanthaceae
Aristolochia bracteolate	Worm killer	Leaves	Aristolochiaceae
Azadirachta indica	Neem	Leaves, flowers	Meliaceae
Brassica juncea	Chinese mustard	Seeds	Cruciferae
Cajanus cajan	Pigeon pea	Seeds	Fabaceae
Carica papaya	Papaya	Seeds, leaves	Caricaceae
Cassia auriculata	Tanner's cassia	Flowers	Caesalpiniaceae
Catharanthus roseus	Nayantara	Flowers	Apocynaceae
Capparis deciduas	Telacucha	Leaves	
Centella asiatica	Murakami	Leaves	Apiaceae
Coccinia grandis	Ivy gourd	Fruits	Cucurbitaceae
Colocasia esculenta	Yam	Leaves	Araceae
Costus igneus	Spiral flag	Leaves	Costaceae
Cuminum cyminum	Cumin	Seeds	Apiaceae
Curcuma longa	Turmeric	Rhizomes, leaves	Zingiberaceae
Eclipta alba	Bhringaraj	Leaves	Asteraceae
Emblica officinalis	Indian gooseberry	Fruit	Phyllanthaceae
Eugenia jambolana	Black plum	Seed	Myrtaceae
Euphorbia hirta	Asthma weed	Leaves	Euphorbiaceae
Ficus benghalensis	Indian banyan	Bark	Moraceae
Ficus racemose	Cluster fig	Root	Moraceae

(Continued)

TABLE 3.1
(Continued)

Scientific Name	Common Name	Parts Used	Family
Gymnema sylvestre	Cow plant	Leaves	Asclepiadaceae
Hibiscus rosa sinensis	China rose	Leaves	Malvaceae
Mangifera indica	Mango	Leaves	Anacardiaceae
Marsilea minuta	Dwarf waterclover	Leaves	Marsileaceae
Melia azedarach	Chinaberry tree	Seeds	Meliaceae
Momordica charantia	Bitter gourd	Fruit, seeds, leaves	Cucurbitaceae
Moringa oleifera	Moringa	Fruit, leaves, flowers	Moringaceae
Murraya koenigii	Curry leaf tree	Leaves	Rutaceae
Ocimum sanctum	Holy basil	Leaves	Lamiaceae
Phyllanthus amarus	Gale of wind	Leaves	Euphorbiaceae
Phyllanthus emblica	Amla	Fruit	Euphorbiaceae
Psidium guajava	Guava	Fruit	Myrtaceae
Punica granatum	Pomegranate	Fruit	Lythraceae
Solanum nigrum	Garden nightshade	Leaves	Solanaceae
Spermacoce hispida	Shaggy button weed	Leaves	Rubiaceae
Swertia chirayita	Cherotha	Stems, bark	Gentianaceae
Syzygium cumini	Blackberry	Fruit, seeds	Rosaceae
Trigonella foenum-graecum	Fenugreek	Seed	Fabaceae
Tinospora cordifolia	Guduchi	Whole plant	Menispermaceae
Vinca rosea	Madagascar periwinkle	Leaves	Apocynaceae
Withania somnifera	Ashwagandha	Leaves	Solanaceae
Zingiber officinalis	Ginger	Rhizomes	Zingiberaceae

Sources: Adapted from Alqahtani et al. (2022); Behera et al. (2021); Bouyahya et al. (2021); Daharia et al. (2022); Mishra et al. (2019).

TABLE 3.2
Chemical Constituents of Plants Used in the Treatment of Diabetes

Scientific Name	Chemical Constituents
Aegle marmelos	Coumarin, imperatorin, xanthotoxol, marmeline aegeline
Aloe barbadensis	Proteins, amino acids, lipids, enzymes, vitamins, inorganic compounds and small organic compounds
Allium sativum	Sulfur-containing compounds such as allicin, vinyldithiins, alliin, ajoenes, and sulfides
Allium cepa	Quercetin, allicin, fisetin, other sulphurous compounds: diallyl disulphide and diallyl trisulphide
Andrographis paniculate	14-deoxy-11,12-didehydroandrographolide, neoandrographolide, 14-deoxyandrographolide, andrograpanin, 14-deoxy-14,15-dehydroandrographolide, isoandrographolide, 3,19-isopropylideneandrographolide, 14-acetylandrographolide
Aristolochia bracteolate	Aristolactams, aristolochic acids and esters, isoquinolines, aporphines, protoberberines, benzylisoquinolines, lignans, amides, coumarins, flavonoids, benzenoids, steroids biphenyl ethers, tetralones, terpenoids
Azadirachta indica	Azadirachtin, nimbin, nimbolinin, nimbidol, nimbidin, nimbandiol, nimbolide, salannin, sodium nimbinate, quercetin, gedunin, nimbanene, 6-desacetylnimbinene, ascorbic acid, 7-desacetyl-7-benzoylgedunin, n-hexacosanol, 7-desacetyl-7-benzoylazadiradione, 17-hydroxyazadiradione

Scientific Name	Chemical Constituents
Brassica juncea	Vitamins, dietary fiber, glucosinolates (and their degradation products), minerals, chlorophylls, polyphenols, volatile components (allyl isothiocyanate, 3-butyl isothiocyanate)
Cajanus cajan	α-himachalene, β-himachalene, γ-himachalene, α-humulene, α-copaene, sesquiterpenes
Carica papaya	Vitamins A, B, and C, carbohydrates, alkaloids (carpaine and pseudocarpaine), proteins, proteolytic enzymes (papain and quimiopapain), benzyl isothiocyanate
Cassia auriculata	Alkaloids, terpenoids, flavonoids, phenols, steroids, tannins, sugar saponins, quinines, proteins
Catharanthus roseus	Vinblastine, alkaloids, tryptamine, strictosidine, antineoplastic agents, phytochemicals, secologanin, vinca alkaloids
Capparis deciduas	Alkaloids (isocodonocarpine, stachydrine, capparisinine, capparisine), fatty acids, phenolics, sterols, flavonoids
Centella asiatica	Isoprenoids (plant sterols, sesquiterpenes, saponins, pentacyclic triterpenoids), phenylpropanoid derivatives (caffeoylquinic acids, eugenol derivatives, flavonoids)
Coccinia grandis	Heptacosane, cephalandrol, β-sitosterol, β-amyrin acetate, alkaloids cephalandrins A and B, lupeol, cucurbitacin B, taraxerone, taraxerol, β-carotene, lycopene, cryptoxanthin, xyloglucan, carotenoids, β-sitosterol, stigma-7-en-3-one, starch, fatty acids, carbonic acid, triterpenoid, saponin, coccinoside, flavonoid glycoside
Colocasia esculenta	Calcium oxalate, minerals (calcium phosphorus, etc.), fibers, starch, vitamin A, B, C, etc., flavones, apigenin, luteolin, anthocyanins
Costus igneus	Carbohydrates, tannins, saponins, triterpenoids, flavonoids, steroids, proteins, alkaloids, appreciable amounts of trace elements
Cuminum cyminum	Alkaloid, flavonoid, glycoside, coumarin, protein, resin, anthraquinone, saponin, tannin, steroid
Curcuma longa	Curcumin, demethoxycurcumin, bisdemethoxycurcumin, curlone, α-turmerone, β-turmerone, terpilonene
Eclipta alba	Wedololactone, demethylwedelolactone, β-amyrin, luteolin-7-O-glucoside, desmethyl-wedelolactone-7-glucoside, ecliptal hentriacontanol, heptacosanol, stigmasterol
Emblica officinalis	Gallic acid, ellagic acid, rutin, ascorbic acid, quercetin, catechol
Eugenia jambolana	Oleanolic acid, β-sitosterol, gallic acid, ellagic acid, ursolic acid, cornusiin B, oenothein C, valoneic acid dilactone
Euphorbia hirta	Alkanes, polyphenols, flavonoids triterpenes, phytosterols, tannins
Ficus benghalensis	Carbohydrates, steroids, saponins, tannins, flavonoids, amino acids/proteins, rutin, friedelin, taraxosterol, bergapten, β-sisterol, lupeol, quercetin-3-galactoside
Ficus racemose	Tannin, β-sitosterol (A), wax, leucopelargonidin-3-O-β-D-glucopyranoside, saponin gluanol acetate, ceryl behenate, lupeol acetate, leucocyanidin-3-O-β-D-glucopyranoside, leucopelargonidin-3-O-α-L-rhamnopyranoside, leucoanthocyanin, lupeol (C), α-amyrin acetate (B), leucoanthocyanidin, stigmasterol
Gymnema sylvestre	Gurmarin, gymnemic acid, flavonoids, phenols, gymnemasaponins, tannin, quinones
Hibiscus rosa sinensis	Tannins, quinines, phenols, anthraquinones, terpenoids, saponins, flavonoids, alkaloids, protein, free amino acids, reducing sugars, mucilage, cardiac glycosides, carbohydrates, essential oils, steroids
Mangifera indica	Carbohydrates, lipid, fatty acids, organic acids, vitamins, minerals, protein, amino acids, phenolic compounds, flavonoids and other polyphenols, chlorophyll, carotenoids, volatile compounds
Marsilea minuta	Tannins, saponins, steroids, terpenoids, triterpenoids, flavonoids, alkaloids, proteins, anthraquinones, carbohydrates, phenolic compounds, phytosterol
Melia azedarach	Alkaloid, a steroidal glycoside, saponin, carbohydrate, chlorogenic acid, flavonoids tannin, phenol, tannins

(Continued)

TABLE 3.2
(Continued)

Scientific Name	Chemical Constituents
Momordica charantia	Water, mineral matters, charantin, fat, carbohydrates, fiber, alkaloids, momordium, glucosides, a steroidal saponin, carbohydrates, ascorbic acid
Moringa oleifera	Flavonoids, saponins, tannins, alkaloids, phenols, proteins, glycosides, vitamins, minerals, glucosinolates, isothiocyanates, terpenes, 9-octadecenoic acid, L-(+)-ascorbic acid-2,6-dihexadecanoate, 14-methyl-8-hexadecenal, 4-hydroxyl-4-methyl-2-pentanone, 3-ethyl-2, 4-dimethyl-pentane, phytol, octadecamethyl-cyclononasiloxane, 1,2-benzene dicarboxylic acid, 3,4-epoxy-ethanone, N-(-1-methylethyllidene)-benzene ethanamine, 4,8,12,16-tetramethylheptadecan-4-olide, 3–5-bis (1, 1-dimethylethyl)-phenol, 1-hexadecanol, 3,7,11,15-tetramethyl-2 hexadecene-1-ol, hexadecanoic acid, 1,2,3-propanetriyl ester-9 octadecenoic acid
Murraya koenigii	Alkaloids, terpenoids, flavonoids, polyphenol, protein, carbohydrate, total sugars, starch, vitamin A (B carotene), vitamin B3 (niacin), vitamin B1 (thiamin)
Ocimum sanctum	Oleanolic acid, rosmarinic acid, eugenol, carvacrol, ursolic acid, linalool, β-caryophyllene
Phyllanthus amarus	Alkaloids, lignans, sterols, flavonoids, tannins, triterpenes, volatile oils
Phyllanthus emblica	Triacontanol, daucosterol, lupeol acetate, triacontanoic acid, β-amyrin ketone, betulonic acid, β-amyrin-3-palmitate, ursolic acid, gallic acid, betulinic acid, oleanolic acid, quercetin, rutin
Psidium guajava	Quercetin, apigenin, guaijaverin, avicularin, kaempferol, gallic acid, catechin, hyperin, myricetin, epicatechin, chlorogenic acid, caffeic acid, epigallocatechin gallate
Punica granatum	Alkaloid, tannin, flavonoids, triterpenic acid, polyholosides, sitosterol, asiatic acid, maslinic acid, alkanes, punicic acid, estrogenic, flavonols, flavones, anthocyanidins, anthocyanins
Solanum nigrum	Alkaloids, flavonoids, saponins, terpenoids, steroids, phenols, gentisic acid, apigenin, kaempferol, luteolin, m-coumaric acid
Spermacoce hispida	Saponins, flavonoids, tannins, steroids, phenolics, essential oils, terpenoids
Swertia chirayita	Xanthones, flavonoids, iridoid glycosides, triterpenoids
Syzygium cumini	Anthocyanins, glucoside, kaempferol ellagic acid, isoquercetin, myricetin, alkaloid, jambosine, glycoside jambolin
Trigonella foenum-graecum	Carbohydrates, alkaloids, flavonoids, proteins, lipids, fibers, steroidal saponins, vitamins, saponins, minerals
Tinospora cordifolia	Alkaloids, aliphatic compounds, glycosides, polysaccharides, steroids, phenolics, protein, calcium, phosphorus, clerodane furono diterpene glucoside (amritoside A, B, C, and D)
Vinca rosea	Vincristine, vinblastine, ajmalicine, serpentine, lochnerine, catharanthine, vindoline
Withania somnifera	Alkaloids (isopelletierine, anaferine), withanolides with glucose, saponins containing an additional acyl group (sitoindoside VII and VIII), steroidal lactones (withanolides, withaferins)
Zingiber officinalis	Volatiles oil, gingerol, diarylheptanoids, proteins, amino acids, sugars, organic acids, inorganic elements

Sources: Adapted from Alqahtani et al. (2022); Behera et al. (2021); Bouyahya et al. (2021); Daharia et al. (2022); Mishra et al. (2019).

TABLE 3.3

Pharmacological Activities of Plants Used in the Treatment of Diabetes

Scientific Name	Pharmacological Activities
Aegle marmelos	Anti-diabetic, anticancer, antifertility, antimicrobial, immunogenic, insecticidal activities
Aloe barbadensis	Promotion of wound healing, hypoglycemic or anti-diabetic effects, immunomodulatory, antifungal activity, anti-inflammatory, anticancer, gastroprotective properties
Allium sativum	Anticarcinogenic, anti-inflammatory, antioxidant, anti-diabetic, renoprotective, anti-atherosclerotic, antiprotozoal, antibacterial, antiviral, antifungal, antihypertensive activities
Allium cepa	Antimicrobial, antioxidant, anticholesterolemic, antihyperuricemia, anti–heavy metal toxicity, anti–gastric ulcer, anticancer activities
Andrographis paniculate	Anti-atherosclerotic, immunostimulatory, anti-infective, anti-inflammatory, antihepatotoxic, immunomodulatory, anti-atherosclerotic, tumor-suppressive activities
Aristolochia bracteolate	Antimicrobial, insecticidal and repellent, antiproliferative, anti-allergic, antiplasmodial, anti–scorpion venom, antimycobacterial activities
Azadirachta indica	Antioxidant, anticancer, tumor suppressive, anti-inflammatory, hepatoprotective, wound healing, anti-diabetic, antimicrobial, antiviral, antifungal, antimalarial, antinephrotoxicity, neuroprotective activities
Brassica juncea	Antioxidant, anti-inflammation, bacteriostatic, anticancer, antiviral, anti-obesity, antidepressant, antihyperglycemia activities
Cajanus cajan	Hepatoprotective, antioxidant, anti-inflammatory, anti-ulcer, antitumor, hypotensive activities
Carica papaya	Anthelmintic, antioxidant, cytoprotective, anticancer activities
Cassia auriculata	Anti-diabetic, antihyperlipidemic, antioxidant, anticancer, hepatoprotective, anti-inflammatory activities
Catharanthus roseus	Antitumor, antimicrobial, anti-diabetic, antioxidant, antimutagenic activities
Capparis deciduas	Anti-diabetic, analgesic, anthelmintic, antifungal, antibacterial, anti-atherosclerotic, antioxidant, antinociceptive, hepatoprotective, anti-inflammatory, antirheumatic, hypolipidemic, antitumor, antigiardial, anticonvulsant activities
Centella asiatica	Antidepressant, anti-epileptic, antioxidant, anti-inflammatory, antinociceptive activities
Coccinia grandis	Analgesic, anti-diabetic, antipyretic, antimalarial, hepatoprotective, anti-inflammatory, hypoglycemic, antimicrobial, anti-ulcer, antioxidant, antidyslipidemic, mutagenic, anticancer, antitussive activities
Colocasia esculenta	Analgesic, antifungal, anticancer, anti-inflammatory, hypolipidemic activities
Costus igneus	Hypolipidemic, antioxidant, antimicrobial, diuretic, anticancer activities
Cuminum cyminum	Antimicrobial, anticancer, anti-diabetic, insecticidal, hypotensive, bronchodilatory, anti-inflammatory, analgesic, contraceptive, anti-amyloidogenic antioxidant, antiplatelet aggregation, immunological, anti-osteoporotic activities
Curcuma longa	Anti-inflammatory, antibacterial, antioxidant, anti-HIV, antiparasitic, nematocidal, antispasmodic, anticarcinogenic activities
Eclipta alba	Anticancer, analgesic, antioxidant, antileprotic, antihemorrhagic, antihepatotoxic, antimyotoxic, antiviral, antibacterial, spasmogenic, hypotensive activities
Emblica officinalis	analgesic, antipyretic, anticancer, antioxidant, antivenom, antitussive, antimicrobial, antibacterial, antifungal, antitumor, anti-ulcerogenic, hepatoprotective, cytoprotective, antidiarrheal Analgesic, antioxidant, anticancer, antivenom, antipyretic, antibacterial, antifungal, antitumor, antidiarrheal, hepatoprotective activities
Eugenia jambolana	Antioxidant, anti-allergic, anti-diabetic, antimicrobial, antihyperlipidemic, hepatoprotective, anticancer, gastroprotective, cardioprotective, radioprotective activities
Euphorbia hirta	Antibacterial, antifertility, anti-amoebic, antimalarial, galactogenic, anti-inflammatory, anticancer, antioxidant, anti-asthmatic, antidiarrheal, antifungal activities
Ficus benghalensis	Antioxidant, analgesic, anti-inflammatory, antidiarrheal, anti-anthelmintic, antistress, anti-allergic, anti-diabetic, immunomodulatory, anticancer, antibacterial activities

(Continued)

TABLE 3.3
(Continued)

Scientific Name	Pharmacological Activities
Ficus racemose	Antidiuretic, antitussive, anthelmintic, antibacterial, antipyretic, antifilarial, antidiarrheal, anti-inflammatory, anti-ulcer, analgesic, antifungal, larvicidal, antioxidant activities
Gymnema sylvestre	Antioxidant, gastro and hepatoprotective, antibiotic, anti-inflammatory, antiviral, anticancer, lipid-lowering activities
Hibiscus rosa sinensis	Anti-diabetic, antipyretic, analgesic, fibrinolytic, hypolipidemic, antioxidant, cytotoxic, antimicrobial, anti-inflammatory, immuno-modulatory, dermatological, antihemolytic, anticonvulsant, neuroprotective, antitussive, antidepressant, memory enhancement, antiparasitic, urinary, hepatoprotective activities
Mangifera indica	Antioxidant, anti-inflammatory, antimicrobial, anticancer activities
Marsilea minuta	Antipyretic, analgesic, anti-aggressive, antimicrobial, anti-diabetic, anti-amnesia, hepatoprotective, antifertility, antitumor, antitussive, expectorant, antioxidant activities
Melia azedarach	Insecticidal, antifeedant, growth-regulating activities
Momordica charantia	Antioxidant, anti-inflammatory, antimicrobial, antiparasitic, wound healing activities
Moringa oleifera	Antioxidant, antimicrobial, anti-bacterial, anticancer, anti-inflammatory, anti-apoptotic, cytotoxic, anti-ulcer, anti-allergic, antifertility activities
Murraya koenigii	Antioxidant, antitumor, anti-diabetic, anti-inflammatory, neuroprotective, antifungal, immunomodulatory activities
Ocimum sanctum	Antimicrobial, arthritis, chronic fever, antifertility, antifungal, anticancer, eye disease, analgesic, anti-emetic, hepatoprotective, antispasmodic activities
Phyllanthus amarus	Antiviral, antihepatoxic, antibacterial, anti-diabetic, antifungal, and anti-inflammatory activities
Phyllanthus emblica	Anti-inflammatory, anticancer, antiviral, antioxidant, anti-diabetic, anti-inflammatory, antipyretic activities
Psidium guajava	Anticestodal, analgesic, hepatoprotective, antioxidant, antidiarrheic, anti-inflammatory, cough sedative, antihypertension
Punica granatum	Antioxidant, anti-inflammatory, anti-analgesic, hepatoprotective, anti-diabetic, antimicrobial, antibacterial, antiviral, antifungal, antiplasmodium, anti-obesity, antitumor, neuroprotective, nephroprotective activities
Solanum nigrum	Antitumor, anticancer, antifungal, antilarvicidal, antistress, antioxidant, anti-allergic, hepatoprotective, estrogenic, anti-diabetic, immunostimulant, antimicrobial, anti-ulcer, cardioprotective, analgesic, antidiarrheal, anti-inflammatory activities
Spermacoce hispida	Anti-diabetic, hepatoprotective, antihypertensive, anti-inflammatory, analgesic, antihyperlipidemic, anticancer, antifungal and antioxidant activities
Swertia chirayita	Hepatoprotective, anti-inflammatory, antihepatotoxic, antileprosy, antimicrobial, anticarcinogenic, anticholinergic, hypoglycemic, antimalarial, antioxidant, central nervous system depressant, mutagenicity activities
Syzygium cumini	Antihyperglycemic, neuropsycho-pharmacological, antioxidant, anti-inflammatory, anti-HIV, antileishmanial antimicrobial, antibacterial, and antifungal, antifertility, anorexigenic, antidiarrheal, gastroprotective, anti-ulcerogenic activities
Trigonella foenum graecum	Anti-diabetic, antioxidant, antitumor, anticarcinogenic, hypocholesterolemia, antigenotoxic, anti-inflammatory, antimicrobial, gastroprotective activities
Tinospora cordifolia	Antioxidant, antimicrobial, anticancer, anti-HIV, antibacterial, hypolipidemic, antiosteoporotic, antitoxic, antifungal, anti-diabetic, antistress, wound healing, anticomplementary, immunomodulating activities
Vinca rosea	Antibacterial, antioxidant, antihypertensive, antihyperglycemic, anticancer, anti-diabetic, wound healing activities
Withania somnifera	Antioxidant, antimicrobial, cytotoxic, antistress, anti-inflammatory, anti-rheumatoid arthritis, anxiolytic, adaptogenic, chemoprotective activities
Zingiber officinalis	Antioxidant, antimicrobial, anticancer, anti-inflammatory, respiratory protective, anti-obesity, neuroprotective, cardiovascular protective, anti-diabetic, antinausea, anti-emetic activities

Sources: Adapted from Alqahtani et al. (2022); Behera et al. (2021); Bouyahya et al. (2021); Daharia et al. (2022); Mishra et al. (2019).

REFERENCES

Airaodion, A. I., Akaninyene, I. U., Ngwogu, K. O., Ekenjoku, J. A., & Ngwogu, A. C (2020). Hypolipidaemic and antidiabetic potency of Allium cepa (Onions) Bulb in alloxan-induced diabetic rats. *Acta Scientific Nutritional Health*, 4(3), 1–8. ISSN: 2582-1423.

Alamgir, A. N. M. (2018). *Therapeutic Use of Medicinal Plants and Their Extracts: Volume 2. Phytochemistry and Bioactive Compounds*. Springer Cham, Springer International Publishing AG, part of Springer Nature. 1 (XXV), 826. ISBN: 978-3-319-92387-1.

Alqahtani, A. S., Ullah, R., & Shahat, A. A. (2022). Bioactive constituents and toxicological evaluation of selected antidiabetic medicinal plants of Saudi Arabia. *Evidence-Based Complementary and Alternative Medicine*, 2022, 1–23.

Amiri-Ardekani, E., Askari, H., Khademian, S., Hemmati, S., & Mohagheghzadeh, A. (2021). Ethnopharmacological survey of Bavi tribe (Kohgiluyeh and Boyer-Ahmad Province, Iran). *Journal of Islamic and Iranian Traditional Medicine*, 11(4), 311–330.

Aradhna, S., Mishra, A. K., Rath, S. K., & Kumar, S. (2021). Plants used in diabetes by the tribal communities of Mayurbhanj district of Odisha state, India. In *Rajkumari Supriya Devi, Padma Mahanti and Sanjeet Kumar*. Medcio-Biowealth of India, Volume-IV, APRF Publishers, Odisha, pp. 35–43.

Arzati, M. M., Honarvar, N. M., Saedisomeolia, A., Anvari, S., Effatpanah, M., Arzati, R. M., & Djalali, M. (2017). The effects of ginger on fasting blood sugar, hemoglobin A1c, and lipid profiles in patients with type 2 diabetes. *International Journal of Endocrinology and Metabolism*, 15(4).

Babu, S. N., Govindarajan, S., & Noor, A. (2021). Aloe vera and its two bioactive constituents in alleviation of diabetes – proteomic & mechanistic insights. *Journal of Ethnopharmacology*, 280, 114445.

Behera, K., Mandal, U., Panda, M., Mohapatra, M., Mallick, S. K., Routray, S., Routray, S., Parida, S., & Mahalik, G. (2021). Ethnobotany and folk medicines used by the local healers of Bhadrak, Odisha, India. *Egyptian Journal of Botany*, 61(2), 375–389.

Bhattacharya, S., Maji, U., Khan, G. A., Das, R., Sinha, A. K., Ghosh, C., & Maiti, S. (2019). Anti-diabetic role of a novel protein from garlic via NO in expression of Glut-4/insulin in liver of alloxan induced diabetic mice. *Biomedicine & Pharmacotherapy*, 111, 1302–1314.

Bouyahya, A., El Omari, N., Elmenyiy, N., Guaouguaou, F. E., Balahbib, A., Belmehdi, O., Salhi, N., Imtara, H., Mrabti, H. N., El-Shazly, M., & Bakri, Y. (2021). Moroccan anti-diabetic medicinal plants: Ethnobotanical studies, phytochemical bioactive compounds, preclinical investigations, toxicological validations and clinical evidences; challenges, guidance and perspectives for future management of diabetes worldwide. *Trends in Food Science & Technology*, 115, 147–254.

Chen, L. X., He, H., Xia, G. Y., Zhou, K. L., Qiu, F. (2014). A new flavonoid from the aerial parts of *Andrographis paniculata*. *Natural Product Research*, 28(3), 138–143.

Chinsembu, K. C. (2019). Diabetes mellitus and nature's pharmacy of putative anti-diabetic plants. *Journal of Herbal Medicine*, 15, 100230.

Christian, E. O., Felicia, E. C., Helen, I. N., Nneka, S. V., Vivian, C. U., & Ogochukwu, A. P. (2019). Anti-diabetic property and antioxidant potentials of aqueous extract of *Azadirachta indica* leaves in strepto-zotocin-induced diabetic rats. *Journal of Medicinal Plants*, 7(6), 18–23.

Daharia, A., Jaiswal, V. K., Royal, K. P., Sharma, H., Joginath, A. K., Kumar, R., & Saha, P. (2022). A comparative review on ginger and garlic with their pharmacological Action. *Asian Journal of Pharmaceutical Research and Development*, 10(3), 65–69.

DiMeglio, L. A., Evans-Molina, C., & Oram, R. A. (2018). Type 1 diabetes. *The Lancet*, 391(10138), 2449–2462.

D'souza, J. J., D'souza, P. P., Fazal, F., Kumar, A., Bhat, H. P., & Baliga, M. S. (2014). Anti-diabetic effects of the Indian indigenous fruit *Emblica officinalis* Gaertn: Active constituents and modes of action. *Food & Function*, 5(4), 635–644.

Dsouza, M. R., Athoibi, S., & Prabha, S. (2020). Pharmacognostical investigation of *Andrographis paniculata* (Green Chiretta) and crystallization of the bioactive component andrographolide. *International Journal of PharmTech Research*, 13(2), 10.

Essa, R., El Sadek, A. M., Baset, M. E., et al. (2019). Effects of turmeric (*Curcuma longa*) extract in streptozocin-induced diabetic model. *Journal of Food Biochemistry*, 43.

Gautam, S., Thakur, M., Aggarwal, M., & Vatsa, E. (2021). *Azadirachta Indica*: A review as a potent anti-diabetic drug. *Journal of Scienc Aliment Agrícola*, 1(10), 1–6.

Geberemeskel, G. A., Debebe, Y. G., & Nguse, N. A. (2019). Antidiabetic effect of fenugreek seed powder solution (*Trigonella foenum-graecum* L.) on hyperlipidemia in diabetic patients. *Journal of Diabetes Research*. https://doi.org/10.1155/2019/8507453

Gulhane, N. S., Ghode, C. D., Jadhao, A. G., & Patil, P. A. (2021). Study of medicinal uses of *Ocimum sanctum* (Tulsi). *Journal of Pharmacognosy and Phytochemistry*, 10(2), 1427–1431.

Hartajanie, L., Fatimah-Muis, S., Heri-Nugroho Hs, K., Riwanto, I., & Sulchan, M. (2020). Probiotics fermented bitter melon juice as promising complementary agent for diabetes type 2: Study on animal model. *Journal of Nutrition and Metabolism*, 2020, Article ID 6369873, 7 pages.

Irfan, H. M., Asmawi, M. Z., Khan, N.A.K., Sadikun, A., & Mordi, M. N. (2017). Anti-diabetic activity-guided screening of aqueous-ethanol *Moringa oleifera* extracts and fractions: Identification of marker compounds. *Tropical Journal of Pharmaceutical Research*, 16(3), 543–552.

Khadayat, K., Marasini, B. P., Gautam, H., Ghaju, S., & Parajuli, N. (2020). Evaluation of the alpha-amylase inhibitory activity of Nepalese medicinal plants used in the treatment of Diabetes mellitus. *Clinical Phytoscience*, 6, 1–8.

Kilambi, P., & Shah, P. A. (2021). Fenugreek: A wonder spice with versatile pharmacological activities and clinical applications. In *Fenugreek* (pp. 395–445). Springer, Singapore.

Mahmood, N., Muazzam, M. A., Ahmad, M., Hussain, S., & Javed, W. (2021). Phytochemistry of *Allium cepa* L. (Onion): Its nutritional and pharmacological importance. *Scientific Inquiry and Review*, 5(3).

Mishra, J., Mahalik, G., & Parida, S. (2019). Ethnobotanical study of traditional medicinal plants used in the management of diabetes in the urban areas of Khurda, Odisha, India. *Asian Journal of Pharmaceutical and Clinical Research*, 12(9), 73–78.

Muñiz-Ramirez, A., Perez, R. M., Garcia, E., & Garcia, F. E. (2020). Antidiabetic activity of *Aloe vera* leaves. *Evidence-Based Complementary and Alternative Medicine*.

Nam, S., Chesla, C., Stotts, N. A., Kroon, L., & Janson, S. L. (2011). Barriers to diabetes management: Patient and provider factors. *Diabetes Research and Clinical Practice*, 93(1), 1–9.

Nazarian-Samani, Z., Sewell, R. D., Lorigooini, Z., & Rafieian-Kopaei, M. (2018). Medicinal plants with multiple effects on Diabetes mellitus and its complications: A systematic review. *Current Diabetes Reports*, 18(10), 1–13.

Paikra, B. K., & Gidwani, B. (2017). Phytochemistry and pharmacology of Moringa oleifera Lam. *Journal of Pharmacopuncture*, 20(3), 194. https://doi.org/10.3831%2FKPI.2017.20.022

Powers, M. A., Bardsley, J. K., Cypress, M., Funnell, M. M., Harms, D., Hess-Fischl, A., Hooks, B., Isaacs, D., Mandel, E. D., Maryniuk, M. D., Norton, A., & Uelmen, S. (2020). Diabetes self-management education and support in adults with type 2 diabetes: A consensus report of the American diabetes association, the association of diabetes care & education specialists, the academy of nutrition and dietetics, the American academy of family physicians, the American academy of PAs, the American association of nurse practitioners, and the American pharmacist association. *Diabetes Care*, 43(7), 1636–1649.

Rafi, M., Devi, A. F., Syafitri, U. D., Heryanto, R., Suparto, I. H., Amran, M. B., & Lim, L. W. (2020). Classification of *Andrographis paniculata* extracts by solvent extraction using HPLC fingerprint and chemometric analysis. *BMC Research Notes*, 13(1), 1–6.

Riaz, S., Hussain, S., Syed, S. K., & Anwar, R. (2021). Chemical characteristics and therapeutic potentials of *Aloe vera*. *Magnesium*, 1(11), 48.

Salleh, N. H., Zulkipli, I. N., Mohd Yasin, H., Ja'afar, F., Ahmad, N., Wan Ahmad, W.A.N., & Ahmad, S. R. (2021). Systematic Review of Medicinal Plants Used for Treatment of Diabetes in Human Clinical Trials: An ASEAN Perspective. *Evidence-Based Complementary and Alternative Medicine*. https://doi.org/10.1155/2021/5570939

Shival, A., Bornare, A., Shinde, A., & Musmade, D. (2020). General introduction, classification, morphology, phytoconstituents, traditional & medicinal uses, pharmacological activities of tulsi (*Ocimum Sanctum*). *World Journal of Pharmaceutical Research*, 9(9), 701–713. https://doi.org/10.20959/wjpr20209-18465

Srinivasan, A., Selvarajan, S., Kamalanathan, S., Kadhiravan, T., Prasanna Lakshmi, N. C., & Adithan, S. (2019). Effect of *Curcuma longa* on vascular function in native Tamilians with type 2 diabetes mellitus: A randomized, double-blind, parallel arm, placebo-controlled trial. *Phytotherapy Research: PT*, 33(7), 1898–1911. https://doi.org/10.1002/ptr.6381

Srinivasan, P., Vijayakumar, S., Kothandaraman, S., & Palani, M. (2018). Anti-diabetic activity of quercetin extracted from *Phyllanthus emblica* L. fruit: In silico and in vivo approaches. *Journal of Pharmaceutical Analysis*, 8(2), 109–118.

Thirumalai, T., Beverly, C. D., Sathiyaraj, K., Senthilkumar, B., & David, E. (2012). Ethnobotanical study of anti-diabetic medicinal plants used by the local people in Javadhu hills Tamilnadu, India. *Asian Pacific Journal of Tropical Biomedicine*, 2(2), S910–S913. https://doi.org/10.1016/S2221-1691(12)60335-9

Tjeck, O. P., Souza, A., Mickala, P., Lepengue, A. N., & M'Batchi, B. (2017). Bio-efficacy of medicinal plants used for the management of Diabetes mellitus in Gabon: An ethnopharmacological approach. *Journal of Intercultural Ethnopharmacology*, 6(2), 206.

Tshabalala, T., Ndhlala, A. R., Ncube, B., Abdelgadir, H. A., & Van Staden, J. (2020). Potential substitution of the root with the leaf in the use of *Moringa oleifera* for antimicrobial, anti-diabetic and antioxidant properties. *South African Journal of Botany*, 129, 106–112.

Verma, S., Gupta, M., Popli, H., & Aggarwal, G. (2018). Diabetes mellitus treatment using herbal drugs. *International Journal of Phytomedicine*, 10(1), 1–10.

Wei, C. K., Tsai, Y. H., Korinek, M., Hung, P. H., El-Shazly, M., Cheng, Y. B., & Chang, F. R. (2017). 6-paradol and 6-shogaol, the pungent compounds of ginger, promote glucose utilization in adipocytes and myotubes, and 6-paradol reduces blood glucose in high-fat diet-fed mice. *International Journal of Molecular Sciences*, 18(1), 168.

Zhao, X. X., Lin, F. J., Li, H., Li, H. B., Wu, D. T., Geng, F., & Gan, R. Y. (2021). Recent advances in bioactive compounds, health functions, and safety concerns of onion (*Allium cepa* L.). *Frontiers in Nutrition*, 8.

4 Jordanian Medicinal Plants in the Treatment of Diabetes

*Wamidh H. Talib, Reem Fawaz Abutayeh, Samar Thiab,
Safa Daoud, Leena Omer and Asma Ismail Mahmod*

CONTENTS

4.1 INTRODUCTION

Jordan is home to a variety of medicinal plants due to its diverse climate. Herbal therapy has been used by Jordanians since ancient times as antioxidants, antimicrobial, antiviral, and antifungal agents, as well as for the prevention and treatment of several chronic illnesses such as hypertension, diabetes, and even cancer (Afifi and Kasabri 2013). Despite its growing popularity, the use of plants in medicine has yet to undergo proper scientific analysis. Recent studies have found that out of 250,000 plants suspected to have a hypoglycemic effect, only less than 1% have been investigated for their potential use in pharmaceutical antidiabetic agents (Abu-Odeh and Talib 2021).

Diabetes mellitus (DM) is a chronic metabolic disease that is associated with abnormalities regarding the insulin hormone which is mainly responsible for regulating glucose blood level. Over the past few years, the global incidence of DM has increased significantly to the point where 1 in 11 adults has DM (Shah et al. 2021). The situation in not different in Jordan, where DM prevalence reached 30% according to various surveys conducted between 1994 and 2017 (Awad et al. 2020). If

DOI: 10.1201/9781003220930-5

left uncontrolled, DM can lead to the development of serious complications including neuropathy, nephropathy, retinopathy, diabetic foot ulcers, and many others (Abu-Odeh and Talib 2021).

Unlike type 1 diabetes mellitus (T1DM), which is completely dependent on insulin therapy, most cases of type 2 diabetes mellitus (T2DM) are managed through the use of oral antidiabetic agents. However, in many cases, antidiabetic drugs alone are not enough to properly manage T2DM; therefore, the addition of complementary alternative medicines, of which medicinal herbs constituted 26.4% alongside conventional therapy, has massively helped T2DM patients in maintaining their glucose blood levels around an acceptable range (Raja et al. 2019).

In this chapter, a discussion of Jordanian medicinal plants with antidiabetic effects is presented, covering the traditional use of each plant along with a detailed description of its activity as an antidiabetic, as well as their general biological activity. Full classification, geographical distribution, mechanisms of action, and pure active compounds isolated from the plants are also mentioned.

4.2   DIABETES AS A METABOLIC DISEASE

DM is a widespread chronic metabolic disorder related to the malfunction of carbohydrate metabolism caused by abnormalities associated with a hormone called insulin, released by pancreatic β islet cells (Galicia-Garcia et al. 2020). T2DM, which constitutes 90% of diabetic cases worldwide, is caused by the inability of insulin receptors to respond properly to the hormone (insulin tolerance), accompanied by the insufficient release of insulin that is unable to keep up with the decreased sensitivity toward the hormone (Galicia-Garcia et al. 2020; Yau et al. 2021). As for T1DM, there is a complete lack of insulin due to a destructive autoimmune attack on pancreatic β islet cells (Espona-Noguera et al. 2019). All this leads to the accumulation of glucose in the blood instead of entering different body cells, causing glucose blood levels to rise above the average (hyperglycemia) (Mishra et al. 2021).

In addition, some women might experience peripheral insulin resistance and hyperglycemia during pregnancy. This condition termed "gestational diabetes" is temporary and although it disappears after birth in most cases, it can cause serious long-term complications for both the mother and the fetus (Olmos-Ortiz et al. 2021).

4.3   THERAPEUTIC TARGETS IN DIABETES

4.3.1   Glucagon-Like Peptide 1 (GLP-1)

GLP-1 is an intestinal hormone composed of 30 amino acid peptides and belongs to a family of hormones called incretins (Müller et al. 2019). GLP-1 has multiple biological activities, including regulation of glycemia, glucose-dependent stimulation of insulin production, controlling of β cell proliferation, suppression of glucagon release, as well as gastric emptying and food intake reduction (Müller et al. 2019). Besides, GLP-1 receptor agonists have been approved for the treatment of T2DM demonstrating a reduction in A_{1C} and body weight as a single therapy or as a combination with other antidiabetic therapies (Hinnen 2017).

4.3.2   Dipeptidyl Peptidase 4 (DPP-4)

DPP-4 is a glycoprotein exopeptidase of 110 kDa, which shows biological activities via pleiotropic actions. The ability of the DPP-4 enzyme to cleave many substrates explains its multifunctional effect. It is associated with signaling process, immune cell stimulation, suppressing tumors, and regulation of glucose level (Röhrborn et al. 2015). Moreover, incretin hormones (GLP-1) and glucose-dependent insulinotropic polypeptide (GIP) are the main regulators of postprandial insulin secretion, as well as one of the DPP-4 substrates. Thus, inhibiting DPP-4 activity will suppress the inactivation of incretin hormones and affect glucose control through different mechanisms, including improvement of glucose-dependent insulin secretion, slowed gastric emptying, and decreasing the level of postprandial glucagon and food intake (Makrilakis 2019).

4.3.3 G-Protein-Coupled Receptors (GPCRs)

GPCRs are a large family of plasma membrane receptors that regulate several intracellular signaling through binding to different ligands associated with extracellular stimuli, including light, odorants, neurotransmitters, and hormones (Talukdar et al. 2011). Moreover, about 850 human GPCRs are found, which have a particular cell type and take part in different physiological and clinical pathways (Talukdar et al. 2011). In T2DM, free fatty acids (FFAs) exert dual effects on insulin secretion and promote both hyper- and hypo-insulinemia during the development of the disease (Talukdar et al. 2011). Since FFAs have represented ligands of many GPCRs, including GPR119, GPR84, GPR120, GPR40, GPR43, and GPR41, GPCRs play a direct role in the occurrence of insulin resistance and β cell dysfunction (Talukdar et al. 2011, Riddy et al. 2018).

4.3.4 Sodium-Glucose Linked Transporters (SGLTs)

Glucose, amino acids, vitamins, and other ions are transported via special membrane proteins called sodium-coupled glucose transporters. There are two types of SGLT: SGLT1 is mainly found in the gastrointestinal tract, and SGLT2 is considered as high-capacity, low-affinity transporter. It is present in the kidney and is responsible for the majority of glucose reabsorption (Vallon and Sharma 2010). SGLT2 regulates almost all glucose reabsorption in the glomerular filtrate; however, this might induce hyperglycemia in diabetic patients (Vallon and Sharma 2010). Interestingly, SGLT2 inhibitors have improved glucose excretion and enhanced glycemic control without increasing insulin secretion in T2DM (Vallon and Sharma 2010).

4.3.5 Diacylglycerol Acyltransferase (DGAT-1)

DGAT1 is a lipid modulator, which helps in the synthesis of triacylglycerol (or triglycerides [TAG]) by working as a catalyst in the esterification reaction that binds acyl-CoA to diacylglycerol (DAG) to finally form TAG (Hong et al. 2020; Gastaldelli et al. 2021). This enzyme is mainly found in the liver, small intestine, and adipose tissue (Hong et al. 2020). Researchers found that a deficiency of DGAT-1 is highly related to an increase in insulin sensitivity; therefore, the use of selective DGAT-1 inhibitors as antidiabetic agents has been studied (Hong et al. 2020, Gastaldelli et al. 2021).

4.3.6 11β-Hydroxysteroid Dehydrogenase-1 (11β-HSD1)

11β-HSD1 is a glucocorticoid (GC) regulator that acts intracellularly by the activation of the inactive form of glucocorticoids. It is usually found in the liver and adipose tissue (Koike et al. 2019; Gant et al. 2018). Studies suggest that there is an increase in the activity of 11β-HSD1 in patients with T2DM compared to non-diabetic individuals (Koike et al. 2019; Gant et al. 2018). This leads to an increased amount of active GC, which can aggravate the condition by increasing glycogenolysis as well as inducing insulin resistance. Thus, 11β-HSD1 inhibitors have the potential to be used as antidiabetic agents (Koike et al. 2019; Cheng et al. 2021).

4.3.7 Peroxisome Proliferator-Activated Receptors (PPARs)

PPARs are ligand-activated nuclear transcription factors involved in various physiological processes, including lipid and energy metabolism (Takada and Makishima 2020). Moreover, PPARs have three known subtypes: PPARα, PPARδ, and PPARγ. A high level of PPARγ is expressed in fat to enhance glucose and lipid ingestion, mediate glucose oxidation, reduce FFA content, and improve

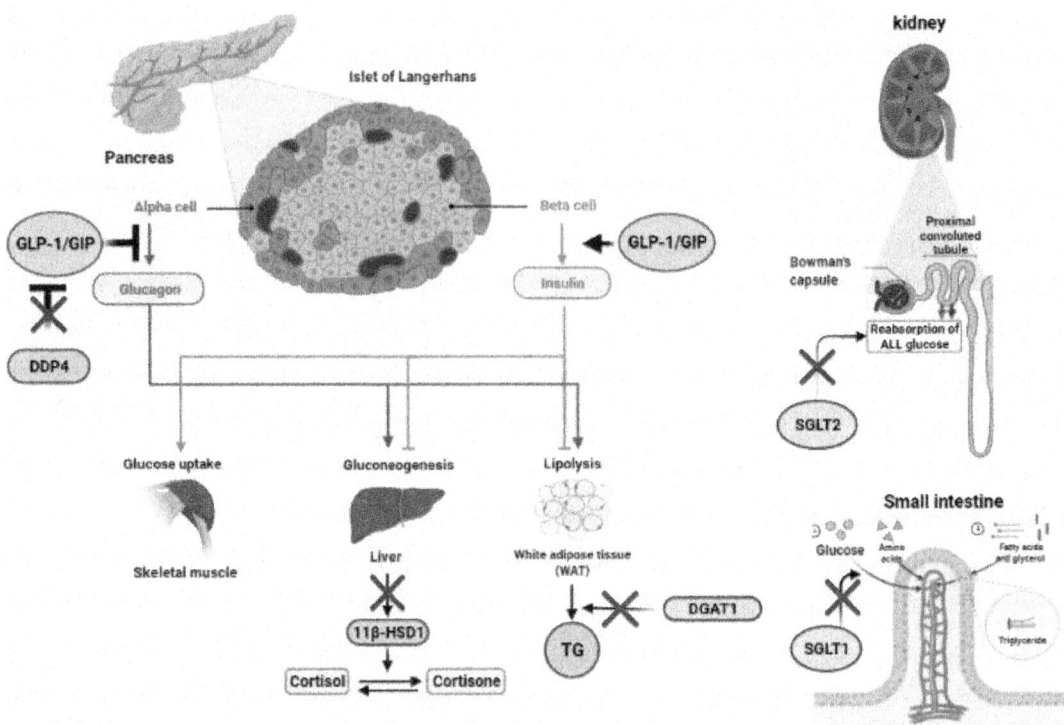

FIGURE 4.1 Therapeutic targets in diabetes. DPP4, dipeptidyl peptidase 4; DGAT, diacylglycerol acyltransferase; 11β-HSD1, 11β-hydroxysteroid dehydrogenase-1; GIP, gastric inhibitory polypeptide; GLP-1, glucagon-like peptide 1; SGLT, sodium-glucose–linked transporter; TG, triglyceride.

insulin resistance (Jay and Ren 2007). Interestingly, PPARs can be potential drug targets in many metabolic and inflammatory diseases like obesity, T2DM, dyslipidemia, and inflammatory bowel syndrome (Takada and Makishima 2020). Figure 4.1 demonstrates the most important therapeutic targets in diabetes.

4.4 JORDANIAN PLANTS IN THE TREATMENT OF DIABETES

4.4.1 *ARTEMISIA HERBA-ALBA*

A. herba-alba is a medicinal and aromatic dwarf shrub belonging to the Asteraceae (Compositae) family, known as desert wormwood or *shih* (Arabic name). It grows in dry and semi-dry climates including the deserts of North Africa, Middle East, Spain, northwestern Himalayas, and India (Réggami et al. 2019). In Jordan, the plant is common in dry regions such as Karak, Tafila, Shaubak, Ras an-Naqab, Mafraq, Zarka, and the Eastern Desert (Hudaib and Aburjai 2006). Herbal infusion and decoction of this plant has been extensively used in folk medicine by many civilizations to treat colds, coughing, bronchitis, diarrhea, diabetes, hypertension, snake bites, neuralgias, and parasitic infections (Jaleel et al. 2016; Réggami et al. 2019).

Various secondary metabolites have been isolated from *A. herba-alba*. Sesquiterpene lactones are the most important constituents found in *Artemisia* species and are largely responsible for the biological activity of these plants. Eudesmanolides and germacranolides seem to be the most abundant types of lactones found in this species. Additionally, many flavonoids with large structural variations have been identified in *A. herba-alba* ranging from common flavone and flavonol glycosides to more unusual highly methylated flavonoids (Abou El Hamd et al. 2010). It was reported that

A. herba-alba oil, called *"scheih* oil," is composed of monoterpenoids, mainly oxygenated, such as 1,8-cineole, chrysanthenone, chrysanthenol, α/β-thujones, and camphor as the major components. In *A. herba-alba* oil collected from Jordan, regular monoterpenes were predominant (39.3%) and the principal components were α- and β-thujones (27.7%). The other major identified components were sabinyl acetate (5.4%), germacrene D (4.6%), α-eudesmol (4.2%) and caryophyllene acetate (5.7%) (Abou El Hamd et al. 2010; Hudaib and Aburjai 2006).

Interestingly, many clinical and experimental studies in literature reported the crucial role of *A. herba-alba* in lowering serum glucose (Réggami et al. 2019). One of the proposed mechanisms to explain the hypoglycemic effect of this plant is its ability to stimulate pancreatic β cells to release more insulin into the blood stream, thus increasing glycogen deposition in the liver causing a reduction of glucose levels (Iriadam et al. 2006).

4.4.2 ACHILLEA SANTOLINA

A. santolina is a flowering wild plant from the family Asteraceae. It is distributed in temperature regions of the Northern Hemisphere, especially in Europe and Asia (Salem et al. 2017). In Jordan, it grows in waste grounds and edges of cultivated lands including Amman, Ajloun, Jerash, Irbid, and Madaba. Locals in Jordan use an infusion of the leaves as a carminative and for the treatment of dysentery and intestinal colic (Ahmed et al. 2020). This plant is also used traditionally as an antidiabetic, anti-inflammatory, and to relieve stomach pain and to relieve symptoms of common cold (Al-Snafi 2013). The phytochemical screening showed that *A. santolina* contained many secondary metabolites including terpenoids (monoterpenes, sesquiterpenes, diterpenes, and triterpenes), lignans, flavonoids, alkaloids, and saponins. The oil of *A. santolina* contains 54 volatile components (Faisal et al. 2020; Al-Snafi 2013). Ahmad et al. reported that eucalyptol was the chief oil constituent of *A. santolina* oil (25.2%) (Ahmed et al. 2020). Recently, Faisal et al. suggested that plants having alkaloids, terpenoids, glycosides, and flavonoids exhibit antioxidant properties, which are responsible for driving their hypoglycemic actions by regenerating the damaged β pancreatic cells in addition to saponin-induced inhibition of SGLT1 in the intestine (Faisal et al. 2020). This suggestion is supported by Yazdanparast et al. who revealed that the hypoglycemic effect of *A. santolina* extract is due to the antioxidative potential of this plant which was shown by significant quenching impact on the extent of lipid peroxidation and protein oxidation along with enhancement of antioxidant defense systems leading to a protective effect against pancreatic damage in streptozotocin (STZ)-treated diabetic rats (Yazdanparast et al. 2007). Additionally, another study conducting in Jordan implies the promising effect of *A. santolina* on β cell mass expansion resulting in restoration of pancreatic dysfunction. This allow T1DM patients to regenerate residual remaining β cells and regain control over blood sugar levels (Kasabri et al. 2012).

4.4.3 CRATAEGUS ARONIA

C. aronia is one of the most dominant hawthorn species that belongs to the family of Rosaceae. It grows in the mountains of the Mediterranean region (Omairi et al. 2020). In Jordan, it can be found in Ajloun, Al-Salt, and Amman (Al-Hallaq et al. 2013). *C. aronia* has been utilized in traditional medicine against many diseases like sexual weakness, cardiovascular diseases, diabetes, obesity, hyperlipidemia, and cancer (Omairi et al. 2020). A decoction of leaves and unripe fruits prepared from *C. aronia* is used to treat diabetes in Arab traditional medicine. Ljubuncic et al. reported that *C. aronia* normalizes plasma lipid peroxide levels and lowers blood glucose levels in diabetic rats (Ljubuncic et al. 2006).

A chemical composition study of the leaves and flowers of *C. aronia* identified different secondary metabolites including phenolics such as oligomeric proanthocyanidin; flavonoids such as vitexine-2-O-rhamnoside, hyperoside, rutin, and quercetin; and polyphenols such as chlorogenic acid (Mostafa et al. 2018).

Many mechanisms are proposed to explain the antidiabetic activity of *C. aronia*: Mostafa et al. highlighted the important role of chlorogenic acid and polyphenols as antioxidants and in lowering glucose and lipid levels in different animal disease models (Mostafa et al. 2018). Another study in Jordan demonstrated that *C. aronia* exerts respective inhibitory activity against crucial gastro-intestinal enzymes that are involved in carbohydrate and lipid digestion and absorption, namely α-amylase, α-glucosidase, and pancreatic lipase as an explanation for the antihyperglycemic and anti-obesity effects of this plant (Al-Hallaq et al. 2013). Moreover, it is well-known that quercetin and its derivatives exert antidiabetic effects by acting through various mechanisms, including inhibition of intestinal starch digestion and hepatic glucose production by enhancing hepatic glucose kinase activity, improving skeletal muscle uptake of glucose, and protecting against pancreatic islet damage (Mostafa et al. 2018).

4.4.4 *TEUCRIUM POLIUM*

The genus *Teucrium* belongs to the Lamiaceae family (Jaradat 2015). The genus includes more than 300 mostly perennial plants with worldwide distribution; however, some species are endemic to the Mediterranean region (Jaradat 2015; Afifi et al. 2005; Aburjai et al. 2006). It is found in Egypt, Iraq, Saudi Arabia, and Palestine (Afifi et al. 2005), and is widely distributed in Jordan, where it is known as *germander*, or *jaa'deh* (Aburjai et al. 2006). *T. polium* is a polymorphous, perennial about 10–35 cm in height (Afifi et al. 2005; Jaradat 2015). It has a yellow or white corolla in a small globular inflorescence and white sessile, linear, or oblong leaves (Afifi et al. 2005). The fruits are different shades of brown (Jaradat 2015).

The plant is edible and is used in traditional medicine as an antispasmodic, anti-inflammatory, antibacterial, anthelmintic, hypotensive, and hypoglycemic. It is also used to alleviate pain and headache as well as treat ulcers and renal stones (Aburjai et al. 2006; Afifi et al. 2005). It is usually drunk as a tea after infusion or decoction of the aerial parts (Jaradat 2015; Aburjai et al. 2006). The antidiabetic activity of the plant was suggested to be due to its ability act via different suggested mechanisms, such as increasing insulin secretion and regenerating of the pancreatic β cells, enhancing glucose uptake by skeletal muscles by increasing the translocation of glucose transporter 4 (GLUT4) (Kadan et al. 2018) and inhibiting α-amylase activity; inhibiting dietary carbohydrate digestion and absorption; increasing the activation of adenosine monophosphate-activated protein kinase (AMPK), which has a role in maintaining cellular energy homeostasis; and improving oxidative damage and thus preventing complication of diabetes (Mahmoudabady et al. 2020; Jaradat 2015).

T. polium contains a complex mixture of compounds belonging to different phytochemical classes. Those include volatile oils, saturated and unsaturated fatty acids, terpenoids, iridoid glycosides, flavonoids, and phenolic compounds (Mahmoudabady et al. 2020; Aburjai et al. 2006; Jaradat 2015; Kadan et al. 2018). Some compounds that were reported to have antidiabetic activity are found in *T. polium*, including palmitic acid, cis-vaccenic acid, eugenol, carvacrol, and thymol (Kadan et al. 2018).

4.4.5 *PISTACIA ATLANTICA*

The genus *Pistacia* belongs to the Anacardiaceae family and includes more than 600 species (Mahjoub et al. 2018). It is widely distributed to the Mediterranean and Middle Eastern region, particularly central Asia, and is found in Iran, Turkey, Iraq, Saudi Arabia, and Jordan (Mahjoub et al. 2018; Kasabri et al. 2011a; Ben Ahmed et al. 2021). *P. atlantica* (wild pistachio) is one of the most famous species of this genus and is named *butm* in Arabic (Mahjoub et al. 2018). The tree is tall and can reach 20 m with grayish-white branches carrying leaves composed of 7–11 leaflets. The tree has a striated, dark gray bark and unisex flowers clustered in inflorescences (Ben Ahmed et al. 2021; Mahjoub et al. 2018).

P. atlantica is used a source of food and is used in traditional medicine as a sedative, anxiolytic, antipyretic, anti-inflammatory, antimicrobial, anticancer, hepatoprotective, antihypertensive, and antidiabetic (Ahmed et al. 2018; Peksel et al. 2010). It is also used to treat stomachache, dyspepsia, peptic ulcer, renal stones, musculoskeletal disorders, asthma, and topically to treat eczema and wounds. In addition, the mastic resin has been used as a respiratory and urinary antiseptic (Peksel et al. 2010; Mahjoub et al. 2018). The antidiabetic activity of the plant was suggested to be due to the inhibition of α-amylase and α-glucosidase leading to slowing down of carbohydrates metabolism and absorption from the small intestine (Ben Ahmed et al. 2021; Kasabri et al. 2011a).

P. atlantica contains a mixture of phytochemical compounds including volatile oils, terpenoids, flavonoids, coumarins, phenolic compounds, fatty acids, and sterols (Mahjoub et al. 2018; Peksel et al. 2010; Ben Ahmed et al. 2021). Compounds with known antidiabetic activity were identified in *P. atlantica* such as quinic acid, glucogallin, and galloylquinic acid, which are believed to have α-amylase inhibition activity. Methyl gallate and tetragalloylglucoside were also identified and believed to have α-glucosidase inhibition activity. Finally, gallic acid, gentisic acid, and digalloylquinic acid were also identified in *P. atlantica* and are believed to have the ability to inhibit both enzymes (Ben Ahmed et al. 2021).

4.4.6 PHASEOLUS VULGARIS

The genus *Phaseolus* belongs to the Fabaceae family and includes about 70 species. *P. vulgaris* seeds are among the most consumed foods worldwide (M Devi et al. 2020). The plant is grown in Africa, China, Europe, the United States, Canada, Latin America, and the Middle East including Jordan (M Devi et al. 2020). *P. vulgaris* is an annual plant; its leaves are composed of leaflets and its flowers composed of inflorescences of white, yellowish, purple, or pale pink (M Devi et al. 2020).

P. vulgaris has important medicinal value and is widely used in traditional medicine as antimicrobial, analgesic, antioxidant, anti-inflammatory, anti-obesity, antifertility, anticancer, antidiabetic, hepatoprotective, and hypolipidemic, as well as to treat renal stones (Loko et al. 2018). The antidiabetic activity of *P. vulgaris* is suggested to be due to inhibiting α-glucosidase and carbohydrate metabolism and absorption (He et al. 2018). Several phytochemical compounds were found in *P. vulgaris* including fatty acids, saponins, flavonoids, phenolic compounds, and tannins (M Devi et al. 2020). The phytochemicals with α-glucosidase inhibitory activity are classified as triacylglycerols, including trilinolenin and 1,3-dilinolenoyl-2-linoleoyl glycerol (Sutedja et al. 2020).

4.4.7 ERYNGIUM CRETICUM

Eryngium L. is a rich genus of the Apiaceae family as it comprises approximately 250 species distributed in regions of moderate climate all over the world (Kikowska et al. 2016). There are three species of *Eryngium* found in Jordan: *E. creticum* Lam., *E. falcatum* Laroche, and *E. glomeratum* Lam. (Afifi et al. 1990; Jaghabir 1991).

E. creticum is an edible plant used raw in salads and appetizers (Kikowska et al. 2016). It commonly grows in the wild in the Eastern Mediterranean region, including Lebanon, Palestine, Syria (Kikowska et al. 2016), and the northern parts of Jordan (Afifi et al. 1990). In Arabic it is called *kursannih*, and in English it has several names such as snake root (Nusair and Ahmad 2019), eryngo, flat holly, and blue sea holly (Kikowska et al. 2016). *E. creticum* has been used traditionally in many disorders including diabetes, liver and renal ailments, poisoning cases, and as a remedy for scorpion stings. The main medicinal parts used of *E. creticum* are the roots, leaves, and seeds (Afifi et al. 1990; Kikowska et al. 2016; Nusair and Ahmad 2019). A number of studies have shown various bioactivities of *E. creticum* including antidotal activities against scorpion and snake venoms (Nusair and Ahmad 2019), antimicrobial activities, antihyperglycemic (Jaghabir 1991; Kasabri et al. 2012), and antioxidant effects (Kikowska et al. 2016).

The antidiabetic activity of *E. creticum* was tested in streptozocin-induced hyperglycemic rat models and normoglycemic rat models using orally administered aqueous extract of aerial parts. Results have shown it to decrease the glucose level in both test and control groups, yet the effect was significant for the streptozocin-induced diabetic rats (Jaghabir 1991). In addition, an antihyperglycemic effect was shown for *E. creticum* bolus treatment in starch-fed rats despite the lack of *in vitro* inhibitory activity of α-amylase and α-glucosidase. However, *E. creticum* aqueous extract was found to regulate the pancreatic mode of action *in vitro* through potentiation of glucose responsive insulin-releasing pancreatic MIN6 β cells, by modulating Ca^{2+} regulated exocytosis. This makes *E. creticum* a good candidate for further investigation in T1DM (Kasabri et al. 2012).

The phytochemical screenings of different (aqueous, ethanolic, and methanolic) extracts of *E. creticum* indicated the presence of different bioactive compounds, mainly sesquiterpenes, monoterpenes, aldehydes, coumarins, sitosterols, tannins, resins, and sugars. In addition, screening for metal displayed that it contains silver, zirconium, selenium, niobium, nickel, iron, calcium, manganese, molybdenum, and copper. Nine compounds were isolated and characterized from the roots of *E. creticum* grown in Jordan, including: two coumarins (deltion and marmesin), cyclic alcohol quercitol, monoterpeneglycoside 3-(β-D-glucopyranosyloxymethyl)-2,4,4-trimethyl-2,5-cyclohexadien-1-one, phloroglucinol glycoside (1-(β-D-glucopyranosyloxy-3-methoxy-5-hydroxybenzene)), β-sitosterol and its glycoside (β-sitosterol-β-D-glucopyranose), and two sugars, mannitol and dulcitol (Kikowska et al. 2016).

4.4.8 GERANIUM GRAVEOLENS

G. graveolens is better known as *Pelargonium graveolens* L'Her ex Ait. (family Geraniaceae). It is commonly known as rose-scented geranium, and it grows in temperate areas of the world including Jordan (Afifi et al. 2014; Boukhris et al. 2012). It is one of the herbs that has been used traditionally in Jordanian folk medicine as antidiabetic as well as diuretic, antispasmodic, and as a throat gargle. The commonly used preparation in traditional medicine is the decoction of leaves (Afifi et al. 2014). Geranium oil is known for its pleasant odor and its safety, and this is why it is increasingly used in cosmetic preparations, perfumery, and food industries (Afifi et al. 2014; Boukhris et al. 2012). A number of studies have reported various biological activities for *P. graveolens* including fumigant, antioxidant, antimicrobial, and insect repellant activities. In addition, immunostimulant effect has been reported for *P. graveolens* when administered to cancer patients treated with chemotherapy and/or radiotherapy. Still its antidiabetic activity is the main bioactivity that has been described (Afifi and Kasabri 2013).

The antidiabetic activity of the aqueous extracts of the aerial parts of *P. graveolens* (*G. graveolens*) was tested *in vitro* for its starch digestion activity and was confirmed with *in vivo* study applied to healthy female Sprague-Dawley rats fed with starch. The *in vitro* assay weighed the inhibitory activity of aldohexose release from polymeric cornstarch, and *P. graveolens* was found to be active in concentrations of 5–100 mg/mL. This finding was confirmed by the *in vivo* experiment, where *P. graveolens* significantly induced hyperglycemia ($p < 0.001$) at 250 mg/kg dose, 45 minutes post–oral administration of starch. The result was comparable with that of acarbose at the same point of determination time. This indicates that *P. graveolens* has a dual inhibitory activity against α-amylase and α-glucosidase *in vitro* confirmed by its *in vivo* antihyperglycemic activity in starch-fed animals. Furthermore, *P. graveolens* had no hypoglycemic effect on fasting animals (Kasabri et al. 2011b). Aqueous extracts of leaves of *P. graveolens* considerably retarded glucose efflux in a dialysis model *in vitro* at concentrations of 25 and 50 mg/mL; still it was not as effective as guar gum (natural oral antidiabetic), which was used as a positive control. The extract also demonstrated an expansion modulatory activity on pancreatic MIN6 β cells (Kasabri et al. 2013). Essential oils hydrodistilled from the leaves of *P. graveolens* were tested on an alloxan-induced diabetic model using male Wistar rats at two doses (75 and 150 mg/kg body weight). The oil significantly decreased blood glucose level and restored perturbed antioxidant activity comparable to glibenclamide activity (Boukhris et al. 2012).

The basis of the antidiabetic activity of *P. graveolens* lies within its essential oils, which contain more than 220 compounds (Rao 2009), including aliphatic, aromatic terpene, and sesquiterpene hydrocarbons; terpene alcohols such as geraniol, linalool, and citronellol; aliphatic, aromatic, and terpene esters such as citronellyl formate and geranyl formate; terpene ketones such as l-menthone; among other constituents of aliphatic, aromatic terpene and sesquiterpene alcohols, and terpene and sesquiterpene oxides (Boukhris et al. 2012; Rao 2009).

4.4.9 *CICHORIUM PUMILUM*

C. pumilum Jacq. (Family: Asteraceae, subfamily: Cichorioideae) has been recommended as an antidiabetic well before there were any reports for *in vivo* or *in vitro* hypoglycemic activities (Al-Aboudi and Afifi 2011). The common name for *C. pumilum* is chicory, a bushy perennial herb that grows wildly in Jordan in plains and hills. The *Cichorium* genus includes *C. intybus*, *C. endivia*, *C. bottae*, *C. spinosum*, *C. calvum*, and *C. pumilum* (Al Khateeb et al. 2012).

C. pumilum is known as *hindbah* in Arabic and is usually taken as a hot beverage derived from the roots or flowers, It is used in folklore medicine as antiseptic, antidiabetic, and as treatment in cases of eczema (Oran and Al-Eisawi 2015). It has been studied for its biological activity in which it displayed antimicrobial (Al Khateeb et al. 2012) and antidiabetic activity (Alkofahi et al. 2017) of its extracts. The ethanolic extract of *C. pumilum* leaves showed significant antihyperglycemic activity in alloxan-induced rat models, but the mechanism of action is still unknown (Alkofahi et al. 2017).

C. pumilum has been found to contain phenolic and sesquiterpene lactone phytochemicals. Phenolics include flavonoids, coumarins, and caffeic acid derivatives (Alkofahi et al. 2017).

Table 4.1 summarizes the above-mentioned plants with their traditional uses and mechanisms of action.

TABLE 4.1
Jordanian Plants with Antidiabetic Effect

Plant Name	Traditional Use	Mechanism of Action	Model of Study	References
Artemisia herba-alba	Used to treat colds, cough, bronchitis, diarrhea, diabetes, hypertension, snake bites, neuralgia, and parasitic infections	↑ Stimulation of β cells to release more insulin ↑ Glycogen deposition in the liver ↓ Glucose level ↑ Insulin receptors	*In vivo* study	Jaleel et al. 2016; Réggami et al. 2019; Iriadam et al. 2006
Achillea santolina	Antidiabetic, anti-inflammatory, to relieve stomach pain and symptoms of the common cold	↓ Glucose level ↑ Stimulation of β cells	*In vivo* study *In vitro* study	Yazdanparast et al. 2007; Kasabri et al. 2012
Crataegus aronia	Used to treat sexual weakness, cardiovascular diseases, diabetes, obesity, hyperlipidemia, and cancer	Normalized plasma lipid peroxide levels ↓ Glucose level ↓ α-Amylase, α-glucosidase, and pancreatic lipase	*In vitro* study *In vitro* and *in vivo* study	Omairi et al. 2020; Ljubuncic et al. 2006; Al-Hallaq et al. 2013

(Continued)

TABLE 4.1
(Continued)

Plant Name	Traditional Use	Mechanism of Action	Model of Study	References
Teucrium polium	Antispasmodic, anti-inflammatory, antibacterial, anthelmintic, hypotensive, and hypoglycemic To alleviate pain, headache, and to treat ulcers and renal stones	↑ Stimulation of β cells to release more insulin ↑ Translocation of (GLUT 4) ↑ Glucose uptake ↓ α-Amylase ↑ AMPK	*In vitro* study *In vivo* study	Aburjai et al. 2006; Afifi et al. 2005; Kadan et al. 2018; Mahmoudabady et al. 2020; Jaradat 2015
Pistacia atlantica	Sedative, anxiolytic, antipyretic, anti-inflammatory, antimicrobial, anticancer, hepatoprotective, antihypertensive, and antidiabetic Used to treat stomachache, dyspepsia, peptic ulcer, renal stones, musculoskeletal disorders, asthma, and topically to treat eczema and wounds	↓ α-Amylase, α-glucosidase ↓ Glucose level	*In vitro* study	Ahmed et al. 2018; Peksel et al. 2010; Peksel et al. 2010; Mahjoub et al. 2018; Ben Ahmed et al. 2021; Kasabri et al. 2011a
Phaseolus vulgaris	Antimicrobial, analgesic, antioxidant, anti-inflammatory, anti-obesity, antifertility, anticancer, antidiabetic, hepatoprotective, and hypolipidemic, as well as to treat renal stones	↓ α-Glucosidase ↓ Carbohydrate metabolism and absorption	*In vivo* study	Loko et al. 2018; He et al. 2018
Eryngium creticum	Used to treat diabetes, liver and renal ailments, poisoning cases, and scorpion stings	↓ Glucose level ↑ Glucose responsive insulin-releasing pancreatic MIN6 β cells	*In vivo* study *In vitro* study	Afifi et al. 1990; Kikowska et al. 2016; Nusair and Ahmad 2019; Jaghabir 1991; Kasabri et al. 2012
Geranium graveolens	Antidiabetic, diuretic, antispasmodic, and throat gargle	↓ α-Amylase, α-glucosidase ↓ Glucose efflux in dialysis model ↓ Glucose level	*In vitro* and *in vivo* study *In vitro* study *In vivo* study	Afifi et al. 2014; Kasabri et al. 2011b; Kasabri et al. 2013; Boukhris et al. 2012
Cichorium pumilum	Antiseptic, antidiabetic, and to treat eczema	↓ Glucose level	*In vivo* study	Oran and Al-Eisawi 2015; Alkofahi et al. 2017

4.5 TOXICITY AND CAUTIONARY NOTES

Herbal medicine and natural compounds are believed to be safe and potent agents. Nowadays, a wide range of the world population is consuming diverse forms of herbal remedies to treat health issues and maintain good health (Ekor 2014). Despite some herbal medicine being effective and widely used, still there is a shortage of knowledge about their quality, safety, and reliability (Ardalan and Rafieian-Kopaei 2013). As reported in the literature, many medicinal plants can be toxic intrinsically or have herb-drug interactions, or may contain contaminants (Mensah et al. 2019; Ardalan and Rafieian-Kopaei 2013). As well, other factors such as misidentification of medicinal herbs, intake overuse, and mislabeling of herbal medicinal products are associated with the occurrence of adverse effects (Ekor 2014). Moreover, to reduce the incidence of toxicity some recommendations can be followed, including obtaining herbal medicines from a registered herbalist, avoiding consuming herbal remedies along with drugs having a narrow therapeutic window, and monitoring herbal intake in case of pregnancy and breastfeeding mothers (Fatima and Nayeem 2016).

4.6 SUMMARY POINTS

- Jordan is rich in medicinal plants that are used to treat different diseases including diabetes.
- Nine Jordanian plants are commonly used to treat diabetes in traditional medicine with multiple mechanisms of action.
- *Teucrium polium* is the most commonly used plant in the treatment of diabetes.
- Regenerating pancreatic β cells and inactivating α-amylase enzyme are the main mechanisms for the antidiabetic effects of Jordanian plants.
- Further studies are needed to fully understand the antidiabetic activity of Jordanian plants.

REFERENCES

Abu-Odeh, A. M., and W. H. Talib. 2021. "Middle east medicinal plants in the treatment of diabetes: A review." *Molecules* no. 26 (3). doi:10.3390/molecules26030742.

Aburjai, Talal, Mohammad Hudaib, and Vanni Cavrini. 2006. "Composition of the essential oil from Jordanian germander (Teucrium polium L.)." *Journal of Essential Oil Research* no. 18 (1):97–99. doi:10.1080/10 412905.2006.9699398.

Afifi, F. U., S. Al-Khalil, M. Aqel, M. H. Al-Muhteseb, M. Jaghabir, M. Saket, and A. Muheid. 1990. "Antagonistic effect of Eryngium creticum extract on scorpion venom *in vitro*." *Journal of Ethnopharmacology* no. 29 (1):43–49.

Afifi, F. U., B. Al-Khalidi, and E. Khalil. 2005. "Studies on the *in vivo* hypoglycemic activities of two medicinal plants used in the treatment of diabetes in Jordanian traditional medicine following intranasal administration." *Journal of Ethnopharmacol* no. 100 (3):314–318. doi:10.1016/j.jep.2005.03.016.

Afifi, Fatma U., and Violet Kasabri. 2013. "Pharmacological and phytochemical appraisal of selected medicinal plants from Jordan with claimed antidiabetic activities." *Scientia Pharmaceutica* no. 81 (4):889–932.

Afifi, F. U., V. Kasabri, R. Abu-Dahab, and I. M. Abaza. 2014. "Chemical composition and *in vitro* studies of the essential oil and aqueous extract of Pelargonium graveolens growing in Jordan for hypoglycaemic and hypolipidemic properties." *European Journal of Medicinal Plants*:220–233.

Ahmed, Wesam, Talal Aburjai, Mohammad Hudaib, and Nehaya Al-Karablieh. 2020. "Chemical composition of essential oils hydrodistilled from aerial parts of Achillea fragrantissima (Forssk.) Sch. Bip. and Achillea santolina L.(Asteraceae) growing in Jordan." *Journal of Essential Oil Bearing Plants* no. 23 (1):15–25.

Ahmed, Z. B., M. Yousfi, J. Viaene, B. Dejaegher, K. Demeyer, D. Mangelings, and Y. Vander Heyden. 2018. "Potentially antidiabetic and antihypertensive compounds identified from Pistacia atlantica leaf extracts by LC fingerprinting." *Journal of Pharmaceutical and Biomedical Analysis* no. 149:547–556. doi:10.1016/j.jpba.2017.11.049.

Al-Aboudi, Amal, and Fatma U. Afifi. 2011. "Plants used for the treatment of diabetes in Jordan: A review of scientific evidence." *Pharmaceutical Biology* no. 49 (3):221–239.

Al-Hallaq, Entisar K., Violet Kasabri, Shtaywy S. Abdalla, Yasser K. Bustanji, and Fatma U. Afifi. 2013. "Anti-obesity and antihyperglycemic effects of Crataegus aronia extracts: *In vitro* and *in vivo* evaluations." *Food and Nutrition Sciences* no. 4 (9).

Al Khateeb, Wesam, Emad Hussein, Lolita Qouta, Muhammad Alu'datt, Baker Al-Shara, and Ahmed Abu-Zaiton. 2012. "*In vitro* propagation and characterization of phenolic content along with antioxidant and antimicrobial activities of Cichorium pumilum Jacq." *Plant Cell, Tissue and Organ Culture (PCTOC)* no. 110 (1):103–110.

Alkofahi, Ahmad S., Khalid K. Abdul-Razzak, Karem H. Alzoubi, and Omar F. Khabour. 2017. "Screening of the Anti-hyperglycemic activity of some medicinal plants of Jordan." *Pakistan Journal of Pharmaceutical Sciences* no. 30 (3).

Al-Snafi, Ali Esmail. 2013. "Chemical constituents and pharmacological activities of Milfoil (Achillea santolina): A review." *International Journal of PharmTech Research* no. 5 (3):1373–1377.

Ardalan, Mohammad-Reza, and Mahmoud Rafieian-Kopaei. 2013. "Is the safety of herbal medicines for kidneys under question?" *Journal of Nephropharmacology* no. 2 (2):11–12.

Awad, S. F., P. Huangfu, S. R. Dargham, K. Ajlouni, A. Batieha, Y. S. Khader, J. A. Critchley, and L. J. Abu-Raddad. 2020. "Characterizing the type 2 diabetes mellitus epidemic in Jordan up to 2050." *Scientific Reports* no. 10 (1):21001. doi:10.1038/s41598-020-77970-7.

Ben Ahmed, Z., M. Yousfi, J. Viaene, B. Dejaegher, K. Demeyer, and Y. V. Heyden. 2021. "Four Pistacia atlantica subspecies (atlantica, cabulica, kurdica and mutica): A review of their botany, ethnobotany, phytochemistry and pharmacology." *Journal of Ethnopharmacology* no. 265:113329. doi:10.1016/j.jep.2020.113329.

Boukhris, Maher, Mohamed Bouaziz, Ines Feki, Hedya Jemai, Abdelfattah El Feki, and Sami Sayadi. 2012. "Hypoglycemic and antioxidant effects of leaf essential oil of Pelargonium graveolens L'Hér. in alloxan induced diabetic rats." *Lipids in Health and Disease* no. 11 (1):1–10.

Cheng, Y. C., Y. Guerra, M. Morkos, B. Tahsin, C. Onyenwenyi, L. Fogg, and L. Fogelfeld. 2021. "Insulin management in hospitalized patients with diabetes mellitus on high-dose glucocorticoids: Management of steroid-exacerbated hyperglycemia." *PLoS ONE* no. 16 (9):e0256682. doi:10.1371/journal.pone.0256682.

Devi, M., Dhanalakshmi S. Dhanalakshmi, G. E. Thillai Govindarajan, Tanisha B. Tanisha, Talluri Sonalika, Ruth Je Ruth, Avinash T. Avinash, C. Jethendra Sri, Logeswaran K. Logeswaran, and M. Nithish Ramasamy. 2020. "A review on phaseolus vulgaris linn." *Pharmacognosy Journal* no. 12 (5):1160–1164. doi:10.5530/pj.2020.12.163.

Ekor, Martins. 2014. "The growing use of herbal medicines: Issues relating to adverse reactions and challenges in monitoring safety." *Frontiers in Pharmacology* no. 4. doi:10.3389/fphar.2013.00177.

Espona-Noguera, A., J. Ciriza, A. Cañibano-Hernandez, G. Orive, R.M.M. Hernandez, L. Saenz Del Burgo, and J. L. Pedraz. 2019. "Review of advanced hydrogel-based cell encapsulation systems for insulin delivery in type 1 diabetes mellitus." *Pharmaceutics* no. 11 (11). doi:10.3390/pharmaceutics11110597.

Faisal, Muhammad Saleh, Asad Inayat, Muhammad Nabi, Waqar Hayat, Muhammad Sajid Khan, and Waheed Iqbal. 2020. "Screening of achillea santolina for anti-diabetic activity and its comparison with caralluma tuberculata." *The Professional Medical Journal* no. 27 (7):1414–1419.

Fatima, Nudrat, and Naira Nayeem. 2016. "Toxic effects as a result of herbal medicine intake." In *Toxicology-New Aspects to This Scientific Conundrum*. London: InTech Open:193–207.

Galicia-Garcia, U., A. Benito-Vicente, S. Jebari, A. Larrea-Sebal, H. Siddiqi, K. B. Uribe, H. Ostolaza, and C. Martin. 2020. "Pathophysiology of type 2 diabetes mellitus." *International Journal of Molecular Sciences* no. 21 (17). doi:10.3390/ijms21176275.

Gant, C. M., I. Minovic, H. Binnenmars, L. de Vries, I. Kema, A. van Beek, G. Navis, S. Bakker, and G. D. Laverman. 2018. "Lower renal function is associated with derangement of 11-beta hydroxysteroid dehydrogenase in type 2 diabetes." *Journal of the Endocrine Society* no. 2 (7):609–620. doi:10.1210/js.2018-00088.

Gastaldelli, A., N. Stefan, and H. U. Haring. 2021. "Liver-targeting drugs and their effect on blood glucose and hepatic lipids." *Diabetologia* no. 64 (7):1461–1479. doi:10.1007/s00125-021-05442-2.

He, S., B. K. Simpson, H. Sun, M. O. Ngadi, Y. Ma, and T. Huang. 2018. "Phaseolus vulgaris lectins: A systematic review of characteristics and health implications." *Critical Reviews in Food Science and Nutrition* no. 58 (1):70–83. doi:10.1080/10408398.2015.1096234.

Hinnen, Deborah. 2017. "Glucagon-like peptide 1 receptor agonists for type 2 diabetes." *Diabetes Spectrum* no. 30 (3):202. doi:10.2337/ds16-0026.

Hong, D. J., S. H. Jung, J. Kim, D. Jung, Y. G. Ahn, K. H. Suh, and K. H. Min. 2020. "Synthesis and biological evaluation of novel thienopyrimidine derivatives as diacylglycerol acyltransferase 1 (DGAT-1) inhibitors." *Journal of Enzyme Inhibition and Medicinal Chemistry* no. 35 (1):227–234. doi:10.1080/14756366.2019.1693555.

Hudaib, Mohammad M., and Talal A. Aburjai. 2006. "Composition of the essential oil from Artemisia herba-alba grown in Jordan." *Journal of Essential Oil Research* no. 18 (3):301–304.

Iriadam, Mehmet, Davut Musa, H. Gumushan, and Füsun Baba. 2006. "Effects of two Turkish medicinal plants Artemisia herba-alba and Teucrium polium on blood glucose levels and other biochemical parameters in rabbits." *The Journal Cellular and Molecular Biology* no. 5 (1):19–24.

Jaghabir, Madi. 1991. "Hypoglycemic effects of eryngium creticum." *Archives of Pharmacal Research* no. 14 (4):295–297.

Jaleel, Gehad Abdel Raheem Abdel, Heba Mohammed Ibrahim Abdallah, and Nawal E. L. Sayed Gomaa. 2016. "Pharmacological effects of ethanol extract of Egyptian Artemisia herba-alba in rats and mice." *Asian Pacific Journal of Tropical Biomedicine* no. 6 (1):44–49.

Jaradat, Nidal Amin. 2015. "Review of the taxonomy, ethnobotany, phytochemistry, phytotherapy and phytotoxicity of germander plant (Teucrium polium L.)." *Asian Journal of Pharmaceutical and Clinical Research* no. 3:4.

Jay, M. A., and J. Ren. 2007. "Peroxisome proliferator-activated receptor (PPAR) in metabolic syndrome and type 2 diabetes mellitus." *Current Diabetes Reviews* no. 3 (1):33–39. doi:10.2174/157339907779802067.

Kadan, Sleman, Yoel Sasson, Raed Abu-Reziq, Bashar Saad, Shoshana Benvalid, Thomas Linn, Guy Cohen, and Hilal Zaid. 2018. "Teucrium polium extracts stimulate GLUT4 translocation to the plasma membrane in L6 muscle cells." *Advancement in Medicinal Plant Research* no. 6 (1):1–8. doi:10.30918/ampr.61.17.028.

Kasabri, V., F. U. Afifi, and I. Hamdan. 2011a. "*In vitro* and *in vivo* acute antihyperglycemic effects of five selected indigenous plants from Jordan used in traditional medicine." *Journal of Ethnopharmacology* no. 133 (2):888–896. doi:10.1016/j.jep.2010.11.025.

Kasabri, Violet, Rana Abu-Dahab, Fatma U. Afifi, Randa Naffa, and Lara Majdalawi. 2012. "Modulation of pancreatic MIN6 insulin secretion and proliferation and extrapancreatic glucose absorption with Achillea santolina, Eryngium creticum and Pistacia atlantica extracts: *In vitro* evaluation." *Journal of Experimental and Integrative Medicine* no. 2:245–254.

Kasabri, Violet, Rana Abu-Dahab, Fatma U. Afifi, Randa Naffa, Lara Majdalawi, and Hazar Shawash. 2013. "*In vitro* effects of Geranium graveolens, Sarcopoterium spinosum and Varthemia iphionoides extracts on pancreatic MIN6 proliferation and insulin secretion and on extrapancreatic glucose diffusion." *International Journal of Diabetes in Developing Countries* no. 33 (3):170–177.

Kasabri, Violet, Fatma U. Afifi, and Imad Hamdan. 2011b. "Evaluation of the acute antihyperglycemic effects of four selected indigenous plants from Jordan used in traditional medicine." *Pharmaceutical Biology* no. 49 (7):687–695.

Kikowska, Małgorzata, Marzena Dworacka, Izabela Kędziora, and Barbara Thiem. 2016. "Eryngium creticum – ethnopharmacology, phytochemistry and pharmacological activity. A review." *Revista Brasileira de Farmacognosia* no. 26:392–399.

Koike, T., R. Shiraki, D. Sasuga, M. Hosaka, T. Kawano, H. Fukudome, K. Kurosawa, A. Moritomo, S. Mimasu, H. Ishii, and S. Yoshimura. 2019. "Discovery and biological evaluation of potent and orally active human 11beta-hydroxysteroid dehydrogenase type 1 inhibitors for the treatment of type 2 diabetes mellitus." *Chemical and Pharmaceutical Bulletin (Tokyo)* no. 67 (8):824–838. doi:10.1248/cpb.c19-00211.

Ljubuncic, Predrag, Hassan Azaizeh, Uri Cogan, and Arieh Bomzon. 2006. "The effects of a decoction prepared from the leaves and unripe fruits of Crataegus aronia in streptozotocin-induced diabetic rats." *Journal of Complementary Integrative Medicine* no. 3 (1).

Loko, L.E.Y., J. Toffa, A. Adjatin, A. J. Akpo, A. Orobiyi, and A. Dansi. 2018. "Folk taxonomy and traditional uses of common bean (Phaseolus vulgaris L.) landraces by the sociolinguistic groups in the central region of the Republic of Benin." *Journal of Ethnobiology and Ethnomedicine* no. 14 (1):52. doi:10.1186/s13002-018-0251-6.

Mahjoub, F., K. Akhavan Rezayat, M. Yousefi, M. Mohebbi, and R. Salari. 2018. "Pistacia atlantica Desf. A review of its traditional uses, phytochemicals and pharmacology." *Journal of Medicine and Life* no. 11 (3):180–186. doi:10.25122/jml-2017-0055.

Mahmoudabady, Maryam, AliAkbar Asghari, Amin Mokhtari-Zaer, Saeed Niazmand, and Kathleen McEntee. 2020. "Anti-diabetic properties and bioactive compounds of Teucrium polium L." *Asian Pacific Journal of Tropical Biomedicine* no. 10 (10). doi:10.4103/2221-1691.290868.

Makrilakis, Konstantinos. 2019. "The role of DPP-4 inhibitors in the treatment algorithm of type 2 diabetes mellitus: When to select, what to expect." *International Journal of Environmental Research and Public Health* no. 16 (15). doi:10.3390/ijerph16152720.

Mensah, M. L., Gustav Komlaga, Arnold D. Forkuo, Caleb Firempong, Alexander K. Anning, and Rita A. Dickson. 2019. "Toxicity and safety implications of herbal medicines used in Africa." *Herbal Medicine* no. 63:1992–0849.

Mishra, V., P. Nayak, M. Sharma, A. Albutti, A.S.S. Alwashmi, M. A. Aljasir, N. Alsowayeh, and M. M. Tambuwala. 2021. "Emerging treatment strategies for diabetes mellitus and associated complications: An update." *Pharmaceutics* no. 13 (10). doi:10.3390/pharmaceutics13101568.

Mohamed, Abou El Hamd H., Magdi A. El-Sayed, Mohamed E. Hegazy, Soleiman E. Helaly, Abeer M. Esmail, and Naglaa S. Mohamed. 2010. "Chemical constituents and biological activities of Artemisia herba-alba." *J Records of Natural Products* no. 4 (1):1–25.

Mostafa, Dalia G., Eman F. Khaleel, and Ghada A. Abdel-Aleem. 2018. "Inhibition of the hepatic glucose output is responsible for the hypoglycemic effect of Crataegus aronia against type 2 diabetes mellitus in rats." *Archives of Biological Sciences* no. 70 (2):277–287.

Müller, T. D., B. Finan, S. R. Bloom, D. D'Alessio, D. J. Drucker, P. R. Flatt, A. Fritsche, F. Gribble, H. J. Grill, J. F. Habener, J. J. Holst, W. Langhans, J. J. Meier, M. A. Nauck, D. Perez-Tilve, A. Pocai, F. Reimann, D. A. Sandoval, T. W. Schwartz, R. J. Seeley, K. Stemmer, M. Tang-Christensen, S. C. Woods, R. D. DiMarchi, and M. H. Tschöp. 2019. "Glucagon-like peptide 1 (GLP-1)." *Molecular Metabolism* no. 30:72–130. doi:10.1016/j.molmet.2019.09.010.

Nusair, Shreen Deeb, and Mohammad Ibrahim Ahmad. 2019. "Toxicity of Vipera palaestinae venom and antagonistic effects of methanolic leaf extract of Eryngium creticum lam." *Toxicon* no. 166:1–8.

Olmos-Ortiz, A., P. Flores-Espinosa, L. Diaz, P. Velazquez, C. Ramirez-Isarraraz, and V. Zaga-Clavellina. 2021. "Immunoendocrine dysregulation during gestational diabetes mellitus: The central role of the placenta." *International Journal of Molecular Sciences* no. 22 (15). doi:10.3390/ijms22158087.

Omairi, Islam, Firas Kobeissy, and Salam Nasreddine. 2020. "Anti-oxidant, anti-hemolytic effects of crataegus aronia leaves and its anti-proliferative effect enhance cisplatin cytotoxicity in A549 human lung cancer cell line." *Asian Pacific Journal of Cancer Prevention: APJCP* no. 21 (10):2993.

Oran, S. A., and D. Al-Eisawi. 2015. "Ethnobotanical survey of the medicinal plants in the central mountains (North-South) in Jordan." *Journal of Biodiversity and Environmental Sciences* no. 6 (3):381–400.

Peksel, Aysegul, Inci Arisan-Atac, and Refiye Yanardag. 2010. "Evaluation of antioxidant and antiacetylcholinesterase activities of the extracts of pistacia atlantica desf. leaves." *Journal of Food Biochemistry* no. 181:1199–1200. doi:10.1111/j.1745-4514.2009.00290.x.

Raja, R., V. Kumar, M. A. Khan, K. A. Sayeed, S.Z.M. Hussain, and A. Rizwan. 2019. "Knowledge, attitude, and practices of complementary and alternative medication usage in patients of type II diabetes mellitus." *Cureus* no. 11 (8):e5357. doi:10.7759/cureus.5357.

Rao, B. R. Rajeswara. 2009. "Chemical composition and uses of Indian rose-scented Geranium (Pelargonium species) essential oil: A review." *Journal of Essential Oil Bearing Plants* no. 12 (4):381–394.

Réggami, Yassine, Abderrahim Benkhaled, Amel Boudjelal, Hajira Berredjem, Amani Amamra, Halima Benyettou, Nadia Larabi, Abderrahmane Senator, Laura Siracusa, and Giuseppe Ruberto. 2019. "Artemisia herba-alba aqueous extract improves insulin sensitivity and hepatic steatosis in rodent model of fructose-induced metabolic syndrome." *Archives of Physiology*:1–10.

Riddy, Darren M., Philippe Delerive, Roger J. Summers, Patrick M. Sexton, and Christopher J. Langmead. 2018. "G protein–coupled receptors targeting insulin resistance, obesity, and type 2 diabetes mellitus." *Pharmacological Reviews* no. 70 (1):39. doi:10.1124/pr.117.014373.

Röhrborn, Diana, Nina Wronkowitz, and Juergen Eckel. 2015. "DPP4 in diabetes." *Frontiers in Immunology* no. 6:386–386. doi:10.3389/fimmu.2015.00386.

Salem, Mohamed L., Reda M. Gaafar, Reham N. Mohasseb, and Mohamed A. Abd-Elbaseer. 2017. "Apoptotic effects of the medicinal plants Achillea santolina and Raphanus sativus extracts on different cancer cell lines." *Journal of Cancer and Biomedical Research* no. 1 (1):24–32.

Shah, N., M. A. Abdalla, H. Deshmukh, and T. Sathyapalan. 2021. "Therapeutics for type-2 diabetes mellitus: A glance at the recent inclusions and novel agents under development for use in clinical practice." *Therapeutic Advances in Endocrinology and Metabolism* no. 12:20420188211042145. doi:10.1177/20420188211042145.

Sutedja, A. M., E. Yanase, I. Batubara, D. Fardiaz, and H. N. Lioe. 2020. "Antidiabetic components from the hexane extract of red kidney beans (Phaseolus vulgaris L.): Isolation and structure determination." *Bioscience, Biotechnology, and Biochemistry* no. 84 (3):598–605. doi:10.1080/09168451.2019.1691911.

Takada, Ichiro, and Makoto Makishima. 2020. "Peroxisome proliferator-activated receptor agonists and antagonists: A patent review (2014-present)." *Expert Opinion on Therapeutic Patents* no. 30 (1):1–13.

Talukdar, Saswata, Jerrold M. Olefsky, and Olivia Osborn. 2011. "Targeting GPR120 and other fatty acid-sensing GPCRs ameliorates insulin resistance and inflammatory diseases." *Trends in Pharmacological Sciences* no. 32 (9):543–550. doi:10.1016/j.tips.2011.04.004.

Vallon, V., and K. Sharma. 2010. "Sodium-glucose transport: Role in diabetes mellitus and potential clinical implications." *Current Opinion in Nephrology and Hypertension* no. 19 (5):425–431. doi:10.1097/MNH.0b013e32833bec06.

Yau, B., S. Naghiloo, A. Diaz-Vegas, A. V. Carr, J. Van Gerwen, E. J. Needham, D. Jevon, S. Y. Chen, K. L. Hoehn, A. E. Brandon, L. Macia, G. J. Cooney, M. R. Shortreed, L. M. Smith, M. P. Keller, P. Thorn, M. Larance, D. E. James, S. J. Humphrey, and M. A. Kebede. 2021. "Proteomic pathways to metabolic disease and type 2 diabetes in the pancreatic islet." *iScience* no. 24 (10):103099. doi:10.1016/j.isci.2021.103099.

Yazdanparast, Razieh, Amin Ardestani, and Shirin J. Jamshidi. 2007. "Experimental diabetes treated with Achillea santolina: Effect on pancreatic oxidative parameters." *Journal of Ethnopharmacology* no. 112 (1):13–18.

5 The Use of Medicinal Plant–Derived Signaling Molecules for the Improvement of Mesenchymal Stromal Cells (MSCs) Antidiabetic Properties

Lynda Bourebaba, Nabila Bourebaba and Krzysztof Marycz

CONTENTS

ABBREVIATIONS

ACC	acetyl-CoA carboxylase
ADMSCs	adipose tissue–derived mesenchymal stem cells
AKT	protein kinase B
AMPK	adenosine monophosphate-activated protein kinase
Ang-1	angiopoietin 1
aP2	adipocyte fatty acid binding protein
BMSCs	bone marrow–derived mesenchymal stromal cells
C/EBP	CCAAT/enhancer-binding protein
CCND1	cyclin D1

DOI: 10.1201/9781003220930-6

CREB	cAMP-responsive element binding protein
DM	diabetes mellitus
DMED	diabetic mellitus erectile dysfunction
DVL2	disheveled 2
ECM	extracellular matrix
EKN	*Epimedium koreanum* Nakai
eNOS	endothelial nitric oxide synthase
ER	endoplasmic reticulum
ERK	extracellular signal-regulated kinase
FABP4	fatty acid binding protein
FAS receptor	tumor necrosis factor receptor superfamily member 6
FAS	fatty acid synthase
FFAs	free fatty acids
FoxO1	forkhead box O1
FoxP3	forkhead box P3
G6PC	glucose-6-phosphatase
GATA-2	GATA-binding factor 2
GLP-1	glucagon-like protein 1
GLUT4	glucose transporter type 4
GPDH	glycerol-3-phosphate dehydrogenase
GSK3β	glycogen synthase kinase 3β
HGF	hepatocyte growth factor
HMGR	hydroxymethylglutaryl-coenzyme A reductase
ICA	icariin
IDO	indoleamine-2,3-dioxygenase
IFN-γ	interferon γ
IKKβ	inhibitor of nuclear factor κB kinase subunit β
IL-10	interleukin-10
IL-1β	interleukin-1β
IL-6	interleukin-6
INSR	insulin receptor
IPCs	insulin-producing cells
JNK	c-Jun N-terminal kinase
KLF	Krüppel-like factor
LDL	low-density lipoprotein
LDLR	low-density lipoprotein receptor
LPL	lipoprotein lipase
LRP6	low-density lipoprotein receptor–related protein 6
MCE	mitotic clonal expansion
MCP-1	monocyte chemoattractant protein-1
MMP-9	matrix metalloproteinase-9
MSCs	mesenchymal stromal cells
mTOR	mammalian target of rapamycin
NF-κB	nuclear factor κB
NLRP3	NOD-, LRR- and pyrin domain-containing 3
NOAEL	no observed adverse effect level
NPY	neuropeptide Y
P38 MAPK	P38 mitogen–activated protein kinase
PD-1	programmed death ligand 1
PGE2	prostaglandin E2
Pi3K	phosphoinositide 3-kinase

PPARγ	peroxisome proliferator-activated receptor γ
pref-1	preadipocyte factor-1
Rap1	Ras-association proximate 1
ROS	reactive oxygen species
SCD	stearoyl-CoA desaturase
SIRT1	sirtuin-1
SOD	superoxidase dismutase
SREBP-1c	sterol regulatory element binding protein-1c
STZ	streptozotocin
T1DM	type 1 diabetes mellitus
T2DM	type 2 diabetes mellitus
TC	total cholesterol
TG	triglyceride
TGF-β	transforming growth factor β
TLR2	toll-like receptor 2
TLR4	toll-like receptor 4
TNF-α	tumor necrosis factor-α
TSA	trichostatin-A
VEGF	vascular endothelial growth factor
WJMSCs	Warton jelly–derived mesenchymal stromal cells

5.1 INTRODUCTION

Diabetes mellitus (DM) is one of the most prevalent chronic metabolic disorders worldwide that poses a real public health burden due to its constant and alarming expansion. DM is defined as a cluster of endocrine metabolic diseases characterized by dysregulated glucose and lipid metabolism, underlying inadequate insulin production and/or action, which triggers various subsequent macrovascular complications (Mohamed et al., 2015; Pal et al., 2014). DM is typically classified into two main categories on the basis of the underlying pathophysiological mechanisms as well as etiologic factors. Type 1 diabetes mellitus (T1DM) is an autoimmune related disease characterized by the selective destruction of pancreatic insulin secreting β cells as a result of critical self-tolerance loss and excessive inflammatory responses, that lead to the establishment of a drastic insulin deficiency (Cañibano-Hernández et al., 2018). Type 2 diabetes mellitus (T2DM) is the more common type of diabetes, accounting for nearly 90% of global cases worldwide. It arises from concomitant loss of insulin sensitivity of the peripheric insulin-responsive tissues and impairment of insulin-producing pancreatic β cells (Goyal and Jialal, 2022).

The evolution of T1DM and T2DM is largely determined by the progressive failure and destruction of pancreatic β cells that attempt to overcome the reduced insulin levels and resulting hampered glucose uptake (Donath and Shoelson, 2011). Chronic inflammation has been demonstrated to play a pivotal role in the pancreatic β cell destruction process. Infiltration of pancreatic islets by adaptive and innate immune cells engenders a severe insulitis that culminates in long-term mass decline of β cells and consequent elevation in blood glucose levels, driving to hyperglycemia and clinical diabetes onset (Clark et al., 2017). Therewith, persistent hyperglycemia further triggers β cell metabolic distress and apoptosis through the activation of pro-apoptotic signals including FAS receptor and the pro-inflammatory cytokine IL-1β (Rojas et al., 2018). Systemic low-grade inflammation is also promoted by obesity and its underlying glucose intolerance and insulin resistance, metabolic perturbation events that trigger chronic hyperinsulinemia and further onset of diabetes (Després et al., 2008). Ectopic adiposity leads to a simultaneous increase in nutrient intake and insufficient energetic expenditure resulting in adipocyte hyperplasia accompanied by macrophage infiltration, ECM remodeling, fibrosis, and excessive ROS generation – all of which contribute to increased pro-inflammatory cytokine production and insulin signaling failure (Jakab et al., 2021).

Current available treatment strategies involve the administration of oral antidiabetic drugs such as the hypoglycemic metformin, exogenous insulin injection, and a controlled diet that enables the temporary maintenance of appropriate blood glucose levels and attenuation of hyperglycemia-related symptoms, but these are yet unable to permanently reverse the characteristic metabolic imbalance. It is therefore imperative to explore new therapeutic alternatives that can ensure a better control of the disease progression (Huang et al., 2021).

Insofar as insulin deficiency represents one of the most salient diabetes defects, the regeneration of insulin-secreting cells seems to be a rather promising approach. Moreover, the highly inflammatory macro- and microenvironment of the pancreatic tissue and other peripheral tissues represents an interesting target for limiting the disease progression. Mesenchymal stromal cells (MSCs) are characterized over other cell types by their self-renewing and multilineage differentiation potential. They exhibit a high ability to regenerate various types of injured tissues and possess important immunomodulatory and anti-inflammatory properties, so that they are able to release a wide range of reactive mediators, as well as microvesicles capable of modulating several molecular processes involved in the progression of various diseases (Via et al., 2012). Previous research has already reported on the efficacy of syngeneic or allogeneic MSC transplantation in preventing and/or delaying DM development. Intravenous infusion of MSCs has been demonstrated to lower hyperglycemia and contribute to the repair and regeneration of deteriorated pancreatic islets in the course of T1DM (Ezquer et al., 2008). Although the use of MSCs cells seems to be a revolutionary approach offering different treatments axes, these cells may in some cases lose their properties and can thus be confronted with various intrinsic limiting factors including apoptosis or senescence. To overcome this issue, different preconditioning methods have been developed for the enhancement of MSC functions (Hu and Li, 2018). Thus, the pre-treatment of MSCs with various pharmacological agents including medicinal plant derivatives has been reported to greatly improve the therapeutic properties of MSCs and their transplantation efficacy in various regenerative medicine applications (Saud et al., 2019).

Traditional medicinal plants have been used for decades in the treatment of a number of human ailments in various forms, such as decoctions, ointments, and fumigations. Later, advances and progress in science highlighted the presence of various secondary metabolites in these natural remedies, such as polyphenols, alkaloids, and terpenes with innumerable therapeutic virtues that can improve or correct a certain number of molecular pathways crucial to the proper functioning of cell and tissue. Extracts from different plant parts (root, bark, flower, leaf, and seed) have been tested for their proliferative, antioxidant, anti-inflammatory, and antidiabetic effects and regulatory potential on the metabolism (Wink, 2015). In regenerative medicine, preconditioning of MSCs with plant extract derivatives has been proven to promote proliferation and multilineage differentiation, suggesting that the use of bioactive molecules in combination with MSCs may offer attractive option for proper DM management (Kornicka et al., 2017).

This chapter will present examples of known traditional medicinal plants rich in active secondary metabolites that have been tested for their beneficial effects on antidiabetic properties of MSCs. Particular emphasis will be given to the underlying molecular pathways of diabetes including inflammation, adiposity, and tissue regeneration.

5.2 ANTIDIABETIC POTENTIAL OF MESENCHYMAL STROMAL CELLS

Stem cell–based therapies have gained more attention during the past few years in applications for the treatment of various degenerative diseases including neuropathies, orthopedic conditions, and endocrine and metabolic disorders. The use of stem cells in regenerative medicine has thus offered many new prospects in the proper management of malfunctioning organs and tissues.

MSCs represent one of the most attractive types of stem cells due to the limited ethical restrictions. MSCs are fibroblast-like cells characterized by their self-renewal capacity, multipotency, and ability to differentiate into the three germ layers, and are considered as being potent immunomodulatory cells. Furthermore, MSC transplantation showcases the advantage of being

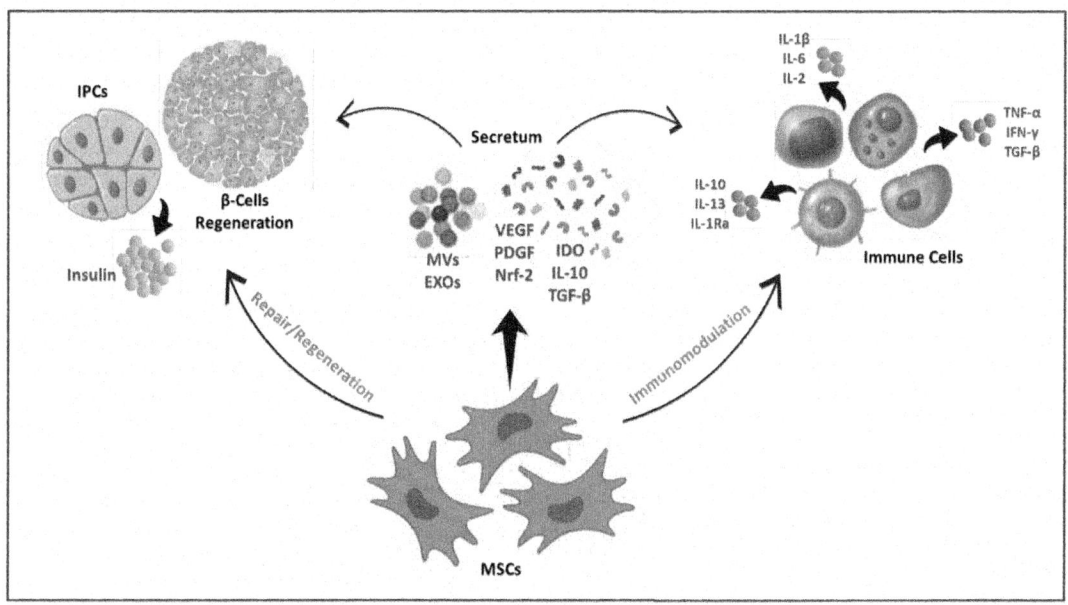

FIGURE 5.1 Main MSC antidiabetic molecular mechanisms. MSCs secrete various bioactive mediators and extracellular vesicles mediating various signaling pathways. MSCs are able to differentiate into insulin producing cells (IPCs) that can produce and release insulin hormone and C-peptide. In a pro-inflammatory milieu, MSCs release factors and cytokines that regulate and suppress innate immune cells activation and reduce the excessive release of pro-inflammatory cytokines, all of which participate in the attenuation of pancreatic islet degeneration and insulin resistance.

non-immunogenic, well tolerated, and at some extent immune privileged, making them good candidates for the *in-situ* repair and replacement of damaged tissues.

Antidiabetic properties of MSCs cells have been previously reported as being most likely attributable to either their pro-regenerative potential, multipotency ability, and their strong immunomodulatory activity (Figure 5.1) (Li et al., 2021).

Insulitis is one of the salient hallmarks of both T1DM and T2DM, which are characterized by the progressive destruction of the pancreatic tissue under highly pro-inflammatory conditions, due to either the activation of the innate immune system or the increased circulating levels or inflammatory mediators arising from the metaflammation characterizing T2DM (Böni-Schnetzler et al., 2008).

Cytokines including IFN-γ, TNF-α, and IL-1β have been identified as being involved in the progressive development of diabetic pancreatitis. Upon activation, they trigger various subsequent molecular events ranging from oxidative stress and increased ROS generation, insulin signaling disruption, β cell apoptosis, and ultimately insulin resistance (Tsalamandris et al., 2019). Accumulating evidence further suggest that high glucose levels and associated oxidative stress induce the overexpression of IL-1β via the selective priming and activation of NOD-, LRR-, and pyrin domain–containing 3 (NLRP3) inflammasome pathway, which initiates caspase 1 activation and pro–IL-1β maturation (Zhou et al., 2010). Besides, nutrients excess such as free fatty acids (FFAs) and their metabolites have also been shown to strongly stimulate pro-inflammatory mediators release via the direct interaction with toll-like receptors 2 and 4 (TLR2 and TLR4), which subsequently stimulate the stress-induced kinases IκB kinase-β (IKKβ) and Jun N-terminal kinase (JNK) to promote transcription factor nuclear factor-κB (NF-κB) expression, pro-inflammatory cytokines production, and insulin resistance development (Cai et al., 2005; Lee et al., 2004).

MSCs have been extensively studied for their immunomodulatory properties; these cells have been found to significantly mitigate acute inflammatory responses through the secretion of various soluble anti-inflammatory molecules or extracellular vesicles loaded in active mediators, the suppression of proinflammatory cytokines, and regulation of immune cell activation and infiltration. The activity of MSCs has been shown to be intimately linked to the microenvironment in which they evolve. Increased inflammatory signals such as TNF-α, IL-1β, and IFN-γ mediate the immunosuppressive phenotype shift of MSCs that tend to modulate inflammation thought the release of IDO, PGE2, Rap1, IL-10, TGF-β, and HGF anti-inflammatory mediators (Shrestha et al., 2021). Furthermore, MSCs have been found to efficiently regulate innate immune system activation via the suppression of T cell proliferation and migration through programmed death 1 (PD-1) release, while enhancing T CD4+CD25+ cells or CD4+CD25+FoxP3+ T regulatory cells maturation (Selmani et al., 2008).

The ultimate consequence of chronic metaflammation lies in gradual pancreatic tissue destruction and loss of β cells, that culminate in insufficient insulin production, pancreas exhaustion, and overall poor glycemic control. MSCs are capable of trans-differentiation to various somatic cell types including β-like cells. Previous researches have reported on the successful *in vitro* differentiation of various types of MSCs, namely BMSCs, ADMSCs, and WJMSCs to insulin-producing cells (IPCs) using either exendin-4, a glucagon-like protein-1 (GLP-1) receptor agonist, or trichostatin-A (TSA)/GLP-1, that efficiently produced high levels of both insulin and C-peptide in response to high glucose level challenge and expressed all the relevant pancreatic endocrine genes (Kassem et al., 2016; Khorsandi et al., 2017; Tayaramma et al., 2006). Moreover, transplantation of human BMSCs-derived IPCs to nude mice with STZ-induced diabetes enabled to maintain euglycemia within 7 days posttransplantation; therewith, transplanted animals exhibited elevated circulating levels of human insulin and C-peptide with negligible levels of mouse insulin (Gabr et al., 2013). In addition to being able to replace β cells, MSCs offer the unique property to repair damaged pancreatic tissue and promote islet survival. Recently, co-transplantation of MSCs with neonatal islets resulted in improved islet cell proliferation and maturation, increased insulin secretion, and potentiated engraftment that have been attributed to the paracrine effect of MSCs. Furthermore, MSCs greatly ameliorated the posttransplantation revascularization due to their known pro-angiogenic ability that takes place via the release of angiogenic mediators including VEGF, FGF, TGF-β, and Ang-1. Likewise, treated mice with co-encapsulated islets and MSCs enabled a proper maintenance of normoglycemia and an overall improvement of the metabolic functions of almost 71% of total transplanted mice within 6 weeks of experimentation. Similar outcomes were observed following the co-culture of human islets with human MSCs that sustained elevated insulin secretion and cell survival, attributable to tight N-cadherin interactions between adjacent cells (Koehler et al., 2022).

Increased adiposity that is accompanied with a raise in pro-inflammatory cytokines, unsaturated lipids, hormones, and pro-fibrotic mediators' levels greatly contribute to the onset of insulin resistance and metabolic failure. MSCs have been reported to reverse obesity-related phenotype by reducing body weight, abdominal fat accumulation, and adipose tissue hypertrophy. The observed effects have been suggested to be associated to an enhanced mitochondrial activity and energy metabolism, diminished oxidative stress, and insulin resistance of peripheral tissues (Zhu et al., 2016). In like manner, other study established that MSCs derived from adipose tissue infusion positively corrected dyslipidemia and associated lipid metabolism dysregulation in obese mice while inducing white fat tissue browning and activation of adenosine monophosphate–activated protein kinase and hormone-sensitive lipase, which overall restored adequate adipose lipid turnover and dynamics (Liu et al., 2016).

5.3 MSCs PRECONDITIONING WITH PLANT DERIVATIVES IMPROVES THEIR ANTIDIABETIC PROPERTIES

MSC-based therapies have already proven their effectiveness in the treatment of various conditions due to their manifold intrinsic properties and their unique ability to regenerate and restore the functions of injured tissues. However, some limitations to the use of MSCs have raised from the various clinical trials that reported poor engraftment and homing ability, as well as low survival and differentiation rates. Moreover, as most MSCs functions have been attributed to their paracrine properties, changes in the composition of their secretum may partly explain the observed defaults (Holthaus et al., 2022).

Traditional medicinal plants have been long used for the curation of plenty of diseases worldwide. Ayurveda, Southeast and Middle East Asian, and Chinese traditional medicines represent the foundation of the natural product–based therapies. These plants have been found to produce a large variety of bioactive molecules such as polyphenols, flavonoids, alkaloids, and terpenoids capable of modulating pathology-associated molecular pathways. Previously, the preconditioning of MSCs cells with different bioactive substances and plant extracts was shown to critically improve their properties, including proliferation, multilineage differentiation, and immunomodulation.

5.3.1 *HYOSCYAMUS ALBUS*

5.3.1.1 Botanic Description

White henbane (*Hyoscyamus albus*), also called hog bean or stinking nightshade, is a highly poisonous plant belonging to the Solanaceae family; indeed, it has been reported as being fatal in the event of direct consumption. All parts of the plant are very toxic, and the most common symptoms of poisoning include impaired vision, convulsions, coma, and death from heart or respiratory failure (Bown and Royal Horticultural Society, 1995). The name henbane means "chicken killer," from the Anglo-Saxon "hen" (chicken) and "bana" (murderer), because when poultry eat its seeds, they become paralyzed and die (Alizadeh et al., 2014a).

This herb is native to Eurasia and grows most often native to southern Europe and can be found in disturbed sites, in Asia and even in the Mediterranean and naturalized in much of the world. Henbane has a branching taproot and large leaves arranged alternately with irregular lobes. Stems and leaves are covered in glandular hairs (trichomes), and the whole plant gives off a strong foul odor. The flowers are recognizable by their distinctive funnel shape, which comprises five petals to dark yellow with purple veins and dark centers. The fruit is a capsule containing numerous small seeds (Swamy et al., 2015).

5.3.1.2 Traditional Use and Plant Extract Description

Formerly, henbane was used to help cultivate prophecies by oracles and diviners. Indeed, this plant was known by different names and terms such as the dragon plant, the Zeus bean, the oracle of the ancient earth, Zeus Ammon, and the plant of Apollo. At that time, the seeds were burned to form a ritual incense and the leaves were used as an additive to wine. Through inhaling the smoke from the seeds and drinking the wine from its leaves, soothsayers and prophetesses believed they could invoke the deity Apollo. In addition, henbane is a genus very rich in tropane alkaloids which give it pharmacological activities such as antispasmodic, mydriatic effect, anticholinergic, and antiemetic. Dried leaves of the plant produce three medicinal alkaloids – atropine, hyoscyamine, and scopolamine – which can be purified for use in pharmaceuticals. The plants are also sometimes used in herbal and traditional medicine (Bown and Royal Horticultural Society, 1995).

5.3.1.3 Calystegines and Their Therapeutic Uses

Lately, a new polyhydroxy nortropane alkaloids group called calystegines, or iminosugars, has been isolated from different species of Solanaceae including *Hyoscyamus*. Calystegines are new allelochemical tropane alkaloids characterized by the absence of N-methylation, a high degree of hydroxylation, and an unusual aminoketal functionality at the bridgehead position. From certain species of the plant families Convolvulaceae, Solanaceae and species of Morus (family Moraceae), a total of seven calystegines that differ in the number, position, and stereochemistry of the substituents of the hydroxyl group on the tropane ring have been identified. Known members of the class have been subdivided into three

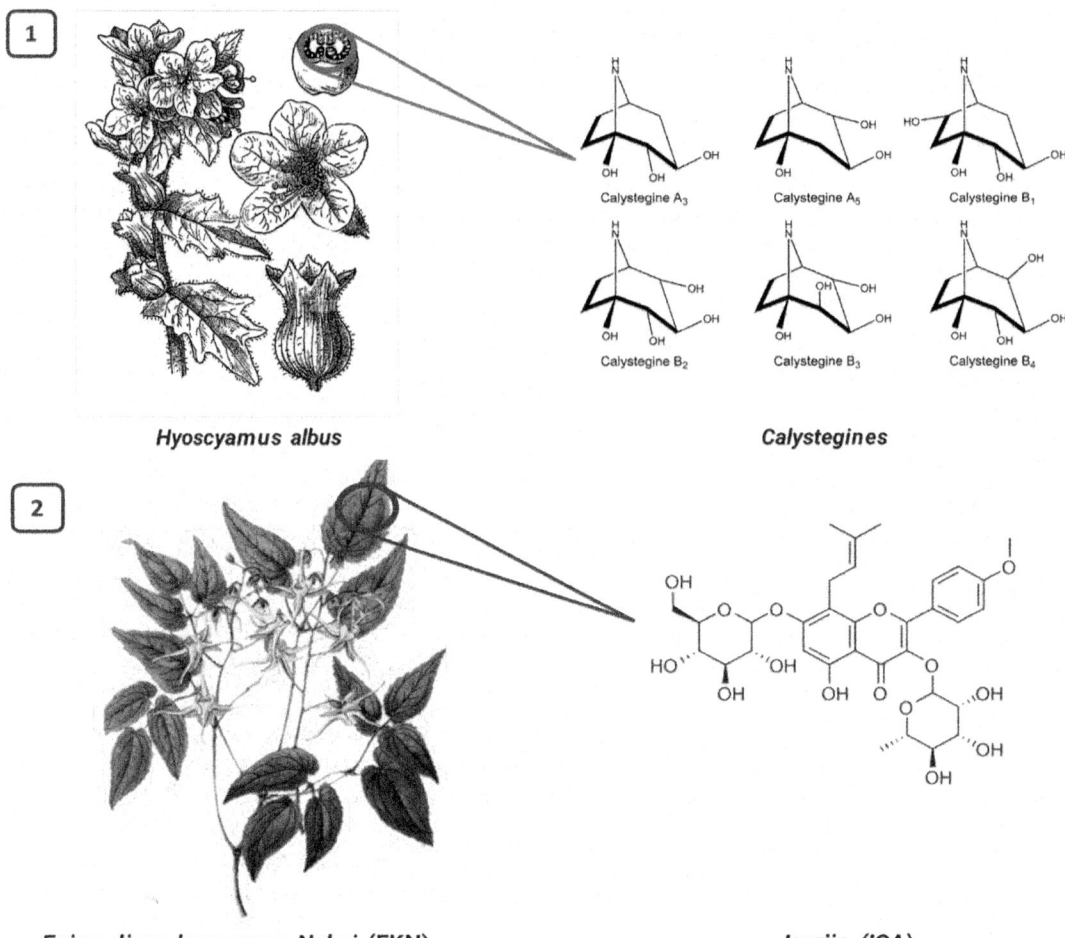

FIGURE 5.2 Representation of the bioactive compound of each plant. (1) The structure of the six calystegines extracted from *Hyoscyamus albus* seeds (the increasing degree of hydroxylation is indicated by the letters; structural isomers and stereoisomers are designated with numbers) (European Food Safety Authority [EFSA] et al., 2019). (2) The chemical structure of Icariin (ICA) extracted from *Epimedium koreanum* Nakai (EKN) leaves (Dygai et al., 2016).

groups based on the number of hydroxyl groups, namely calystegines A, B, and C. Calystegines A3, A5, and A6 each have three –OH moieties; calystegines B1, B2, and B3 exhibit four –OH groups; and calystegine C1 display five hydroxyl groups (Figure 5.2) (Goldmann et al., 1996).

The polyhydroxylated alkaloids arouse important interest thanks to their structural similarities with carbohydrates, as they can inhibit various glycosidases in a reversible and competitive manner by mimicking the pyranosyl or furanosyl moiety of their natural substrates, making them excellent candidates for the treatment of diabetes mellitus (Bourebaba et al., 2016).

Recently, Kowalczuk et al. aimed at investigating the therapeutic effect of *Hyoscyamus albus* calystegines on human adipose–derived mesenchymal stem cell (HuASC) metabolism. In this regard, the study was carried out on an experimental model of hyperglycemia induced on HuASCs in order to mimic the physiological condition of type 2 diabetes associated with insulin resistance. Calystegines at doses of 125 and 250 µg/mL were found to significantly regulate the overall metabolic activity of treated stem cells. The norptopan alkaloids promoted the immunomodulatory properties of cells by upregulating the anti-inflammatory cytokines expression, namely IL-10, IL-13 and TGF-β, while reducing the expression and secretion of IL-1β and TNF-α. Moreover, the alkaloids have been demonstrated to diminish the characteristic oxidative stress underlying glucotoxicity and to boost the endogenous cellular antioxidant defenses, by increasing the activity of SOD and catalase enzymes. The authors also highlighted the beneficial effects of the plant caly-stegines on the mitochondrial dynamics of the HuASCs, suggesting an enhancement of their differentiation abilities. What is more, calystegines treatment led to a restoration of the impaired Akt/Pi3K/mTOR signaling which relates to the improved insulin sensitizing effect of the calystegines (Kowalczuk et al., 2022). In another study, Bourebaba et al. reported on the beneficial outcomes of calystegine application on equine adipose–derived stromal stem cells (EqASCs), which played the role of pharmacological chaperones. Similarly, the alkaloids demonstrated potent ability to improve the proliferation, viability, morphology, and multipotency of EqASCs cells. Moreover, the molecules showed positive impact on mitochondrial membrane potential, ER stress, and insulin signaling via the upregulation of IRS1 and GLUT4. Interestingly, calystegines exerted a stimula-tory effect on autophagy process, suggesting their involvement in the regulation of cellular homeo-stasis (Bourebaba et al., 2019).

5.3.2 Epimedium (*Epimedium koreanum* Nakai)

5.3.2.1 Botanical Description

Epimedium is a genus of 52 species that belongs to the Buttercup family. It is a woody, pungent ornamental herb widely distributed in western and eastern Asia and the Mediterranean. Various hybrids of this plant are grown elsewhere in the world and are most often used as ground cover, especially in shady areas. The grass is also known as horny goat weed and horn grass. The Chinese call it *yin yang huo*, which means "licentious goat plant" (Ma et al., 2011).

Epimedium is a 0.5 m tall perennial herbaceous plant with a long creeping, branching rhizome up to 0.2 cm in diameter. Its leaves are basal, cauline and trifoliate; the leaflets are narrowly ovate-deltoid to lanceolate and are 3.7–8.2 cm × 2.2–3.4 cm in diameter. It has a long, acuminate apex, a deep bottom whose leaflet is cordate and terminal with equal round lobes. This grass also presents spiny-tight, under leather margins, with a glabrous adaxial and abaxial surface densely furnished with fairly large appressed short hairs. Its flowering stem measures 40 cm or more and is furnished with two opposite leaves. Its flowers are yellow in color and are between 2 and 3 cm in diameter (Ma et al., 2011; Zhang et al., 2021).

The plant was named *Epimedium* in relation to a plant found in the ancient southwest Asian kingdom of Media, now part of Iran. Species used for medicinal purposes include *E. sagittatum, E. brevicornum, E. wushanense, E. koreanum*, and *E. pubescens*. The grass is harvested in summer or early fall and then dried in the sunlight. Some use it plain, while others cook it with mutton fat. The herb is usually ingested as a tea infusion, and the recommended dosage is one to three cups daily with meals. Also, a powdered form can be prepared by combining 100 kg of dried *Epimedium* leaves with 20 kg of refined tallow, then popping the concoction. *Epimedium* can also be combined with *Lycium* fruits to make a tea concoction that stimulates the kidneys and the reproductive system (Liang et al., 2012; Li et al., 2016).

5.3.2.2 Traditional Use and Plant Extract Description

The use of *Epimedium* as a medicinal herb date back thousands of years. Indeed, this odorless and bitter herb has been used as a kidney tonic to help relieve problems with frequent urination and cor-rect dizziness and weakness associated with improper body fluid volumes; a reproductive system tonic to treat impotence and premature ejaculation; and a rejuvenating tonic as an aphrodisiac or to relieve fatigue. In addition, this plant has dilating effects on blood vessels, explaining its use in the treatment of coronary heart disease, asthma, bronchitis, and sinusitis. It also serves as an expectorant to control cough. It can be used to lower blood pressure. On the other hand, studies have shown that *Epimedium* increases the levels of adrenaline, noradrenaline, serotonin, and dopamine in certain animals; this is why the herb is used as a reproductive tonic, as the increase in dopamine levels in the body triggers a chain reaction that leads to a release of testosterone, the male sex hormone. Other evidence suggests that the herb increases the sensitivity of nerve endings, which may explain why it is prescribed as an aphrodisiac (Wei et al., 2017; Zhai et al., 2013).

Nowadays, five species of *Epimedium* (*E. brevicornum, E. sagittatum, E. pubescens, E. wushanense*, and *E. koreanum*) are mainly used as medicinal plants and supplements, and have been developed in much more practical formats (capsules, tablets, ointments, and creams), notably in Korea, Japan and China. *E. koreanum* Nakai (EKN), known as *sam-ji-goo-yep-cho* among Koreans, has been recently reported for its immunomodulatory, anti-osteoporotic, antitumor, and antiviral effects. Indeed, this herb is known to contain phenolic acids, lignin, and prenylated flavonoid glycosides. Prenylated flavonoid glycosides (such as icariin and epimedin A, B, C), represent major molecules of EKN; these components also possess various biological activities similar to those of the EKN plant (Hwang et al., 2017).

5.3.2.3 Icariin (ICA) and Its Therapeutic Effects on MSCs

Icariin (ICA) is one of the most common bioactive compounds in *Epimedium*. ICA is a prenylated flavonoid consisting of a glucosyl group at C-3, a methoxyl group at C-4, a prenyl group at position C-8 (the main active site for its pharmacological effect), and a rhamnosyl group at C-7 (Figure 5.2). Furthermore, metabolic enzymes have the ability to modify icariin into glucuronide conjugates of isoflavonoids and flavonoid aglycones (He et al., 2020).

The involvement of inflammatory cells in the pathogenesis of many chronic diseases including those of the pancreatic gland is undeniable. Type 1 diabetes is the direct consequence of the auto-immune deterioration of insulin-producing β cells in the pancreatic endocrine islets. In addition, examinations carried out on pancreas and islets from donors with type 1 diabetes revealed that the interferon-mediated inflammatory response was altered (Roberts et al., 2017). Moustafa et al. recently investigated the combined effect of icariin and MSCs in restoring acinar cells from the pancreas of rats with chronic pancreatitis. The obtained results demonstrated that icariin promotes the proliferation of MSCs by increasing their metabolism through the regulation of the TGF-β/PDGF axis and the stimulation of PDX-1 and MafA release, which are crucial for pancreatic tissue regeneration, as they mediate the recruitment of stem/progenitor cells into the injured tissue. In addition, a significant decrease in pro-inflammatory cytokines (IL-8 and TNF-α) was observed, suggesting the beneficial effect of icariin on the immunomodulatory properties of MSCs (Moustafa et al., 2020). Additionally, another study performed on rats with diabetes mellitus erectile dysfunction (DMED) examined the activity of icariin on the enhancement of the therapeutic effects of mesenchymal stem cells derived from adipose tissue (ADSC). DMED was induced in rats by intraperitoneal injection of streptozotocin that selectively destroys pancreatic β cells. Subsequently, the rats received treatment with ADSC, icariin, or ADSC combined with ICA. The obtained data demonstrated an intensification of the transplanted ADSC survival, a reduction in their apoptosis and a decrease in the level of reactive intracellular oxygen species (ROS) together with an increase in the activity of superoxidase dismutase (SOD), via the regulation of the PI3K/Akt-STAT3 signal pathway. Another investigation further confirmed the involvement of icariin in the stimulation of pro-regenerative potency of MSCs. Application of icariin to BMSCs resulted in the promotion of their migratory and survival potential, as well as the reduction of ROS and nitric oxide (NO) generation. More interestingly, the compound enabled to stimulate and increase the angiogenic differentiation of the BMSCs through the regulation of the VEGFR-2/PI3K/Akt-PKB axis (Tang et al., 2015). These studies therefore suggest that icariin represents a powerful functional adjuvant in stem cell therapy for the management of cellular degeneration associated with type 1 and type 2 diabetes (Wang et al., 2017).

5.4 OTHER MEDICINAL PLANTS THAT IMPROVED MSCS ANTIDIABETIC AND ANTI-OBESITY EFFECTS

Many other medicinal plants, herbs, and spices contain a wide range of bioactive molecules (Figure 5.3) that can regulate MSCs signaling governing lipid metabolism and turnover that have been suggested to participate in obesity and diabetes progression (Table 5.1).

As an example, resveratrol (3, 4', 5 trihydroxystilbene) a polyphenolic compound mostly present in grapes (*Vitis vinifera*), is known for its potent anti-inflammatory effects. This molecule has been reported as a meaningful adipogenesis and lipogenesis regulator, as it participates in lowering lipids accumulation, as well as the downregulation of C/EBPα, PPARγ, LPL, FAS, and SREBP-1c expression in progenitor cells exposed to 20–80 µM resveratrol by initiating the AMP-activated protein kinase (AMPK). Genistein is a bioactive isoflavone found in soybeans (*Glycine max*) that possess antidiabetic and anti-obesity activities. Several researches reported the anti-adipogenic effect of

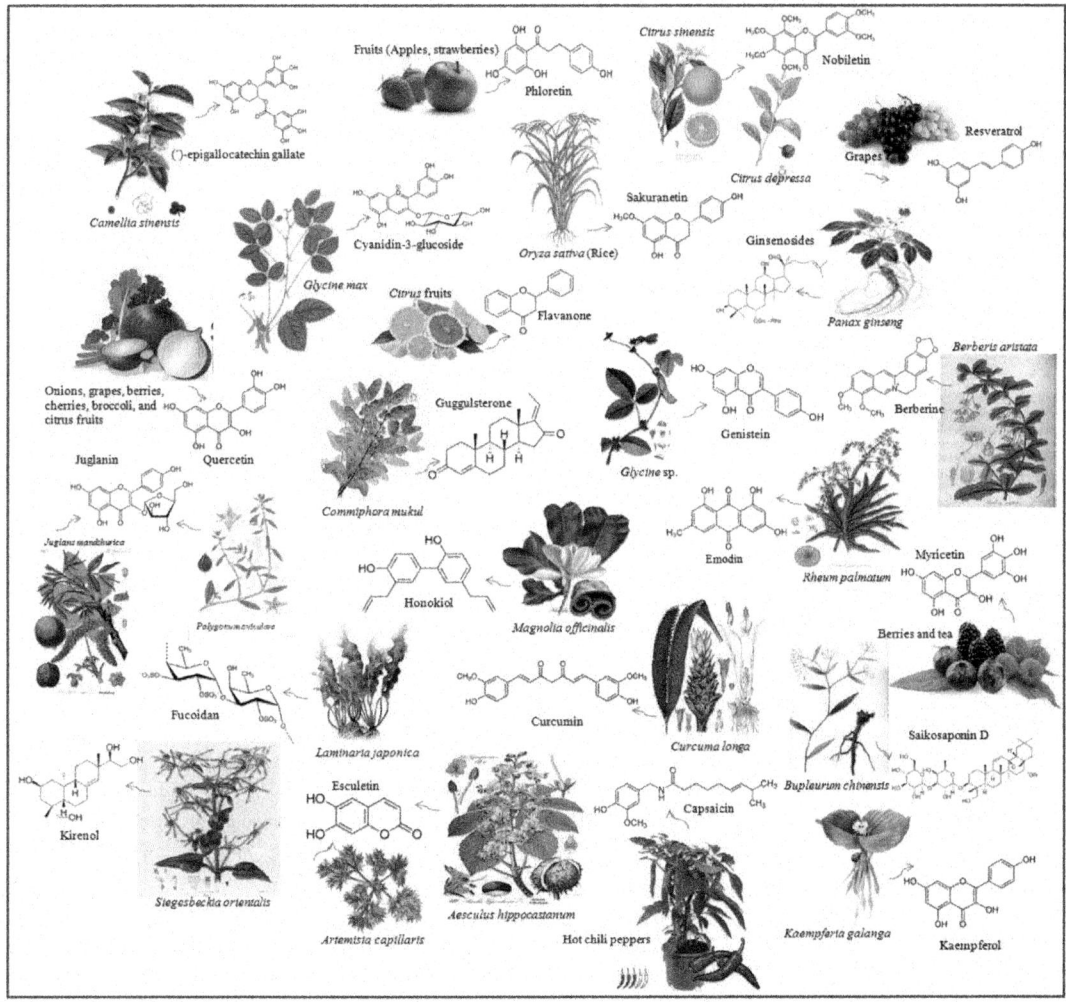

FIGURE 5.3 The various medicinal plants, herbs and foods and their associated bioactive molecules listed in Table 5.1 that have been tested for their beneficial effect of MSCs' antidiabetogenic and anti-obesogenic properties.

TABLE 5.1

Medicinal Plants, Herbs, and Dietary Vegetables with Their Bioactive Compounds Affecting the Antidiabetic and Anti-Obesity Potential of MSCs

Plant Name	Traditional Uses	Bioactive Compound	Effect on MSCs	References
Camellia sinensis (green tea)	Anti-obesogenic	(')-epigallocatechin gallate	↓ Adipogenesis ↓ Body weight and fat deposition Inhibits PPARγ and C/EBPα expression Induces apoptosis, lipolysis, and thermogenesis AMPK activation Wnt/β-catenin pathway	(Yang et al., 2014)
Glycine max (black soybean)	Anti-inflammatory Anti-obesity Antioxidative effect Antidiabetes	Cyanidin-3-glucoside	↓ NPY expression ↑ Adiponectin secretion ↓ MCP-1, IL-6, and TNF-α levels JNK/FoxO1 pathway inhibition Prevents adipocyte hypertrophy ↑ PPARγ expression, TG accumulation, and GPDH activity ↑ C/EBPα, GLUT4 genes and insulin receptor protein expression	(Matsukawa et al., 2015)
Fruits (apples, strawberries, etc.)	Anti-inflammatory Antioxidant activity Hypoglycemic effect	Phloretin	↑ PPARγ and C/EBPα transcriptional activity ↑TG accumulation and GPDH activity ↑ Adiponectin expression and secretion Promote lipolysis ERK1/2 and JNK signals suppression p 38 MAPK activation ↑ AMPK phosphorylation	(Takeno et al., 2018)
Onions, grapes, berries, cherries, broccoli, and citrus fruits	Osteoporosis Lung cancer Cardiovascular disease	Quercetin	Inhibits mRNA expression of PPARγ and C/EBPα Inhibits PPARγ protein expression ↓ Lipid accumulation Suppresses mRNA expression of cyclin A	(Swick et al., 2012)
Citrus depressa *Citrus sinensis*	Anti-inflammatory Hypoglycemic activity	Nobiletin	↑ Lipid droplets accumulation ↑ PPARγ gene expression CREB and ERK activation Inhibits GPDH activity Stimulates lipolysis by cAMP pathway	(Lee et al., 2014)

Plant Name	Traditional Uses	Bioactive Compound	Effect on MSCs	References
Grapes	Anti-inflammatory	Resveratrol	↓ Lipid accumulation ↓ C/EBPα, LPL, FAS, and SREBP-1c expression AMPK activation ↓ MMP-9 activity ↓ ATP content by glucose transport and/or metabolism inhibition ↓ Plasma total cholesterol, LDL cholesterol, hepatic fatty acids, TG contents	(Kang et al., 2012)
Citrus fruits	Anti-inflammatory	Flavanone	↑ PPARγ transcriptional activity Lipid droplets accumulation ↑ GPDH activity ↓ ERK1/2 phosphorylation	(Saito et al., 2009)
Panax ginseng (ginseng)	Anti-obesity Controls glycemia Immunomodulatory	Ginsenosides	↓ Lipid accumulation ↓ PPARγ and C/EBPα expression	(Yang and Kim, 2015)
Oryza sativa (rice) *Polyomnia fruticosa*	Maintains glucose homeostasis Anti-inflammatory Antidiabetic	Sakuranetin	↑ TG accumulation and GPDH activity Induce PPARγ2 expression independently of C/EBPβ ↓ GATA-2 expression Stimulate glucose uptake	(Saito et al., 2008; Stompor, 2020)
Glycine sp. (soybean)	Anti-obesity Antidiabetes	Genistein	Inhibits PPARγ and C/EBPα gene expression Promotes lipolysis ↑ C/EBP homologous protein expression ↓ C/EBPβ transcription AMPK activation Improves eNOS and inhibits P38 MAPK Inhibits GPDH activity Inhibits aP2, SREBP 1 and FAS genes PPARγ, GLUT-4 and SREBP-1 inhibition	(Zhang et al., 2009)
Commiphora mukul (gum guggul)	Anti-obesity	Guggulsterone	↓ PPARγ2, C/EBPα, and C/EBPβ Cholesterol-lowering activity ↓ Adiponectin mRNA levels	(Yang et al., 2008)
Juglans mandshurica *Polygonum aviculare*	Anti-inflammatory Antioxidant effects Anti-obesity	Juglanin	↓ Lipid accumulation ↓ GLUT4 expression ↓ C/EBPα and C/EBPβ expression without affecting PPARα or PPARγ expression ↓ SREBP-1c expression	(Wang et al., 2020)

(Continued)

TABLE 5.1
(Continued)

Plant Name	Traditional Uses	Bioactive Compound	Effect on MSCs	References
Rheum palmatum L.	Anticancer Hepatoprotective Anti-inflammatory Antioxidant Antimicrobial activities	Emodin	↑ GPDH activity ↑ Adipocyte aP2 mRNA expression ↑ TG accumulation ↑ C/EBPα and PPARγ2 expression levels ↑ GLUT1 and GLUT4 mRNA expression	(Dong et al., 2016)
Magnolia officinalis *Magnolia obovata*	Anti-angiogenic Antitumor properties	Honokiol	↑ PPARγ2 and PPARγ expression Adiponectin and GLUT4 genes induction ↑ PI3K/Akt signaling pathway	(Choi et al., 2011)
Curcuma longa	Anti-angiogenic and chemopreventive properties	Curcumin	↓ PPARγ and C/EBPα expression MCE inhibition ↓ Lipid accumulation Activating AMPK ↓ MAPKs phosphorylation	(Ahn et al., 2010)
Laminaria japonica Marine brown algae Jelly coat from sea urchin eggs Sea cucumber body wall	Anti-inflammatory Immunomodulatory Antitumor Antibacterial Antiviral Antioxidant	Fucoidan	↑ Inhibiting fat accumulation ↓ PPARγ expression gene Inhibits adipocyte differentiation ↓ C/EBPα, PPARγ, and aP2 adipogenic transcription factors Inhibits the early activation of p 38 MAPKs, ERK, and JNK	(Kim et al., 2010)
Bupleurum chinensis	Inflammation Fever Liver diseases Anti-obesity	Saikosaponin A Saikosaponin D	Inhibited lipid accumulation PPARγ, C/EBPα, SREBP-1c, and adiponectin expression suppression Repressed expression of lipogenic genes (FABP4, FAS, and LPL) ↑ Phosphorylation of AMPK and its substrate, ACC Inhibited the phosphorylation of ERK1/2 and p 38, but not JNK	(Lim et al., 2021)
Berberis aristata	Inflammatory disorders Skin diseases and wound healing Reducing fevers Antitumors Digestive and respiratory diseases	Berberine	Inhibits adipogenesis ↓ Weight gain, food intake and serum glucose, TG, and TC levels ↑ GATA-3 expression ↓ SREBP1, FAS, PPARγ, C/EBPα, SREBP2, LDLR, and HMGR genes expression ↓ SREBP1, SREBP2, and LDLR protein levels ↑ GATA-2 and GATA3 mRNA and protein expression levels	(Li et al., 2016)

Plant Name	Traditional Uses	Bioactive Compound	Effect on MSCs	References
Pigmented fruits and vegetables	Antioxidant Anti-inflammatory Anti-obesity Anti-atherosclerosis Anticancer bioactivities	Delphinidin	↓ Expression of adipogenesis and lipogenesis markers Inhibits lipid accumulation ↑ Fatty acid metabolism gene expression ↓ C/EBPβ and C/EBPδ, C/EBPα, PPARγ, and the PPARγ-target adipocyte markers adiponectin and aP2 (FABP4) expression	(Park et al., 2019)
Siegesbeckia orientalis	Anti-inflammatory Antioxidant Antirheumatic	Kirenol	Prevents intracellular lipid accumulation ↓ PPARγ, C/EBPα, and SREBP-1c ↓ Lipid biosynthesis-related enzymes (FAS, ACC) ↓ Adipocytokines (adiponectin and leptin) Activates the Wnt/β-catenin signaling pathway ↑ LRP6, DVL2, β-catenin, and CCND1 expression Inactivate GSK3β by ↑ its phosphorylation	(Kim et al., 2014)
Aesculus hippocastanum Artemisia capillaris Euphorbia lathyris Citrus limonia Fraxinus rhynchophylla	Antioxidant Anticancer Hepatoprotective activities Anti-inflammatory	Esculetin	Inhibits lipid accumulation ↓ c-fos and c-jun gene expression Suppresses PPARγ, C/EBPα, and aP2 expression ↑ AMPK and ACC phosphorylation ↑ Intracellular ROS production	(Kim and Lee, 2017)
Hot chili peppers	Anti-obesity Chronic neuropathic pain disorders Antioxidant Anti-obesity Antidiabetic	Capsaicin	Suppresses fat deposition ↓ PPARγ, C/EBPα, FABP4, and *SCD* expression ↑ Apoptotic cells ↑ Apoptotic genes expression levels	(Jeong et al., 2014)
Kaempferia galanga Opuntia ficus indica var. *saboten*	Antioxidant Anti-inflammatory Anticancer Anti-obesity	Kaempferol	Inhibits lipid accumulation ↓ Intracellular lipid droplets ↓ C/EBPβ, KLFs 4 and KLFs5 ↑ KLF2 and pref-1 ↓ C/EBPα and PPARγ	(Lee et al., 2015)
Plant leaves and seeds	Antimutagenic Anticancer Antioxidant Anti-inflammatory	Apigetrin	Inhibit lipid accumulation Inhibit cell proliferation during mitotic clonal expansion Suppress C/EBP-α, PPARγ, SREBP-1c, and FAS mRNA levels TNF-α and IL-6 suppression	(Hadrich and Sayadi, 2018)
Vegetables, fruits, nuts, berries and tea	Antioxidant Anti-inflammatory Anticancer effects	Myricetin	↓ Accumulation of intracellular lipid droplets ↓ C/EBP-α, PPARγ, LPL, aP2, and adiponectin mRNA levels	(Bin and Choi, 2012)

genistein by inhibiting adipogenic genes like PPARγ and C/EBPα. Moreover, other plants with bioactive compounds like Fruits (Phloretin), *Camellia sinensis* ((′)-epigallocatechin gallate), *Rheum palmatum* L. (emodin), *Curcuma longa* (curcumin), Pigmented fruits and vegetables (Delphinidin), and *Siegesbeckia orientalis* (Kirenol) can be also implicated in the adipogenesis process through the regulation of key markers involved in adipose tissue hypertrophy such as like PPARγ and C/EBPα, and the prevention of fat accumulation and resulting lipotoxicity.

5.5   TOXICITY AND CAUTIONARY NOTES

5.5.1   *HYOSCYAMUS ALBUS*

This plant was once widely cultivated to meet the demand for its use. Being a very poisonous plant, it should be used with great caution and only under the supervision of a qualified practitioner (Chevallier, 1996). Henbane intoxication usually manifests as symptoms derived from atropine or scopolamine overdose and include mydriasis, tachycardia, arrhythmia, agitation, convulsion, and coma. Other common symptoms may manifest as hallucinations, restlessness, and skin flushing (Alizadeh et al., 2014b). By contrast, previous studies demonstrated the nontoxicity of calystegines that are expected to be well tolerated as they can be found in many dietary Solanaceae (Bourebaba et al., 2016).

5.5.2   *EPIMEDIUM*

Several studies have been conducted in the past on the phytopharmacological aspects of *Epimedium*; however, there are no reported toxicological effects of these herbs as they have been used for a long time. Nevertheless, in 2010, Kim et al. evaluated the possible toxicity of an aqueous extract of EKN leaves. The study was conducted on healthy models of Sprague Dawley rats; the latter were administered orally doses of 10, 100 and 1000 mg/kg/day for 4 weeks. According to the obtained hematology and serum chemistry results, some changes were observed, however, these remained within the normal ranges. Furthermore, the histological examination reported mild to moderate changes. However, these results suggest that no adverse effect was detected following the oral administration of EKN and therefore demonstrate that the latter induces no toxicological effect and that the unobserved adverse effect level (NOAEL) of the aqueous extract of EKN in SD rats is 1000 mg/kg/day (J. Kim et al., 2010).

5.6   CONCLUDING REMARKS

- MSCs preconditioning with medicinal plant derivatives represents an attractive approach for the improvement of their antidiabetic properties.
- Calystegines isolated from *Hyoscyamus albus* improve the viability, proliferation, and immunomodulatory abilities of human adipose–derived MSCs.
- Calystegines further sustain MSCs homeostasis by regulating autophagy and restoring insulin signaling pathways.
- *Epimedium koreanum* Nakai, rich in icariin, substantially improves the regenerative potential of MSCs via the stimulation of their migratory, their survival, proliferation, and angiogenic potential.
- Many other ancient traditional plants and herbs including curcuma, grapes, and *Siegesbeckia orientalis* have also been demonstrated to promote the antidiabetic potential of MSCs mainly though the regulation and the enhancement of their anti-obesogenic ability.

5.7   SUMMARY POINTS

- Diabetes mellitus is an endocrine disorder that spreads exponentially worldwide.
- Whether type 1 or type 2, the involved pathophysiological mechanisms include progressive degeneration of pancreatic tissue, drop in insulin levels, and chronic metaflammation leading to the onset of insulin resistance.
- Mesenchymal stromal cell (MSC)-based therapy has gained particular attention in the past few years due to their versatile properties and ability to regenerate injured tissues and restore their functions.
- MSCs have been reported to sustain metabolic homeostasis through their immunomodulatory and paracrine actions, and via their potency to generate insulin producing cells.
- The use of medicinal plants derivatives for the preconditioning of MSCs, and thus the improvement of their activities has been suggested to offer new prospects in the development of effective antidiabetic therapies.
- The calystegines of *Hyoscyamus albus* and *Epimedium*-derived icariin have demonstrated great potential in promoting MSCs' antidiabetic potential essentially by improving their immunomodulatory, migratory, survival, regenerative, and angiogenic ability, and overall, their metabolic homeostasis including insulin signaling pathways.

REFERENCES

Ahn, J., Lee, H., Kim, S., Ha, T., 2010. Curcumin-Induced Suppression of Adipogenic Differentiation is Accompanied by Activation of Wnt/β-Catenin Signaling. *Am J Physiol Cell Physiol* 298, C1510–C1516. https://doi.org/10.1152/ajpcell.00369.2009

Alizadeh, A., Moshiri, M., Alizadeh, J., Balali-Mood, M., 2014a. Black Henbane and Its Toxicity – A Descriptive Review. *Avicenna J Phytomed* 4, 297–311.

Alizadeh, A., Moshiri, M., Alizadeh, J., Balali-Mood, M., 2014b. Black Henbane and Its Toxicity – A Descriptive Review. *Avicenna J Phytomed* 4, 297–311.

Bin, H.-S., Choi, U.-K., 2012. Myricetin Inhibits Adipogenesis in Human Adipose Tissue-derived Mesenchymal Stem Cells. *Food Sci Biotechnol* 21, 1391–1396. https://doi.org/10.1007/s10068-012-0183-1

Böni-Schnetzler, M., Ehses, J.A., Faulenbach, M., Donath, M.Y., 2008. Insulitis in Type 2 Diabetes. *Diabetes Obes Metab* 10, 201–204. https://doi.org/10.1111/j.1463-1326.2008.00950.x

Bourebaba, L., Bedjou, F., Röcken, M., Marycz, K., 2019. Nortropane alkaloids as pharmacological chaperones in the rescue of equine adipose-derived mesenchymal stromal stem cells affected by metabolic syndrome through mitochondrial potentiation, endoplasmic reticulum stress mitigation and insulin resistance alleviation. *Stem Cell Res Ther* 10, 178. https://doi.org/10.1186/s13287-019-1292-z

Bourebaba, L., Saci, S., Touguit, D., Gali, L., Terkmane, S., Oukil, N., Bedjou, F., 2016. Evaluation of antidiabetic effect of total calystegines extracted from Hyoscyamus albus. *Biomed Pharmacother* 82, 337–344. https://doi.org/10.1016/j.biopha.2016.05.011

Bown, D., Royal Horticultural Society (Eds.), 1995. *Encyclopedia of Herbs & Their Uses*. A Dorling Kindersley Book. Dorling Kindersley, London and Stuttgart.

Cai, D., Yuan, M., Frantz, D.F., Melendez, P.A., Hansen, L., Lee, J., Shoelson, S.E., 2005. Local and Systemic Insulin Resistance Resulting from Hepatic Activation of IKK-β and NF-κB. *Nat Med* 11, 183–190. https://doi.org/10.1038/nm1166

Cañibano-Hernández, A., Sáenz del Burgo, L., Espona-Noguera, A., Ciriza, J., Pedraz, J.L., 2018. Current Advanced Therapy Cell-based Medicinal Products for Type-1-Diabetes Treatment. *Int J Pharm* 543, 107–120. https://doi.org/10.1016/j.ijpharm.2018.03.041

Chevallier, A., 1996. *The Encyclopedia of Medicinal Plants*. A Dorling Kindersley Book. Dorling Kindersley, London.

Choi, S.-S., Cha, B.-Y., Iida, K., Sato, M., Lee, Y.-S., Teruya, T., Yonezawa, T., Nagai, K., Woo, J.-T., 2011. Honokiol Enhances Adipocyte Differentiation by Potentiating Insulin Signaling in 3T3-L1 Preadipocytes. *J Nat Med* 65, 424–430. https://doi.org/10.1007/s11418-011-0512-3

Clark, M., Kroger, C.J., Tisch, R.M., 2017. Type 1 Diabetes: A Chronic Anti-Self-Inflammatory Response. *Front Immunol* 8, 1898. https://doi.org/10.3389/fimmu.2017.01898

Després, J.-P., Lemieux, I., Bergeron, J., Pibarot, P., Mathieu, P., Larose, E., Rodés-Cabau, J., Bertrand, O.F., Poirier, P., 2008. Abdominal Obesity and the Metabolic Syndrome: Contribution to Global Cardiometabolic Risk. *ATVB* 28, 1039–1049. https://doi.org/10.1161/ATVBAHA.107.159228

Donath, M.Y., Shoelson, S.E., 2011. Type 2 Diabetes as an Inflammatory Disease. *Nat Rev Immunol* 11, 98–107. https://doi.org/10.1038/nri2925

Dong, X., Fu, J., Yin, X., Cao, S., Li, X., Lin, L., Huyiligeqi, Ni, J., 2016. Emodin: A Review of its Pharmacology, Toxicity and Pharmacokinetics: Emodin: Pharmacology, Toxicity and Pharmacokinetics. *Phytother Res* 30, 1207–1218. https://doi.org/10.1002/ptr.5631

Dygai, A.M., Skurikhin, E.G., Pershina, O.V., Ermakova, N.N., Krupin, V.A., Ermolaeva, L.A., Stakheeva, M.N., Choinzonov, E.L., Goldberg, V.E., Reikhart, D.V., Ellinidi, V.N., Kravtsov, V.Y., 2016. Role of Hematopoietic Stem Cells in Inflammation of the Pancreas during Diabetes Mellitus. *Bull Exp Biol Med* 160, 474–479. https://doi.org/10.1007/s10517-016-3200-1

European Food Safety Authority (EFSA), Binaglia, M., Baert, K., Schutte, M., Serafimova, R., 2019. Overview of Available Toxicity Data for Calystegines. *EFS2* 17. https://doi.org/10.2903/j.efsa.2019.5574

Ezquer, F.E., Ezquer, M.E., Parrau, D.B., Carpio, D., Yañez, A.J., Conget, P.A., 2008. Systemic Administration of Multipotent Mesenchymal Stromal Cells Reverts Hyperglycemia and Prevents Nephropathy in Type 1 Diabetic Mice. *Biol Blood Marrow Transplant* 14, 631–640. https://doi.org/10.1016/j.bbmt.2008.01.006

Gabr, M.M., Zakaria, M.M., Refaie, A.F., Ismail, A.M., Abou-El-Mahasen, M.A., Ashamallah, S.A., Khater, S.M., El-Halawani, S.M., Ibrahim, R.Y., Uin, G.S., Kloc, M., Calne, R.Y., Ghoneim, M.A., 2013. Insulin-Producing Cells from Adult Human Bone Marrow Mesenchymal Stem Cells Control Streptozotocin-Induced Diabetes in Nude Mice. *Cell Transplant* 22, 133–145. https://doi.org/10.3727/096368912X647162

Goldmann, A., Message, B., Tepfer, D., Molyneux, R.J., Duclos, O., Boyer, F.-D., Pan, Y.T., Elbein, A.D., 1996. Biological Activities of the Nortropane Alkaloid, Calystegine B$_2$, and Analogs: Structure–Function Relationships. *J Nat Prod* 59, 1137–1142. https://doi.org/10.1021/np960409v

Goyal, R., Jialal, I., 2022. *Diabetes Mellitus Type 2*. StatPearls Publishing, Treasure Island (FL).

Hadrich, F., Sayadi, S., 2018. Apigetrin Inhibits Adipogenesis in 3T3-L1 Cells by Downregulating PPARγ and CEBP-α. *Lipids Health Dis* 17, 95. https://doi.org/10.1186/s12944-018-0738-0

He, C., Wang, Z., Shi, J., 2020. Pharmacological Effects of Icariin. In: *Advances in Pharmacology*. Elsevier, San Diego, CA, pp. 179–203. https://doi.org/10.1016/bs.apha.2019.10.004

Holthaus, M., Santhakumar, N., Wahlers, T., Paunel-Görgülü, A., 2022. The Secretome of Preconditioned Mesenchymal Stem Cells Drives Polarization and Reprogramming of M2a Macrophages Toward an IL-10-Producing Phenotype. *IJMS* 23, 4104. https://doi.org/10.3390/ijms23084104

Hu, C., Li, L., 2018. Preconditioning Influences Mesenchymal Stem Cell Properties in vitro and in vivo. *J Cell Mol Med* 22, 1428–1442. https://doi.org/10.1111/jcmm.13492

Huang, Q., Huang, Y., Liu, J., 2021. Mesenchymal Stem Cells: An Excellent Candidate for the Treatment of Diabetes Mellitus. *Int J Endocrinol* 2021, 1–11. https://doi.org/10.1155/2021/9938658

Hwang, Y.-H., Yang, H.J., Yim, N.-H., Ma, J.Y., 2017. Genetic Toxicity of Epimedium Koreanum Nakai. *J Ethnopharmacol* 198, 87–90. https://doi.org/10.1016/j.jep.2016.11.050

Jakab, J., Miškić, B., Mikšić, Š., Juranić, B., Ćosić, V., Schwarz, D., Včev, A., 2021. Adipogenesis as a Potential Anti-Obesity Target: A Review of Pharmacological Treatment and Natural Products. *DMSO* 14, 67–83. https://doi.org/10.2147/DMSO.S281186

Jeong, J.Y., Suresh, S., Park, M.N., Jang, M., Park, S., Gobianand, K., You, S., Yeon, S.-H., Lee, H.-J., 2014. Effects of Capsaicin on Adipogenic Differentiation in Bovine Bone Marrow Mesenchymal Stem Cell. *Asian Australas. J Anim Sci* 27, 1783–1793. https://doi.org/10.5713/ajas.2014.14720

Kang, N.E., Ha, A.W., Kim, J.Y., Kim, W.K., 2012. Resveratrol Inhibits the Protein Expression of Transcription Factors Related Adipocyte Differentiation and the Activity of Matrix metallOproteinase in Mouse Fibroblast 3T3-L1 Preadipocytes. *Nutr Res Pract* 6, 499. https://doi.org/10.4162/nrp.2012.6.6.499

Kassem, D.H., Kamal, M.M., El-Kholy, A.E.-L.G., El-Mesallamy, H.O., 2016. Exendin-4 Enhances the Differentiation of Wharton's Jelly Mesenchymal Stem Cells into Insulin-Producing Cells Through Activation of Various β-Cell Markers. *Stem Cell Res Ther* 7, 108. https://doi.org/10.1186/s13287-016-0374-4

Khorsandi, L., Saremy, S., Khodadadi, A., Dehbashi, F., 2017. Effects of Exendine-4 on The Differentiation of Insulin Producing Cells from Rat Adipose-Derived Mesenchymal Stem Cells. *CellJ* 17. https://doi.org/10.22074/cellj.2016.3844

Kim, J., Lim, M., Kim, H., Ku, S., Chang, H., Oh, T., Lee, K., 2010. Safety Evaluation of Epimedium Koreanum Water Extract in Sprague-Dawley Rats. *J Vet Clin* 27, 163–169.

Kim, K.-J., Lee, O.-H., Lee, B.-Y., 2010. Fucoidan, a Sulfated Polysaccharide, Inhibits Adipogenesis Through the Mitogen-Activated Protein Kinase Pathway in 3T3-L1 Preadipocytes. *Life Sci* 86, 791–797. https://doi.org/10.1016/j.lfs.2010.03.010

Kim, M.-B., Song, Y., Kim, C., Hwang, J.-K., 2014. Kirenol Inhibits Adipogenesis Through Activation of the Wnt/β-Catenin Signaling Pathway in 3T3-L1 Adipocytes. *Biochem Biophys Res Commun* 445, 433–438. https://doi.org/10.1016/j.bbrc.2014.02.017

Kim, Y., Lee, J., 2017. Esculetin Inhibits Adipogenesis and Increases Antioxidant Activity during Adipocyte Differentiation in 3T3-L1 Cells. *Prev Nutr Food Sci* 22, 118–123. https://doi.org/10.3746/pnf.2017.22.2.118

Koehler, N., Buhler, L., Egger, B., Gonelle-Gispert, C., 2022. Multipotent Mesenchymal Stromal Cells Interact and Support Islet of Langerhans Viability and Function. *Front Endocrinol* 13, 822191. https://doi.org/10.3389/fendo.2022.822191

Kornicka, K., Kocherova, I., Marycz, K., 2017. The Effects of Chosen Plant Extracts and Compounds on Mesenchymal Stem Cells-a Bridge Between Molecular Nutrition and Regenerative Medicine – Concise Review: Influence of Plant Extracts on ASC. *Phytother Res* 31, 947–958. https://doi.org/10.1002/ptr.5812

Kowalczuk, A., Bourebaba, N., Panchuk, J., Marycz, K., Bourebaba, L., 2022. Calystegines Improve the Metabolic Activity of Human Adipose Derived Stromal Stem Cells (ASCs) under Hyperglycaemic Condition through the Reduction of Oxidative/ER Stress, Inflammation, and the Promotion of the AKT/PI3K/mTOR Pathway. *Biomolecules* 12, 460. https://doi.org/10.3390/biom12030460

Lee, J.Y., Zhao, L., Youn, H.S., Weatherill, A.R., Tapping, R., Feng, L., Lee, W.H., Fitzgerald, K.A., Hwang, D.H., 2004. Saturated Fatty Acid Activates but Polyunsaturated Fatty Acid Inhibits Toll-like Receptor 2 Dimerized with Toll-like Receptor 6 or 1. *J Biol Chem* 279, 16971–16979. https://doi.org/10.1074/jbc.M312990200

Lee, Y.-J., Choi, H.-S., Seo, M.-J., Jeon, H.-J., Kim, K.-J., Lee, B.-Y., 2015. Kaempferol Suppresses Lipid Accumulation by Inhibiting Early Adipogenesis in 3T3-L1 Cells and Zebrafish. *Food Funct* 6, 2824–2833. https://doi.org/10.1039/C5FO00481K

Lee, Y.-S., Asai, M., Choi, S.-S., Yonezawa, T., Teruya, T., Nagai, K., Woo, J.-T., Cha, B.-Y., 2014. Nobiletin Prevents Body Weight Gain and Bone Loss in Ovariectomized C57BL/6J Mice. *Pharm Pharmacol* 5, 959–965. https://doi.org/10.4236/pp.2014.510108

Li, B., Cheng, X., Aierken, A., Du, J., He, W., Zhang, M., Tan, N., Kou, Z., Peng, S., Jia, W., Tang, H., Hua, J., 2021. Melatonin Promotes the Therapeutic Effect of Mesenchymal Stem Cells on Type 2 Diabetes Mellitus by Regulating TGF-β Pathway. *Front Cell Dev Biol* 9, 722365. https://doi.org/10.3389/fcell.2021.722365

Li, Y., Zhao, X., Feng, X., Liu, X., Deng, C., Hu, C.-H., 2016. Berberine Alleviates Olanzapine-Induced Adipogenesis via the AMPKα–SREBP Pathway in 3T3-L1 Cells. *IJMS* 17, 1865. https://doi.org/10.3390/ijms17111865

Li, Z., Zeng, S., Li, Y., Li, M., Souer, E., 2016. Leaf-Like Sepals Induced by Ectopic Expression of a *SHORT VEGETATIVE PHASE* (*SVP*)-Like MADS-Box Gene from the Basal Eudicot *Epimedium sagittatum*. *Front Plant Sci* 7, 1461. https://doi.org/10.3389/fpls.2016.01461

Liang, Q., Wei, G., Chen, J., Wang, Y., Huang, H., 2012. Variation of Medicinal Components in a Unique Geographical Accession of Horny Goat Weed *Epimedium sagittatum* Maxim. (Berberidaceae). *Molecules* 17, 13345–13356. https://doi.org/10.3390/molecules171113345

Lim, S.H., Lee, H.S., Han, H.-K., Choi, C.-I., 2021. Saikosaponin A and D Inhibit Adipogenesis via the AMPK and MAPK Signaling Pathways in 3T3-L1 Adipocytes. *IJMS* 22, 11409. https://doi.org/10.3390/ijms222111409

Liu, G.-Y., Liu, J., Wang, Y.-L., Liu, Y., Shao, Y., Han, Y., Qin, Y.-R., Xiao, F.-J., Li, P.-F., Zhao, L.-J., Gu, E.-Y., Chen, S.-Y., Gao, L.-H., Wu, C.-T., Hu, X.-W., Duan, H.-F., 2016. Adipose-Derived Mesenchymal Stem Cells Ameliorate Lipid Metabolic Disturbance in Mice. *Stem Cells Transl Med* 5, 1162–1170. https://doi.org/10.5966/sctm.2015-0239

Ma, H., He, X., Yang, Y., Li, M., Hao, D., Jia, Z., 2011. The Genus *Epimedium*: An Ethnopharmacological and Phytochemical Review. *J Ethnopharmacol* 134, 519–541. https://doi.org/10.1016/j.jep.2011.01.001

Matsukawa, T., Inaguma, T., Han, J., Villareal, M.O., Isoda, H., 2015. Cyanidin-3-Glucoside Derived from Black Soybeans Ameliorate Type 2 Diabetes through the Induction of Differentiation of Preadipocytes into Smaller and Insulin-Sensitive Adipocytes. *J Nutr Biochem* 26, 860–867. https://doi.org/10.1016/j.jnutbio.2015.03.006

Mohamed, S.S., AI Ali, E., Hosny, S., 2015. The Antidiabetic Effect of Mesenchymal Stem Cells vs. Nigella Sativa Oil on Streptozotocin Induced Type 1 Diabetic Rats. *J Cell Sci Ther* 6. https://doi.org/10.4172/2157-7013.1000226

Moustafa, E.M., Moawed, F.S.M., Abdel-Hamid, G.R., 2020. Icariin Promote Stem Cells Regeneration and Repair Acinar Cells in L-arginine/Radiation-Inducing Chronic Pancreatitis in Rats. *Dose-Response* 18, 155932582097081. https://doi.org/10.1177/1559325820970810

Pal, P.B., Sinha, K., Sil, P.C., 2014. Mangiferin Attenuates Diabetic Nephropathy by Inhibiting Oxidative Stress Mediated Signaling Cascade, TNFα Related and Mitochondrial Dependent Apoptotic Pathways in Streptozotocin-Induced Diabetic Rats. *PLoS ONE* 9, e107220. https://doi.org/10.1371/journal.pone.0107220

Park, M., Sharma, A., Lee, H.-J., 2019. Anti-Adipogenic Effects of Delphinidin-3-O-β-Glucoside in 3T3-L1 Preadipocytes and Primary White Adipocytes. *Molecules* 24, 1848. https://doi.org/10.3390/molecules24101848

Roberts, F.R., Hupple, C., Norowski, E., Walsh, N.C., Przewozniak, N., Aryee, K.-E., Van Dessel, F.M., Jurczyk, A., Harlan, D.M., Greiner, D.L., Bortell, R., Yang, C., 2017. Possible Type 1 Diabetes Risk Prediction: Using Ultrasound Imaging to Assess Pancreas Inflammation in the Inducible Autoimmune Diabetes BBDR Model. *PLoS ONE* 12, e0178641. https://doi.org/10.1371/journal.pone.0178641

Rojas, J., Bermudez, V., Palmar, J., Martínez, M.S., Olivar, L.C., Nava, M., Tomey, D., Rojas, M., Salazar, J., Garicano, C., Velasco, M., 2018. Pancreatic Beta Cell Death: Novel Potential Mechanisms in Diabetes Therapy. *J Diabetes Res* 2018, 1–19. https://doi.org/10.1155/2018/9601801

Saito, T., Abe, D., Sekiya, K., 2008. Sakuranetin Induces Adipogenesis of 3T3-L1 Cells Through Enhanced Expression of PPARγ2. *Biochem Biophys Res Commun* 372, 835–839. https://doi.org/10.1016/j.bbrc.2008.05.146

Saito, T., Abe, D., Sekiya, K., 2009. Flavanone Exhibits PPARγ Ligand Activity and Enhances Differentiation of 3T3-L1 Adipocytes. *Biochem Biophys Res Commun* 380, 281–285. https://doi.org/10.1016/j.bbrc.2009.01.058

Saud, B., Malla, R., Shrestha, K., 2019. A Review on the Effect of Plant Extract on Mesenchymal Stem Cell Proliferation and Differentiation. *Stem Cells Int* 2019, 1–13. https://doi.org/10.1155/2019/7513404

Selmani, Z., Naji, A., Zidi, I., Favier, B., Gaiffe, E., Obert, L., Borg, C., Saas, P., Tiberghien, P., Rouas-Freiss, N., Carosella, E.D., Deschaseaux, F., 2008. Human Leukocyte Antigen-G5 Secretion by Human Mesenchymal Stem Cells Is Required to Suppress T Lymphocyte and Natural Killer Function and to Induce CD4+CD25highFOXP3+ Regulatory T Cells. *Stem Cells* 26, 212–222. https://doi.org/10.1634/stemcells.2007-0554

Shrestha, M., Nguyen, T.T., Park, J., Choi, J.U., Yook, S., Jeong, J.-H., 2021. Immunomodulation Effect of Mesenchymal Stem Cells in Islet Transplantation. *Biomed Pharmacother* 142, 112042. https://doi.org/10.1016/j.biopha.2021.112042

Stompor, M., 2020. A Review on Sources and Pharmacological Aspects of Sakuranetin. *Nutrients* 12, 513. https://doi.org/10.3390/nu12020513

Swamy, J., Annamma, P.S., Chandra Mohan, K., Rasingam, L., 2015. Hyoscyamus Albus (Solanaceae): A New Distributional Record for India. *Rheedea*, 54–56.

Swick, J., Lee, O.H., Kim, Y.-C., 2012. Quercetin Exerts Anti-Adipogenic Effects Through Modulation of 3T3-L1 Preadipocyte Proliferation and Differentiation. *FASEB J.* 26. https://doi.org/10.1096/fasebj.26.1_supplement.644.11

Takeno, A., Kanazawa, I., Notsu, M., Tanaka, K., Sugimoto, T., 2018. Phloretin Promotes Adipogenesis via Mitogen-Activated Protein Kinase Pathways in Mouse Marrow Stromal ST2 Cells. *IJMS* 19, 1772. https://doi.org/10.3390/ijms19061772

Tang, Y., Jacobi, A., Vater, C., Zou, L., Zou, X., Stiehler, M., 2015. Icariin Promotes Angiogenic Differentiation and Prevents Oxidative Stress-Induced Autophagy in Endothelial Progenitor Cells. *Stem Cells* 33, 1863–1877. https://doi.org/10.1002/stem.2005

Tayaramma, T., Ma, B., Rohde, M., Mayer, H., 2006. Chromatin-Remodeling Factors Allow Differentiation of Bone Marrow Cells into Insulin-Producing Cells. *Stem Cells* 24, 2858–2867. https://doi.org/10.1634/stemcells.2006-0109

Tsalamandris, S., Antonopoulos, A.S., Oikonomou, E., Papamikroulis, G.-A., Vogiatzi, G., Papaioannou, S., Deftereos, S., Tousoulis, D., 2019. The Role of Inflammation in Diabetes: Current Concepts and Future Perspectives. *Eur Cardiol* 14, 50–59. https://doi.org/10.15420/ecr.2018.33.1

Via, A.G., Frizziero, A., Oliva, F., 2012. Biological Properties of Mesenchymal Stem Cells from Different Sources. *Muscles Ligaments Tendons J* 2, 154–162.

Wang, G., Wu, B., Xu, W., Jin, X., Wang, K., Wang, H., 2020. The Inhibitory Effects of Juglanin on Adipogenesis in 3T3-L1 Adipocytes. *DDDT* 14, 5349–5357. https://doi.org/10.2147/DDDT.S256504

Wang, X., Liu, Chuanhai, Xu, Yong, Chen, P., Shen, Y., Xu, Yansheng, Zhao, Y., Chen, W., Zhang, X., Ouyang, Y., Wang, Y., Xie, C., Zhou, M., Liu, Cuilong, 2017. Combination of Mesenchymal Stem Cell Injection with Icariin for the Treatment of Diabetes-associated Erectile Dysfunction. *PLoS ONE* 12, e0174145. https://doi.org/10.1371/journal.pone.0174145

Wei, N., Zhang, Y.-J., Xu, Z., Kamande, E.M., Ngumbau, V.M., Hu, G.-W., 2017. Epimedium Zhaotongense (Berberidaceae), a New Species from Yunnan Province, China. *Phytotaxa* 296, 88. https://doi.org/10.11646/phytotaxa.296.1.7

Wink, M., 2015. Modes of Action of Herbal Medicines and Plant Secondary Metabolites. *Medicines* 2, 251–286. https://doi.org/10.3390/medicines2030251

Yang, J.-W., Kim, S., 2015. Ginsenoside Rc Promotes Anti-Adipogenic Activity on 3T3-L1 Adipocytes by Down-Regulating C/EBPα and PPARγ. *Molecules* 20, 1293–1303. https://doi.org/10.3390/molecules20011293

Yang, J.-Y., Della-Fera, M.A., Baile, C.A., 2008. Guggulsterone Inhibits Adipocyte Differentiation and Induces Apoptosis in 3T3-L1 Cells. *Obesity* 16, 16–22. https://doi.org/10.1038/oby.2007.24

Yang, X., Yin, L., Li, T., Chen, Z., 2014. Green Tea Extracts Reduce Adipogenesis by Decreasing Expression of Transcription Factors C/EBPα and PPARγ. *Int J Clin Exp Med* 7, 4906–4914.

Zhai, Y.-K., Guo, X., Pan, Y.-L., Niu, Y.-B., Li, C.-R., Wu, X.-L., Mel, Q.-B., 2013. A Systematic Review of the Efficacy and Pharmacological Profile of *Herba Epimedii* in Osteoporosis Therapy. *Die Pharmazie* 68, 713–722. https://doi.org/10.1691/ph.2013.2900

Zhang, M., Ikeda, K., Xu, J.-W., Yamori, Y., Gao, X.-M., Zhang, B.-L., 2009. Genistein Suppresses Adipogenesis of 3T3-L1 Cells via Multiple Signal Pathways: Genistein and Adipogenesis. *Phytother Res* 23, 713–718. https://doi.org/10.1002/ptr.2724

Zhang, Y., Li, J., Wang, Y., Liang, Q., 2021. Taxonomy of *Epimedium* (Berberidaceae) with Special Reference to Chinese Species. *Chin Herb Med* 14, 20–35. https://doi.org/10.1016/j.chmed.2021.12.001

Zhou, R., Tardivel, A., Thorens, B., Choi, I., Tschopp, J., 2010. Thioredoxin-Interacting Protein Links Oxidative Stress to Inflammasome Activation. *Nat Immunol* 11, 136–140. https://doi.org/10.1038/ni.1831

Zhu, X.-Y., Ma, S., Eirin, A., Woollard, J.R., Hickson, L.J., Sun, D., Lerman, A., Lerman, L.O., 2016. Functional Plasticity of Adipose-Derived Stromal Cells During Development of Obesity: ASC Function in Obesity. *Stem Cells Transl Med* 5, 893–900. https://doi.org/10.5966/sctm.2015-0240

Section II

Specific Agents, Items and Extracts

6 Gaultheria spp. Berries Use in Diabetes
Molecular, Cellular, and Metabolic Effects

Felipe Jiménez-Aspee

CONTENTS

ABBREVIATIONS

AGEs   advanced glycation end products
AMPK   AMP-activated protein kinase
DPP4   dipeptidyl peptidase 4
GIP   glucose-dependent insulinotropic polypeptide
GLP-1   glucagon-like peptide 1
GLUT   glucose transporter
SGLT   sodium-dependent glucose transporter
T2D   type 2 diabetes

6.1 INTRODUCTION

Gaultheria is a genus of shrubs belonging to the Ericaceae family, comprising more than 135 recognized species (Mabberley 1997). The different species can be found worldwide, but they are originally native to Asia, Australasia, and the Americas (Mabberley 1997). There is no common name that groups all the species worldwide, and thus they are referred to under several local names, the most common being *wintergreen berry, creeping snowberry, moxie-berry, teaberry, salal, chaura*, and *hued-hued* (Teillier and Escobar 2013; McDougall et al. 2016; Mieres-Castro et al. 2020). More than 100 different compounds have been identified in rhizomes, roots, stems, branches, leaves, and fruits of different *Gaultheria* species, including methyl salicylate derivatives, phenolic acids, flavonoids, terpenoids, iridoids, steroids, and others (Liu et al. 2013). Many of the species are used as part of folk medicine to treat inflammation, pain, infections, and even cancer (Liu et al. 2013; Luo

DOI: 10.1201/9781003220930-8

et al. 2018). Some reports from North and South American Indigenous groups point to the role of some *Gaultheria* species to treat symptoms associated with diabetes (e.g., polyurea and polydipsia; Leduc et al. 2006). In recent years, insights into the mechanisms of action and health promoting properties of *Gaultheria* berries have been discovered showing an unrivaled potential for the commercial development of the species.

6.2 BACKGROUND

Nutritional interventions are an essential part of prediabetes and diabetes management and are a key component of a lifestyle intervention program, used in conjunction with medications and surgical interventions (Evert et al. 2014). In a recent review and meta-analysis of prospective studies, it was reported that with each additional 100 g of fruits incorporated into the normal diet, a decrease in the risk of type 2 diabetes (T2D) was observed, up to a maximum of 300 g/day (Schwingshackl et al. 2017). Another review on prospective cohort studies concluded that increasing the consumption of berries by 17 g/day reduces the risk of developing T2D by 5% (Guo et al. 2016). Berries such as blueberries, cranberries, blackberries, raspberries, and strawberries are low in total calories and contain a wide range of micronutrients, vitamins, and secondary plant metabolites, such as anthocyanins, flavonols, flavan-3-ols, proanthocyanidins, tannins, and iridoids (Calvano et al. 2019). Several epidemiological studies have shown an inverse correlation between the dietary intake of polyphenols and the risk of developing several metabolic diseases, including diabetes and its complications (Calvano et al. 2019). The mechanisms described in the literature include the regulation of carbohydrate digestion by inhibition of enzymes such as α-glucosidase and α-amylase, the regulation of the glucose uptake in insulin-sensitive tissues, the promotion of insulin secretion, the reduction of insulin resistance, and the protection of pancreatic β cells against glucose toxicity, among others (Hanhineva et al. 2010; Babu et al. 2013; Kazeem and Davies 2016; Papuc et al. 2020). The present chapter summarizes the research carried out in recent years on a particular genus of berries, *Gaultheria* spp., which has been recognized along with the *Vaccinium* genus, as a source of bioactive compounds of interest for the prevention and complementary treatment of T2D (Luo et al. 2018).

6.3 *GAULTHERIA*: BOTANICAL DESCRIPTION AND
CHEMICAL COMPOSITION

Gaultheria spp. are normally cultivated for their ornamental characteristics due to their attractive foliage, colorful striking red stems, and glossy berries, but some species also produce edible fruits with importance for wildlife and local economies. The members of this genus can be shrubs or subshrubs that can be no taller than 15 cm, such as *G. hispidula* and *G. poeppigii* (Mabberley 1997; Teiller and Escobar 2013). Some other species, under shade and good soil conditions, can reach up to 2.5–3 m tall, such as *G. shallon*, *G. phillyreifolia*, and *G. mucronata* (Mabberley 1997; Teiller and Escobar 2013). The more than 100 species described in this genus have botanical characteristics that differentiate them, in particular with high variability on their leaves (e.g., blade ovate, elliptic, orbiculate, reniform, coriaceous, margins serrate, crenate or ciliate, surface glabrous or hairy), inflorescence (axillary, racemes, 2–12 flowered, sometimes flowers solitary), flowers (e.g., white or cream to pink, corolla urceolate to campanulates, 8–10 stamens, filaments straight, flattened, usually widest proximally, glabrous or hairy) and fruits (capsular, five-valved, globose, fleshy, and surrounded by persistent and fleshy calyx). Some of the main representative species of this genus are depicted in Figure 6.1.

The extensive investigation carried out in recent years on the chemical constituents of the *Gaultheria* genus has led to the identification of more than 100 compounds in the roots, stems, leaves, aerial parts, flowers, fruits, and seeds, which were last summarized by Liu et al. (2013). An update on the composition of *Gaultheria* species reported between 2013 and 2022 is presented in Table 6.1. The main compounds include methyl salicylate and its glycosides, phenylpropanoids,

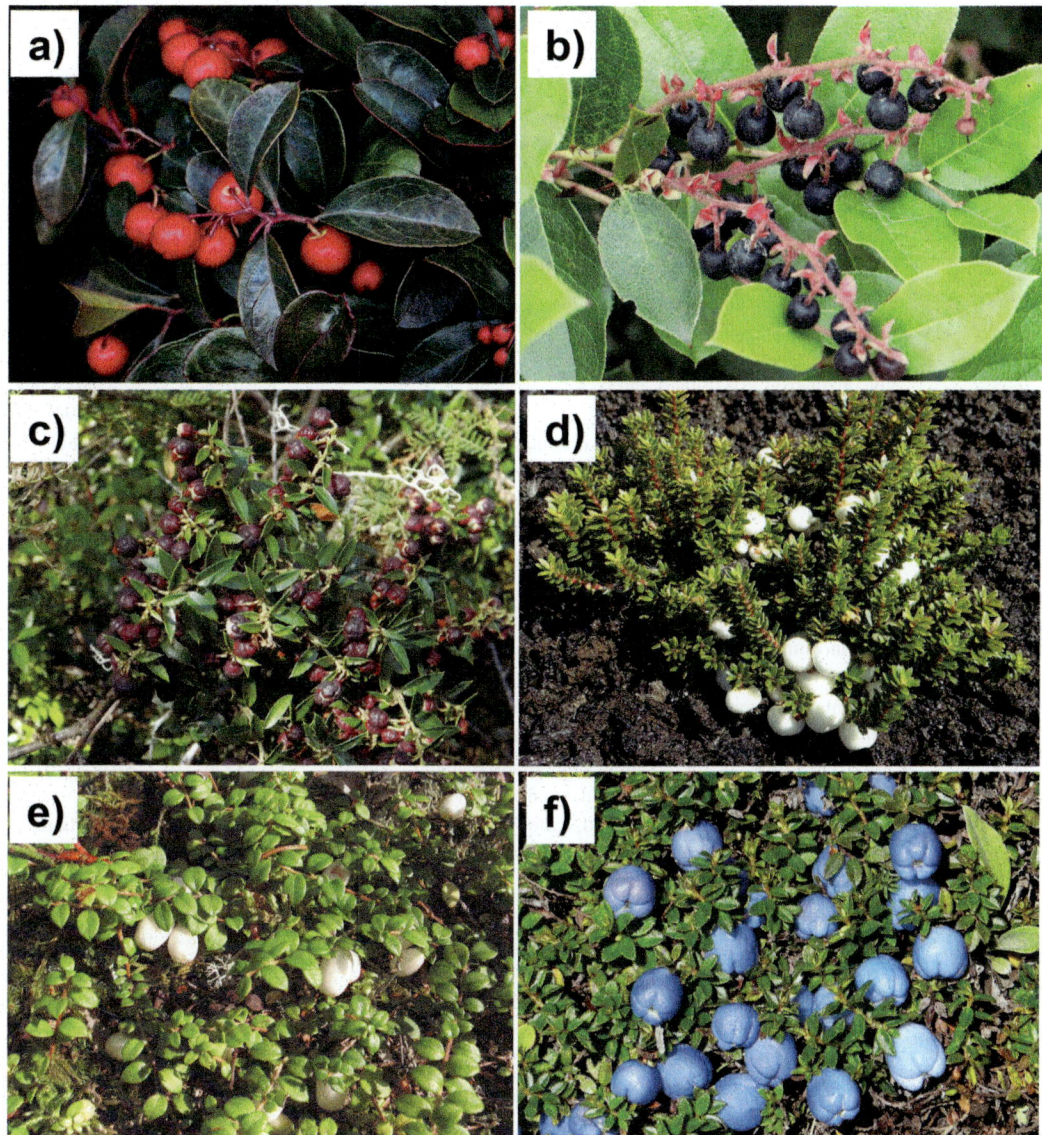

FIGURE 6.1 Some *Gaultheria* species with antidiabetic properties: (a) *G. procumbens*; (b) *G. shallon*; (c) *G. phillyreifolia*; (d) *G. poeppigii*; (e) *G. hispidula*; (f) *G. tricophylla*.

Sources: (a, b) Purchased from iStock.com with license permit; (c, d) original photos from the author; (e) reproduced with permission of owner, Mrs. Marilee Lovit; (f) reproduced with permission of owner, Dr. Gurinder Goraya.

flavonoids, lignans, terpenoids, steroids, alkaloids, anthraquinones, and dilactones (Liu et al. 2013). In the edible fruits, the main compounds are anthocyanins (mainly cyanidin and delphinidin glycosides); iridoids (mainly p-coumaroyl monotropein esters); flavonols (glycosides and glucuronides of quercetin, kaempferol, myricetin, and isorhamnetin); and phenylpropanoids (3-caffeoylquinic acid) (Liu et al. 2013; Ruiz et al. 2015; McDougall et al. 2016; Ferguson et al. 2018; Mieres-Castro et al. 2019; Oyarzún et al. 2020; Fernández-Galleguillos et al. 2021). Some species present high methyl salicylate contents in their fruit (Nikolić et al. 2013; Mieres-Castro et al. 2020).

TABLE 6.1

Chemical Constituents of *Gaultheria* spp.

Group	Representatives	References From 2013–2022
Anthocyanins	Delphinidin-3-O-galactoside, delphinidin-3-O-arabinoside, delphinidin-3-O-glucoside, cyanidin-3-O-galactoside, cyanidin-3-O-arabinoside, cyanidin-3-O-glucoside, cyanidin-3-O-lathyroside, cyanidin-3-O-sambubioside, petunidin-3-O-glycoside, malvidin-3-O-glycoside, peonidin-3-O-glycoside, cyanidin diglycoside	Ruiz et al. 2013; McDougall et al. 2016; Ferguson et al. 2018; Mieres-Castro et al. 2019; Mieres-Castro et al. 2020; Oyarzún et al. 2020; Fernández-Galleguillos et al. 2021
Salicylates	Methylsalicylate, methylsalicylate-2-O-glycoside, gaultherin, methylsalicilate-2-O-lactoside, methylbenzoate-2-O-glucopyranosyl-glycoside A and B, salicylic acid	Cong et al. 2015; Xu et al. 2016; Michel et al. 2019; Mieres-Castro et al. 2020; Olszewska et al. 2021; Luo et al. 2021
Flavonoids	Avicularin, apigenin, isoschaftoside, dhasingreoside, myricetin, myricetin glucuronide, myricetin pentoside, myricetin rhamnoside, myricetin hexoside, kaempferol-3-O-glucuronide, kaempferol-3-O-rutinoside, kaempferol-3-O-rhamnoside, kaempferol pentoside; quercetin, quercetin-3-O-glucuronide, quercetin-3-O-rhamnoside, quercetin-3-O-galactoside, quercetin-3-O-glucoside, quercetin-3-O-sulfate, quercetin-3-O-arabinoside, quercetin-3-O-rutinoside, hyperin, homoeridictyol, hesperetin, hesperidin, ginkgetin, luteolin-7-O-glucoside, luteolin-7-glucuronide, naringenin, naringenin-7-O-glucoside, isorhamnetin-3-O-rutinoside, isorhamnetin rhamnoside, irigenin hexoside	Ruiz et al. 2015; Cong et al. 2015; McDougall et al. 2016; Ferguson et al. 2018; Mieres-Castro et al. 2019; Michel et al. 2019; Mieres-Castro et al. 2020; Olszewska et al. 2021; Oyarzún et al. 2020; Fernández-Galleguillos et al. 2021
Phenolic acids	Caffeoyl hexoside, 3-caffeoylquinic acid, 4-caffeoylquinic acid, 5-caffeoylquinic acid, coumaric acid, coumaric acid hexoside, 5-caffeoylshikimic acid, caffeic acid, caffeoylferuloyl tartaric acid, caffoylglucaric acid, gallic acid, dihydroxybenzoic acid, ferulic acid, sinapic acid, gentisic acid	Ruiz et al. 2015; Xu et al. 2016; McDougall et al. 2016; Ferguson et al. 2018; Mieres-Castro et al. 2019; Mieres-Castro et al. 2020; Olszewska et al. 2021; Oyarzún et al. 2020; Fernández-Galleguillos et al. 2021
Flavan-3-ols and procyanidins	Catechin, epicatechin, gallocatechin, epicatechin-epicatechin, epigallocatechin, epigallocatechin-epicatechin, procyanidin B1, procyanidin B2, procyanidin B3, procyanidin B4, procyanidin A2, B-type procyanidin dimers, B-type procyanidin trimers, A-type prodelphinidin	McDougall et al. 2016; Ferguson et al. 2018; Michel et al. 2019; Mieres-Castro et al. 2019; Mieres-Castro et al. 2020; Olszewska et al. 2021; Fernández-Galleguillos et al. 2021
Iridoids and terpenoids	Gauleucin A, gauleucin B, gauleucin C, gauleucin D, gauleucin E, gauleucin F, gauleucin G, gaultheronoterpene, gaultheric acid, 3β,12dihydroxy-13-acetyl-8,11,13-podocarpatriene, 12,19-dihydroxy-13-acetyl-8,11,13-podocarpatriene, 12,19-dihydroxyabieta-8,11,13-trien-8-one, margoclin, hinokiol, 19-hydroxyferruginol, (4aS,6cS)-8-hydroxy-9-isopropyl-4,4,6c-trimethyl-1,2,3,4,4a,5,6,6c-octahydrophenanthren-3-one, abieta-6,8, oleanolic acid, α-amyrin, β-amyrin, β-sitosterol, campesterol, p-coumaroyl dihydromonotropein, monotropein-10-trans-p-coumarate (vaccinoside), monotropein-10-trans-p-cinnamate, 6-hydroxy-dihydromonotroepin-10-trans-coumarate, dihydromonotropein-10-trans-cinnamate, swertiamarin, methoxygeniposidic acid, 6,7-dihydro-6β-hydroxymonotropein, nuzhenal B, enmenol, scupolin I, dictamnoside	Michel et al. 2017; Mieres-Castro et al. 2019; Mieres-Castro et al. 2020; Fernández-Galleguillos et al. 2021; Hu et al. 2022

Note: A full list of constituents can be found in Liu et al. (2013).

6.4 ETHNOPHARMACOLOGICAL USES OF *GAULTHERIA* SPP.

Over 1200 species of plants have been reported worldwide as traditional medicine for diabetes, with over 80% of these species having reported benefits in *in vitro* and *in vivo* studies (Marles and Farnsworth 1995). Moreover, secondary metabolites from plants are the inspiration of many current treatments of diabetes, such as the biguanide metformin from the high guanidine content in *Galega officinalis*, or 4-deoxyphlorizin derivatives such as canagliflozin, inspired by the phlorizin content of the bark of different fruit trees (Sun et al. 2020). Berries have shown to be good sources of health-promoting phytochemicals with antidiabetic potential among other activities (Schreckinger et al. 2010). The supplementation of diet with berries significantly improves postprandial hyperglycemia and hyperinsulinemia in overweight and obese adults and can improve glycemic and lipid profiles (Calvano et al. 2019). Different botanical parts of *Gaultheria* spp. are used worldwide in traditional medicine. In China, most *Gaultheria* species are used to treat rheumatic arthritis and other inflammatory diseases due to the high methyl salicylate content (Luo et al. 2018). In India, there are reports of consumption of *Gaultheria* berries as food and in herbal teas, as well as part of the folk medicine (Liu et al. 2013; Luo et al. 2018). In South America, there is evidence of the consumption of the fruits of *Gaultheria* by the Mapuche people of Chile and Argentina and the Selk'nam and Yamana tribes of southern Patagonia, either as food or medicine against headaches (Mösbach 1992). *Gaultheria* berries are usually included by the local people in the lists of berries used to treat symptoms that can be associated with diabetes. For example, people from the Cree tribe of northern Canada used the fruits and leaves of *G. hispidula* (L). Muhl to treat diabetes (Leduc et al. 2006; Tam et al. 2009; Harbilas et al. 2009). The Iroquois, Ojibwa, Algonquin, and Cree Indigenous people from North American boreal forests used the leaves of *G. procumbens* L. for the treatment of the symptoms of diabetes and its complications (McCune and Johns 2002; Patel et al. 2012). Similarly, both species were reported as antidiabetic plants by the Eeyou Istchee Cree First Nations of North America (Saleem et al. 2010). It is interesting to note that those fruits with high methyl salicylate content, such as *G. fragrantissima, G. yunnanensis, G. tenuifolia,* and *G. griffithiana* have ethnopharmacological importance in inflammatory diseases but with less information regarding its consumption as foods, while those with less wintergreen flavor, such as *G. hispidula, G. procumbens, G. phillyreifolia,* and *G. poeppigii* are mostly consumed fresh or processed due to their sweet taste and pleasant aroma.

6.5 MOLECULAR, CELLULAR, AND METABOLIC EVIDENCE

The traditional uses of medicinal plants against symptoms that can be attributed to diabetes are well described in literature (Patel et al. 2012). However, many times the mechanisms that explain the observed effects are unknown. The medicinal plants usually contain several bioactive compounds that can affect multiple targets in the physiopathology of diabetes. As recently reviewed, for example, they can delay gastric emptying, inhibit digestive and glucose metabolizing enzymes, regulate intestinal flora, protect pancreatic β cells, improve insulin signaling pathways and its secretion, and attenuate oxidative stress and the generation of advanced glycation end products (AGEs), among others (Sun et al. 2020). In addition, due to the high diversity of secondary metabolites, the synergistic effect cannot be overlooked. The evidence on the direct effects of *Gaultheria* species is more limited, and only a few studies have been published trying to disclose the mechanisms explaining the potential of these berries to prevent and/or treat diabetes. A graphic summary of the evidence so far regarding the potential of *Gaultheria* species is presented in Figure 6.2.

6.5.1 INHIBITION OF CARBOHYDRATE DIGESTIVE AND DIPEPTIDYL PEPTIDASE 4 ENZYMES

Carbohydrate digestibility is directly associated with postprandial glycemia, and thus, one of the strategies to reduce the hyperglycemia and associated hyperinsulinemia observed in prediabetes or T2D is to inhibit the activity of carbohydrate digestive enzymes in the gastrointestinal tract.

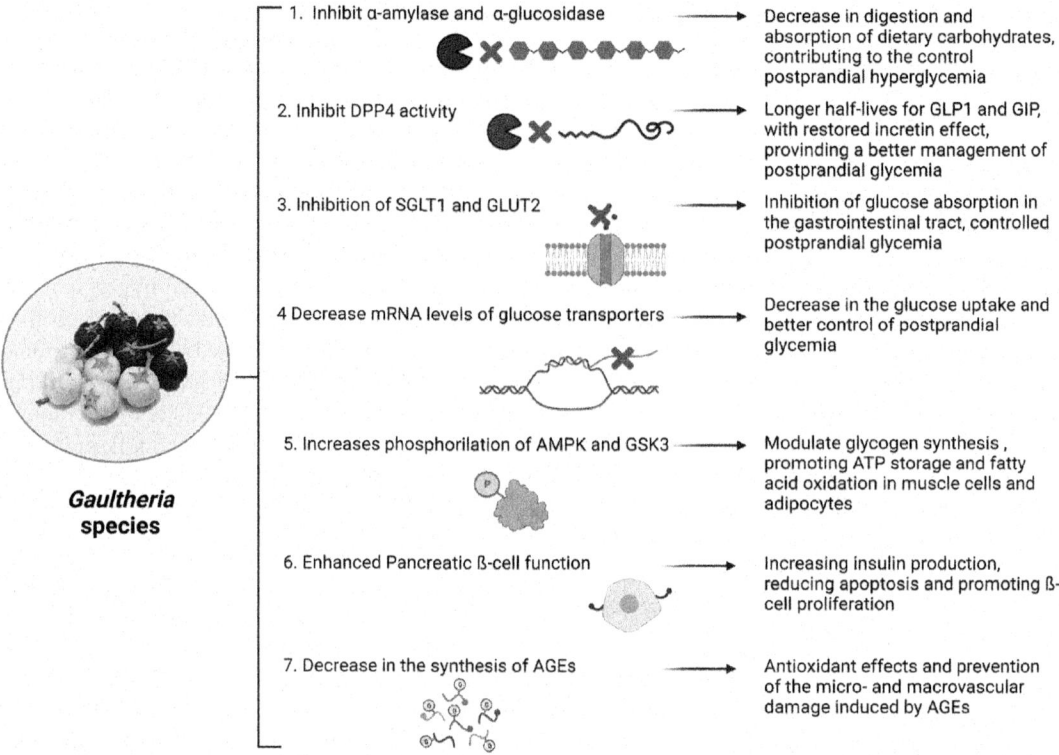

FIGURE 6.2   Scheme representing the reported mechanisms on how *Gaultheria* species can exert antidiabetic effects (created with www.Biorender.com).

Throughout the digestive system different metabolizing enzymes are associated with the digestion of complex carbohydrates into mono- and disaccharides, which then can be absorbed at intestinal level (Gong et al. 2020). The key enzymes involved are the pancreatic α-amylase (EC 3.2.1.1) and the intestinal α-glucosidases (EC 3.2.1.20). α-Amylase degrades starch, maltodextrins, and other polysaccharides into short oligomers by catalyzing the hydrolysis of α-1,4-glucan linkages to a large number of maltose units. α-Glucosidase is present in the brush border of human intestinal cells and hydrolyzes the α-1,4-glycosidic bond from disaccharides to free glucose units. Inhibitors of both enzymes, such as acarbose or miglitol, are commercially available as part of the battery of therapeutic products available for T2D management (ADA 2021). Although the risk of hypoglycemia is low compared to other drugs, both drugs have the disadvantage of inducing gastrointestinal discomfort and bowel sounds.

Some of the different *Gaultheria* spp. worldwide have demonstrated inhibitory effects toward these carbohydrate metabolizing enzymes. The methanol extract of *G. tricophylla* plants had inhibitory effects on α-glucosidase, with an IC_{50} value of 17.5 ± 0.1 μg/mL, while the chloroform and hexane extracts had no effect on the enzyme activity (Alam and Saqib 2017). The fruit extracts of *G. phillyreifolia* and *G. poeppigii* showed strong inhibition against α-glucosidase at a concentration of 100 μg/mL, with IC_{50} values ranging between 0.66 and 3.14 μg/mL (Mieres-Castro et al. 2022). Authors reported an increase in the IC_{50} value after *in vitro* gastrointestinal digestion, with new values ranging between 2.76 and 24.9 μg/mL. In the same study, the authors reported that the main compounds responsible for this activity were cyanidin-3-O-arabinoside, quercetin, and different *p*-coumaroyl iridoids present in high concentrations in the fruits. In another study, seven new abietane diterpenoids were isolated from the aerial parts of *G. leucocarpa* var. *yunnanensis*. Among them, the compounds gauleucin E, 12,19-dihydroxyabeta-8,11,13-trien-7-one, and margoclin presented inhibitory effects against α-glucosidase, with IC_{50} values of 319 ± 8.5, 539 ± 5.9, and 327 ± 5.5 µM, respectively, while under the same conditions, the positive control acarbose presented an IC_{50} value of 387 ± 10.7 µM (Hu et al. 2022). In another study, the berries of *G. shallon* were extracted with pure water and incorporated at 20% into a yogurt and fermented until a pH of 4.5 was reached. An aqueous extract of the yogurt was evaluated as an inhibitor of α-amylase, and it was observed that the inhibitory capacity increased from 20% up to 60% after 7 days of fermentation. In the same way, the inhibitory capacity against α-glucosidase increased from 0 to almost 50% after 28 days of storage at 4°C (Ni et al. 2018). The authors suggested that the fruit extract induces changes in milk protein conformation, affecting its susceptibility to lactic fermentation, which results in the release of casein-derived peptides that can inhibit both enzymes (Ni et al. 2018).

Dipeptidyl peptidase 4 (DPP4, EC 3.4.14.5) is an important enzyme ubiquitously expressed on numerous cell types, whose main known substrates are the incretin hormones, the glucagon-like peptide 1 (GLP-1) and the glucose-dependent insulinotropic polypeptide (GIP) (Nauck and Meier 2018). Incretins are secreted from K and L intestinal cells and play an important role in promoting insulin secretion, biosynthesis, β cell proliferation and survival, and decreasing gastric emptying, food intake, and body weight (Nauck and Meier 2018). Several studies have shown that incretin secretion is reduced in T2D, and an important pharmacological strategy is to decrease the degradation of these peptides by inhibiting the catabolic action of DPP4. The inhibition of DPP4 by the gliptin family of drugs are important members of the therapeutical arsenal, and their efficacy as a first line of treatment in addition to metformin was recently demonstrated (ADA 2021). In the study of Ni et al. (2018), the lactic fermentation of the yogurt supplemented with a *G. shallon* aqueous fruit extract produced different peptides with DPP4 inhibitory activity, reaching up to 60% inhibition of the enzyme after 28 days of fermentation. In a continuation of their study, the authors showed that the *G. shallon* extract increased the degree of hydrolyzation of whey proteins by 41%, facilitating the release of peptides with DPP4 inhibitory activity. Moreover, it was observed that the phenolics present in the fruit extract may be responsible for the susceptibility of α-lactalbumin, but not β-lactoglobulin, to the proteolytic activity of peptidases (Ni et al. 2019).

6.5.2 Glucose Uptake and Metabolism

The transport of glucose from the intestinal lumen to the systemic circulation is a complex process regulated by many factors, most of them not clearly understood to this day. What is clear is that the gut provides not only a barrier that limits glucose passage but also acts as an important endocrine organ in modulating postprandial glycemia through different regulatory mechanisms (Gromova et al. 2021). The role of different glucose transporters and hormones secreted from the gut to the pancreas – and even more, the role of gut microbiome – are all interconnected processes that work in harmony to maintain homeostasis (Kazakos 2011; Chen et al. 2021). Any imbalance in these mechanisms can affect the overall picture and lead to different diseases, including metabolic syndrome and T2D.

Once monosaccharides reach the small intestine, glucose absorption actively occurs across the apical membrane of the enterocytes through the sodium-dependent glucose transporter (SGLT1). From the enterocytes, glucose is released to the portal vein through the basolateral membrane via the glucose transporter 2 (GLUT2). Several studies have shown that the expression and activity of glucose transporters is increased in diabetes, suggesting an important role in hyperglycemia (Koepsell 2020). Berry extracts have been shown to modify postprandial plasma glycemia in healthy subjects (Törrönen et al. 2010), and some reports indicate that the effect can be through direct inhibition of the SGLT1 (Castro-Acosta et al. 2017) or by a decrease in the expression of the glucose transporter and metabolizing genes (Alzaid et al. 2013).

Gaultheria species have demonstrated effects on the glucose uptake of different cell lines, as well as effects on the activity and expression of the glucose transporters. Harbilas et al. (2009) showed that an ethanol extract prepared with the leaves of *G. hispidula* at a working concentration of 25 μg/mL increased the glucose uptake in differentiated C2C12 skeletal muscle cells and in differentiated 3T3-L1 adipocytes, but the effects were only observed after 1 hour treatment and not at 18 hours. In the same article, the *G. hispidula* extract increased the PC212-AC cell viability when they were exposed to glucose deprivation (1.1 mM) and glucose toxicity (150 mM). In the intestinal Caco-2 cell model, the same *G. hispidula* extract significantly inhibited the intestinal glucose absorption in a dose-dependent manner (25–100 μg/mL) after 10 min of co-incubation, but failed to have effects in the long term, indicating a direct inhibition of the glucose uptake mechanisms (Nistor-Baldea et al. 2010). In another study, the *G. hispidula* extract increased by 300% the phosphorylation of AMP-activated protein kinase (AMPK) in rat H4IIE hepatoma cells, thus promoting ATP synthesis and fatty acid oxidation (Nachar et al. 2013). Moreover, the extract also increased the ratio of glycogen synthase kinase-3 that was phosphorylated (p-GSK3/GSK3) in HepG2 cells and thus promoting the less active form of the enzyme. Both observations indicate that the *G. hispidula* extract could modulate the glycogen synthesis at the hepatic level (Nachar et al. 2013).

In a recent study, *G. phillyreifolia* and *G. poeppigii* white and pink fruit extracts were subjected to *in vitro* gastrointestinal digestion, and the resulting micellar solution was evaluated for its potential to modulate glucose uptake in a differentiated Caco-2 cell model (Mieres-Castro et al. 2022). After overnight incubation with 200 μg/mL of the fruit extracts, the glucose uptake was reduced by 28.2%, 17.6%, and 22.4% for *G. phillyreifolia*, *G. poeppigii* pink fruits, and *G. poeppigii* white fruits, respectively. The authors showed that the effects could be attributed to the anthocyanins and monotropein esters present in the digested samples (Mieres-Castro et al. 2022). In addition, the digested *G. phillyreifolia* and white *G. poeppigii* fruit extracts decreased the relative mRNA expression of SGLT1 by 92% and 78%, respectively. The effects were higher than those observed for the main secondary metabolites found in the digested extracts. In the same way, the digested *G. phillyreifolia* fruit extract decreased the relative mRNA expression of GLUT2 and GLUT5 by 90% and 85%, respectively. To a lesser extent, the pink fruits of *G. poeppigii* reduced the relative mRNA expression of GLUT2 and GLUT5 by 45% and 28%, respectively. The relative mRNA levels of the enzyme sucrose-isomaltase were affected by the pre-treatment with the fruit extracts, with decreases in the range of 82% to 93% (Mieres-Castro et al. 2022).

The *in vivo* antidiabetic potential of *G. tricophylla* was evaluated in alloxan-induced diabetic mice (Alam and Saquib 2017). The rodents were divided into five groups: (1) normal saline, (2) diabetic control, (3) diabetic model + 500 mg of *G. tricophylla* methanolic extract/kg, (4) normal mice + 500 mg of *G. tricophylla* methanolic extract/kg, and (5) a reference control of animals treated with glibenclamide. Animals were weighed and blood samples were collected every 3 days to study different biochemical parameters for 15 days until their sacrifice. The authors found that the body weight of rats treated with the *G. tricophylla* extract did not decrease to the degree observed for the non-treated diabetic rats, at a rate like that achieved by glibenclamide. Similarly, the *G. tricophylla* group and the glibenclamide group presented a significant reduction in the fasting blood glucose, compared to the non-treated diabetes control. Likewise, the *G. tricophylla* and glibenclamide groups presented lower total cholesterol, total triglyceride, low-density lipoprotein, creatinine, and urea levels, as well as higher levels of high-density lipoprotein compared to the non-treated diabetes rats. The authors suggested that the observed effects could be attributed to the prevention of β cell death induced by alloxan, as well as a reduction in the absorption of glucose from the intestinal tract (Alam and Saquib 2017).

6.5.3 Effects on Advanced Glycation End Products (AGEs)

Micro- and macrovascular diabetes complications are multifactorial and may occur as a result of chronic hyperglycemia that leads to the biochemical process of advanced glycation (Gho and Cooper 2008). AGEs are formed through non-enzymatic reactions between the amine residue of proteins, nucleic acids, or lipids and the reducing end of carbohydrates such as glucose and fructose (Kuzan 2021). AGEs, such as pentosidine and *N*(carboxymethyl)lysine (CML), can activate specific receptors (RAGEs) that in turn activate proinflammatory pathways implicated in the initiation and progression of diabetic vascular damage (Stern et al. 2002). In addition, receptor-independent effects, such as cross-linking with extracellular matrix proteins, can contribute to the microvascular damage observed in diabetes (Goh and Cooper 2008). As a consequence, the inhibition of AGE formation is considered a potential therapeutic target to decrease and prevent the complications of diabetes (Singh et al. 2014). Due to their antioxidant capacity, plant phenolics are of particular interest in the prevention of the damage exerted by AGEs (Wu and Yen 2005; Jiménez-Aspee et al. 2016).

An ethanol extract from the leaves of *Gaultheria hispidula* was assayed for its capacity to prevent AGE formation (Harris et al. 2011). The extract inhibited the formation of AGEs by 30%–60% in a serum bovine albumin/glucose + fructose model at concentrations ranging from 0.39 to 10 µg/mL, respectively. Interestingly, the inhibitory effects were partially lost at concentrations higher than 10 µg/mL. The authors evaluated by Western blot the presence of CML-BSA adducts and observed that the *G. hispidula* extract decreased the adduct formation in a concentration-dependent manner, achieving its maximum effect of 67.8 ± 5.7% inhibition at 25 µg/mL. AGEs formation was also quantified based on their fluorescent properties (λ_{exc} 355 nm, λ_{em} 460 nm), and IC_{50} values were calculated. The *G. hispidula* extract presented an IC_{50} of 1.5 ± 0.2 µg/mL, which was in the same range than that exerted by the positive control quercetin (1.8 ± 0.7 µg/mL) and ranked fourth among 17 different plant extracts evaluated (Harris et al. 2011). The authors reported that the antiglycation activity observed was positively correlated with the total phenolic content and the antioxidant activity of the extract.

6.6 TOXICITY AND CAUTIONARY NOTES

The *Gaultheria* species are normally considered safe for human consumption as food and as herbal medicine. An exception is *G. insana*, whose fruits have been traditionally considered as "bad, with bad taste and even poisonous" (Mösbach 1992). Additionally, due to the high content of methyl salicylate in some species, such as *G. tenuifolia* and *G. procumbens*, the strong wintergreen flavor can be overwhelming for consumption.

Cytochromes P450 are a superfamily of enzymes functioning as monooxygenases that are essential for the biosynthesis of cholesterol, steroids, and prostaglandins. They are also important for the detoxification of xenobiotics and can be inhibited or induced by different substrates leading to interactions of clinical importance. The inhibition of the cytochrome P450 enzyme complex by the leaf extract of *G. procumbens* was reported (Scott et al. 2006). The extract inhibited the activity of CYP3A4 and CYP19 by 72% and 41%, respectively, at a concentration of 55 µg/mL. The extract ranked first as an inhibitor of CYP3A4 and sixth as an inhibitor of CYP19 among ten species studied. In another study, the ethanol extract of *G. hispidula* also showed inhibitory activities against CYP1A2 (15.3 ± 3.9%), 2C9 (25.3 ± 4.1%), 2C19 (23.7 ± 1.1%), 2E1 (34.6 ± 4.3%), 19 (11.7 ± 3.2%), 3A4 (65.1 ± 8.6), 3A5 (57.6 ± 11.3), and 3A7 (49.2 ± 2.5%) (Tam et al. 2009). In addition, the extract showed inhibitory activity against flavin-containing monooxygenase 3 (FMO3) by 64.0 ± 0.8% (Tam et al. 2009). Unlike the previous study, the *G. hispidula* ranked 14th among 17 species studied. In another study, the same extract inhibited by almost 70% the metabolism of repaglinide in a human liver microsome-mediated assay but did not affect the activity of UDP-glucuronosyltransferase (UDPG) (Cieniak et al. 2013). Altogether, the findings of both studies are of clinical importance since the parallel use of *Gaultheria* berries with antidiabetic drugs could potentially influence the bioavailability and pharmacokinetics of drugs, thus affecting the outcomes of pharmacological therapy and increase the incidence of side effects such as hypoglycemia for sulfonylureas, glitazones, and other substrates of CYP450.

Regarding the cytotoxic effects of *Gaultheria* species, since the 1930s several studies have shown their potential for the treatment of different types of cancer (Luo et al. 2018). Most of the studies are focused on the essential oil and fractions rich in terpenes, dilactones, and saponins obtained from *G. iotana, G. yunnanensis,* and *G. tricophylla* against different cancer cell lines (Chen et al. 2009;

Li et al. 2010; Li et al. 2018). The fruit extracts from *G. phillyreifolia*, *G. poeppigii*, and *G. tenuifolia* showed a lack of cytotoxic effect against AGS and Caco-2 cells up to concentrations of 200 μg/mL (Mieres-Castro et al. 2019; Mieres-Castro et al. 2020).

Hence, the evidence regarding the potential toxicity of *Gaultheria* species is limited to *in vitro* assays in cell culture and some studies carried out in *Artemia salina* (Plazas González 2015). It is important to take into consideration the effects on the cytochrome enzyme complex and the potential pharmacokinetic/pharmacodynamic interactions. *In vivo* studies on the antidiabetic effects of *Gaultheria* species should be designed while taking these observations into consideration.

6.7   SUMMARY POINTS

- This chapter focuses on the antidiabetic potential of *Gaultheria* species.
- Asian, North, and South American Indigenous populations have used the *Gaultheria* species in traditional medicine.
- Leaves and berries of *Gaultheria* species have inhibitory activities against α-amylase, α-glucosidase, and DPP4.
- Leaves and berries of *Gaultheria* species inhibit the glucose uptake and metabolism in intestinal, hepatic, and muscle cells.
- Leaves and berries of *Gaultheria* species can decrease the mRNA levels of glucose transporters in intestinal cells.
- Animal studies show that *Gaultheria* species can help normalize the glycemia and the biochemical profile of diabetes-induced animals.
- *In vitro* evidence shows that *Gaultheria* species are nontoxic but can affect the activity of phase I enzymes and thus potentially have pharmacokinetic interactions with drugs and other herbs.
- Therefore, the effect of *Gaultheria* species for the prevention and treatment of diabetes is still not completely understood but has promising potential worthy of future research.

REFERENCES

Alam, Fianz, and Qazi Najam us Saquib. 2017. Anti-diabetic potential of *Gaultheria tricophylla* in mice. *Bangladesh Journal of Pharmacology* 12, 292–298.

Alzaid, Fawaz, Hoi-Man Cheung, Victor R. Preedy, and Paul A. Sharp. 2013. Regulation of glucose transporter expression in human intestinal Caco-2 cells following exposure to an anthocyanin-rich berry extract. *PLoS ONE* 8, e78932.

American Diabetes Association (ADA). 2021. 9. Pharmacologic approaches to glycemic treatment: Standards of medical care in diabetes – 2021. *Diabetes Care* 44, S111–S124.

Babu, Pon Velayutham, Dongmin Liu, and Elizabeth R. Gilbert. 2013. Recent advances in understanding the anti-diabetic actions of dietary flavonoids. *Journal of Nutritional Biochemistry* 24, 1777–1789.

Calvano, Aaron, Kenneth Izuora, Edwin C. Oh, Jeffrey L. Ebersole, Timothy J. Lyons, and Arpita Basu. 2019. Dietary berries, insulin resistance and type 2 diabetes: An overview of human feeding trials. *Food and Function* 10, 6227–6243.

Castro-Acosta, Monica L., Stephanie G. Stone, Jonathan E. Mok, Rhia K. Mhajan, Chi-leng Fu, Georgia N. Lenihan-Geels, Christopher P. Corpe, and Wendy L. Hall. 2017. Apple and blackcurrant polyphenol-rich drinks decrease postprandial glucose, insulin and incretin response to a high-carbohydrate meal in healthy men and women. *Journal of Nutritional Biochemistry* 49, 53–62.

Chen, Chun-Yin, Rong-Jyh Lin, Jin-Cherng Huang, Yi-Hung Wu, Ming-Jen Cheng, His-Chou Hung, and Wen-Li Lo. 2009. Chemical constituents from the whole plant of *Gaultheria itoana* Hayata. *Chemistry and Biodiversity* 6, 1737–1743.

Chen, Zhangling, Djawad Radjabzadeh, Lianmin Chen, Alexander Kurilshikov, Maryam Kavousi, Fariba Ahmadizar, M. Arfan Ikram, et al. 2021. Association of insulin resistance and type 2 diabetes with gut microbial diversity: A microbiome-wide analysis from population studies. *JAMA Network Open* 4, e2118811.

Cieniak, Carolina, Rui Liu, Alexandra Fottinger, Sheila A.M. Smiley, Jose A. Guerrero Analco, Steffany A.L. Bennett, Pierre S. Haddad, et al. 2013. In vitro inhibition of metabolism but not transport of glicazide and repaglinide by Cree medicinal plant extracts. *Journal of Ethnopharmacology* 150, 1087–1095.

Cong, Fei, Khem Raj Joshi, Hari Prasad Devkota, Takashi Watanabe, and Shoji Yahara. 2015. Dhasingreoside: New flavonoid from the stems and leaves of *Gaultheria fragantissima*. *Natural Product Research* 29, 1442–1448.

Evert, Alison B., Jackie L. Boucher, Marjorie Cypress, Stephanie A. Dunbar, Marion J. Franz, Elizabeth J. Mayer-Davis, Joshua J. Neumiller, et al. 2014. Nutrition therapy recommendations for the management of adults with diabetes. *Diabetes Care* 37, S120–S143.

Ferguson, Andrew, Elisabete Carvalho, Geraldine Gourlay, Vincent Walker, Stefan Martens, Juha-Pekka Salminen, and C. Peter Constabel. 2018. Phytochemical analysis of salal berry (*Gaultheria shallon* Pursh.), a traditionally-consumed fruit from western North America with exceptionally high proanthocyanidin content. *Phytochemistry* 147, 203–210.

Fernández-Galleguillos, Carlos, Luisa Quesada-Romero, Adrián Puerta, José M. Padrón, Ernane Souza, Javier Romero-Parra, and Mario J. Simirgiotis. 2021. UHPLC-MS chemical fingerprinting and antioxidant, antiproliferative, and enzyme inhibition potential of *Gaultheria pumila* berries. *Metabolites* 11, 523.

Goh, Su-Yen, and Mark E. Cooper. 2008. The role of advanced glycation end products in progression and complications of diabetes. *The Journal of Clinical Endocrinology & Metabolism* 93, 1143–1152.

Gong, Lingxiao, Danning Feng, Tianxi Wang, Yuqin Ren, Yingli Liu, and Jing Wang. 2020. Inhibitors of α-amylase and α-glucosidase: Potential linkage for whole cereal foods on prevention of hyperglycemia. *Food Science and Nutrition* 8, 6320–6337.

Gromova, Lyudmila V., Serguei O. Fetissov, and Andrey A. Gruzdkov. 2021. Mechanisms of glucose absorption in the small intestine in health and metabolic diseases and their role in appetite regulation. *Nutrients* 13, 2474.

Guo, Xiao-Fei, Bo Yang, J. Tan, and D. Li. 2016. Association of dietary intakes of anthocyanins and berry fruits with risk of type 2 diabetes mellitus: A systematic review and meta-analysis of prospective cohort studies. *European Journal of Clinical Nutrition* 70, 1360–1367.

Hanhineva, Kati, Riitta Törrönen, Isabel Bondia-Pons, Jenna Pekkinen, Marjukka Kolehmainen, Hannu Mykkänen, and Kaisa Poutanen. 2010. Impact of dietary polyphenols on carbohydrate metabolism. *International Journal Molecular Science* 11, 1365–1402.

Harbilas, Despina, Louis C. Martineau, Cory S. Harris, Danielle C.A. Adeyiwola-Spoor, Ammar Saleem, Jennifer Lambert, Dayna Caves, et al. 2009. Evaluation of the antidiabetic potential of selected medicinal plant extracts from the Canadian boreal forest used to treat symptoms of diabetes: Part II. *Canadian Journal of Physiology and Pharmacology* 87, 479–492.

Harris, Cory S., Louis-Philippe Beaulieu, Marie-Hélene Fraser, Kristina L. McIntyre, Patrick L. Owen, Louis C. Martineau, Alain Cuerrier, et al. 2011. Inhibition of advanced glycation end products formation by medicinal plant extracts correlates with phenolic metabolites and antioxidant activity. *Planta Medica* 77, 196–204.

Hu, Ya-Jie, Qian Lan, Bao-Jun Su, Zhen-Feng Chen, and Dong Liang. 2022. Structurally diverse abietane-type diterpenoids from the aerial parts of *Gaultheria leucocarpa var. yunnanensis*. *Phytochemistry* 201, 113255.

Jiménez-Aspee, Felipe, Cristina Theoduloz, Mariana Neves Vieira, Miriam A. Rodríguez-Werner, Eva Schmalfuss, Peter Winterhalter, and Guillermo Schmeda-Hirschmann G. 2016. Phenolics from the Patagonian currants *Ribes* spp: Isolation, characterization and cytoprotective effect in human AGS cells. *Journal of Functional Foods* 26, 11–26.

Kazakos, Kyriakaos. 2011. Incretin effect: GLP-1, GIP, DPP4. *Diabetes Research and Clinical Practice* 93S, S32–S36.

Kazeem, Mutiu I., and Theophilus C. Davies. 2016. Anti-diabetic functional foods as sources of insulin secreting, insulin sensitizing and insulin mimetic agents. *Journal of Functional Foods* 20, 122–138.

Koepsell, Hermann. 2020. Glucose transporters in the small intestine in health and disease. *European Journal of Physiology* 472, 1207–1248.

Kuzan, Aleksandra. 2021. Toxicity of advanced glycation end products (review). *Biomedical Reports* 14, 46.

Leduc, Charles, Jason Coonishish, Pierre S. Haddad, and Alain Cuerrier. 2006. Plants used by the Cree nation of Eeyou Istchee (Quebec, Canada) for the treatment of diabetes: A novel approach in quantitative ethnobotany. *Journal of Ethnopharmacology* 105, 55–63.

Li, Jun, Fu Li, Yuan-Yuan Lu, Xiao-Jiang Su, Cui-Ping Huang, and Xue-Wen Lu. 2010. A new dilactone from the seeds of *Gaultheria yunnanensis. Fitoterapia* 81, 35–37.

Li, Shilin, Sarah Pasquin, Hoda M. Eid, Jean-Francois Gauchat, Ammar Saleem, and Pierre S. Haddad. 2018. Antiapoptotic potential of several antidiabetic medicinal plants of the eastern James Bay Cree pharmacopoeia in cultured kidney cells. *BMC Complementary and Alternative Medicine* 18, 37.

Liu, Wei-Rui, Wen-Lin Qiao, Zi-Zhen Liu, Xiao-Hong Wang, Rui Jiang, Shu-Yi Li, Ren-Bing Shi, Gai-Me She. 2013. *Gaultheria*: Phytochemical and pharmacological characteristics. *Molecules* 18, 12071–12108.

Luo, Bin-Sheng, Rong-Hui Gu, Edward J. Kennelly, and Chun-Lin Long. 2018. *Gaultheria* ethnobotany and bioactivity: Blueberry relatives with anti-inflammatory, antioxidant, and anticancer constituents. *Current Medicinal Chemistry* 25, 51168.

Luo, Bin-Sheng, Ertan Kastrat, Taylan Morcol, Haiping Cheng, Edward J. Kennelly, Chun-Lin Long. 2021. *Gaultheria longibracteolata*, an alternative source for wintergreen oil. *Food Chemistry* 342, 128244.

Mabberley, David J. 1997. *The Plant-Book*, 2nd ed. Cambridge: Cambridge University Press, p. 295.

Marles, Robin J., and Norman R. Farnsworth. 1995. Antidiabetic plants and their active constituents. *Phytomedicine* 2, 137–189.

McCune, Letitia M., and Timothy Johns. 2002. Antioxidant activity in medicinal plants associated with the symptoms of diabetes mellitus used by the indigenous peoples of the North American boreal forest. *Journal of Ethnopharmacology* 82, 197–205.

McDougall, Gordon, Ceri Austin, E. Van Schayk, and Peter Martin. 2016. Salal (*Gaultheria shallon*) and aronia (*Aronia melanocarpa*) fruits from Orkney: Phenolic content, composition and effect of wine making. *Food Chemistry* 205, 239–247.

Michel, Piotr, Sebastian Granica, Anna Magiera, Karolina Rosinska, Malgorzata Jurek, Lukasz Poraj, and Monika A. Oleswska. 2019. Salicylate and procyanidin-rich stem extracts of *Gaultheria procumbens* L. inhibit pro-inflammatory enzymes and suppress pro-inflammatory and pro-oxidant functions of human neutrophiles *ex vivo. International Journal of Molecular Sciences* 20, 1753.

Michel, Piotr, Aleksandra Owczarek, Magdalena Matczak, Martyna Kosno, Pawel Szymanski, Elzbieta Mikiciuk-Olasik, Anna Kilanowcicz, Wiktor Wesolowski, and Monika A. Olszewska. 2017. Metabolite profiling of eastern teaberry (*Gaultheria procumbens* L.) lipophilic leaf extracts with hyaluronidase and lipoxygenase inhibitory activity. *Molecules* 22, 412.

Mieres-Castro, Daniel, Guillermo Schmeda-Hirschmann, Cristina Theoduloz, Sergio Gómez-Alonso, José Pérez Navarro, Katherine Márquez, and Felipe Jiménez-Aspee. 2019. Antioxidant activity and isolation of polyphenols and new iridoids from Chilean *Gaultheria phillyreifolia* and *G. poeppigii* berries by counter-current chromatography. *Food Chemistry* 291, 167–179.

Mieres-Castro, Daniel, Guillermo Schmeda-Hirschmann, Cristina Theoduloz, Ana Rojas, Daniela Piderit, and Felipe Jiménez-Aspee. 2020. Isolation and characterization of secondary metabolites from *Gaultheria tenuifolia* berries. *Journal of Food Science* 85, 2792–2802.

Mieres-Castro, Daniel, Cristina Theoduloz, Nadine Sus, Alberto Burgos-Edwards, Guillermo Schmeda-Hirschmann, Jan Frank, and Felipe Jiménez-Aspee. 2022. Iridoids and polyphenols from Chilean gaultheria spp. Berries decrease the glucose uptake in caco-2 cells after simulated gastrointestinal digestion. *Food Chemistry* 369, 130940.

Mösbach, Ernest W. 1992. *Botánica Indígena de Chile*. Ed. C. Aldunate and C. Villagrán. Santiago de Chile: Editorial Andrés Bello, pp. 94–95.

Nachar, Abrir, Diane Vallerand, Lina Musallam, Louis Lavoie, Alaa Badawi, John Arnason, and Pierre S. Haddad. 2013. The action of antidiabetic plants of the Canadian James Bay Cree traditional pharmacopoeia on key enzymes of hepatic glucose metabolism. *Evidence-Based Complementary and Alternative Medicine*, ID 189819.

Nauck, Michael A., and Juris J. Meier. 2018. Incretin hormones: Their role in health and disease. *Diabetes, Obesity and Metabolism* 20, 5–21.

Ni, He, Helen E. Hayes, David Stead, Guang Liu, Huaijie Yang, Haihang Li, and Vassilios Raikos. 2019. Interaction of whey protein with polyphenols from salal fruits (*Gaultheria shallon*) and the effects on protein structure and hydrolysis by Flavourzyme®. *International Journal of Food Science and Technology* 55, 1281–1288.

Ni, He, Helen E. Hayes, David Stead, and Vassilios Raikos. 2018. Incorporating salal berry (*Gaultheria shallon*) and blackcurrant (*Ribes nigrum*) pomace in yogurt for the development of a beverage with antidiabetic properties. *Heliyon* 4, e00875.

Nikolić, Miloš, Tatjana Marković, Miloš Mojović, Boris Pejin, Aleksandar Savić, Tamara Perić, Dejan Marković, Tatjana Stević, and Marina Soković. 2013. Chemical composition and biological activity of *Gaultheria procumbens* L. essential oil. *Industrial Crops and Products* 49, 561–567.

Nistor Baldea, Lidia A., Louis C. Martineau, Ali Benhaddou-Andaloussi, John T. Arnason, Émile Lévz, and Pierre S. Haddad. 2010. Inhibition of intestinal glucose absorption by anti-diabetic medicinal plants derived from the James Bay Cree traditional pharmacopoeia. *Journal of Ethnopharmacology* 132, 473–482.

Olszewska, Monika A., Aleksandra Owczarek, Anna Magiera, Sebastian Granica, and Piotr Michel. 2021. Screening for the active anti-inflammatory and antioxidant polyphenols of *Gaultheria procumbens* and their application for standardization: From identification through cellular studies to quantitative determination. *International Journal of Molecular Sciences* 22, 11532.

Oyarzún, Paulina, Pablo Cornejo, Sergio Gómez-Alonso, and Antonieta Ruiz. 2020. Influence of profiles and concentrations of phenolic compounds in the coloration and antioxidant properties of *Gaultheria poeppigii* fruits from southern Chile. *Plant Foods for Human Nutrition* 75, 532–539.

Papuc, Camelia, Gheorghe V. Goran, Corina N. Predescu, Liliana Tudoreanu, and Georgeta Stefan. 2020. Plant polyphenols mechanism of action on insulin resistance and against the loss of pancreatic beta cells. *Critical Reviews in Food Science and Nutrition* 62, 325–352.

Patel, Dinesh K., Raj Kumar, Damiki Laloo, and Siva Hemalatha. 2012. Natural medicines from plant sources used for therapy of diabetes mellitus: An overview of its pharmacological aspects. *Asian Pacific Journal of Tropical Disease* 2, 239–250.

Plazas González, Erika A. 2015. Preliminary phytochemical screening, antioxidant, and toxic activity evaluation of six species of Colombian Ericaeas. *Revista Cubana de Plantas Medicinales* 19, 182–199.

Ruiz, Antonieta, Luis Bustamante, Carola Vergara, Dietrich von Baer, Isidro Hermosín-Gutiérrez, Luis Obando, and Claudia Mardones. 2015. Hydroxycinnamic acids and flavonoids in native edible berries of South Patagonia. *Food Chemistry* 167, 84–90.

Ruiz, Antonieta, Isidro Hermosín-Gutiérrez, Carola Vergara, Dietrich von Baer, Moisés Zapata, Antonieta Hitschfeld, Luis Obando, and Claudia Mardones. 2013. Anthocyanin profiles in south Patagonian wild berries by HPLC-DAD-ESI-MS/MS. *Food Research International* 51, 706–713.

Saleem, Ammar, Cory S. Harris, Muhammad Asim, Alain Cuerrier, Louis Martineau, Pierre S.-Haddad, and John T. Arnason. 2010. A RP-HPLC-DAD-APCI/MSD method for the characterization of medicinal Ericaceae used by the Eeyou Istchee Cree First Nations. *Phytochemical Analysis* 21, 328–339.

Schreckinger, Maria Elisa, Jennifer Lotton, Mary Ann Lila, and Elvira González de Mejía. 2010. Berries from South America: A comprehensive review on chemistry, health potential, and commercialization. *Journal of Medicinal Food* 13, 233–246.

Schwingshackl, Lukas, Georg Hoffmann, Anna-Maria Lampousi, Sven Knüppel, Khalid Iqbal, Carolina Schwedhelm, Angela Bechthold, Sabrina Schlesinger, and Heiner Boeing. 2017. Food groups and risk of type 2 diabetes mellitus: A systematic review and meta-analysis of prospective studies. *European Journal of Epidemiology* 32, 363–375.

Scott, Ian M., Renée I. Leduc, Andrew J. Burt, Robin J. Marles, John T. Arnason, and Brian C. Foster. 2006. The inhibition of human cytochrome P450 by ethanol extracts of North American botanicals. *Pharmaceutical Biology* 44, 315–327.

Singh, Varun P., Anjana Bali, Nirmal Singh, and Amteshwar S. Jaggi. 2014. Advanced glycation end products and diabetic complications. *The Korean Journal Physiology & Pharmacology* 18, 1–14.

Stern, David M., Shi Du Yan, Shi Fang Yan, and Ann Marie Schmidt. 2002. Receptor for advanced glycation end products (RAGE) and the complications of diabetes. *Ageing Research Reviews* 1, 1–15.

Sun, Chongde, Chao Zhao, Esra Capanoglu Guven, Paolo Paoli, Jesús Simal-Gandara, Kunka Mohanram Ramkumar, Shengpeng Wang, et al. 2020. Dietary polyphenols as antidiabetic agents: Advances and opportunities. *Food Frontiers* 1, 18–44.

Tam, Teresa W., Rui Liu, John T. Arnason, Anthony Krantis, William A. Staines, Pierre S. Haddad, and Brian C. Foster. 2009. Actions of ethnobotanically selected Cree anti-diabetic plants on human cytochrome P450 isoforms and flavin-containing monooxygenase 3. *Journal of Ethnopharmacology* 126, 119–126.

Teillier, Sebastián, and Felipe Escobar. 2013. Revision of the genus *Gaultheria* L. (Ericaceae) in Chile. *Gayana Botanica* 70, 136–153.

Törrönen, Riitta, Essi Sarkkinen, Niina Tapola, Elina Hautaniemi, Kyllikki Kilpi, and Leo Niskanen. 2010. Berries modify the postprandial plasma glucose response to sucrose in healthy subjects. *British Journal of Nutrition* 103, 1094–1097.

Wu, Chi-Hao, and Gow-Chin Yen. 2005. Inhibitory effect of naturally occurring flavonoids on the formation of advanced glycation endproducts. *Journal of Agricultural and Food Chemistry* 53, 3167–3173.

Xu, G.L., Z.Z. Liu, M. Xie, X. Zhang, Y. Yang, C. Yan, W.L. Qiao, et al. 2016. Salicylic acid derivatives and other components from *Gaultheria trichoclada*. *Chemistry of Natural Compounds* 52, 301–303.

7 Arjuna (*Terminalia arjuna*), the Natural Dipeptidyl Peptidase IV Inhibitor, Offers Cardiometabolic Protection

*Ipseeta Ray Mohanty, Manjusha Borde,
Selvaa Kumar C and Rajesh Kumar Suman*

CONTENTS

ABBREVIATIONS

AI	atherogenic index
ALT	alanine aminotransferase
AST	aspartate aminotransferase
BNP	brain natriuretic peptide
CPK-MB	creatinine phosphokinase
DPP-IV	dipeptidyl peptidase-IV
ECG	electrocardiography
HbA_{1c}	glycosylated hemoglobin

DOI: 10.1201/9781003220930-9

HDL-C	high-density lipoprotein cholesterol
hs-CRP	high-sensitivity C-reactive protein
IDDM	insulin-dependent diabetes mellitus
LDL-C	low-density lipoprotein cholesterol
LPO	lipid peroxidation
MDA	malondialdehyde
MI	myocardial infarction
NaF	sodium fluoride
NIDDM	non–insulin-dependent diabetes mellitus
TBARS	thiobarbituric acid reactive substances
TC	total cholesterol
TG	triglyceride
TNF-α	tumor necrosis factor-α
TUNEL	terminal deoxynucleotidyl transferase nick end labeling

7.1 INTRODUCTION

Terminalia arjuna, popularly known as *arjuna* in many local Indian languages, is a deciduous tree found throughout the country. The bark of *T. arjuna* is widely used as a cardiotonic in Ayurveda, the Indian system of medicine (Dwivedi and Chopra 2014). Its bark decoction is used in the Indian sub-continent for anginal pain, hypertension, congestive heart failure, and dyslipidemia, based on the observations of ancient physicians for centuries. The scientific description of *T. arjuna* is depicted in Table 7.1.

  I. Description
    a. Macroscopic
       Market samples up to 10 cm in length and 7 cm in width, outer surface somewhat smooth and gray, inner surface somewhat fibrous and pinkish, transversely cut smooth-ened bark shows pinkish surface, fracture, short in inner and laminated in outer section; taste, bitter and astringent (Ayurvedic Pharmacopoeia of India 2016).
    b. Microscopic
       Cork cambium and secondary cortex not distinct, and medullary rays observed travers-ing almost to outer bark; secondary phloem occupies a wide zone, consisting of sieve tubes, companion cells, phloem parenchyma, and phloem fibers, traversed by phloem rays, usually uniseriate but biseriate rays also occasionally seen. In a tangential cut, the uniseriate phloem rays 2–10 cells high and biseriate, 4–12 cells high; in a longitudinal section, rosette crystals of calcium oxalate discovered in the form of strands in the phloem parenchyma are observed (missing in *T. alata*).
    c. Powder
       Reddish-brown; pieces of cork cells, uniseriate phloem rays, fibers, a few rhomboi-dal crystals, starch grains simple and compound, round to oval, elliptic, containing 2–3 components with concentric striations and short narrow hilum, measuring 5–13 in diameter.
 II. Habitat and distribution: *Arjuna* trees grow to be about 60–80 feet tall. The arjuna is commonly seen growing in abundance near ponds and rivers in the Indo–Sub-Himalayan regions of Uttar Pradesh, South Bihar, Madhya Pradesh, Delhi, and the Deccan region. It may grow in virtually every soil type but prefers damp, fertile loam and red lateritic soils. It is also found in the forests of Sri Lanka, Burma, and Mauritius.
III. Botanical distribution: The tree is roughly 60–80 feet tall, according to botanists. *Arjuna* is a large evergreen shrub with a spreading crown and limbs that drop. The tree grows to enormous proportions in ideal locations, especially along stream banks. The leaves are

TABLE 7.1
Scientific Description of *Terminalia arjuna*

Kingdom	Plantae
Division	Magnoliophyta
Class	Magnoliopsida
Order	Myrtales
Family	Combretaceae
Genus	*Terminalia*
Species	*T. arjuna*
Common (Indian) Names	Arjun, arjuna, koha, kahu, arjan
Sanskrit	Kakubha, partha, svetavaha
Assamese	Arjun
Bengali	Arjuna
Gujrati	Sadad, arjuna, sajada
Hindi	Arjuna
Kannada	Matti, bilimatti, neermatti, mathichakke, kudare kivimase
Malayalam	Nirmasuthu, vellamaruthi, kellemasuthu, mattimora, torematti
Marathi	Arjuna, sadada
Oriya	Arjuna
Urdu	Arjun
Punjabi	Arjon
Tamil	Marudam
Telugu	Maddi
Plant parts used	Stem bark, fruit and leaves
Constituents	Tannins
	Triterpenoids, Glycosides, Flavonoids, Alkaloids

Terminalia arjuna plant photograph

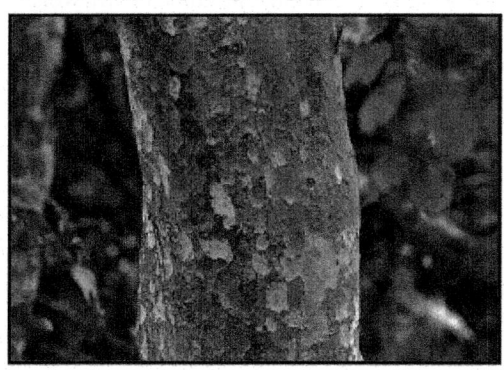

Terminalia arjuna stem bark photograph

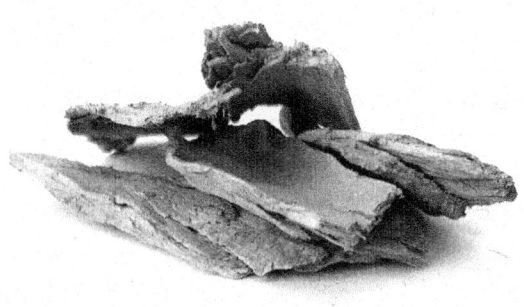

subopposite, oblong or elliptic, coriaceous, cordate, apex acute or obtuse. Flowers have panicle spikes and 2.5–5 cm long ovoid or ovoid-oblong fruits.

IV. Phytochemical constituents: Phytochemical constituents of various stem bark extracts revealed the presence of triterpenoids (such as arjunic acid, arjunolic acid, arjungenin, arjunetin, arjunoside, arjunolitin, arjugenin); tannins (pentagalloyl glucose, ellagic acid, hexaadroxdiphenyl galloyl glucose, tetragalloyl glucose); glycosides (arjunetin, arjunoside I, arjunoside II); and very high levels of flavonoids (arjunone, arjunolone, gallic acid, baicalein). The major chemical constituents present in stems include triterpenoids, glycosides, flavonoids, tannins and β-sitosterol. In the roots, triterpenoids, glycosides, and β-sitosterol. In the leaves, flavonoids, alkaloids, tannins, and steroids (Dwivedi and Chopra 2014).

V. Identity, purity and strength
- Foreign matter not more than 2%
- Total ash not more than 25%
- Acid–insoluble ash not more than 1%
- Alcohol–soluble extractive not less than 20%
- Water–soluble extractive not less than 20%

7.2 BACKGROUND

7.2.1 HISTORICAL USE OF *TERMINALIA ARJUNA* IN AYURVEDA

The bark of the *T. arjuna* tree is used in Ayurveda for treatment of various cardiac ailments. *T. arjuna* the miracle herb has been utilized during ancient times to cure heart problems. Its bark decoction is used in the Indian subcontinent for anginal pain, hypertension, congestive heart failure, and dyslipidemia, based on the observations of ancient physicians for centuries. Arjuna has been reported to be a beneficial herb in treating heart problems since 1200 BC. In the *Rigveda*, the word *arjuna* was used for the first time. Both Carakacharya and Sushrutacharya have mentioned this plant in their Samhitas but have not indicated its use for heart diseases. It was Vagbhatta who for the first time mentioned this in his book *Astang Hridayam* written some 1200 years ago for the use of Arjuna in the treatment of heart diseases, and the same was endorsed by Cakradattam and Bhavamisram (Kuleshwar 2021).

The bark has been used to treat fractures, ulcers, leukorrhea, diabetes, anemia, cardiopathy, and cirrhosis and has been described as an astringent, demulcent, expectorant, cardiotonic, styptic, antidysenteric, and urinary astringent (Jain et al. 2009). The eminent physician Chakradatta suggested it to be used as a bark decoction with milk or as a *ghrita* (a preparation with ghee or butter). Decoction of the bark has been used as ulcer wash, while bark ashes have been prescribed for snakebite and scorpion sting. Traditional healers from Kancheepuram district, Tamil Nadu boil the bark powder of *T arjuna* with water and inhale it to cure headache and to kill worms (Muthu et al. 2006). They also use fruit paste topically on wounds. Fresh leaf juice is used for the treatment of earache and bark powder for treating heart ailments by the Malabar tribe in Kerala. Tribes in the Sundargarh District, Orissa, cure hematuria with dried bark powder and rice-washed water, whereas tribes in Malkangiri chew the fresh bark and take the juice as an antacid (Dwivedi and Chopra 2014).

7.2.1.1 Medicinal Properties of Arjuna

Various extracts of the stem bark of arjuna have been shown to possess many pharmacological properties including inotropic, anti-ischemic, antioxidant, hypotensive, antiplatelet, hypolipidemic, anti-atherogenic, and antihypertrophic (Maulik and Talwar 2012; Amalraj and Gopi 2017).

- *Hypolipidemic*: enhances the elimination of cholesterol by accelerating the turnover of LDL-C in the liver. Lowers β-lipoprotein lipids and the recovery of HDL-C components in hyperlipidemia.
- *Cardiac stimulant*: Strengthens the heart muscles and maintains the heart functioning properly.
- *Hypotensive*: Due to its hypolipidemic activity and also the diuretic property, it acts against hypertension.
- *Astringent and hemostatic*: Has prostaglandin-enhancing and coronary risk modulating properties.
- *Antioxidant*: *T. arjuna* augments endogenous antioxidant enzyme activities, inhibiting lipid peroxidation and cytokine levels (Amalraj and Gopi 2016).

7.2.2 PROPERTIES OF ARJUNA MENTIONED IN AYURVEDIC PHARMACOPEIA, GOVERNMENT OF INDIA

Ayurvedic energetics: Arjuna possess the following properties:

- *Rasa (taste)*: Kasaya (astringent, bitter)
- *Guna (quality)*: Ruksa (light, dry)
- *Virya (action)*: Sita (cooling)
- *Vipaka (postdigestive effect)*: Katu (pungent)
- *Karma*: Bhagnasandhanakara, Hridya, Kaphahara, Pittahara, Vranasana, Vyanga Hara

Therapeutic uses: Medoroga, Vrana, Hrdroga, Ksataksaya, Prameha, Trsa, Vyanga.
Important formulations: Parthadyarista, Nagarjunabhra Rasa, Arjuna Ghrta.
Dose: 3–6 g of the drug in powder (Ayurvedic Pharmacopoeia of India 2016).

7.2.3 TOXICITY AND SIDE EFFECTS

Mild adverse effects have been recorded with *Terminalia arjuna*, including nausea, gastritis, headache, bodyache, constipation, and insomnia. Even after more than 24 months of use, no hematological, renal, or metabolic damage has been recorded (Dwivedi et al. 1989). However, Parmar et al. discovered that giving arjuna to euthyroid rats resulted in a decrease in thyroid hormone levels while increasing hepatic lipid peroxidation (LPO). As a result, large doses of the plant extract should be avoided because they can cause hepatotoxicity and hypothyroidism (Parmar et al. 2006). The results of a recent acute and oral toxicological research in animals revealed that giving ethanolic extract to animals at a limit dose of 2000 mg/kg orally did not cause toxicity or death (Patil et al. 2011).

7.3 STATUS OF RESEARCH OF *TERMINALIA ARJUNA*

7.3.1 EXPERIMENTAL STUDIES

The benefits of *T. arjuna* on diabetes mellitus and cardiovascular illnesses have been scientifically shown. *T. arjuna* extract were found to have antidiabetic properties in both HFD/STZ and alloxan-induced diabetes mellitus in several studies (Parveen et al. 2011a). In addition, arjunarishta, a hydroalcoholic preparation of *T. arjuna*, has been shown to have an antihyperglycemic and antihyperlipidemic impact in a high-fat diet model, which could be mediated by decreased TNF-α and elevated PGC-1α and IRS-1 (Sushant et al. 2018). An *in vitro* investigation found that *T. arjuna* bark extract stimulated insulin production, improved insulin action, blocked starch digestion, and prevented protein glycation at the cellular level (Thomson et al. 2014). The impact of *T. arjuna* 500 mg/kg extract to diabetic rats was found to be nearly identical to that of standard therapy glimepiride (Kumar et al. 2013).

T. arjuna protects the rat heart from isoproterenol-induced myocardial ischemic reperfusion injury by boosting endogenous antioxidant compounds (Karthikeyan et al. 2003). In addition, *T. arjuna* has been shown to protect against caffeine-induced coronary heart disease (Asha and Taju 2012). In isoproterenol-induced chronic heart failure, *T. arjuna* extract has preventive and therapeutic potential, probably via preserving endogenous antioxidant enzyme activities and suppressing lipid peroxidation and cytokine levels. *T. arjuna* improves cardioprotection against oxidative stress associated with IR injury by activating myocardial heat shock protein 72 and increasing endogenous antioxidants in rats without causing cellular damage (Karunakaran 2015). Similarly, *in vivo* ischemia-reperfusion injury–induced oxidative stress, heart tissue injury, and hemodynamic effects were all mitigated in rabbit hearts treated with *T. arjuna*, providing scientific support for its putative therapeutic benefit in ischemic heart disease (Gauthaman et al. 2005).

An ethanol extract of *T. arjuna*, antioxidant properties have been proven to protect mouse hearts against sodium fluoride (NaF)-induced oxidative damage (Sinha et al. 2008). *T. arjuna* has been shown to restore the gene regulatory network in the rat heart that has been disrupted by ISO treatment, indicating that it is effective in preventing ISO-induced cardiac hypertrophy (Kumar et al. 2019). Furthermore, hypotension and bradycardia were also observed after injection of the extract into the lateral cerebral ventricle and vertebral artery, indicating that beneficial effects are primarily of central origin (Singh et al. 1982). Thyroid hormones were investigated for their possible involvement in the amelioration of cardiac and hepatic lipid peroxidation by a bark extract of *T. arjuna* in albino rats, implying that the drug action could be mediated through an inhibition of thyroid function (Parmar et al. 2006) In anesthetized dogs, intravenous injection of *T. arjuna* caused dose-dependent hypotension. The observed impact could be attributable to adrenergic 2-receptor agonistic and/or direct action on the heart, confirming its historic use in cardiovascular diseases (Nammi et al. 2003).

7.3.2 CLINICAL STUDIES

The efficacy of *Terminalis arjuna* bark in cardiac diseases has been studied in a variety of ways. Patients with ischemic cardiomyopathy exhibited considerable symptomatic improvement in coronary heart failure with *T. arjuna*. Following that, it was revealed in an open-label trial that monotherapy with *T. arjuna* is fairly helpful in people with stable angina but has a partial role in patient with unstable angina (Dwivedi and Jauhari 1997). Patients with chronic stable angina with evidence of provocable ischemia on treadmill test were given *T. arjuna* (500 mg, every 8 hours) and isosorbide mononitrate (40 mg/day) for 1 week each in a randomized, double-blind, crossover study. When compared to placebo management, *T. arjuna* improved clinical and treadmill exercise parameters in individuals with stable angina and provocable ischemia during treadmill exercise (Bharani et al. 2002). The effectiveness of the *T. arjuna*–based herbal product Hartone was tested in ten patients with stable angina. The findings were compared to those of ten patients with stable angina who were given 20 mg of isosorbide mononitrate twice a day. Hartone was found to provide excellent tolerability and symptomatic relief in 80% of patients compared to 70% in those treated with isosorbide mononitrate (Kumar et al. 1999).

It was documented that the impact of *T. arjuna* on left ventricular hypertrophy regression in hypertensive individuals was due to its negatively chronotropic and ionotropic qualities (Rao et al. 2001). *T. arjuna* has a favorable impact in people with severe refractory heart failure. There was a substantial improvement in left ventricular metrics and functional capacity when patients with dilated cardiomyopathy and lower left ventricular ejection fraction received *T. arjuna* (500 mg every 8 hours) in addition to their standard medication, according to a recent open design trial. In a two-phase, double-blind, placebo-controlled study including 12 patients with refractory congestive heart failure, the effect of *T. arjuna* (500 mg every 8 hours) was studied. The echo–left ventricular end-diastolic and end-systolic volume indices both decreased, whereas the left ventricular stroke volume index and left ventricular ejection fraction both increased, indicating improvement (Bharani et al. 1995). *T. arjuna* has been shown to improve cardiovascular endurance while also lowering systolic blood pressure in healthy subjects. Furthermore, *T. arjuna* bark extract was found to have beneficial effects on blood pressure in patients with coronary artery disease (Sandhu et al. 2010). *T. arjuna* was observed to reduce ischemic mitral regurgitation and anginal frequency in patients with ischemic mitral regurgitation after an acute MI in a randomized, double-blind, placebo-controlled study. In addition, the diastolic dysfunction was much improved (Dwivedi et al. 2005). The efficacy of *T. arjuna* in decompensated rheumatic heart disease was studied in a double-blind study in which 30 patients with congestive heart failure and rheumatic valvular heart disease were given 200 mg *T. arjuna* three times daily. Significant improvements in left ventricular ejection fraction, exercise duration, and heart size were found (Antani et al. 1991).

7.3.3 LABORATORY FINDINGS (IN SILICO, IN VITRO AND IN VIVO STUDIES) WITH TERMINALIS ARJUNA

7.3.3.1 In Silico Study Results with Active Ingredients of *Terminalia arjuna*

Availability of voluminous chemical compounds from plant derivatives and drug molecules in both 2D and 3D format has made protein-ligand docking and virtual screening possible. In addition to this, in silico–based methods help in identifying the active site pocket required for docking with the selected chemical compounds with the help of docking software. Conversely, crystallized and modeled proteins can be energy minimized to optimize them to the near-native state. All these bioinformatics-based methods were converged to identify the active ingredients of medicinal plants having DPP-IV binding activity. The DPP-IV inhibitory activity of the active ingredients of the medicinal plants was directly proportional to the binding affinity for the DPP-IV enzyme. In this study, some selective medicinal active compounds were computationally designed, and potential binding affinity studies and binding sites against the crystal structure of DPP-IV were carried out (Karthik 2004).

The crystal structure of human DPP-IV (PDB ID: 2QT9) was downloaded from the Protein Databank which has a resolution of 2.1 Å in complex with 4-aryl cyclohexylalanine inhibitor. This was considered as a receptor for docking studies. In this crystal structure, 38 amino acids were missing. All the ligands and water molecules were deleted and were further subjected to energy minimization using CHIMERA standalone software. Within the parameters, the steepest descent steps were maintained at 100 and the conjugate gradient steps were at 10 with an update interval of 10. The optimized structure was further structurally validated using ProSA-Web and PROCHECK-Ramachandran plot analysis and considered for docking with the available ligands (Wiederstein 2007). The chemical compounds considered for protein-ligand docking included the active ingredients of *Terminalia arjuna* (arjunetin, arjungenin, arjunic acid arjunone, ellagic acid, and gallic acid), sitagliptin, and vildagliptin. A search was initiated to download the ten ligands from the PubChem database, which listed all of them except arjunic acid; these nine ligands were downloaded (Kim et al. 2021). Arjunic acid was obtained from ChemFaces (www.chemfaces.com). Ligands available in SDF file format were further subjected to stable conformer generation using Frog v2.14 (FRee Online druG conformation generation) wherein the 2D format is converted into 3D PDB format (Miteva et al. 2010).

In the Frog2 online server, the input was maintained as "1D to 2D" and the input drug description was "SDF." In the calculation parameters the output format was maintained as "PDB." The minimize option was opted as "yes." In the produce option we selected "single" because the "multiple" option gives many conformers. The total number of conformers generated was kept as 100, while the rest of the options were left at the default. A single conformer generated from each chemical compound was selected for docking with the receptor protein. The active site residues required for docking the ligands against DPP-IV were retrieved through literature search and also predicted based on the CASTp online server (Binkowski et al. 2003) to identify potential pockets. Additionally, the downloaded PDB ID: 2QT9 with their inhibitor 4-aryl cyclohexylalanine in complex state was considered as the reference pose for the docking of DPP-IV of *Homo sapiens* against all the available chemical compounds. Now the energy minimized receptor and the optimized 3D generated ligands were considered for docking using Hex software 8.0.0 (Ritchie 2005). This interactive molecular graphics program was used for calculating and displaying feasible docking modes which uses spherical polar Fourier (SPF) correlations to accelerate the calculations. While docking, within the docking parameter settings, "shape and electro" was selected for correlation type. The sampling method was maintained at "range angles." Postprocessing was kept at "OPLS minimization." The rest of the options were left at the default. Each run generated top ten docked poses, which were downloaded and considered for further analysis using Swiss-PdbViewer (Guex and Peitsch 1997) and CHIMERA software.

In this study, the energy minimized DPP-IV receptor and the stable conformers were considered for protein-ligand docking. The available chemicals in 2D format were converted into 3D format and further minimized using Frog2 software. Based on the CASTp report, there were 198 pockets listed, of which the largest pocket displayed an area of 6086.4 Å^2 and a volume of 16471 Å^3. The second largest pocket had an area of 574.3 Å^2 with a volume of 1171.8 Å^3. The largest pocket was in accordance with the binding site of 4-aryl cyclohexylalanine inhibitor binding site from 2QT9 crystal structure. The active site cavity is well guarded by residues including W659, Y631, Y547, P550, W629, Y752, F357, Y666, E205, E206, Y662, N710, R125, V656, S630, and V711. This site forms a deep cleft in DPP-IV which can be accessed via the opening of the propeller domain or through a side opening formed at the interface of the β-propeller and hydrolase domains. The β-propeller forms a funnel-shaped tunnel which extends toward the active site (Figure 7.1).

The propeller domain is well packed against the hydrolase domain and the catalytic triad (S630, H740, and D708) which is at the interface of the two domains. Docking chemical compounds

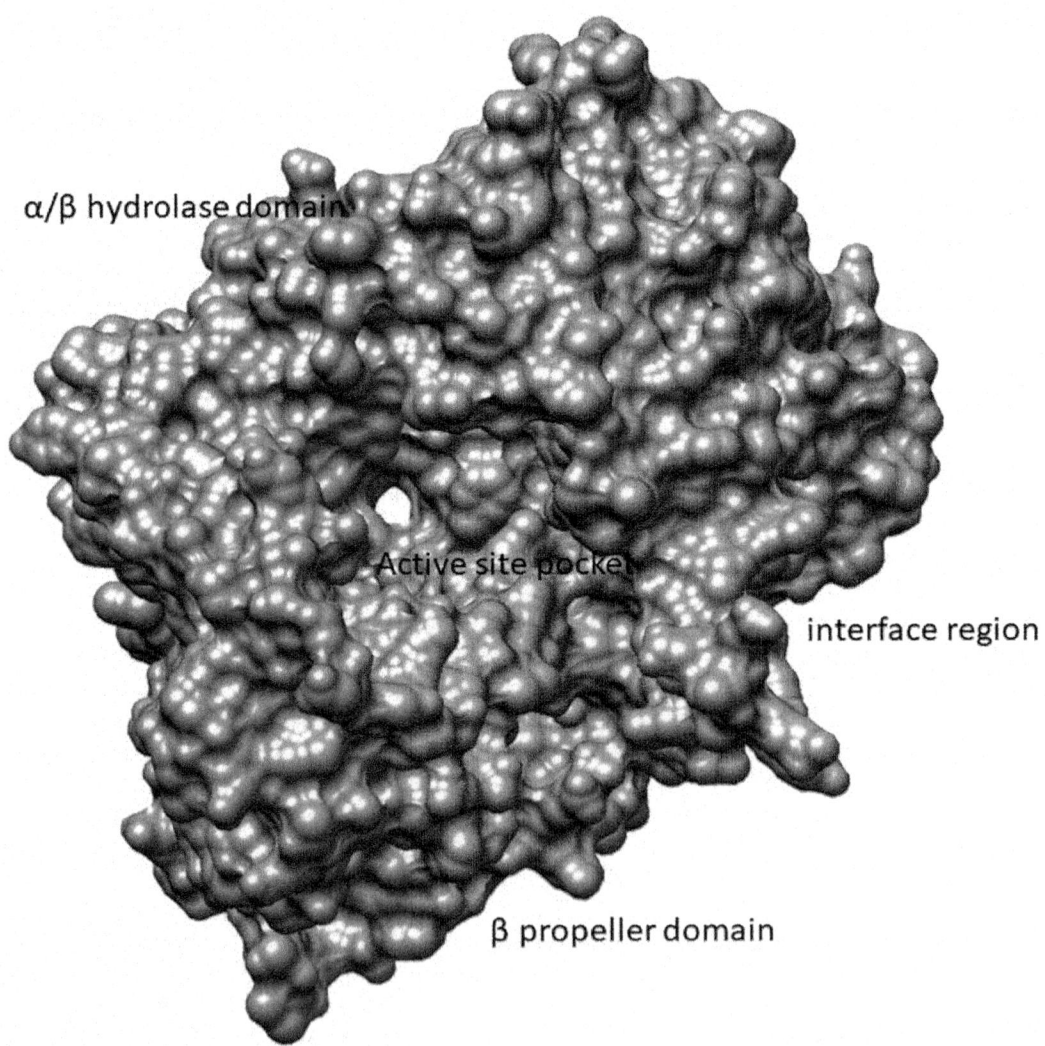

FIGURE 7.1   The molecular surface of the modeled human DPP-IV showing their distinct domains and the active site pocket.

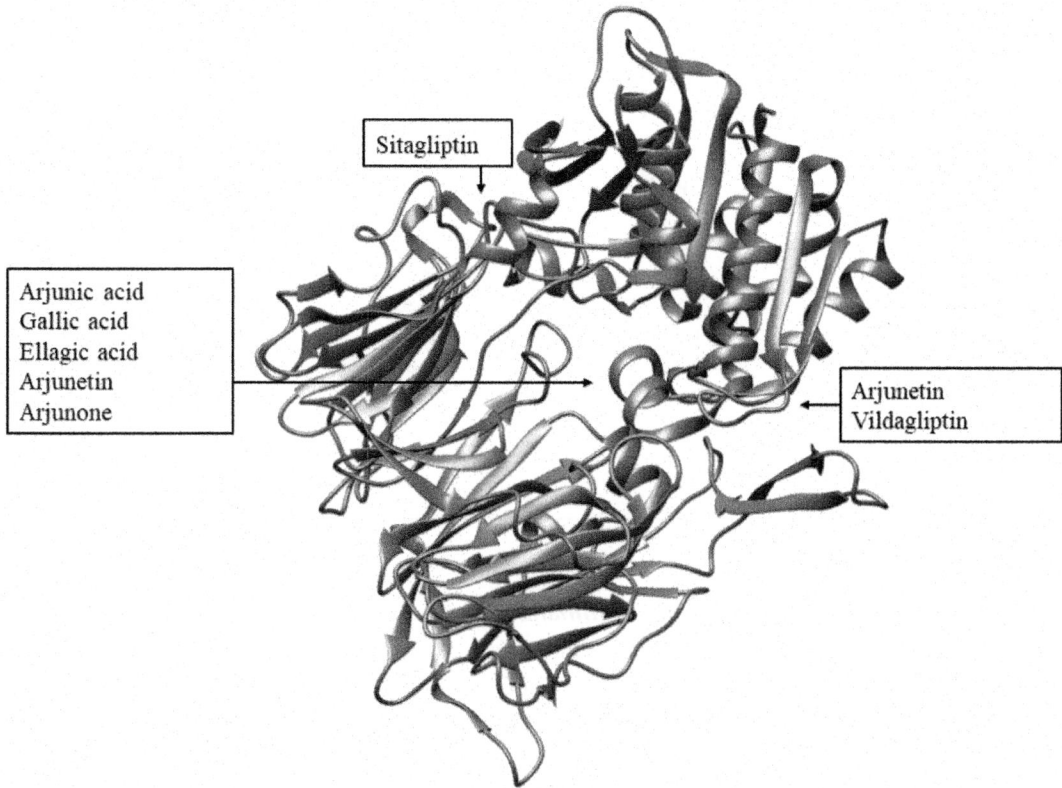

FIGURE 7.2   The three drug binding sites (α/β hydrolase domain, interface region, and β-propeller domain) occupied by drug molecules shown in ribbon format.

like arjunic acid, arjunone, and ellagic acid prefer to interact within the active site pocket. In particular, arjunone interacts in proximity with residues such as Glu205 and Glu206. Arjunetin and vildagliptin prefer to interact with the interface region. Sitagliptin interacts close to the α/β hydrolase domain. Gallic acid prefers to interact between the α/β hydrolase and β-propeller domains. However, as per CASTp prediction, in addition to the active site, the region of interface and the α/β hydrolase and β-propeller domain combo is also considered part of the largest active site pocket (Figure 7.2).

In summary, compounds like arjunic acid, arjunone, and ellagic acid prefer to bind within the active site pocket (the largest pocket), whereas sitagliptin prefers to bind in the second largest pocket (Table 7.2).

The availability of voluminous chemical compounds from plant derivatives and drug molecules in both 2D and 3D formats has made protein-ligand docking and virtual screening possible. In addition, in silico–based methods using docking software help identify the active site pocket required for docking with the selected chemical compounds. Conversely, crystallized and modeled proteins can be energy minimized to optimize them to the near-native state. All these bioinformatics-based methods were converged to identify the active ingredients of medicinal plants having DPP-IV binding activity. The DPP-IV inhibitory activity of the active ingredients of the medicinal plants was directly proportional to the binding affinity for the DPP-IV enzyme. In this study, some selective medicinal active compounds were computationally designed, and potential binding affinity studies and binding sites against the crystal structure of DPP-IV were carried out (Karthik 2004).

TABLE 7.2

Details of Active Ingredients of *Terminalia arjuna* with Their IC$_{50}$ Value, Binding Energy, and Interacting Residues against DPP-IV

Chemical compound	IC$_{50}$ (μM)	Binding energy (kcal/mol)	Amino acids
Terminalia arjuna			
Arjunetin	>50	−388.63	Asp737, Asp739
Arjungenin	>50	−348.95	Ile107
Arjunic acid	>50	−315.80	Arg358
Gallic acid	0.36	−182.63	Arg382
Arjunone	NA	−242.85	Ser209, Phe357
Ellagic acid	18.8	−270.42	Arg382
Standard DPP-IV Inhibitors			
Sitagliptin	18 nm	−139.91	Glu452
Vildagliptin	3 nm	−237.57	Asp739

7.3.3.2 *In Vitro* Study Results with *Terminalia arjuna*

The potential of manufacturing DPP-IV inhibitors from natural sources such as medicinal plants must be explored in order to uncover new sources of DPP-IV inhibitors. In our laboratory setting, the 1% hydroalcoholic extract of medicinal plant *T. arjuna* was screened for DPP-IV inhibitory activity by *in vitro* assay using an ELISA kit as per the Al-Masri 2009 approach with minor modifications (Al-Masri et al. 2009). According to the findings of our investigation, *T. arjuna* (86.39 ± 7.58%), exhibited significant DPP-IV inhibitory effect. DPP-IV inhibitors derived from synthetic sources are commercially available and have been employed in clinical trials as antidiabetic medicines. As a result, comparing the DPP-IV inhibitory efficacy of medicinal plants (natural DPP-IV inhibitor) to synthetic DPP-IV inhibitor proved intriguing. The 1% hydroalcoholic extract of medicinal plant extracts *Terminalia arjuna* was compared with the synthetic DPP-IV inhibitors vildagliptin and sitagliptin using *in vitro* DPP-IV assay. DPP-IV inhibitory activity of *T. arjuna* was comparable to marketed synthetic DPP-IV inhibitors (vildagliptin, 90.42 ± 7.84%; sitagliptin, 84.67 ± 8.21%), reflecting the potential benefits of developing an Indigenous DPP-IV inhibitor (Figure 7.3).

There was no statistically significant difference in DPP-IV inhibitory activity between the groups. The antidiabetic action of *T. arjuna* has been described in several study, but this is the first report of DPP-IV inhibitory efficacy. Therefore, it is selected for further studies in the experimental model of MI coexisting with diabetes mellitus.

7.3.4 In Vivo Study Results with Terminalia arjuna

DPP-IV–based therapeutics may represent novel antidiabetic drugs, the cardioprotective actions of which may translate into demonstrable therapeutic benefits in diabetes with coexisting cardiovascular diseases. With this point of view, the present study was designed to evaluate the DPP-IV inhibitory activity and cardioprotective efficacy of *T. arjuna* in an experimental model of MI coexisting with diabetes mellitus, and also to generate experimental evidence for possible placement of natural DPP-IV inhibitors in therapy by comparing their cardioprotective efficacy with standard antidiabetic drugs.

Monotherapy and combination therapy (with metformin 100 mg/kg) of *T. arjuna* (500 mg/kg) and synthetic DPP-IV inhibitor vildagliptin (10 mg/kg) were given to experimental rats for 4 weeks as per treatment protocol. The Streptozotocin (45 mg/kg body weight, i.p.) was injected to induce diabetes at 0 weeks. Subsequently, the rats were challenged with

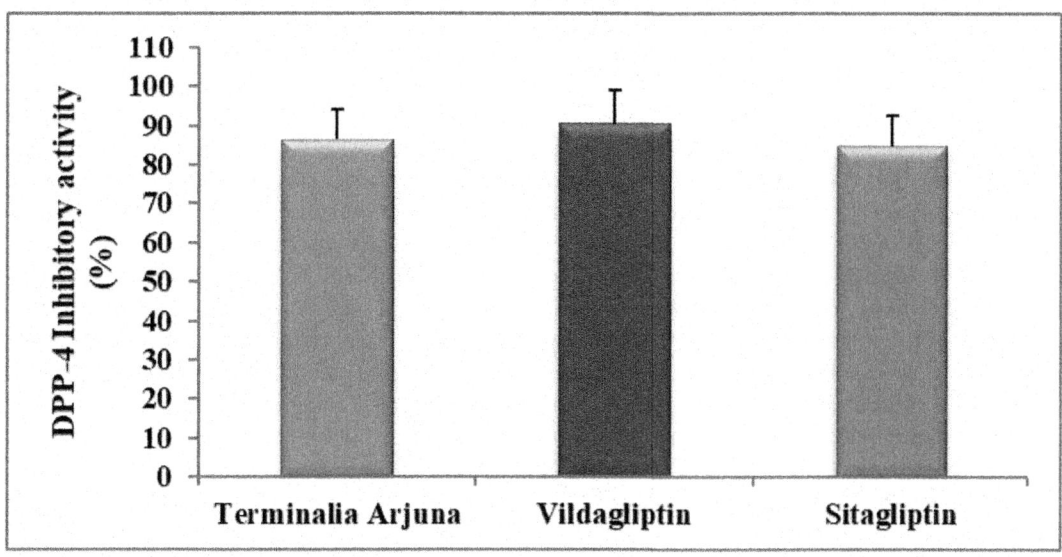

Each vertical bar represents the mean ± SD.

FIGURE 7.3 Comparative *in vitro* DPP-IV inhibitory activity.

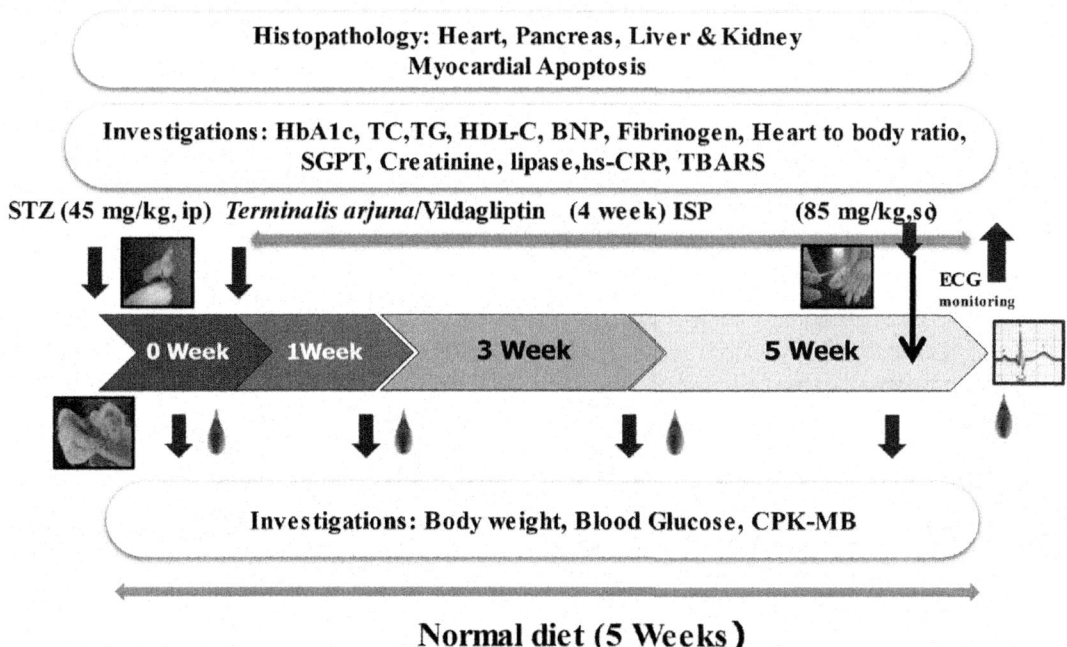

FIGURE 7.4 Experimental protocol of myocardial infarction coexisting with diabetes mellitus.

isoproterenol (85 mg/kg body weight sc) 24 and 48 hours prior to scarification to produce myocardial infarction (MI) (Figure 7.4).

The study provides evidence that the present experimental model can be used for studying myocardial changes associated with diabetes using a combination of inducing agents (isoproterenol and streptozotocin, which resulted in an altered DPP-IV pathway, prothrombotic state (fibrinogen), and marked apoptosis along with changes in functional (ECG), biochemical (CPK-MB, hs-CRP, BNP), and metabolic (lipid profile, atherogenic potential) parameters, as well as histopathological changes.

The present study for the first time described the cardioprotective efficacy of the natural DPP-IV inhibitor *T. arjuna* in the setting of diabetes based on the heart to body weight ratio, myocardial CPK-MB, hs-CRP, and atherogenic index parameters. However, the cardioprotective efficacy of the marketed synthetic DPP-IV inhibitor vildagliptin was found to be superior than *T. arjuna* monotherapy ($p < 0.01$). Furthermore, serum DPP-IV levels were found to be favorably correlated with *T. arjuna*, implying that modulation of the DPP-IV pathway contributes to their cardioprotective efficacy. A light microscopic analysis of the myocardium validated the myocardial salvaging effect in the setting of diabetes. Cardioprotective efficacy of *T. arjuna* combination therapy with metformin was found to be superior to metformin monotherapy. Myocardial salvaging effects of *T. arjuna* + metformin were found to be comparable to metformin + vildagliptin combination therapy.

Experimental evidence supports the benefits of *T. arjuna* as an adjuvant to metformin therapy in the setting of diabetes with MI. The following properties of *T. arjuna* contributed to the cardioprotective efficacy in context of diabetes: antidiabetic (blood glucose, HbA$_{1c}$); DPP-IV inhibition (serum DPP-IV); hypolipidemic activity (TG, TC, HDL-C, LDL-C, AI); reduction in volume overload (heart to body weight ratio, BNP); improvement of left ventricular function (ECG); antithrombotic (fibrinogen level); anti-inflammatory (hs-CRP); and antioxidant (TBARS). In the present study, TUNEL positivity was studied to delineate the involvement of apoptosis in the setting of myocardial injury coexisting with diabetes. *T. arjuna* monotherapy (13.2 ± 1.46%) and combination with metformin (7.92 ± 0.88%) protected diabetic rats from myocardial injury through attenuation of myocardial apoptosis (Figure 7.5).

It was found that *T. arjuna* treatment did not adversely affect pancreatic, liver, and kidney function in MI coexisting with diabetes rats, as evidenced by biochemical markers (pancreatic function [lipase], liver function [SGPT], and kidney function [creatinine]) of injury and histopathological architecture of the vital organs.

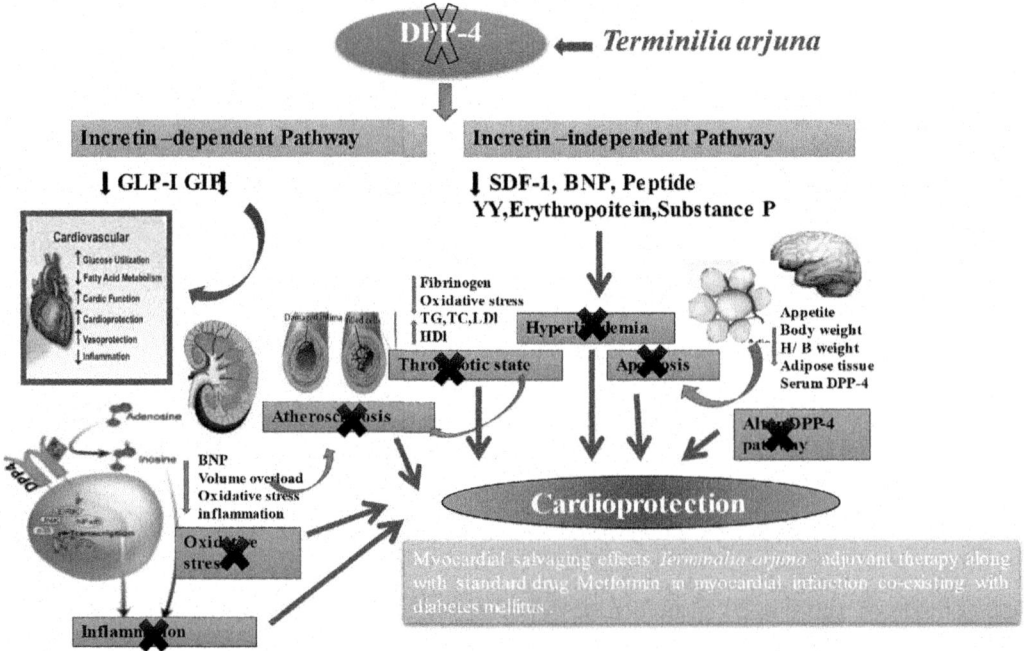

FIGURE 7.5 Cardiometabolic mechanisms of *Terminalia arjuna* in experimental diabetes.

The highlight of the study is that the myocardial salvaging effects of *T. arjuna* + metformin were found to be comparable to vildagliptin + metformin combination therapy. Interestingly, combination therapy was found to be superior compared to metformin monotherapy. Thus, results demonstrate the cardiovascular beneficial effects of *T. arjuna* adjuvant therapy in combination with standard drug metformin in experimentally induced MI coexisting with diabetes mellitus. DPP-IV–based therapeutics may represent novel targets, the cardioprotective actions of which may translate into demonstrable therapeutic benefits in diabetes with coexisting cardiovascular diseases.

7.3.5 POLYHERBAL FORMULATION WITH *TERMINALIA ARJUNA* PATENTED

A plain, uncoated polyherbal tablet of medicinal plants (*T. arjuna, Commiphora mukul,* and *Phyllanthus emblica*) in the ratio of 2.5:1:1.5 was formulated and bio-standardization of the polyherbal combination was undertaken using the HPTLC method. The polyherbal formulation was also patented and the patent has been published (Patent Application No. 201921053266A).

The DPP-IV inhibitory activity of the synthetic inhibitors vildagliptin and sitagliptin was compared to that of the polyherbal tablet. The synthetic drugs were found to have DPP-IV inhibitory activity of $90.42 \pm 7.34\%$ and $84.67 \pm 8.11\%$, respectively. When compared to these reference drugs, the polyherbal combination demonstrated superior DPP-IV percent inhibition of $96.85 \pm 7.35\%$, suggesting the possible benefits of developing the polyherbal formulation as a DPP-IV inhibitor.

The polyherbal formulation was studied in various experimental models of prediabetes and diabetes and demonstrated significant antidiabetic and cardioprotective efficacy. Although the polyherbal combination's antidiabetic efficacy was comparable to metformin, its myocardial salvaging effect was found to be superior than metformin. The hypolipidemic β cell–preserving, DPP-IV–inhibitory, and insulin-stimulatory properties of the polyherbal combination contribute to its cardioprotective and antidiabetic efficacy. Its protection was verified by biochemical markers of myocardial damage (CPK-MB), kidney (creatinine), and liver (SGPT). Histopathological studies supported the effectiveness of the combination.

7.3.6 OTHER FOODS, HERBS, SPICES, AND BOTANICALS USED IN DIABETES

A description of studies using various foods, herbs, spices, and botanicals used in diabetes is depicted in Table 7.3.

TABLE 7.3
Other Foods, Herbs, Spices, and Botanicals Used in Diabetes

Botanical Name	Common Name	Parts of Plant to Be Taken	Reported Activity
Acacia arabic	Babul	Seed	The experimental study was conducted at King Fahd Research Center, King Abdulaziz University (KAU), Jeddah, Kingdom of Saudi Arabia, from December 2012 to January 2013. A significant decrease in levels of serum glucose, insulin resistance, TC, TG, LDL-C, MDA, and a significant increase in HDL-C and Co-Q10 were observed (Hegazy et al. 2013).
Allium sativum L.	Lahasun	Aqueous Garlic	The antidiabetic effect of garlic ethanolic extract (*A. sativum* L.) was investigated in normal and streptozotocin-induced diabetic rats. Oral administrations of the garlic extract significantly decreased serum glucose, total cholesterol, triglycerides, urea, uric acid, creatinine, AST, and ALT levels (Eidi et al. 2005).

(Continued)

TABLE 7.3
(Continued)

Botanical Name	Common Name	Parts of Plant to Be Taken	Reported Activity
Aloe vera	Ghee kunwar	Leaves	*A. vera* leaf pulp extract showed hypoglycemic activity on IDDM and NIDDM rats, the effectiveness being enhanced for type 2 diabetes in comparison with glibenclamide (Okyar et al. 2001).
Artemisia pallens	Davana	Aerial part	Oral administration of the methanol extract of the aerial parts of *A. pallens* Wall. (used in Indian folk medicine for the treatment of diabetes mellitus) led to a significant blood glucose–lowering effect in glucose-fed hyperglycemic and alloxan-induced diabetic rats (Subramoniam et al. 1996).
Brassica juncea	Rai	Seed	The hypoglycemic activity of *B. juncea* (seeds) aqueous extract was evaluated an found that aqueous seed extract of *B. juncea* has potent hypoglycemic activity in male albino rat (Thirumalai et al. 2011).
Caesalpinia bonducella	Kantikaranja	Seed	*C. bonducella*, widely distributed throughout the coastal region of India and used ethnically by the tribal people of India for controlling blood sugar, was earlier reported by us to possess hypoglycemic activity in animal models. This prompted us to undertake a detail study with the aqueous and ethanolic extracts of the seeds of this plant in both type 1 and 2 diabetes mellitus in Long Evans rats. Significant blood sugar lowering effect of *C. bonducella* was observed in type 2 diabetic models (Chakrabarti et al. 2003).
Cajanus cajan	Tuvar	Seed	This antioxidant activity of extract of germinated pigeon pea (*C. cajan*) was studied in alloxan-induced diabetic rats. Consumption of germinated pigeon pea extract gave rise to a reduced fasting blood glucose level in diabetic rats (Uchegbu and Ishiwu 2016).
Momordica charantia	Karela	Dry fruit	*M. charantia* has significant antidiabetic and hypolipidemic activity. It can be used as an adjuvant along with allopathic treatments for diabetes as well as to delay late diabetic complications (Joseph and Jini 2013).
Eucalyptus globulus	Safeda	Leaves	*E. globulus* is used as a traditional treatment for diabetes. In this study, incorporation of eucalyptus in the diet (62.5 g/kg) and drinking water (2.5 g/L) reduced the hyperglycemia and associated weight loss of streptozotocin-treated mice (Gray and Flatt 1998).
Syzygium cumini	Jamun	Dry leaves	*S. cumini* (L.) Skeels (syn. *S. jambolanum* DC, *Eugenia jambolana* Lam.) is among the medicinal plants most often recommended as adjuvant therapies in type 2 diabetes. The plant was extensively studied during the last 125 years; approximately 100 case reports were reported already before the discovery of insulin. After the Second World War, research was concentrated on animal studies. Many of them reported some success in reducing type 2 diabetes symptoms (Helmstädter 2008).
Ipomoea batatas	Mitha aalu	Tuberous root	Sweet potato (WSSP; *I. batatas* L.) peel was selected to find out its antidiabetic potential as well as to explore the effects on selected biochemical parameters in diabetes-induced Wistar rats. It was found that WSSP (*I. batatas* L.) peel significantly decreased blood glucose level, protein glycation level, total cholesterol, triglycerides, and LDL-C (Akhtar et al. 2018).

Botanical Name	Common Name	Parts of Plant to Be Taken	Reported Activity
Murraya koenigii	Curry patta	Leaves	The medicinal plant *M. koenigii* was shown to have a wide variety of pharmacological activities (hypoglycemic and hypolipidemic). The antidiabetic and hypolipidemic properties of *M. koenigii* in experimentally induced diabetes in rats was evaluated. It was found that *M. koenigii* significantly decreases blood glucose and lipid parameters (Suman et al. 2019).
Musa sapientum	Kela (banana)	Fresh flower decoction	The antihyperglycemic effect of ethanolic extract of flowers of *M. sapientum*, an herb used in Indian folklore medicine for the treatment of diabetes mellitus, in alloxan-induced diabetic rats. Oral administration of the ethanolic extract showed significant blood glucose–lowering effects (Dhanabal et al. 2005).
Nelumbo nucifera	Kamal (lotus)	Rhizome	Oral administration of the ethanolic extract of rhizomes of *N. nucifera* markedly reduced the blood sugar level of normal, glucose-fed hyperglycemic and streptozotocin-induced diabetic rats. The extract improved glucose tolerance and potentiated the action of exogenously injected insulin in normal rats (Mukherjee et al. 1997).
Punica granatum	Anar	Flowers	*P. granatum* L. is a well-known traditional herbal remedy in Iran due to its positive effects on ameliorating blood glucose homeostasis. *P. granatum* administration contributes to the modulation of both hyperglycemia and hyperlipidemia in alloxan-diabetic Wistar rats (Gharib and Kouhsari 2019).
Swertia bimaculate	Chirata	Hexane fraction	The antidiabetic activity of *S. bimaculata* is well established. One potent mechanism attributes to the protection of pancreatic β cells and liver tissues by ameliorating lipid metabolism and oxidative stress. *S. bimaculata* could be considered an alternative agent against diabetes mellitus (Zhaoxia Liu et al. 2013).

7.3.7 TOXICITY AND CAUTIONARY NOTES

The effect of any drug on an individual may be different than expected because that drug may interact with another drug (drug-drug interaction); a food, beverage, or dietary supplement the person is consuming (drug-nutrient/food interaction); or another disease the individual has (drug-disease interaction). These interactions may occur out of accidental misuse or due to lack of knowledge about the active ingredients involved in the relevant substances. Regarding food-drug interactions, physicians and pharmacists recognize that some foods and drugs, when taken simultaneously, can alter the body's ability to utilize a particular food or drug or cause serious side effects. Clinically significant drug interactions, which pose potential harm to the patient, may result from changes in pharmaceutical, pharmacokinetic, or pharmacodynamic properties.

Grapefruit juice interacts with almost all types of drugs. In 2007 Taniguchi reported a case of purpura associated with concomitant ingestion of cilostazol, aspirin, and grapefruit juice in a 79-year-old man. His purpura disappeared upon cessation of grapefruit juice ingestion (Kirby and Unadkat 2007). Antibiotics are widely prescribed in medical practice. Many of them induce or are subject to interactions that may diminish their anti-infectious efficiency or elicit toxic effects. Azithromycin absorption is decreased when taken with food, resulting in a 43% reduction in bioavailability (Størmer et al. 1993).

Herbal medicines are mixtures of more than one active ingredient. The multitude of pharmacologically active compounds obviously increases the likelihood of interactions taking place. Hence, the likelihood of herb-drug interactions is theoretically higher than drug-drug interactions. St. John's wort is a popular herbal supplement widely used to help with symptoms of depression. There are more than 500 drug interactions with St. John's wort, and some can be dangerous. It has been shown to lower the plasma concentration and/or the pharmacological effects of a number of conventional drugs, including cyclosporine, indinavir, irinotecan, nevirapine, oral contraceptives, and digoxin (Angelo A. Izzo 2005).

7.4 SUMMARY POINTS

The chapter focused on the DPP-IV inhibitory activity of arjuna (*Terminalia arjuna*) responsible for its beneficial cardiometabolic effects.

- For the first time, the DPP-IV inhibitory activity and cardioprotective efficacy of *T. arjuna* in setting of diabetes was reported.
- DPP-IV inhibitory activity of *T. arjuna* was comparable to marketed synthetic DPP-IV inhibitors, vildagliptin and sitagliptin.
- Experimental evidence supports the benefits of *T. arjuna* as an adjuvant to metformin, a standard antidiabetic therapy in the setting of diabetes with cardiovascular co-morbidity (myocardial infarction).
- The myocardial salvaging effects of *T. arjuna* + metformin were found to be comparable to metformin + vildagliptin combination therapy.
- The following properties of *T. arjuna* contributed to its cardiometabolic efficacy:
  - Antidiabetic (blood glucose, HbA_{1c})
  - Cardioprotective (CPK-MB, histopathology)
  - DPP-IV inhibition (serum DPP-IV)
  - Hypolipidemic activities (TG, TC, HDL-C, LDL-C, AI)
  - Reduction in volume overload (heart to body weight ratio, BNP)
  - Improvement of left ventricular function (ECG)
  - Antithrombotic (fibrinogen level)
  - Anti-inflammatory (hs-CRP)
  - Antioxidant (TBARS)
  - Anti-apoptotic (TUNEL assay)
- *T. arjuna* treatment did not adversely affect the pancreatic, hepatic, and renal function in the experimental model of MI coexisting with diabetes, as evidenced by biochemical markers of injury and histopathological studies.
- To determine the active principles in the medicinal plant *T. arjuna* responsible for the DPP-IV inhibitory activities, in silico studies were conducted. The active ingredients of *T. arjuna* (arjunetin, arjungenin, arjunic acid, arjunone, ellagic acid, and gallic acid) demonstrated significant inhibition of the DPP-IV enzyme.
- Results demonstrated that arjunic acid and arjunone prefer to bind the active site pocket of DPP-IV enzyme. Compounds like arjunetin and vildagliptin prefer to bind near the interface region of the DPP-IV as their biological active forms are homodimer. Sitagliptin binds near the α/β hydrolase domain.
- Arjunetin, arjungenin, ellagic acid, and arjunic acid showed superior DPP-IV inhibitory activity as compared to synthetic DPP-IV inhibitors (sitagliptin and vildagliptin).
- *T. arjuna* has the potential to be developed as a natural alternative to synthetic DPP-IV inhibitors with cardiometabolic benefits to be used as adjuvant therapy along with the standard drug metformin.

REFERENCES

Akhtar, N., Akram, M., Daniyal, M., Ahmad, S. 2018. Evaluation of antidiabetic activity of Ipomoea batatas L. extract in alloxan-induced diabetic rats. *Int J Immunopathol Pharmacol* 32: 2058738418814678.

Al-Masri, I.M., Mohammad, M.K., Tahaa, M.O. 2009. Inhibition of dipeptidyl peptidase IV (DPP-IV) is one of the mechanisms explaining the hypoglycemic effect of berberine. *J Enzyme Inhib Med Chem* 24(50): 1061–1066.

Amalraj, A., Gopi, S. 2016. Medicinal properties of Terminalia arjuna (Roxb.) Wight & Arn. A review. *J Tradit Complement Med*: 1–14.

Amalraj, A., Gopi, S. 2017. Medicinal properties of Terminalia arjuna (Roxb.) Wight & Arn: A review. *J Traditional Complement Med* 7(1): 65–78.

Antani, J.A., Gandhi, S., Antani, N.J. 1991. Terminalia arjuna in congestive heart failure. *J Assoc Physicians India* 39: 809.

Asha, S., Taju, G. 2012. Cardioprotective effect of terminalia arjuna on caffeine induced coronary heart disease. *IJPSR* 3(1): 150–153.

Bharani, A., Ganguli, A., Mathur, L.K., Jamra, Y., Raman, P.G. 2002. Efficacy of Terminalia arjuna in chronic stable angina: A double-blind, placebo-controlled, crossover study comparing Terminalia arjuna with isosorbide mononitrate. *Indian Heart J* 54(2): 170–175.

Bharani, A., Ganguly, A., Bhargava, K.D. 1995. Salutary effect of Terminalia arjuna in patients with severe refractory heart failure. *Int J Cardiol* 49(3): 191–199.

Binkowski, T.A., Naghibzadeh, S., Lianga, J. 2003. CASTp: Computed atlas of surface topography of proteins. *Nucleic Acids Res* 31(13): 3352–3355.

Chakrabarti, S., Biswas, T.K., Rokeya, B., Ali, L., Mosihuzzaman, M., Nahar, N., Khan, A.K., Mukherjee, B. 2003. Advanced studies on the hypoglycemic effect of Caesalpinia bonducella F. in type 1 and 2 diabetes in Long Evans rats. *J Ethnopharmacol* 84(1): 41–46.

Dhanabal, S.P., Sureshkumar, M., Ramanathan, M., Suresh, B. 2005. Hypoglycemic effect of ethanolic extract of Musa sapientum on alloxan induced diabetes mellitus in rats and its relation with antioxidant potential. *J Herb Pharmacother* 5(2): 7–19.

Dwivedi, S., Aggarwal, A., Agarwal, M.P., Rajpal, S. 2005. Role of Terminalia arjuna in ischaemic mitral regurgitation. *Int J Cardiol* 100: 507–508.

Dwivedi, S., Chansouria, J.P., Somani, P.N., Udupa, K.N. 1989. Effect of Terminalia arjuna on ischaemic heart disease. *Altern Med* 3: 115–122.

Dwivedi, S., Chopra, D. 2014. Revisiting *Terminalia arjuna* – An ancient cardiovascular drug. *J Tradit Complement Med* 4(4): 224–231.

Dwivedi, S., Jauhari, R. 1997. Beneficial effects of Terminalia arjuna in coronary artery disease. *Indian Heart J* 49(5): 507–510.

Gauthaman, K., Banerjee, S.K., Dinda, A.K., Ghosh, C.C., Maulik, S.K. 2005. Terminalia arjuna (Roxb.) protects rabbit heart against ischemic-reperfusion injury: Role of antioxidant enzymes and heat shock protein. *J Ethnopharmacol* 96(3): 403–409.

Gharib, E., Kouhsari, M.S. 2019. Study of the antidiabetic activity of Punica granatum L. fruits aqueous extract on the alloxan-diabetic Wistar rats. *Iran J Pharm Res* 18(1): 358–368.

Gray, A.M., Flatt, P.R. 1998. Antihyperglycemic actions of Eucalyptus globulus (Eucalyptus) are associated with pancreatic and extra-pancreatic effects in mice. *J Nutr* 128(12): 2319–2323.

Guex, N., Peitsch, M.C. 1997. SWISS-MODEL and the Swiss-PdbViewer: An environment for comparative protein modeling. *Electrophoresis* 18: 2714–2723.

Hegazy, G.A., Alnoury, A.M., Gad, H.G. 2013. The role of Acacia Arabica extract as an antidiabetic, antihyperlipidemic, and antioxidant in treptozotocin-induced diabetic rats. *Saudi Med J* 34(7): 727–733.

Helmstädter, A. 2008. Syzygium cumini (L.) SKEELS (Myrtaceae) against diabetes–125 years of research. *Pharmazie.* 63(2): 91–101.

Izzo, A.A. 2005. Herb-drug interactions: An overview of the clinical evidence. *Fundam Clin Pharmacol* 19(1): 1–16.

Jain, S., Yadav, P.P., Gill, V., Vasudeva, N., Singla, N. 2009. Terminalia arjuna a sacred medicinal plant: Phytochemical and pharmacological profile. *Phytochem Rev* 8: 491–502.

Joseph, B., Jini, D. 2013. Antidiabetic effects of Momordica charantia (bitter melon) and its medicinal potency. *Asian Pac J Trop Dis* 3(2): 93–102.

Karthik, D. 2014. In-silico docking analysis of Dipeptidylpeptidase-4 (DPP-IV or CD26) with some selective bioflavonoids using Genetic Lamarckian Algorithm. *J Comput Methods Mol Des* 4(2): 24–31.

Karthikeyan, K., Bai, B.R., Gauthaman, K., Sathish, K.S., Devaraj, S.N. 2003. Cardioprotective effect of the alcoholic extract of Terminalia arjuna bark in an in vivo model of myocardial ischemic reperfusion injury. *Life Sci* 73(21): 2727–2739.

Karunakaran, G. 2015. Cardioprotective role of methanolic extract of bark of Terminalia arjuna against in-vitro model of myocardial ischemic-reperfusion injury. *Anc Sci Life* 35(2): 79–84.

Kim, S., Chen, J., Cheng, T. 2021. PubChem in 2021: New data content and improved web interfaces. *Nucleic Acids Res* 49(D1): D1388–D1395.

Kirby, B.J., Unadkat, J.D. 2007. Grapefruit juice, a glass full of drug interactions. *Clin Pharmacol Ther* 81(5): 631–633.

Kuleshwar, J.K., Thakur, T., Mishra, N., Kumar, A. 2021. Pharmacological approach of terminalia arjuna: A review. *Plant Cell Biotechnol Mol Biol* 22(57&58): 1–15.

Kumar, C., Nehar, S. 2013. Hypoglycemic effect of acetone extract of terminalia arjuna roxb. Bark on type-2 diabetic albino rats. *Bioscan* 8(2): 709–712.

Kumar, G., Saleem, N., Kumar, S., Maulik, S.K., Ahmad, S., Sharma, M., Goswami, S.K. 2019. Transcriptomic validation of the protective effects of aqueous bark extract of Terminalia arjuna (Roxb.) on isoproterenol-induced cardiac hypertrophy in rats. *Front Pharmacol* 10: 1443.

Kumar, P.U., Adhikari, P., Pereira, P., Bhat, P. 1999. Safety and efficacy of hartone in stable angina pectoris – an open comparative trial. *J Assoc Physicians India*: 685–689.

Maulik, S.K., Talwar, K.K. 2012. Therapeutic potential of Terminalia arjuna in cardiovascular disorders. *Am J Cardiovasc Drugs* 12: 157–163.

Miteva, M.A., Guyon, F., Tufféry, P. 2010. Frog2: Efficient 3D conformation ensemble generator for small compounds. *Nucleic Acids Res* 38(Web Server issue): W622–W627. http://doi.org/10.1093/nar/gkq325

Mukherjee, P.K., Saha, K., Pal, M., Saha, B.P. 1997. Effect of Nelumbo nucifera rhizome extract on blood sugar level in rats. *J Ethnopharmacol* 58(3): 207–213.

Muthu, C., Ayyanar, M., Raja, N., Ignacimuthu, S. 2006. Medicinal plants used by traditional healers in Kancheepuram District of Tamil Nadu, India. *J Ethnobilol Ethnomed* 2: 43.

Nammi, R.G., Behara, S., Babu, R., Lodagala, D., Boini, K. 2003. Possible mechanisms of hypotension produced 70% alcoholic extract of Terminalia arjuna (L.) in anaesthetized dogs Srinivas. *BMC Complement Altern Med*: 3–5.

Okyar, A., Can, A., Akev, N., Baktir, G., Sütlüpinar, N. 2001. Effect of Aloe vera leaves on blood glucose level in type I and type II diabetic rat models. *Phytother Res* 15(2): 157–161.

Parmar, H.S., Panda, S., Jatwa, R., Kar, A. 2006. Cardio-protective role of Terminalia arjuna bark extract is possibly mediated through alterations in thyroid hormones. *Pharmazie* 61: 793–795.

Parveen, A., Babbar, R., Agarwal, S., Kotwani, A., Fahim, M. 2011a. Mechanistic clues in the cardioprotective effect of Terminalia arjuna bark extract in isoproterenol-induced chronic heart failure in rats. *Cardiovasc Toxicol.* 11(1): 48–57.

Parveen, K., Khan, R., Siddiqui, W.A. 2011b. Antidiabetic effects afforded by Terminalia arjuna in high fat-fed and streptozotocin-induced type 2 diabetic rats. *Int J Diabetes & Metab* 19: 23–33.

Patil, R.H., Prakash, K., Maheshwari, V.L. 2011. Hypolipidemic effect of Terminalia arjuna (L.) in experimentally induced hypercholesteremic rats. *Acta Biol Szeged.* 55: 289–293.

Rao, B.C.S., Singh, R.H., Tripathi, K. 2001. Effect of Terminalia arjuna (W&A) on regression of LVH in hypertensives: A clinical study. *J Res Ayurveda Sidhha* 3–4: 216–227.

Ritchie, D.W. 2005. High order analytic translation matrix elements for real space six-dimensional polar fourier correlations. *J Appl Cryst* 38: 808–818.

Sandhu, J.S., Shah, B., Shenoy, S., Chauhan, S., Lavekar, G.S., Padhi, M.M. 2010. Effects of withania somnifera (Ashwagandha) and Terminalia arjuna (Arjuna) on physical performance and cardiorespiratory endurance in healthy young adults. *Int J Ayurveda Res*: 144–149.

Singh, N., Kapur, K.K., Singh, S.P., Shanker, K.J., Sinha, N., Kohli, R.P. 1982. Mechanism of cardiovascular action of Terminalia arjuna. *Planta Med* 45: 102–104.

Sinha, M., Manna, P., Sil, P.C. 2008. Terminalia arjuna protects mouse hearts against sodium fluoride-induced oxidative stress. *J Med Food* 11(4): 733–740.

Størmer, F.C., Reistad, R., Alexander, J. 1993. Glycyrrhizic acid in liquorice – evaluation of health hazard. *Food Chem Toxicol* 31(4): 302–312.

Subramoniam, A., Pushpangadan, P., Rajasekharan, S., Evans, D.A., Latha, P.G., Valsaraj, R. 1996. Effects of artemisia pallens wall on blood glucose levels in normal and alloxan-induced diabetic rats. *J Ethnopharmacol* 50(1): 13–17.

Suman, R.K., Ray, I., Borde, M.K., Deshmukh, Y.A., Pathak, A., Adhikari, A.K. 2019. Evaluation of antidiabetic efficacy of Murraya koenigii on Streptozotocin induced diabetes in experimental rats. *Int J Basic Clin Pharmacol* 8: 1906–1910.

Sushant, A.S., Mishra, S., Joshi, K., Apte, K., Patil, P.K., Shah, T., Deshpande, M., Puran, A. 2018. Anti-hyperglycemic and anti-hyperlipidaemic effect of Arjunarishta in high-fat fed animals. *J Ayurveda Integr Med* 9(1): 45–52.

Thirumalai, T., Therasa, S.V., Elumalai, E.K., David, E. 2011. Hypoglycemic effect of Brassica juncea (seeds) on streptozotocin induced diabetic male albino rat. *Asian Pac J Trop Biomed* 1(4): 323–325.

Thomson, H.A.J., Ojo, O.O., Flatt, P.R., Abdel-Wahab, Y.H.A. 2014. Aqueous bark extracts of Terminalia arjuna stimulates insulin release, enhances insulin action and inhibits starch digestion and protein glycation in vitro. *Austin J Endocrinol Diabetes* 1(1): 1001.

Uchegbu, N.N., Ishiwu, C.N. 2016. Germinated Pigeon Pea (Cajanus cajan): A novel diet for lowering oxidative stress and hyperglycemia. *Food Sci Nutr* 4(5): 772–777.

Wiederstein, S. 2007. ProSA-web: Interactive web service for the recognition of errors in three-dimensional structures of proteins. *Nucleic Acids Research* 35: W407–W410.

Zhaoxia, L., Luosheng, W., Yuedong, Y., Zuoqi, X., Yutang, Z., Yonglong, W., Cuiping, C., Qiuxia, M., Jiachun, C. 2013. Hypoglycemic activity and antioxidative stress of extracts and corymbiferin from swertia bimaculata in vitro and in vivo. *Evid Based Complement Altern Med* 125416: 12.

8 Banana (*Musa paradisiaca*) as a Functional Food for Managing Diabetes

Mohammed Abdel-Gabbar, Sarah M. Abdel Aziz, Sanaa M. Abd El-Twab and Osama M. Ahmed

CONTENTS

LIST OF ABBREVIATIONS

AGE	advanced glycation end product
Akt	serine/threonine kinase
ATP	adenosine triphosphate
CAP	c-Cbl-associating protein
CETP	cholesteryl ester transfer protein
DM	diabetes mellitus
FA	fatty acid
FFA	free fatty acid
FOX	forkhead family of transcription factors
FRAP/mTOR	mammalian target of rapamycin
GDM	gestational diabetes mellitus
GLUT	glucose transporter proteins
GPx	glutathione peroxidase
GSH	glutathione (reduced form)
GST	glutathione S-transferase
GSK3	glycogen synthase kinase 3

DOI: 10.1201/9781003220930-10

HDL	high-density lipoprotein
HLA	human leukocyte antigen
IA-2	islet-cell antigen-2 (ICA512)
ICA-1	β-cell surface protein
IDF	International Diabetes Federation
IDL	intermediate-density lipoprotein
IGF-1	insulin-like growth factor 1
IL	interleukin
IRS	insulin receptor substrate
JNK	c-Jun N-terminal kinases
LDL	low-density lipoprotein
LPO	lipid peroxidation
MAP	mitogen-activated protein
MAPK	MAP kinase, MEK, MAP/ERK kinase
MDA	malondialdehyde
mTOR/FRAP	mammalian target of rapamycin
NA/STZ	nicotinamide/streptozotocin
NF-κB	nuclear factor κ-light-chain-enhancer of activated B cells
NKT	natural killer T cells
PI3-K	phosphatidylinositol 3-kinase
PKB/Akt	protein kinase B
PPAR	peroxisome proliferator-activated receptor
RNS	reactive nitrogen species
ROS	reactive oxygen species
SHP-2	Src homology 2
SOD	superoxide dismutase
SREBP	sterol regulatory element binding protein
TGs	triglycerides
TNFα	tumor necrosis factor α
T1DM	type 1 diabetes (IDDM)
T2DM	type 2 diabetes (NIDDM)
VLDL	very-low-density lipoprotein
WHO	World Health Organization
ZnT-8	pancreatic β cell–specific zinc-transporter

8.1 BACKGROUND

Current hypoglycemic drugs usually have adverse risk effects and reduced efficacy over time. Though different kinds of oral hypoglycemic agents, such as insulin releasers, insulin sensitizers, and glucosidase inhibitors, are available for the treatment of diabetes mellitus (DM), there is an increment demand by patients to utilize herbal medicines with lesser side effects (Chauhan et al., 2010). Thus, renewed recognition and scientific interest is now booming throughout the world in the study of medicinal plants due to their perceived effectiveness, lower side effects in clinical practice, and relatively low treatment costs. Although many plants are used in the world to stop or cure diseases, scientific proof is lacking in most cases. Most plants are rich in carotenoids, flavonoids, terpenoids, alkaloids, and glycosides, so they often have hypoglycemic effects (Afrisham et al., 2015). The anti-diabetic effects of treatment with plants are often attributed to their ability to ameliorate the function of pancreatic tissue, which is done by prompting insulin secretions or decreasing the intestinal absorption of glucose. The number of people with diabetes today has been rising and causing increasing concerns in medical community and the public.

8.1.1 BANANA (*MUSA PARADISIACA*)

M. paradisiaca is a crop in the genus *Musa*, and all members of the genus are native to the tropical and subtropical countries (Plants and Khare, 2007). In addition to having a high amount of dietary fiber, manganese, potassium, and some vitamins, ripe fruit has up to 22% of its weight as carbohydrates. *M. paradisiaca* has been recorded to have valuable impacts on several disease conditions and displays defensive impacts on organs of the body (Vinaykumar et al., 2010). *M. paradisiaca* acts as a good source of several compounds and minerals which regenerate tissues in the body (Imam and Akter, 2011). A study by Kappel et al. (2013b) proved that extracts of various parts of *M. paradisiaca* show potential hypoglycemic activity. The decrease in serum glucose levels, induction of insulin secretion, stimulation of glycogen storage, and inhibition of enzyme activity related to glucose absorption and AGE formation clarify the worthy impacts of *M. paradisiaca* on the regulation of glucose homeostasis. Moreover, phytochemical analysis elucidates presence of flavonoids in crude extract and fractions of *M. paradisiaca*.

Rutin is the main compound which indicates anti-diabetic potential properties (Kappel et al., 2013a, b). The hypoglycemic and hypolipidemic effects of *M. paradisiaca* in streptozotocin-induced diabetic mice and alloxan-induced diabetic mice were illustrated (Ajiboye et al., 2018). Hence, this chapter sheds light on the molecular mechanistic of the anti-diabetic potentials of extracts of various parts of the *M. paradisiaca* plant.

8.2 THE EFFECT OF BANANA ON DIABETES MELLITUS

8.2.1 WHAT IS DIABETES MELLITUS?

DM is a combination of metabolic disorders identified by elevated blood glucose levels and disturbances in carbohydrate, fat, and protein metabolism due to reduction in secretion, action of insulin, or both (Das et al., 2012). As the disease advances, tissue or vascular damage ensues, leading to intense diabetic complications such as retinopathy, neuropathy, nephropathy, cardiovascular complications, and ulceration (Shi et al., 2018).

Diabetes was first certified by the ancient Egyptians, but the Greek physician Aretaeus who coined the term *diabetes mellitus*. In Greek, diabetes means "to pass through" and mellitus is the Latin word for honey (referring to sweetness) (Shamim, 2013).

There are about 400 plants used to treat DM, including *Ferula assafoetida, Allium sativum, Trigonella foenum-graecum, Coccinia grandis, Caesalpinia bonduc*, and *Rosmarinus officinalis*. WHO has indicated that traditional plant treatments are effective and nontoxic with few or no side effects, and are assumed to be excellent candidates for oral therapy (Kumar et al., 2021). One such plant is banana (*Musa paradisiaca*). It has been reported to have pharmacological activities such as antilithiatic, antioxidant, antibacterial, anti-diabetic, anti-ulcer, antidiarrheal, hypocholesterolemic, hepatoprotective, anti–snake venom, wound healing, hair growth–promoting, antifungal, and anti-menorrhagic activity (Lavanya et al., 2016). Lakshmi et al. (2014) recorded the anti-diabetic activity of the different parts of *M. paradisaica*. The hydroethanolic extracts, the hexane and chloroform fractions of leaves and fruit peels, showed promising anti-diabetic activity.

8.2.2 PREVALENCE OF DIABETES MELLITUS

The prevalence of DM is continually rising worldwide at alarming rate. The International Diabetes Federation (IDF) evaluated the worldwide prevalence to be 151 million in 2000 to 629 million of people by 2045 with a prevalence of 9.9% (IDF, 2017). The prevalence is higher in urban in comparison with rural areas (10.2% vs. 6.9%).

Around 8.2 million people in Egypt have diabetes, and it is expected that this number will grow to 16.7 million by 2045. Hence, IDF recorded Egypt as one of the top ten countries in the number of patients with diabetes (IDF, 2017).

8.2.3 Classification of Diabetes Mellitus

The new classification distinguishes four types of diabetes mellitus: type 1, type 2, "other specific types," and gestational diabetes (WHO, 1999). Classification of diabetes mellitus depends on its etiology and clinical presentation.

8.2.3.1 Type 1 Diabetes (T1DM)

T1DM is an autoimmune disorder that involves the destruction of the β cells by activated $CD4^+$ and $CD8^+$ T cells (NKT cells) and macrophages infiltrating the pancreatic islets (Ozougwu et al., 2013). Viral infections and autoimmune diseases such as Graves' disease and Hashimoto thyroiditis have been implicated in the etiology of T1DM (Yeung et al., 2011).

8.3.2.2 Type 2 Diabetes (T2DM)

It is established that the most widely recognized type of diabetes is T2DM, which represents a combination of genetically specified diseases that might be affected by life habitat. The worldwide rise in diabetes happens due to aging, expanding patterns toward unhealthy food, obesity, and stationary lifestyles (Motala et al., 2003).

T2DM is a chronic disease that hinders insulin secretion and/or insulin resistance. Obesity is a common risk factor for this type of diabetes, and most patients with T2DM are obese (Nolte and Karam, 2001).

8.3.3.3 Gestational Diabetes Mellitus (GDM)

GDM is a case of glucose intolerance that occurs usually in the second or third trimester during pregnancy. During pregnancy, the maternal tissues become insensitive to insulin. GDM occurs due to the placental lactogen hormone and other hormones, such as progesterone, cortisol, and growth hormone. Once the baby is born, GDM may disappear. There is chance of recurrence in the following pregnancy or any time after delivery (Bortolon et al., 2016).

8.2.4 Insulin Signaling

The action of insulin is initiated by binding to its cognate receptor to the extracellular α subunit resulting in conformational change enabling ATP to bind to the intracellular component of the β subunit. ATP binding in turn triggers and activates the β subunit protein tyrosine kinase activity, resulting in the phosphorylation of tyrosine residues located in the cytoplasmic face (De Meyts and Whittaker, 2002). This enables tyrosine phosphorylation of intracellular substrate proteins known as insulin receptor substrates (IRS). Activated IRs can then phosphorylate tyrosine deposits of substrate proteins (e.g., IRS1 and Shc), which will proliferate the signaling further downstream (Figure 8.1) (Kido et al., 2001). There are four known IRS proteins. IRS 1 is phosphorylated by both the insulin receptor and insulin like growth factor 1 (IGF-1) receptor and is proposed to be the main IRS in skeletal muscle. IRS 2, proposed to be the principal IRS in liver, intercedes peripheral activities of insulin and development of pancreatic β cells (Kido et al., 2001). IRS 3 exists distinctly in adipose tissue, β cells, and liver, and IRS 4 exists in the thymus, brain, and kidney (Burks and White, 2001). Insulin receptor signaling includes two significant pathways, the phosphatidylinositol 3-kinase (PI3K) pathway and the mitogen-activated protein kinase (MAPK) pathway (Figure 8.1) (White, 2002).

PKB acts as a major hub in the insulin signaling pathway and regulates many cellular processes (Figure 8.1). PKB phosphorylated at Thr308 has been suggested to primarily regulate protein synthesis via mTORC1 activation, whereas PKB phosphorylated at Ser473 by PDK1 has been suggested to regulate glucose uptake via phosphorylation of AS160 and regulate FOXO1 activity (Vadlakonda et al., 2013).

Insulin resistance results from the interplay between genetic and environmental factors as indicated in Figure 8.2 (El-Zayadi, 2010). The genetic factors include abnormal insulin, abnormal

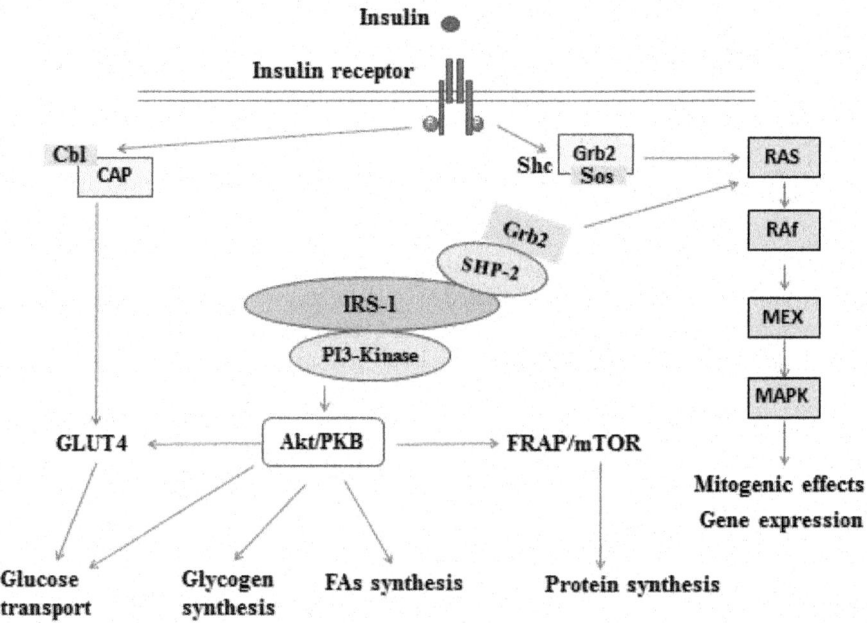

FIGURE 8.1 Scheme of the major insulin signaling pathways. The activated insulin receptor phosphorylates tyrosine residues on IRS proteins, Shc, CAP, and other intracellular substrates. These substrates then bind to various downstream signaling effectors, transmitting the metabolic and mitogenic signal of insulin. CAP: c-Cbl-associating protein; FAs: fatty acids; FRAP/mTOR: mammalian target of rapamycin; MAP: mitogen-activated protein; MAPK: MAP kinase; MEK: MAP/ERK kinase; PI3-kinase: phosphatidylinositol 3-kinase; PKB/Akt: protein kinase B; SHP-2: SH2 containing phosphatase-2; Sos: son of sevenless (Cheng et al., 2002).

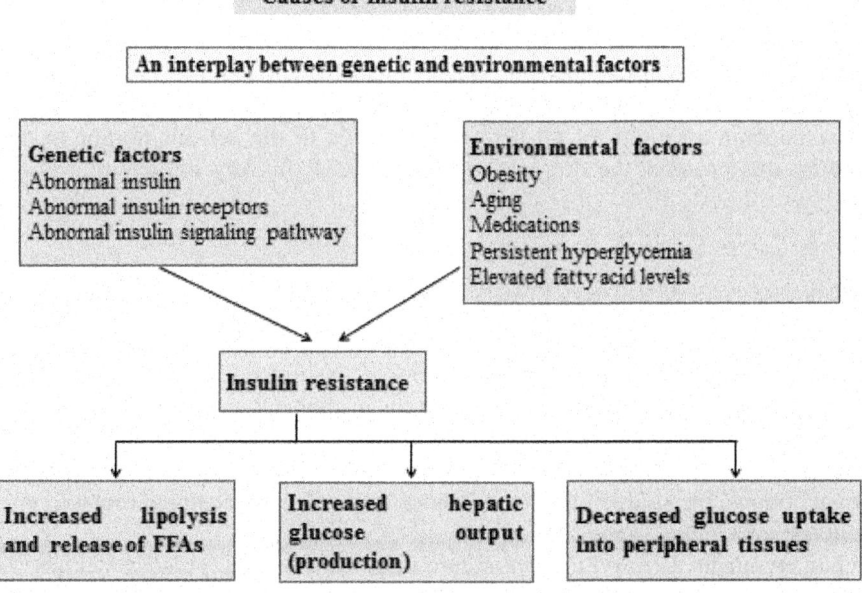

FIGURE 8.2 Causes of insulin resistance (El-Zayadi, 2010).

insulin receptors, and abnormal insulin signaling pathway while the environmental factors include obesity, aging, and effects of medications, persistent hyperglycemia and elevated fatty acids (AFs) levels. The detailed mechanisms by which free fatty acids (FFAs) induce insulin resistance are illustrated in Figure 8.3 (Schenk et al., 2008).

8.2.4.1   Akt Targets

8.2.4.1.1   Glycogen Synthase Kinase-3 (GSK3)

GSK3 was first identified as the kinase responsible for phosphorylating and repressing of glycogen synthase activity, finally antagonizing the storage of glucose as glycogen. Its activity antagonizes the impacts of insulin on glucose metabolism, and Akt is known as one of the key molecules equipped for phosphorylating GSK3 and repressing its activity (Cross et al., 1995).

8.2.4.1.2   Mammalian Target of Rapamycin (mTOR)

Akt triggers mTOR by phosphorylation and repression of tuberous sclerosis complex 2 (TSC2) (Long et al., 2005).

8.2.4.1.3   Forkhead Family of Transcription Factors (FOX)

The FOX family contains more than 100 members, and many of these are critical for insulin activity. FOXO1 activates gluconeogenic genes in liver and inhibits adipogenesis. FOXO2 is a crucial regulator of fasting lipid metabolism (Titchenell et al., 2015).

8.2.4.1.4   Sterol Regulator Element Binding Protein (SREBP)

The group of sterol regulatory element binding proteins (SREBPs) comprises three firmly related members: SREBP1a, SREBP1c, and SREBP2 (Eberle et al., 2004). The biosynthesis of FAs and TGs is governed by SREBP-1c; the upregulation of genes implicated in cholesterol metabolism is specially controlled by SREBP-2; and SREBP-1a is a prompt for both the FA and cholesterol biosynthetic pathways. Insulin signaling through PI3K and Akt brings about stimulation of SREBP-1c expression and assemblage of nuclear SREBP-1c protein (Matsuzaka et al., 2004).

8.2.4.1.5   Glucose Transporter Proteins (GLUTs)

Glucose enters cells in an ATP-independent way by means of GLUTs, of which at least 13 subtypes under three classes have been distinguished (Navale and Paranjape, 2016).

PI3-kinase become essential for GLUT4 translocation to the cell membrane in muscle cells and adipocytes; this prompts the downstream activities of this key intracellular enzyme (Kido et al., 2001).

8.2.5   Treatment with Medicinal Plants

Current hypoglycemic drugs usually have adverse risk effects and reduced efficacy over time. Though different kinds of oral hypoglycemic agents as insulin releasers, insulin sensitizers, and glucosidase inhibitors are available for the treatment of diabetes mellitus. There is an increased demand by patients to utilize herbal medicines with lesser side effects (Chauhan et al., 2010). As a result, due to their perceived efficacy, fewer side effects in clinical practice, and generally affordable treatment options, the study of medicinal plants is once again receiving renewed attention and scientific interest on a global scale.

Although many plants are used to stop or cure diseases, scientific proof is lacking. Most plants are rich in carotenoids, flavonoids, terpenoids, alkaloids, glycosides, so they often have hypoglycemic effects (Afrisham et al., 2015).

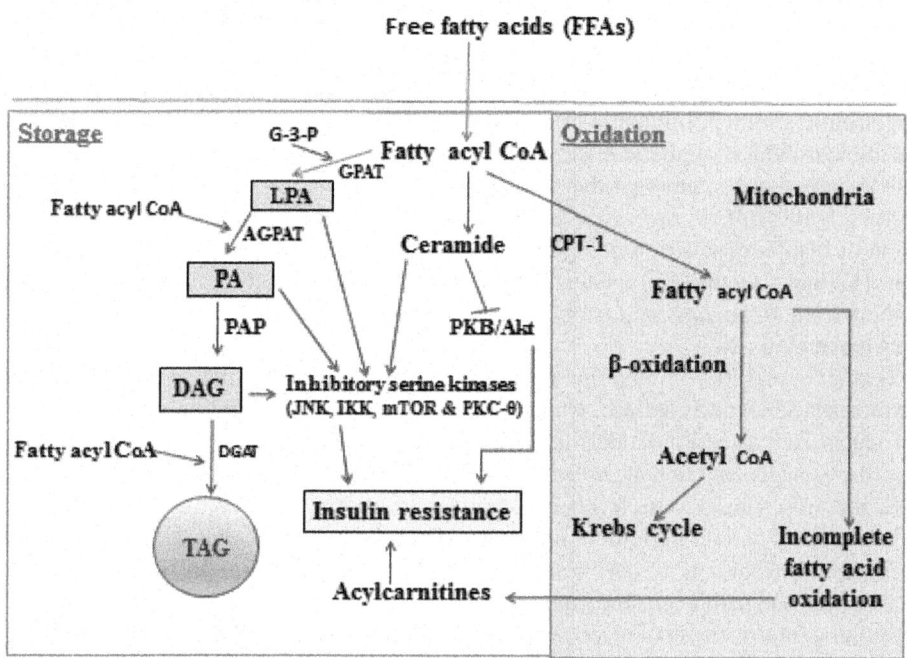

FIGURE 8.3 Fatty acid metabolism and insulin action in skeletal muscle or liver. Increased circulating levels of free fatty acids and myocyte or hepatocyte uptake are brought on by obesity. Fatty acyl-CoAs, or activated fatty acids, are largely "metabolized" through one of two pathways: oxidation or storage. When fatty acid flux exceeds the ability of these pathways to dispose of fatty acyl-CoAs, intermediaries of fatty acid metabolism (e.g., DAG, PA, LPA, and ceramide) accumulate. In turn, these fatty acid intermediates can activate a number of different serine kinases that can negatively regulate insulin action. Ceramide can also impair insulin action through interactions with PKB/Akt. An inability to completely oxidize fatty acids through β-oxidation, which leads to an accumulation of acylcarnitines, has also been hypothesized to cause insulin resistance, although the precise mechanisms leading to insulin resistance are, to date, unknown. AGPAT: acylglycerol-3-phosphate acyltransferase; CPT 1: Carnitine palmitoyl transferase 1; DAG: diacylglycerol; DGAT: DAG acyltransferase; IKK: IκB kinase; LPA: lysophosphatidic acid; mTOR: mammalian target of rapamycin; PA: phosphatidic acid; PAP: PA phosphohydrolase; PKB: protein kinase B; PKC-θ: protein kinase C; TAG: triacylglycerol (Schenk et al., 2008).

8.2.5.1 Treatment with Banana (*Musa paradisiaca*)

Musa paradisiaca (M. paradisiaca) is a crop in the genus *Musa*, and all members of the genus are native to the tropical and subtropical countries (Plants and Khare, 2007). *M. paradisiaca* has been recorded to have valuable impacts on several disease conditions, including atherosclerosis, diabetes mellitus, hypertension, hyperlipidemia, and thyroid dysfunction. Furthermore, it displays defensive effects on organs of the body (Vinaykumar et al., 2010). *M. paradisiaca* promotes healthy digestion, ameliorates affective state, and is a good source of potassium, calcium, phosphorus, and nitrogen, which assemble and regenerate tissues in the body. *M. paradisiaca* also contains iron and vitamins, especially vitamins C and E (Imam and Akter, 2011).

A study by Kappel et al. (2013b) proved that the crude extract n-butanol and aqueous residual fractions of *M. paradisiaca* leaves show potential hypoglycemic activity. The decrease in serum glucose levels, induction of insulin secretion, stimulation of glycogen storage, and inhibition of enzyme activity related to glucose absorption and advanced glycation end product (AGE) formation clarify the worthy impacts observed for *M. paradisiaca* leaves on the regulation of glucose homeostasis.

Moreover, phytochemical analysis elucidates the presence of flavonoids in crude extracts of *M. paradisiaca* leaves, and rutin is the main compound which indicates anti-diabetic potential properties (Kappel et al., 2013a, b).

Hypoglycemic and hypolipidemic effects of *M. paradisiaca* in streptozotocin-induced diabetic mice and alloxan-induced diabetic mice were illustrated (Ajiboye et al., 2018), likely due to its fibers and antioxidant potentials, among others.

The green fruit of *M. paradisiaca* has been reported to possess hypoglycemic effects due to stimulation of insulin production and glucose utilization (Ojewale and Adewunni, 2003). Its high potassium (K) and sodium (Na) content has been associated with the glycemic effect (Rai et al., 2009). Fibers from *M. paradisiaca* fruit prompt glycogenesis in the liver and decrease fasting blood glucose (Ahmed et al., 2021).

Vijayakumar et al. (2008) found that the flavonoids from banana induced the activities of superoxide dismutase (SOD) and catalase, which might be responsible for the decreased level of peroxidation products such as malondialdehyde, hydroperoxides, and conjugated dienes. In light of those outcomes, it was suggested that *M. paradisiaca* has antioxidant activity.

The decline in serum glucose levels is as per the investigations of Wu et al. (2015), who report that the banana peel and its ingredient lupenone demonstrated promising antihyperglycemic properties. Likewise, Lakshmi et al. (2014) state that the ethanolic extracts, the hexane and chloroform portions of leaves and fruit peels, indicated promising antihyperglycemic activity in the STZ model.

The glycemic improvement of *M. paradisiaca* leaf and fruit peel hydroethanolic extracts returned to presence bioactive compounds such as n-hexadecanoic acid, 9, 12-octadecatrienoic acid, phytol, sterols, and vitamin E. These compounds are notable antioxidants and might have contributed to enhance hypoglycemia in the diabetic rats (Bahadoran et al., 2013).

Glycogen levels in different tissues, especially the liver, are a direct indication of insulin activity. It was demonstrated that a significant depletion in hepatic glycogen content was associated with significant increase in glucose-6-phosphatase and glycogen phosphorylase activities in diabetic rats (Ahmed et al., 2017b), enhancing the glycogenolytic and gluconeogenic pathways. On the other side, diabetic rats set on an *M. paradisiaca*–based diet displayed an increase in liver glycogen content, serum insulin, and reduction in activity of glucose-6-phosphatase (Ajiboye et al., 2018; Ahmed et al., 2021). Moreover, the hepatoprotective activity of *M. paradisiaca* may be related to presence of vitamin E and linolenic acid with high amounts in fruit peel and leaf extracts, respectively.

The antihyperglycemic effects of *M. paradisiaca* leaf and fruit peel extracts may be attributed to their ability to enhance insulin secretion and/or insulin action. Phytols, rutin, and vitamin E, which are present in *M. paradisiaca*, were reported to exhibit hypoglycemic activity and are also known for their ability of β cell regeneration in the pancreas (Kurian et al., 2005).

8.2.5.1.1 *The Antihyperlipidemic Effects of Musa paradisiaca*

Lipids play a crucial role in the pathogenesis of DM, and the most common lipid abnormalities in DM are hypercholesterolemia and hypertriglyceridemia, and secondarily the elevation of FFA levels in the blood. Not only quantitative lipid abnormalities, but also qualitative and kinetic lipid abnormalities are included in lipid disorders observed in T2DM (Chahil and Ginsberg, 2006) and are potentially atherogenic.

Increased triglyceride levels are major quantitative abnormalities which relate to an augmented hepatic production of VLDL and a reduction of both VLDL and IDL catabolism, and decreased HDL levels due to an accelerated HDL catabolism (Arvind et al., 2002). In diabetes, the related hyperglycemia, obesity, and insulin changes profoundly quicken the progression to atherosclerosis, the main source of death in patients with T2DM (Eliasson et al., 2011). The high LDL found in hypercholesterolemia rats may be attributed to diminished number of low LDL receptors with consequent delayed clearance (Mustad et al., 1997).

Treatments of diabetic rats with *M. paradisiaca* extracts reversed this abnormality with an increase in HDL concentration, probably by enhancing the insulin secretion and improving the insulin sensitivity as well. The hypolipidemic effect may be due to the presence of polyunsaturated fatty acids, linoleic acid ester, and vitamin E in the extracts (Khizar et al., 2019; Ahmed et al., 2021).

Supplementation with either *M. paradisiaca* leaf or peel hydroethanolic extract might lead to a reduction in the risk of developing vascular and heart diseases. The observed cardioprotective effect of both extracts was further confirmed by the notably decreased serum cardiac markers CK-MB, AST, and LDH (Ahmed et al., 2021).

The serum elevated FFA level in NA/STZ-induced diabetic rats was decreased due to treatments with *M. paradisiaca* (Ahmed et al., 2021). That elevation is due to the chronic rise of lipolysis, which was attributed to lack of insulin. Additionally, critical increase of FFAs might be because of breakdown of membrane phospholipids by free radicals and/or by increased activity of phospholipase (Geetha et al., 2008).

FFAs regulate gene expression, especially those involved in lipid and carbohydrate metabolism. The mechanisms by which the elevated levels of FFAs decrease insulin sensitivity include inhibition of insulin-stimulated glucose transport, flux of FFAs to the non-adipose tissue leading to progression of insulin resistance, reduction of expression of IRS-1, and impairment of the activation of PI3K-AKT signaling (Khorami et al., 2015) in the liver and skeletal muscles, increasing the expression of JNK signaling in the pancreas (Cheon et al., 2010). Thus, the decrease in serum FFAs in the diabetic rats treated with *M. paradisiaca* extracts is participating in their insulin sensitizing effects and improved β cell secretory response.

Adipocytokines are cytokines secreted by adipose tissue that concerned on glucose metabolism (e.g., adiponectin, resistin), lipid metabolism (cholesteryl ester transfer protein [CETP]), inflammation (TNF-α, IL-6), coagulation (PAI-1), blood pressure (angiotensinogen, angiotensin II), and nutrition behavior (leptin), which subsequently impact metabolism and function of many organs and tissues (Ran et al., 2006).

Kwon and Pessin (2013) announced that deregulation of adipokines has been implicated in obesity, T2DM, and cardiovascular disorders. TNF-α, IL-6, and resistin weaken the ability of tissues to accurately sense and respond to insulin. Conversely, adiponectin and leptin improve the response of tissues to insulin and glucose (Blüher and Mantzoros, 2015). Thus, the harmful and defensive cytokines should have been balanced to keep up glucose hemostasis.

8.2.5.1.2 The Anti-Inflammatory Effect of Musa paradisiaca

Haidari et al. (2016) demonstrated that high plasma level of inflammatory cytokines, such as TNF-α and IL-6, are associated with the development of insulin resistance and T2DM. It is worth mentioning that TNF-α is a potent pro-inflammatory cytokine primarily secreted from myeloid cells via activation of MAPK and NF-κB signaling pathways, resulting in the release of other inflammatory cytokines, such as IL-1β and IL-6 (Cheung et al., 2000). TNF-α elicits antagonistic activity toward insulin because of its ability to inhibit IRS-1 and insulin receptor phosphorylation and decrease synthesis/translocation of GLUT4 (Zozulinska and Wierusz-Wysocka, 2006).

TNF-α also downregulates the mRNA level of adiponectin (Hector et al., 2007). The decrease in the FFAs levels, the increase in adipose tissue mRNA expression level of adiponectin, and the enhancement of insulin sensitivity as a result of treatment of NA/STZ-induced diabetic rats with *M. paradisiaca* may be secondary to improvement in the elevated TNF-α level (Ahmed et al., 2021). Moreover, it was suggested that the amelioration of blood IL-6 level may have a role in the improvement of insulin sensitivity which was induced as a result of treatment with *M. paradisiaca* leaf and fruit peel hydroethanolic extracts (Abdel Aziz et al., 2020).

The anti-inflammatory effects of *M. paradisiaca* leaf and fruit peel hydroethanolic extracts may be attributed to the presence of phytochemicals such as phytol, vitamin E, and phytosterols such as β-sitosterol and stigmasterol. These compounds have been reported to exert anti-inflammatory effects (Silva et al., 2014).

In association with the decrease in serum fatty acid level, the treatment of NA/STZ-induced diabetic rats with *M. paradisiaca* extracts also resulted in an increase in the expression of adipose tissue PPARγ, GLUT4, adiponectin, and insulin receptor β-subunit (Ahmed et al., 2021). PPARs may either activate or inhibit transcription and regulate activity of nuclear factors essential for immune-modulatory and inflammatory responses (Semple et al., 2006). Three isoforms of PPAR with distinct tissue-specific distribution and biological activity have been identified, namely PPARα, PPARβ/δ, and PPARγ with two subforms (PPARγ1 and PPARγ2) (Omi et al., 2005).

PPARs modulate expression of the genes involved in lipid metabolism. Their activation stimulates differentiation and insulin sensitivity of adipocytes (Yadav et al., 2013). Therefore, synthetic PPARγ ligands such as thiazolidinediones (TZDs) are applied clinically to control diabetes (Chen et al., 2009). The PPARγ agonists pioglitazone and decreases plasma triglycerides through increase the fractional clearance rate of VLDL triglycerides, increasing lipoprotein lipase mass and decreasing apoC-III. PPARγ increases the expression and translocation of GLUT4 in fat tissue and the catabolism of glucose in the liver decreasing the hepatic glucose output. It also decreases the insulin resistance in muscle and adipose tissue by increasing protein production involved in glucose uptake (Elmazar et al., 2013).

The activity of PPARγ on insulin sensitivity results from its capacity to channel unsaturated fats (FAs) into fat tissue, subsequently diminishing plasma FA concentration and alleviating lipotoxicity in skeletal muscle, liver, and pancreas (Feige et al., 2006). In addition, PPARγ can affect insulin sensitivity by regulating adipocyte hormones, cytokines, and proteins that are involved in insulin resistance. Indeed, PPARγ downregulates the expression of genes encoding resistin and tumor necrosis factor α (TNF-α), whereas it induces adiponectin expression, which increases fatty acid oxidation by activation of the AMPK pathway (Lefebvre et al., 2006). Activated PPARγ decreases inducible nitric oxide synthase synthesis and its subsequent NO production. PPARγ upregulated expression of antioxidant enzymes SOD and CAT (Gong et al., 2012), therefore attenuating oxidative stress.

Upregulation of PPARγ gene expression by *M. paradisiaca* leaf or peel hydroethanolic extracts reflects their hypoglycemic, hypolipidemic, and anti-inflammatory effects (Ahmed et al., 2021; Abdel Aziz et al., 2020).

8.2.5.1.3   Effect of Banana on GLUT4

The increased GLUT4 expression in diabetic rats treated with *Musa paradisiaca* leaf as well as fruit peel hydroethanolic extracts may be due to the enhanced insulin secretory response of β cells and the improved peripheral insulin-sensitizing effects of both agents.

8.2.5.1.4   Effect of Banana on Adiponectin

Adiponectin, one of the most important adipokines, increases β-oxidation of FFAs in muscles and glucose transport mediated by phosphorylation of AMPK and inhibition of acetyl-CoA carboxylase (Lee et al., 2009). Moreover, it decreases hepatic gluconeogenesis secondary to its decrease the expression of phosphoenol pyruvate carboxylase and glucose-6-phosphatase, partly through PPARα activation, leading to decreased triglyceride content in skeletal muscles and liver (Yamauchi et al., 2003).

It is well established that there is a converse relationship between insulin resistance and plasma adiponectin levels, suggesting that adiponectin is a significant stimulator of insulin sensitivity and glucose homeostasis, potentially, through AMPK pathway (Ohashi et al., 2012). Adiponectin has no direct impact on adipose tissue hormone-sensitive lipase (Combs et al., 2001), showing that decrease of plasma FAs results from accelerated tissue uptake rather than restraint of lipolysis. Considering this information, adiponectin was imagined to be a novel therapy target for obesity and insulin resistance. The anti-diabetic effect of hydroethanolic extract of *Musa paradisiaca* leaves and fruit peels in NA/STZ-induced diabetic rats might be explained, at least in part, through its ability to produce a pronounced increase in mRNA expression of adiponectin (Ahmed et al., 2021).

The mechanism of upregulation of adipose tissue PPARγ, GLUT4, and adiponectin induced by hydroethanolic extracts of *M. paradisiaca* leaf and fruit peel extracts may include increased expression of key proteins of insulin receptors, IRS-1 and PI3K that are associated with the insulin signaling processes (Ahmed et al., 2017b)

8.2.5.1.5 Effect of Banana on Resistin

It has been reported that resistin is expressed exclusively in adipocytes and is linked with the traits that are related to obesity and insulin resistance. These findings might be ascribed to resistin-induced impairment of glucose homeostasis and insulin action that modulates one or more steps in the insulin signaling pathway (Muse et al., 2004).

Contrary to that, Savage et al. (2001) reported no correlation between insulin resistance and resistin gene expression in whole abdominal adipose tissue. Different impacts of resistin on insulin sensitivity have been suggested. This include decreasing the phosphorylation of AMPK (Muse et al., 2004), blockade of insulin signal transduction pathways (Sheng et al., 2008), increasing suppressor of cytokine signaling 3 (SOCS-3) expression (Steppan et al., 2005), decreasing activation of PPARγ (Patel et al., 2003), regulating NF-κB expression (Silswal et al., 2005), and suppressing GLUT4 gene expression (Fu et al., 2006).

Resistin induces elevation of endogenous glucose production, as indicated by the upregulation of genes encoding the hepatic gluconeogenic enzymes in liver cells and downregulation of glycogen synthase activity (Banerjee et al., 2004). Likewise, it promotes lipid accumulation in human macrophages by upregulating CD36 cell surface expression, which is one of the scavenger receptors in macrophages associated with modified LDL uptake (Xu et al., 2006). In view of Tsukahara et al. (2009), resistin is supposed to induce atherosclerosis mediating endothelial hyperactivity in response to the systematic inflammatory condition in human.

Hydroethanolic extracts of *Musa paradisiaca* leaf and fruit peel extracts' supplementation to diabetic rats significantly downregulated adipose tissue resistin expression. Therefore, the potent anti-diabetic effect of *M. paradisiaca* could perhaps be attributed, at least in part, to its resistin-modulating effect. The increase in resistin expression in adipose tissue of diabetic rats was related with raised serum TC, TG, and LDL cholesterol and decreased HDL cholesterol, representing a connection between atherogenesis and T2DM. In contrast, Qi et al. (2008) found no critical relationship between resistin levels and lipid profile parameters aside from a negative connection with HDL levels just in patients with metabolic disorder.

It was reported that the renal protective effects of *M. paradisiaca* seems to be mediated by means of hypoglycemic effect, antioxidant activity, and enhancement of Na$^+$,K$^+$-ATPase expression and activity. This further shows the ability of the extracts in treating DM-associated with renal complications (Navghare and Dhawale, 2016).

8.2.5.1.6 Effect of Banana on the Oxidative Stress System

Oxidative stress is the result of an imbalance between the generation and neutralization of reactive oxygen and nitrogen species (ROS and RNS, respectively) overwhelming the antioxidant capacity of cell. These free radicals are thought to contribute to lipid peroxidation, DNA damage, and protein degradation (Jaganjac et al., 2013). Subsequently, this imbalance may evoke tissue deterioration related to DM pathology (Bajaj and Khan, 2012). Oxidative tissue damage in diabetes might be mediated via autoxidation of glucose and glycated proteins, polyol pathway activation, intracellular NADH/NAD$^+$ ratio increase, glutathione alteration, ascorbate redox status, nitric oxide disturbance, and/or prostaglandin metabolism disturbance (Roy et al., 1997; Yoshida et al., 1995).

Chronic hyperglycemia observed in diabetic rats is attributed to accumulation of free radical that declines enzymatic and non-enzymatic antioxidant defense system (Hong et al., 2004). Glutathione contributes to the maintenance of exogenous antioxidants such as vitamins E and C in their active states. The cellular demand for NADPH is increased when the level of GSH is decreased. Thus, in hyperglycemic conditions, the alteration of GSH levels may be linked to increased polyol pathway activity, resulting in NADPH deficiency (Preet et al., 2005).

In view of oxidative stress, liver LPO increased while GSH content and antioxidant enzymes, SOD, GPx, and GST activities decreased in diabetic rats. These are reported by Arulselvan and Subramanian (2007) and Ahmed et al. (2021), who detailed that STZ produces oxidative stress and depletion of antioxidant systems in both blood and tissues. Also, these results were in accordance with other reports revealing an increase in lipid hydroperoxides in the plasma of diabetic subjects (de Souza Bastos et al., 2016) and in animals with experimental DM (Ramesh and Pugalendi, 2005).

It is worth mentioning that the reduction in antioxidant enzymes activities and GSH content along with raised MDA under diabetic conditions could be credited to the glycation of these enzymes and contribute to oxidative stress–induced damage of the diabetic liver (Oyagbemi et al., 2016).

Rats treated with *Musa paradisiaca* leaf and peel hydroethanolic extracts were able to restore the level of GSH and higher activities of GPx, SOD, and GST and successfully produced a significant suppression of LPO in diabetic rats. These results are in line with Mokbel and Hashinaga (2005) and Ahmed et al. (2021). GC-MS results of the *M. paradisiaca* leaf and fruit peel hydroethanolic extract proved the presence of a lot of antioxidant ingredients (Kaplaner et al., 2017).

Hence, our brief review suggests that the extracts of various parts of *M. paradisiaca* such as leaf and fruit peel may be considered as promising candidates for treatment of diabetic patients, pending further investigations in order to trace out their anti-diabetic efficacies and exact mechanistic pathways.

8.3 CONCLUSION

Diabetes mellitus is an endocrinological disorder which is a group of metabolic or heterogeneous afflictions resulting from an irregularity in insulin secretion and/or insulin action consistent with derangement in carbohydrate, protein, and lipid metabolism. Because none of the currently available anti-diabetic drugs can give a long-term glycemic control without producing any unfavorable side effects, medicinal plants which are effective in improving plasma glucose level with minimal side effects are widely used in underdeveloped and developing countries as an alternative therapy. Treatment with either *Musa paradisiaca* leaf or fruit peel hydroethanolic extracts reduced the elevated blood glucose levels at all points of the OGTT significantly. The serum insulin, C-peptide levels, HOMA-IR (as index of insulin resistance) and QUICKI, HOMA-IS and HOMA-β cell function were significantly alleviated. In association, the deteriorated serum lipid profile and FFAs, TNF-α, and IL-6 levels are significantly decreased. It can be concluded that *M. paradisiaca* leaf and fruit peel hydroethanolic extracts have hypoglycemic effects which may be mediated via their insulinotropic and insulin-sensitizing effects.

8.4 SUMMARY POINTS

- This chapter focuses on *Musa paradisiaca*, which is native to tropical and subtropical countries.
- Extracts of various parts of *M. paradisiaca* have both pancreatic (insulinotropic) and extrapancreatic (insulin-mimetic) effects.
- *M. paradisiaca* has improved impaired glucose tolerance and increased serum insulin and C-peptide concentrations.
- Deteriorated HOMA-IR, HOMA-IS, HOMA-β cell function, and QUICK were significantly improved as a result of *M. paradisiaca* treatments.
- Treatment of diabetic rats with either *M. paradisiaca* leaf or fruit peel hydroethanolic extracts had profound ameliorative effects on the disrupted lipid profile, expressing their hypolipidemic effects.
- Serum IL-6 and TNF-α were increased in diabetic rats and decreased after treatments with extracts of *M. paradisiaca*, reflecting their anti-inflammatory effects.
- *M. paradisiaca* extracts supplementations potentially upregulated the diminished PPARγ, adiponectin, GLUT4, and insulin receptor mRNA expression and decreased the elevated expression of resistin.
- The activities of SOD, GPX, and GST, as well as GSH content, were decreased in the livers of diabetic rats and increased as a result of treatment with *M. paradisiaca*.
- *M. paradisiaca* exerted powerful antihyperlipidemic, cardiovascular protective, hepatoprotective, nephroprotective, and antioxidant effects in diabetic rats.

REFERENCES

Abdel Aziz, S. M.; Ahmed, O. M.; Abd El-Twab, S. M.; Al-Muzafar, H. M.; Amin, K. A.; Abdel-Gabbar, M. (2020): Antihyperglycemic effects and mode of actions of musa paradisiaca leaf and fruit peel hydro-ethanolic extracts in nicotinamide/streptozotocin-induced diabetic rats. *Evid Based Complement Alternat Med.* 26: 9276343.

Afrisham, R.; Aberomand, M.; Ghaffari, M. A.; Siahpoosh, A.; Jamalan, M. (2015): Inhibitory effect of heracleum persicum and ziziphus jujuba on activity of alpha-amylase. *J Bot*: 1–8.

Ahmed, O. M.; Abd El-Twab, S. M.; Al-Muzafar, H. M.; Adel Amin, K.; Abdel Aziz, S. M.; Abdel-Gabbar, M. (2021): Musa paradisiaca L. leaf and fruit peel hydroethanolic extracts improved the lipid profile, glycemic index and oxidative stress in nicotinamide/streptozotocin-induced diabetic rats. *Vet Med Sci.* 7(2): 500–511.

Ahmed, O. M.; Hassan, M. A.; Abdel-Twab, S. M.; Azeem, M. N. (2017b): Navel orange peel hydroethanolic extract, naringin and naringenin have anti-diabetic potentials in type 2 diabetic rats. *Biomed Pharmacother.* 94: 197–205.

Ajiboye, B. O.; Oloyede, H.O.B.; Salawu, M. O. (2018): Antihyperglycemic and antidyslipidemic activity of Musa paradisiaca-based diet in alloxan-induced diabetic rats. *Food Sci Nutr.* 6: 137–145.

Arulselvan, P.; Subramanian, S. P. (2007): Beneficial effects of Murraya koenigii leaves on antioxidant defense system and ultra-structural changes of pancreatic β-cells in experimental diabetes in rats. *Chem Biol Interact.* 165: 155–164.

Arvind, K.; Pradeep, R.; Deepa, R.; Mohan, V. (2002): Diabetes and coronary artery diseases. *Indian J Med Res.* 116: 163–176.

Bahadoran, Z.; Mirmiran, P.; Azizi, F. (2013): Dietary polyphenols as potential nutraceuticals in management of diabetes: A review. *J Diabetes Metab Disord.* 12: 43.

Bajaj, S.; Khan, A. (2012): Antioxidants and diabetes. *Indian J Endocrinol Metab.* 16: S267–S271.

Banerjee, R. R.; Rangwala, S. M.; Shapiro, J. S.; Rich, A. S.; Rhoades, B.; Qi, Y.; Wang, J.; Rajala, M. W.; Pocai, A.; Scherer, P. E.; et al. (2004): Regulation of fasted blood glucose by resistin. *Science.* 303: 1195–1198.

Blüher, M.; Mantzoros, C. S. (2015): From leptin to other adipokines in health and disease: Facts and expectations at the beginning of the 21st century. *Metab Clin Exp.* 64: 131–145.

Bortolon, L.N.M.; Triz, L. de P. L.; Faustino, B. de S.; de Sá, L.B.C.; Rocha, D.R.T.W.; Arbex, A. K. (2016): Gestational diabetes mellitus: New diagnostic criteria. *Open J Endocr Metab Dis.* 6: 13–19.

Burks, D. J.; White, M. F. (2001): IRS proteins and beta-cell function. *Diabetes.* 50(Suppl 1): S140–S145.

Chahil, T. J.; Ginsberg, H. N. (2006): Diabetic dyslipidemia. *Endocrinol Metab Clin North Am.* 35: 491–510.

Chauhan, P. K.; Pandey, I. P.; Dhatwalia, V. K. (2010): Evaluation of the anti-diabetic effect of ethanolic and methanolic extracts of Centella asiatica leaves extract on alloxan induced diabetic rats. *Adv Biol Res.* 4: 27–30.

Chen, Y.; Li, Y.; Wang, Y.; Wen, Y.; Sun, C. (2009): Berberine improves free-fatty-acid – induced insulin resistance in L6 myotubes through inhibiting peroxisome proliferator – activated receptor γ and fatty acid transferase expressions. *Metabolism.* 58(12): 1694–1702.

Cheng, A.; et al. (2002): Coordinated action of protein tyrosine phosphatases in insulin signal transduction. *Eur J Biochem.* 69(4): 1050–1059.

Cheon, H.; Cho, J. M.; Kim, S.; Baek, S. H.; Lee, M. K.; Kim, K. W.; Yu, S. W.; Solinas, G.; Kim, S. S.; Lee, M. S. (2010): Role of jnk activation in pancreatic beta-cell death by streptozotocin. *Mol Cell Endocrinol.* 321: 131–137.

Cheung, A. T.; Wang, J.; Ree, D.; Kolls, J. K.; Bryer-Ash, M. (2000): Tumor necrosis factor-alpha induces hepatic insulin resistance in obese Zucker (fa/fa)rats via interaction of leukocyte antigen-related tyrosine phosphatase with focal adhesion kinase. *Diabetes.* 49(5): 810–819.

Combs, T. P.; Berg, A. H.; Obici, S.; Scherer, P. E.; Rossetti, L. (2001): Endogenous glucose production is inhibited by the adipose-derived protein Acrp30. *J Clin Invest.* 108: 1875–1881.

Cross, D. A.; Alessi, D. R.; Cohen, P.; Andjelkovich, M.; Hemmings, B. A. (1995): Inhibition of glycogen synthase kinase-3 by insulin mediated by protein kinase B. *Nature.* 378(6559): 785.

Das, J.; Vasan, V.; Sil, P. C. (2012): Taurine exerts hypoglycemic effect in alloxan-induced diabetic rats, improves insulin-mediated glucose transport signaling pathway in heart and ameliorates cardiac oxidative stress and apoptosis. *Toxicol Appl Pharmacol.* 258(2): 296–308.

De Meyts, P.; Whittaker, J. (2002): Structural biology of insulin and IGF1 receptors: Implications for drug design. *Nat Rev Drug Discov.* 1(10): 769.

de Souza Bastos, A.; Graves, D. T.; de Melo Loureiro, A. P.; et al. (2016): Diabetes and increased lipid peroxidation are associated with systemic inflammation even in well-controlled patients. *J Diabetes Complicat.* 30(8): 1593–1599.

Eberle, D.; Hegarty, B.; Bossard, P.; Ferre, P.; Foufelle, F. (2004): SREBP transcription factors: Master regulators of lipid homeostasis. *Biochimie.* 86: 839–848.

Eliasson, B.; Cederholm, J.; Eeg-Olofsson, K.; Svensson, A. M.; Zethelius, B.; Gudbjornsddottir, S. (2011): Clinical usefulness of different lipid measures for prediction of coronary heart disease in type 2 diabetes: A report from the Swedish National Diabetes Register. *Diabetes Care.* 34: 2095–2100.

Elmazar, M. M.; Hanan, S.; Schaalan, M. F.; Farag, N. A. (2013): Phytol/Phytanic acid and insulin resistance: Potential role of phytanic acid proven by docking simulation and modulation of biochemical alterations. *PLoS ONE.* 8(1):]

El-Zayadi, A. (2010): Insulin resistance. *Arab J Gastroenterol.* 11(2): 66–69.

Feige, J. N.; Gelman, L.; Michalik, L.; Desvergne, B.; Wahli, W. (2006): From molecular action to physiological outputs: Peroxisome proliferator-activated receptors are nuclear receptors at the crossroads of key cellular functions. *Prog Lipid Res.* 45: 120–159.

Fu, Y.; Luo, L.; Luo, N.; Garvey, W. T. (2006): Pro-inflammatory cytokine production and insulin sensitivity regulated by overexpression of resistin in 3T3-L1 adipocytes. *Nutr Metab.* 3(1): 28.

Geetha, G.; Prasanth, K. G.; Samuel, T. B.; Prudence, A. R.; Hari, B. V. (2008): Hypolipidemic effect of achyranthes rubrofusca linn. Whole plant extracts in high fat diet induced hyperlipidemic rats. *Pharmacologyonline.* 1: 466–473.

Gong, P.; Xu, H.; Zhang, J.; Wang, Z. (2012): PPAR expression and its association with SOD and NF-κB in rats with obstructive jaundice. *Biomed Res–India.* 23: 551–560.

Haidari, F.; Zakerkish, M.; Karandish, M.; Saki, A.; Pooraziz, S. (2016): Association between serum vitamin D level and glycemic and inflammatory markers in non-obese patients with type 2 diabetes. *Iran J Med Sci.* 41(5): 367–373.

Hector, J.; Schwarzloh, B.; Goehring, J.; Strate, T. G.; Hess, U. F.; Deuretzbacher, G.; Algenstaedt, P. (2007): TNF-α alters visfatin and adiponectin levels in human fat. *Horm Metab Res.* 39(4): 250–255.

Hong, J. H.; Kim, M. J.; Park, M. R.; Kwang, A. J.; Lee, I. S.; Byun, B. H.; et al. (2004): Effects of vitamin E on oxidative stress and membrane fluidity in brain of streptozotocin-induced diabetic rats. *Clin Chim Acta.* 340: 107–115.

Imam, M. Z.; Akter, S. (2011): Musa paradisiaca L. and Musa sapientum L.: A phytochemical and pharmacological review. *J Appl Pharma Sci.* 1: 14–20.

International Diabetes Federation (2017): *IDF Diabetes Atlas,* 8th ed. International Diabetes Federation, Brussels, Belgium.

Jaganjac, M.; Tirosh, O.; Cohen, G.; Sasson, S.; Zarkovic, N. (2013): Reactive aldehydes–second messengers of free radicals in diabetes mellitus. *Free Radic Res.* 47(Suppl 1): 39–48.

Kaplaner, E.; Singeç, M. H.; Öztürk, M. (2017): Fatty acid composition and antioxidant activity of tricholoma imbricatum and T. Focale. *Turk J Agric Food Sci Technol.* 5(9): 1080–1085.

Kappel, V. D.; Cazarolli, L. H.; Pereira, D. F.; Postal, B. G.; Madoglio, F. A.; Buss, Z.D.S.; Reginatto, F. H.; Silva, F. R. (2013b): Beneficial effects of banana leaves (Musa x paradisiaca) on glucose homeostasis: Multiple sites of action. *Revista Brasileira de Farmacognosia.* 23(4): 706–715.

Kappel, V. D.; Frederico, M. J.; Postal, B. G.; Mendes, C. P.; Cazarolli, L. H.; Silva, F. R. (2013a): The role of calcium in intracellular pathways of rutin in rat pancreatic islets: Potential insulin secretagogue effect. *Eur J Pharmacol.* 702(1–3): 264–268.

Khizar, A.; Rizwani, G. H.; Hina, Z.; Shareef, H.; Taqi, M. M. (2019): *Musa paradisiaca* L. may restore pancreatic morphology and function to trigger its antidiabetic and hypolipidemic activities in alloxon-induce diabetic rats. *Med Aromat Plants (Los Angel).* 8: 333.

Khorami, S.A.H.; Movahedi, A.; Sokhini, A.M.M. (2015): Review article; PI3K/AKT pathway in modulating glucose homeostasis and its alteration in Diabetes. *Ann. Med. Biomed. Sci.* 1(2):

Kido, Y.; Nakae, J.; Accili, D. (2001): The insulin receptor and its cellular targets. *J Clin Endocrinol Metab.* 86: 972–979.

Kumar, S.; Mittal, A.; Babu, D.; Mittal, A. (2021): Herbal medicines for diabetes management and its secondary complications. *Curr Diabetes Rev.* 17(4): 437–456.

Kurian, G. A.; Philp, S.; Varghese, T. (2005): Effect of aqueous extract of Desmodiumgangeticum DC root in the severity of myocardial infarction. *J Ethnopharmacol.* 97: 4557–4561.

Kwon, H.; Pessin, J. E. (2013): Adipokines mediate inflammation and insulin resistance. *Frontier Endocrinol.* 4: 1–11.

Lakshmi, V.; Agarwal, S. K.; Ansari, J. A.; Mahdi, A. A.; Srivastava, A. K. (2014): Antidiabetic potential of Musa paradisiaca in streptozotocin-induced diabetic rats. *J Phytopharmacol.* 3: 77–81.

Lavanya, K.; Abi Beaulah, G.; Vani, G. (2016): Musa paradisiaca-A review on phytochemistry and pharmacology. *World J Pharm Med Res.* 2(6): 163–173.

Lee, C. Y.; Lee, C. H.; Tsai, S.; et al. (2009): Association between serum leptin and adiponectin levels with risk of insulin resistance and impaired glucose tolerance in non-diabetic women. *Kaohsiung J Med Sci.* 25(3): 116–125.

Lefebvre, P.; Chinetti, G.; Fruchart, J. C.; Staels, B. (2006): Sorting out the roles of PPAR alpha in energy metabolism and vascular homeostasis. *J Clin Invest.* 116(3): 571–580.

Long, X.; Lin, Y.; Ortiz-Vega, S.; Yonezawa, K.; Avruch, J. (2005): Rheb binds and regulates the mTOR kinase. *Curr Biol.* 15: 702–713.

Matsuzaka, T.; Shimano, H.; Yahagi, N.; et al. (2004): Insulin-independent induction of sterol regulatory element-binding protein-1c expression in the livers of streptozotocin-treated mice. *Diabetes.* 53: 560–569.

Mokbel, M. S.; Hashinaga, F. (2005): Antibacterial and antioxidant activities of banana (Musa, AAA cv. Cavendish) fruits peel. *Am J Biochem Biotechnol.* 1(3): 125–131.

Motala, A. A.; Pirie, F. J.; Gouws, E.; Amod, A.; Omar, M. K. (2003): High incidence of Type 2 diabetes mellitus in South African Indians: A 10-year follow-up study. *Diabet Med.* 20: 23–30.

Muse, E. D.; Obici, S.; Bhanot, S.; Monia, B. P.; McKay, R. A.; Rajala, M. W.; Scherer, P. E.; Rossetti, L. (2004): Role of resistin in diet-induced hepatic insulin resistance. *J Clin Invest.* 114: 232–239.

Mustad, V. A.; Etherton, T. D.; Cooper, A. D.; Mastro, A. M.; Pearson, T. A.; Jonnalagadda, S. S.; Kris-Etherton, P. M. (1997): Reducing saturated fat intake is associated with increased levels of LDL receptors on mononuclear cells in healthy men and women. *J Lipid Res.* 38(3): 459–468.

Navale, A. M.; Paranjape, A. N. (2016): Glucose transporters: Physiological and pathological roles. *Biophys Rev.* 8(1): 5–9.

Navghare, V.; Dhawale, S. (2016): Suppression of Type-II diabetes with dyslipidemia and nephropathy by peels of Musa cavendish fruit. *Indian J Clin Biochem.* 31(4): 380–389.

Nolte, M. S.; Karam, J. H. (2001): Pancreatic hormones and anti-diabetic drugs. In: *Basic and Clinical Pharmacology*, 8th ed. Katzung B. G. Lange Medical Books, McGraw-Hill, San Francisco, 711–734.

Ohashi, K.; Ouchi, N.; Matsuzawa, Y. (2012): Anti-inflammatory and anti-atherogenic properties of adiponectin. *Biochimie.* 94(10): 2137–2142.

Ojewale, J. A.; Adewunni, C. O. (2003): Hypoglycaemic effect of methanolic extracts of Musa paradisiaca (Musaceae) green fruits in normal and diabetic mice. *Methods Find Exp Clin Pharmacol.* 25(6): 453–456.

Omi, T.; Brenig, B.; Špilar Kramer, Š.; Iwamoto, S.; Stranzinger, G.; Neuenschwander, S. (2005): Identification and characterization of novel peroxisome proliferator-activated receptor-gamma (PPAR-γ) transcriptional variants in pig and human. *J Anim Breed Genet.* 122: 45–53.

Oyagbemi, A. A.; Omobowale, O. T.; Asenuga, E. R.; Akinleye, A. S.; Ogunsanwo, R. O.; Saba, A. B. (2016): Cyclophosphamide-induced hepatotoxicity in wistar rats: The modulatory role of gallic acid as a hepatoprotective and chemopreventive phytochemical. *Int J Prev Med.* 7.

Ozougwu, J. C.; Obimba, K. C.; Belonwu, C. D.; Unakalamba, C. B. (2013): The pathogenesis and pathophysiology of type 1 and type 2 diabetes mellitus. *J Physiol Pathophysiol.* 4 (4): 46–57.

Patel, L.; Buckels, A. C.; Kinghorn, I. J.; et al. (2003): Resistin is expressed in human macrophages and directly regulated by PPAR activators. *Biochem Biophys Res Commun.* 300(2): 472–476.

Plants, I. M.; Khare, B. C. (2007): *An Illustrated Dictionary.* Springer Science+ Business Media, LLC, Spring Street, New York, 1–739.

Preet, A.; Gupta, B. L.; Siddiqui, M. R.; Yadava, P. K.; Baquer, N. Z. (2005): Restoration of ultrastructural and biochemical changes in alloxan-induced diabetic rat sciatic nerve on treatment with Na3VO4 and Trigonella: A promising antidiabetic agent. *Mol Cell Biochem.* 278: 21–31.

Qi, Q.; Wang, J.; Li, H.; Yu, Z.; Ye, X.; Hu, F. B.; Franco, O. H.; Pan, A.; Liu, Y.; Lin, X. (2008): Association of resistin with inflammatory and fibrinolytic markers, insulin resistance, and metabolic syndrome in middle-aged and older Chinese. *Eur J Endocrinol.* 159: 585–593.

Rai, P. K.; Jaiswal, D.; Rai, N. K.; Pandhija, S.; Rai, A. K.; Watal, G. (2009): Role of glycemic elements of Cynodon dactylon and Musa paradisiaca in diabetes management. *Lasers Med Sci.* 24(5): 761.

Ramesh, B.; Pugalendi, K. V. (2005): Impact of umbelliferone on erythrocyte redox status in STZ-diabetic rats. *Yale J Biol Med.* 78(3): 133.

Ran, J.; Hirano, T.; Fukui, T.; et al. (2006): Angiotensin II infusion decreases plasma adiponectin level via its type 1 receptor in rats: An implication for hypertension-related insulin resistance. *Metabolism.* 55(4): 478–488.

Roy, S.; Sen, C. K.; Tritschler, H. J.; Packer, L. (1997): Modulation of cellular reducing equivalent homeostasis by alpha-lipoic acid. Mechanisms and implications for diabetes and ischemic injury. *Biochem Pharmacol.* 53: 393–399.

Savage, D. B.; Sewter, C. P.; Klenk, E. S.; et al. (2001): Resistin/Fizz3 expression in relation to obesity and peroxisome proliferator-activated receptor-action in humans. *Diabetes.* 50: 2199–2202.

Schenk, S.; Saberi, M.; Olefsky, J. M. (2008): Insulin sensitivity: Modulation by nutrients and inflammation. *J Clin Invest.* 118(9): 2992–3002.

Semple, R. K.; Chatterjee, V. K.; O'rahilly, S. (2006): PPAR gamma and human metabolic disease. *J Clin Invest.* 116(3): 581–589.

Shamim A. (2013): *Diabetes: An Old Disease, a New Insight.* Springer New York, NY, XXXIII, 485. https://doi.org/10.1007/978-1-4614-5441-0

Sheng, C. H.; Di, J.; Jin, Y.; Zhang, Y. C.; Wu, M.; Sun, Y.; Zhang, G. Z. (2008): Resistin is expressed in human hepatocytes and induces insulin resistance. *Endocrine.* 33(2): 135–143.

Shi, G. J.; Shi, G. R.; Zhou, J. Y.; et al. (2018): Involvement of growth factors in diabetes mellitus and its complications: A general review. *Biomed Pharmacother.* 101: 510–527.

Silswal, N.; Singh, A. K.; Aruna, B.; Mukhopadhyay, S.; Ghosh, S.; Ehtesham, N. Z. (2005): Human resistin stimulates the pro-inflammatory cytokines TNF-α and IL-12 in macrophages by NF-κB-dependent pathway. *Biochem Biophys Res Commun.* 334(4): 1092–1101.

Silva, R. O.; Sousa, F.B.M.; Damasceno, S. R.; et al. (2014): Phytol, a diterpene alcohol, inhibits the inflammatory response by reducing cytokine production and oxidative stress. *Fundam Clin Pharmacol.* 28(4): 455–464.

Steppan, C. M.; Wang, J.; Whiteman, E. L.; Birnbaum, M. J.; Lazar, M. A. (2005): Activation of SOCS-3 by resistin. *Mol Cell Biol.* 25: 1569–1575.

Titchenell, P. M.; Chu, Q.; Monks, B. R.; Birnbaum, M. J. (2015): Hepatic insulin signalling is dispensable for suppression of glucose output by insulin in vivo. *Nat Commun.* 6: 7078.

Tsukahara, T.; Nakashima, E.; Watarai, A.; et al. (2009): Polymorphism in resistin promoter region at S420 determines the serum resistin levels and may be a risk marker of stroke in Japanese type 2 diabetic patients. *Diab Res Clin Pract.* 84: 179–186.

Vadlakonda, L.; Pasupuleti, M.; Pallu, R. (2013): Role of PI3K-AKT-mTOR and Wnt signaling pathways in transition of G1-S phase of cell cycle in cancer cells. *Front Oncol.* 3: 85.

Vijayakumar, S.; Presannakumar, G.; Vijayalakshmi, N. R. (2008): Antioxidant activity of banana flavonoids. *Fitoterapia.* 79: 279–282.

Vinaykumar, T.; Sunath, M. G.; Suman, L.; Vijayan, V.; Sriniva-Sarao, D.; Sharmila, A. M.; et al. (2010): Renoprotective and testicular protective effect of Musa paradisiaca flower extract in streptozotocin-induced diabetic rats. *JITPS.* 1: 106–114.

White, M. F. (2002): IRS proteins and the common path to diabetes. *Am J Physiol Endocrinol Metab.* 283: E413–422.

World Health Organization. (1999): *Definition, diagnosis and classification of diabetes mellitus and its complications: Report of a WHO consultation. Part 1, Diagnosis and classification of diabetes mellitus (No. WHO/NCD/NCS/99.2).* World Health Organization, Geneva.

Wu, H.; Xu, F.; Hao, J.; Yang, Y.; Wang, X. (2015): Antihyperglycemic activity of banana (Musa nana Lour.) peel and its active ingredients in alloxan-induced diabetic mice. *ICME.* 2015.

Xu, W.; Yu, L.; Zhou, W.; Luo, M. (2006): Resistin increases lipid accumulation and CD36 expression in human macrophages. *Biochem Biophys Res Commun.* 351: 376–382.

Yadav, A.; Kataria, M. A.; Saini, V.; Yadav, A. (2013): Role of leptin and adiponectin in insulin resistance. *Clin Chim Acta.* 417: 80–84.

Yamauchi, T.; Kamon, J.; Ito, Y.; et al. (2003): Cloning of adiponectin receptors that mediate antidiabetic metabolic effects. *Nature.* 423(6941): 762–769.

Yeung, W. C.; Rawlinson, W. D.; Craig, M. (2011): Enterovirus infection and type 1 diabetes mellitus: Systematic review and meta-analysis of observational molecular studies. *BMJ* 342: d35.

Yoshida, K.; Hirokawa, J.; Tagami, S.; Kawakami, Y.; Urata, Y.; Kondo, T. (1995): Weakened cellular scavenging activity against oxidative stress in diabetes mellitus: Regulation of glutathione synthesis and efflux. *Diabetologia.* 38(2): 201–210.

Zozulinska, D.; Wierusz-Wysocka, B. (2006): Type 2 diabetes mellitus as inflammatory disease. *Diabetes Res Clin Prac Suppl.* 74: S12–S16.

9 Beneficial Effects of Bilberry (*Vaccinium myrtillus* L.) in Diabetes and Cardiovascular Disease

Sze Wa Chan and Brian Tomlinson

CONTENTS

ABBREVIATIONS

Apo	apolipoprotein
CAT	catalase
CETP	cholesteryl ester transfer protein
CHD	coronary heart disease
COX	cyclooxygenase
CVD	cardiovascular disease
FRAP	ferric-reducing/antioxidant power
GSH	glutathione
hsCRP	high-sensitivity C-reactive protein
IL	interleukin
LDL	low-density lipoprotein
NF-κB	nuclear factor-κB
NO	nitric oxide
RNS	reactive nitrogen species
ROS	reactive oxygen species
SOD	superoxide dismutase
STZ	streptozotocin
sVCAM-1	soluble vascular cell adhesion molecule-1
TG	triglycerides
TNF	tumor necrosis factor
T2DM	type 2 diabetes mellitus
VLDL	very-low-density lipoprotein

DOI: 10.1201/9781003220930-11

9.1 INTRODUCTION

Bilberry (*Vaccinium myrtillus* L.), also called whortleberry, is a perennial shrub of the heather family (Ericaceae) that is widely distributed across Europe and Northern Asia and also growing in the heaths, meadows, and moist coniferous forests (Judd and Judd 2017). Bilberry leaves are alternate, deciduous, blade elliptic–ovate, bright green, 6–18 mm wide and 10–30 mm long. Bilberry fruits are usually harvested from July to September, when they have ripened and are 5–9 mm in diameter (Upton 2001). Bilberry has a very high content of anthocyanins, which are the important plant polyphenolic compounds that give the berries their red/purple/blue coloration (Dandona et al. 2004). The total amount of anthocyanins per 100 g fresh fruits ranges from 300 to 700 mg, which is the highest among edible berries, including cranberry, elderberry, strawberry, sour cherry, and raspberry (Upton 2001; Kowalczyk et al. 2003; Chu et al. 2011). Bilberry fruits are usually consumed as fresh, frozen, or dried whole berries; however, because of their short shelf life, they are also processed into various food products and beverages, such as jam, infusion, wine, and fresh and pasteurized juices (Zorenc et al. 2018).

9.2 BACKGROUND

The common name bilberry originates from the Danish word *bollebar*, which means "dark berry." Bilberry fruits have been used in traditional European medicine for centuries. In the Middle Ages, the medieval abbess St. Hildegard of Bingen (1098–1179) recommended the bilberry fruit for promoting menstruation (Morazzoni and Bombardelli 1996). Culpeper reported on the use of bilberry for treating a variety of conditions, including scurvy, coughs, tuberculosis, liver, and stomach (Culpeper 1981). Bernstein (1903) reported on the use of bilberry as a remedy in typhoid fever and other infectious diseases of the intestine, including enteric fever and dysentery. From the end of the 19th century, the antidiabetic effects of *Vaccinium* leaf extracts had been reported (Helmstädter and Schuster 2010). During World War II, British Royal Air Force pilots consumed bilberry jam to improve their visual acuity at night. More recently, bilberry fruits and extracts have been used for treating gastrointestinal inflammation, dysentery, diarrhea, hemorrhoids, vaginal discharges, scurvy, urinary disorders, and to dry up breast milk (Grieve 1994).

The usual dietary daily intake of anthocyanins is about 200 mg (Bravo 1998). Fifteen different types of anthocyanins have been identified in bilberry fruit, juice, and extract (Upton 2001; Winefield et al. 2009). Among these anthocyanidins, the percentage contents of delphinidin, cyaniding, petunidin, malvidin, and peonidin are the highest (Figure 9.1). Anthocyanins have characteristic

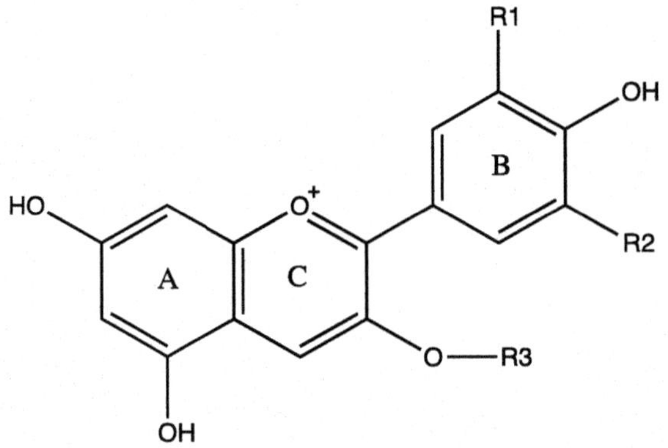

FIGURE 9.1 Chemical structures of bilberry (*Vaccinium myrtillus* L.) anthocyanins. The basic structures of anthocyanins are 2-phenylbenzopyrylium (flavylium cation), which contain two phenyl rings (A and B) separated by a heterocyclic (C) ring, and can have common groups or acyl moieties attached at different positions. R1 and R2 can be H, OH, or OCH_3; R3 can be H or sugar (Upton 2001, Winefield et al. 2009).

colors that can change depending on the pH of the solution. The content of anthocyanin is directly correlated with the antioxidant activity (Upton 2001; Bagchi et al. 2006; Prior et al. 1998). Apart from the antioxidant effects, anthocyanins have been reported to possess anticarcinogenic, anti-inflammatory, antibacterial, antidiabetic, and antidyslipidemic effects (Chan and Tomlinson 2020; Kowalczyk et al. 2003; Kong et al. 2003).

9.3 PHARMACOKINETICS OF ANTHOCYANINS

The majority of ingested anthocyanins are absorbed rapidly in the intact glycosidic form and circulate in the plasma and are eliminated in the urine without undergoing metabolic changes (Pojer et al. 2013). Animal studies have shown that anthocyanins can be detected in the bloodstream 6–20 minutes following consumption and reach maximum levels after 15 to 60 minutes (Pojer et al. 2013). Anthocyanins can be absorbed from both the stomach and small intestine. Anthocyanins have relatively low oral bioavailability, and the factors affecting their bioavailability include pH, digestive enzymes, food matrix, ability of a compound to cross membranes, and their structure (Fernandes et al. 2014). In animal studies, the systemic bioavailability of anthocyanins was estimated to be 0.26%–1.8% (Borges et al. 2007; Felgines et al. 2003; Felgines et al. 2002; Marczylo et al. 2009; Fang 2014). Absorption of anthocyanins through the gastric mucosa varied from 11% for malvidin-3-glucoside to 22% for cyanidin-3-glucoside (Chu et al. 2011). In the intestine, the absorption of anthocyanins mainly occurs in the jejunum, while only limited absorption occurs in the duodenum and no absorption occurs in the ileum and colon (Matuschek et al. 2006). Some anthocyanins can undergo microbiota metabolism in the colon (Fang 2014). Anthocyanins are capable of crossing the blood-brain barrier and localize in brain regions implicated in learning and memory (Andres-Lacueva et al. 2005).

In rats, anthocyanins appear to be taken up rapidly from the blood into the kidneys and liver (Vanzo et al. 2011). The main anthocyanins distributed in the kidneys and liver were malvidin, peonidin, cyanidin, delphinidin, and petunidin glycosides (Ichiyanagi et al. 2006). It has been reported that the amounts of anthocyanins recovered in urine and bile during the first 4 hours following intravenous administration were 30.8% and 13.4%, respectively (Ichiyanagi et al. 2006). In humans, urinary excretion of anthocyanins was very low (0.005%–0.1% of intake), suggesting pronounced biliary excretion or extensive metabolism of the compounds (Manach et al. 2004). Anthocyanins are cleared rapidly with an elimination half-life of about 2 hours (Cao et al. 2001). There is accumulating evidence that consumption of berries improves plasma antioxidant status (Cao et al. 1998; Mazza et al. 2002), suggesting that berry components with antioxidant activity are bioavailable.

9.4 ANTIOXIDANT EFFECTS

Free radical reactive oxygen species (ROS) and reactive nitrogen species (RNS) are generated from normal metabolic processes in the human body or acquired from external sources (Leopold and Loscalzo 2008). A balance among free radicals and antioxidants is crucial in maintaining proper physiological functions. Excessive formation and/or insufficient removal of ROS and RNS, known as "oxidative stress," may play a role in the development of various illnesses, such as diabetes mellitus, heart disease, and cancer (Johansen et al. 2005).

In vitro studies have shown that bilberry extracts have a protective effect against oxidative damage induced by allyl alcohol, tert-butyl hydroperoxide, lipid micelle, and ultraviolet radiation (Valentova et al. 2007; Upton 2001; Calo and Marabini 2014; Ershad et al. 2021), and the effect is probably attributed to their ability to directly eliminate excess ROS, which can trigger an oxidative chain reaction in the lipids in cell membranes, leading to lipid peroxidation (Calo and Marabini 2014), or via upregulation of the activity of the antioxidant enzymes catalase (CAT) and superoxide dismutase (SOD) (Casedas et al. 2018).

The antioxidant effect of bilberry extracts has been demonstrated in animal models of diabetes. In Wistar rats with streptozotocin (STZ) and high-fructose diet–induced diabetes, consumption of bilberry leaf extract (2% solution) for 50 days reduced lipid and glucose levels and also showed an antioxidant effect on diene compounds in the blood serum (Sidorova et al. 2017). In a rat model of nephrotoxicity, consumption of bilberry extract (100 mg/kg/day) for 15 days improved gentamicin-induced nephrotoxicity through modulating the serum malondialdehyde, advanced oxidation protein products, and CAT activity (Veljkovic et al. 2017). Likewise, consumption of the edible berry mixture OptiBerry (20 mg/kg/week) (wild blueberry, bilberry, cranberry, elderberry, raspberry seeds, and strawberry) for 8 weeks prevented hyperbaric oxygen–induced glutathione (GSH) oxidation in the lung and liver of vitamin E–deficient rats (Bagchi et al. 2006).

Bilberry contains ascorbic acid in addition to anthocyanins, and both are powerful antioxidants (Prior and Wu 2006), although studies on various *Vaccinium* species, including highbush blueberries (*V. corymbosum* L.) and lowbush blueberries (*V. angustifolium* Aiton), suggested that ascorbic acid only made a small contribution (0.4%–9.4%) to the overall antioxidant capacity of the fruits (Kalt et al. 1999). Evidence from clinical studies on the effects of berries on antioxidant status and plasma lipids, however, is inconsistent. Supplementation with a 100 g portion of deep-frozen berries (bilberries, lingonberries, or blackcurrants) daily for 8 weeks increased serum ascorbate concentrations and led to a slight increase in serum antioxidant capacity and a slight decrease in LDL diene conjugation, compared with control groups (Marniemi et al. 2000). However, supplementation with anthocyanin-rich cranberry juice (750 ml/day) for 2 weeks had no effect on the blood or cellular antioxidant status or the biomarkers of lipid status pertinent to heart disease in healthy subjects (Duthie et al. 2006). In subjects with at least one risk factor for CVD, supplementation with bilberry juice (330 ml/day) for 4 weeks did not alter the levels of biomarkers of antioxidant status or oxidative stress (Karlsen et al. 2010). In an open-label randomized study involving 50 patients who were within 24 hours of percutaneous coronary intervention, bilberry powder supplementation (40 g/day, equivalent to 480 g fresh bilberries) for 8 weeks reduced significantly the total and LDL cholesterol compared to baseline, although no significant differences were observed between the bilberry and the placebo groups (Arevstrom et al. 2019). In a recent randomized, double-blind, placebo-controlled, crossover study, 20 patients with T2DM who had not yet developed overt vascular complications were randomized to receive either bilberry supplementation (1.4 g/day of extract) daily for 4 weeks followed by 6 weeks of washout and then an additional 4 weeks of matching placebo, or vice versa. Daily supplementation with bilberry had no effect on the ferric-reducing/antioxidant power, ascorbic acid, vitamin E lipid standardization, allantoin, erythrocyte glutathione peroxidase, erythrocyte SOD, urinary 8-oxoguanine, and urinary creatinine, compared with placebo control groups, suggesting that bilberry supplementation did not modify antioxidant status or oxidative stress (Chan et al. 2021). It is noteworthy that the potential effects of bilberry supplementation may vary based on the quantity of the anthocyanins, the length of the intervention, and population baseline, and this may explain the failure of bilberry supplementation to produce significant antioxidant effects in some of the human trials.

9.5   ANTI-INFLAMMATORY EFFECTS

Organ-specific and multisystem chronic inflammation disorders are associated with an increased risk of coronary heart disease (CHD), stroke, and T2DM (Dregan et al. 2014; Donath and Shoelson 2011). Several markers of inflammation, including tumor necrosis factor (TNF)-α, interleukin (IL)-6, IL-1, and high-sensitivity C-reactive protein (hsCRP) have been shown to link with metabolic syndrome, obesity, and the risk of chronic diseases (Nijhuis et al. 2009; Pravenec et al. 2011). Weight loss of obese patients has been shown to be associated with a reduction in inflammation biomarkers (Ziccardi et al. 2002; Abd El-Kader and Al-Dahr 2016; Tajik et al. 2013), resulting in improved metabolic profiles, including insulin resistance, blood pressure, and lipid levels (Kopp et al. 2005; Sjostrom et al. 1999; Blumenthal et al. 2000).

The anti-inflammatory effects of bilberries and anthocyanins have been reported in numerous *in vitro* and *in vivo* studies. Bilberry extract and single anthocyanins significantly inhibited the expression and secretion of inflammatory bowel disease–associated pro-inflammatory mediators in the stimulated human colon epithelial cells T84; the intensity of inflammatory activity depends on the aglycon structure and the sugar moiety of anthocyanins (Triebel et al. 2012). In an acute and chronic dextran sodium sulphate colitis mice model, short-term supplementation with 20% dried bilberries (containing 11.2% anthocyanins) ameliorated colitis by preventing inflammation-induced apoptosis in colonic epithelial cells (Piberger et al. 2011). Furthermore, bilberry extract decreased nitric oxide (NO) generation and reversed pro-inflammatory cytokines, including TNF-α, IL-6, iNOS, and cyclooxygenase (COX)-2 in lipopolysaccharide-induced RAW 264.7 cells (Bayazid et al. 2021).

In a randomized controlled trial in subjects with features of the metabolic syndrome, daily consumption of a diet rich in bilberries (equivalent dose of 400 g fresh fruits) for 8 weeks ameliorated low-grade inflammation, suggesting a protective effect on cardiometabolic risk (Kolehmainen et al. 2012). Nuclear factor-κB (NF-κB) represents a family of inducible transcription factors that is activated by oxidative stress and pro-inflammatory stimuli and plays a key role in the regulation of genes related to inflammatory response. In a parallel-designed, placebo-controlled clinical trial involving 120 healthy volunteers, supplementation with anthocyanins isolated from bilberries and black currants (Medox, 300 mg/d) for 3 weeks inhibited NF-κB transactivation and decreased plasma concentrations of pro-inflammatory mediators, suggesting a protective effect in chronic inflammatory diseases (Karlsen et al. 2007). In subsequent studies, Karlsen et al. (2010) reported that supplementation with bilberry juice (330 ml/day) for 4 weeks in subjects with elevated risk of cardiovascular disease reduced the plasma level of inflammatory cytokines and hsCRP. In a randomized, placebo-controlled, double-blinded trial involving 150 hypercholesterolemia subjects, 24 weeks of supplementation with purified anthocyanin mixture (320 mg/day) derived from bilberries and blackcurrant decreased serum hsCRP, IL-1b, soluble vascular cell adhesion molecule-1 (sVCAM-1), and LDL cholesterol and increased HDL cholesterol level, suggesting an anti-inflammatory effect in hypercholesterolemic subjects (Zhu et al. 2013). Conversely, in a randomized, controlled parallel group human dietary intervention with healthy subjects, 6-week diets either rich or poor in vegetables, berries, and apple did not alter platelet activation or inflammation markers (Freese et al. 2004). Furthermore, in a randomized, double-blind, placebo controlled, crossover study, daily supplementation with bilberry (1.4 g/day of extract) for 4 weeks did not improve inflammatory status compared with control groups (Chan et al. 2021).

9.6 HYPOGLYCEMIC EFFECTS

T2DM is a chronic metabolic disease characterized by hyperglycemia resulting from insulin deficiency, insulin resistance, or defects in both insulin secretion and insulin action. Oxidative stress appears to implicate in the pathogenesis of diabetic complications (Hurrle and Hsu 2017; Dos Santos et al. 2019). Subclinical inflammation is associated with insulin resistance and is linked to the characteristics of metabolic syndrome including hyperglycemia (Crook 2004), which may increase the susceptibility to lipid peroxidation and ultimately contribute to the increased risk of atherosclerosis, a major complication of T2DM (Giugliano et al. 1996).

The mechanism of the hypoglycemic effect of bilberry may be mediated in part by inhibition of intestinal α-glucosidase activity and pancreatic α-amylase activity (Podsedek et al. 2014; McDougall et al. 2008; Belwal et al. 2017). Intestinal α-glucosidase breaks down disaccharides and oligosaccharides into monosaccharides that can be absorbed into the blood circulation, thus bilberry may slow down the release of glucose into the bloodstream (de Sales et al. 2012). Indeed, α-glucosidase inhibitors, for example acarbose, are a class of antidiabetic treatment for T2DM. It has been shown that bilberry extracts (containing 25% anthocyanidins) and anthocyanidins (cyanidin, delphinidin, malvidin, peonidin, and pelargonidin) inhibited the adipocyte differentiation via the insulin signaling pathway in 3T3-L1 cells (Suzuki et al. 2011). Furthermore, ethanol extract of

Vaccinium angustifolium Ait, a low-bush blueberry which belongs to the same family as bilberry, enhanced glucose transport into C2C12 muscle cells and 3T3-L1 adipocytes in the absence of insulin (Martineau et al. 2006).

The hypoglycemic effects of bilberries and anthocyanins have been reported in animal models of diabetes. For instance, in KK-A^y diabetic mice, supplementation with dietary bilberry extract (containing a total anthocyanin concentration of 10 g/kg diet) for 5 weeks decreased blood glucose level and enhanced insulin sensitivity, probably via an activation of AMP-activated protein kinase in the liver, skeletal muscle, and white adipose tissue, and an upregulation of glucose transporter 4 expression and suppression of hepatic gluconeogenesis in these tissues (Takikawa et al. 2010). In STZ-induced diabetic mice, supplementation of a water-alcohol extract of bilberry leaves (3.0 g/kg) for 4 days decreased plasma glucose level, and the effect was accompanied by a decrease in triglycerides (TG) (Cignarella et al. 1996). Ştefănuţ et al. (2013) compared the hypoglycemic effects of bilberry, blackberry, and mulberry ultrasonic extracts in STZ-induced diabetic rats and found that only blackberry extract and mulberry extract, but not bilberry extract, reduced the blood glucose levels significantly. Likewise, bilberry extracts may be associated with delay in onset of early diabetic retinopathy in STZ-induced diabetic rats but had no effect to modulate blood glucose levels and body weight (Kim et al. 2015).

In a randomized, double-blinded, crossover study involving eight male volunteers with T2DM controlled by diet and lifestyle alone, or with impaired glucose tolerance, ingestion of a single oral capsule of 0.47 g standardized bilberry extract (36% w/w anthocyanins), which equates to about 50 g of fresh bilberries, followed by a polysaccharide drink (equivalent to 75 g glucose) decreased postprandial insulin and glucose levels. The reduced glycemic response may be related to a reduced rate of carbohydrate digestion and/or absorption while the decreased plasma insulin may be related to the lower plasma glucose or that the volunteers became more insulin sensitive (Hoggard et al. 2013). In a randomized, double-blind, placebo-controlled trial of 120 overweight dyslipidemic patients, daily supplementation with 320 mg purified anthocyanins from bilberry and black currant decreased LDL cholesterol and increased HDL cholesterol concentrations, and the action was partially mediated via the inhibition of cholesteryl ester transfer protein (CETP). However, anthocyanin supplementation did not modulate glucose concentrations, apolipoprotein (apo) A-I, apo B, total cholesterol, and TG (Qin et al. 2009). A randomized crossover study in overweight women showed that the effects of berries on serum metabolites was associated with the cardiometabolic risk profile at baseline (Larmo et al. 2013). Chan et al. (2021) reported that short-term supplementation with bilberry extract (1.4 g/day) for 4 weeks reduced the hemoglobin A_{1c} (HbA$_{1c}$) by $0.31 \pm 0.58\%$ during bilberry supplementation, but this change was not significantly different from that with placebo in T2DM patients who had not yet developed overt vascular complications.

9.7   EFFECTS ON DYSLIPIDEMIA

Dyslipidemia is characterized by increased levels of TG, apo B, and small dense LDL cholesterol particles and decreased levels of HDL cholesterol. Visceral obesity leads to insulin resistance, which in turn modulates the assembly and secretion of very-low-density lipoprotein (VLDL) particles, resulting in hypertriglyceridemia, which leads to the generation of small dense LDL cholesterol particles and a decreased level in HDL cholesterol (Ginsberg et al. 2006). A clustering of diabetes, obesity, dyslipidemia, and hypertension usually occurs simultaneously in many patients. Epidemiological data suggest that low levels of HDL cholesterol and elevated levels of TG are closely related to the incidence of T2DM (Wilson et al. 2007). The serum TG levels are also the leading predictor of cardiovascular disease, comparable to LDL cholesterol for coronary heart disease in T2DM patients (Sone et al. 2011).

Pharmacological studies have shown that bilberry and anthocyanin supplementation is effective in ameliorating hyperlipidemia. In Zucker diabetic fatty rats, consumption of diet enriched with bilberries (5 g berry powder/day) for 8 weeks reduced total and LDL cholesterol levels partially via altering hepatic liver X receptor-α expression. However, bilberry supplementation did not influence glucose metabolism, blood pressure, or HDL cholesterol. The authors concluded that the effect of bilberries on hypercholesterolemia could probably be attributed to their high anthocyanin content (Brader et al. 2013). Likewise, in a study in alloxan-induced diabetic rats, supplementation with bilberry powder (2 g/day) for 4 weeks elevated insulin and reduced total cholesterol, LDL cholesterol, VLDL cholesterol, and TG levels and prevented HDL cholesterol decline, accompanied with an increase in islet size (Asgary et al. 2016). In mice fed with high-fat diet, supplementation with bilberry extract (5 g freeze-dried berries) for 13 weeks reduced body weight gain, lowered fasting insulin levels, decreased body fat content, hepatic lipid accumulation, and plasma levels of the inflammatory marker plasminogen activator inhibitor-1, suggesting that bilberry has beneficial metabolic effect in high-fat fed mice (Heyman et al. 2014).

The effects of berries on dyslipidemia have also been demonstrated in several clinical trials. In a single-blind, randomized, placebo-controlled trial in 71 subjects with at least one cardiovascular risk factor, consumption of berries for 8 weeks increased serum HDL cholesterol concentrations, reduced systolic blood pressure, and improved platelet function, suggesting that berries may have a potential cardioprotective effect (Erlund et al. 2008). Zhu et al. (2011) reported that supplementation with anthocyanins (320 mg/day) purified from the bilberry and blackcurrant for 12 weeks elevated the brachial artery flow-mediated dilation, cGMP and HDL cholesterol concentrations, but decreased the serum soluble sVCAM-1 and LDL cholesterol concentrations in hypercholesterolemic individuals. In a subsequent study involving 122 hypercholesterolemic subjects, supplementation with anthocyanins (320 mg/day) purified from bilberry and blackcurrant for 24 weeks increased the HDL-associated protein paraoxonase 1 activity, increased the antioxidant effects and enhanced the cholesterol efflux capacity of HDL, resulting in an increased HDL cholesterol and decreased LDL cholesterol concentrations (Zhu et al. 2014). Conversely, a recent randomized, double-blind, placebo-controlled, crossover study in 20 T2DM patients who had not yet developed overt vascular complications found that daily supplementation with bilberry extract (1.4 g/day) had no significant effect on the TC, HCL cholesterol, TG, LDL cholesterol, and uric acid levels, suggesting that short-term supplementation with bilberry extract may not improve lipid profile or cardiovascular risk in patients with T2DM (Chan et al. 2021).

9.8 TOXICITY AND CAUTIONARY NOTES

Bilberry is generally safe and has been recognized as a Class 1 herb by the American Herbal Products Association (Upton 2001). An open pilot trial with a bilberry preparation has included safety, tolerability, side effects, and patient satisfaction in the analysis and reported no serious clinical adverse events or alternations in the safety laboratory parameters (Biedermann et al. 2013). Although bilberry and bilberry extract have no known interactions with other drugs and no known adverse effect of bilberry and bilberry extract has been reported (Karlsen et al. 2010; Arevstrom et al. 2019; Hoggard et al. 2013), patients taking a chronic high dose of concentrated bilberry extract in combination with warfarin and antiplatelet drugs should be monitored for hemorrhagic disorders. The available data from animal or clinical studies are insufficient to assess the safety of bilberry in pregnancy or while nursing, so women who are pregnant, contemplating pregnancy, or breastfeeding should generally be discouraged from consuming high-dose bilberry preparations.

9.9 SUMMARY POINTS

- This chapter focuses on the potential health benefits of bilberry (*Vaccinium myrtillus*) on the metabolic and cardiovascular disease risk.
- The health benefits of bilberry have been attributed to the presence of its high anthocyanin contents.

- The earliest use of bilberry dates back to the Middle Ages, and bilberry is often used to treat gastrointestinal disorders and to improve vision.
- The existing evidence suggests that bilberry/anthocyanin has antioxidant, anti-inflammatory, hypoglycemic, and antidyslipidemic activities.
- The degree of health benefits of bilberry supplementation may vary with baseline health conditions.
- Further research using standardized bilberry extract products is warranted to better understand the potential benefits of bilberry supplementation.

REFERENCES

Abd El-Kader, S. M., and M.H.S. Al-Dahr. 2016. Impact of weight loss on oxidative stress and inflammatory cytokines in obese type 2 diabetic patients. *Afr. Health Sci.* 16 (3):725–733.

American Diabetes Association. 2010. Diagnosis and classification of diabetes mellitus. *Diabetes Care.* 33 (Suppl 1):S62–S69.

Andres-Lacueva, C., B. Shukitt-Hale, R. L. Galli, O. Jauregui, R. M. Lamuela-Raventos, and J. A. Joseph. 2005. Anthocyanins in aged blueberry-fed rats are found centrally and may enhance memory. *Nutr. Neurosci.* 8 (2):111–120.

Arevstrom, L., C. Bergh, R. Landberg, H. X. Wu, A. Rodriguez-Mateos, M. Waldenborg, A. Magnuson, S. Blanc, and O. Frobert. 2019. Freeze-dried bilberry (*Vaccinium myrtillus*) dietary supplement improves walking distance and lipids after myocardial infarction: An open-label randomized clinical trial. *Nutr. Res.* 62:13–22.

Asgary, S., M. Rafieian-Kopaei, A. Sahebkar, F. Shamsi, and N. Goli-malekabadi. 2016. Anti-hyperglycemic and anti-hyperlipidemic effects of *Vaccinium myrtillus* fruit in experimentally induced diabetes (antidiabetic effect of *Vaccinium myrtillus* fruit). *J. Sci. Food Agric.* 96 (3):764–768.

Bagchi, D., S. Roy, V. Patel, G. L. He, S. Khanna, N. Ojha, C. Phillips, S. Ghosh, M. Bagchi, and C. K. Sen. 2006. Safety and whole-body antioxidant potential of a novel anthocyanin-rich formulation of edible berries. *Mol. Cell. Biochem.* 281 (1–2):197–209.

Bayazid, A., E. M. Chun, M. Al Mijan, S. H. Park, S. K. Moon, and B. O. Lim. 2021. Anthocyanins profiling of bilberry (Vaccinium myrtillus L.) extract that elucidates antioxidant and anti-inflammatory effects. *Food Agric. Immunol.* 32 (1):713–726.

Belwal, T., S. F. Nabavi, S. M. Nabavi, and S. Habtemariam. 2017. Dietary anthocyanins and insulin resistance: When food becomes a medicine. *Nutrients.* 9 (10):22.

Bernstein, M. M. 1903. On the bilberry (*Vaccinium myrtillus*) as a remedy in typhoid fever and other infectious diseases of the intestine. *Br. Med. J.* 1 (2197):306–308.

Biedermann, L., J. Mwinyi, M. Scharl, P. Frei, J. Zeitz, G. A. Kullak-Ublick, S. R. Vavricka, M. Fried, A. Weber, H. U. Humpf, S. Peschke, A. Jetter, G. Krammer, and G. Rogler. 2013. Bilberry ingestion improves disease activity in mild to moderate ulcerative colitis – an open pilot study. *J. Crohns Colitis.* 7 (4):271–279.

Blumenthal, J. A., A. Sherwood, E.C.D. Gullette, M. Babyak, R. Waugh, A. Georgiades, L. W. Craighead, D. Tweedy, M. Feinglos, M. Appelbaum, J. Hayano, and A. Hinderliter. 2000. Exercise and weight loss reduce blood pressure in men and women with mild hypertension – effects on cardiovascular, metabolic, and hemodynamic functioning. *Arch. Intern. Med.* 160 (13):1947–1958.

Borges, G., S. Roowi, J. M. Rouanet, G. G. Duthie, M.E.J. Lean, and A. Crozier. 2007. The bioavailability of raspberry anthocyanins and ellagitannins in rats. *Mol. Nutr. Food Res.* 51 (6):714–725.

Brader, L., A. Overgaard, L. P. Christensen, P. B. Jeppesen, and K. Hermansen. 2013. Polyphenol-rich bilberry ameliorates total cholesterol and LDL-cholesterol when implemented in the diet of Zucker diabetic fatty rats. *Rev. Diabet. Stud.* 10 (4):270–282.

Bravo, L. 1998. Polyphenols: Chemistry, dietary sources, metabolism, and nutritional significance. *Nutr. Rev.* 56 (11):317–333.

Calo, R., and L. Marabini. 2014. Protective effect of *Vaccinium myrtillus* extract against UVA- and UVB-induced damage in a human keratinocyte cell line (HaCaT Cells). *J. Photochem. Photobiol. B.* 132:27–35.

Cao, G. H., H. U. Muccitelli, C. Sanchez-Moreno, and R. L. Prior. 2001. Anthocyanins are absorbed in glycated forms in elderly women: A pharmacokinetic study. *Am. J. Clin. Nutr.* 73 (5):920–926.

Cao, G., R. M. Russell, N. Lischner, and R. L. Prior. 1998. Serum antioxidant capacity is increased by consumption of strawberries, spinach, red wine or vitamin C in elderly women. *J. Nutr.* 128 (12):2383–2390.

Casedas, G., E. Gonzalez-Burgos, C. Smith, V. Lopez, and M. P. Gomez-Serranillos. 2018. Regulation of redox status in neuronal SH-SY5Y cells by blueberry (*Vaccinium myrtillus* L.) juice, cranberry (*Vaccinium macrocarpon* A.) juice and cyanidin. *Food Chem. Toxicol.* 118:572–580.

Chan, S. W., T.T.W. Chu, S. W. Choi, I.F.F. Benzie, and B. Tomlinson. 2021. Impact of short-term bilberry supplementation on glycemic control, cardiovascular disease risk factors, and antioxidant status in Chinese patients with type 2 diabetes. *Phytother. Res.* 35 (6):3236–3245.

Chan, S. W., and B. Tomlinson. 2020. Effects of bilberry supplementation on metabolic and cardiovascular disease risk. *Molecules.* 25 (7):15.

Chu, W. K., S.C.M. Cheung, R.A.W. Lau, and I.F.F. Benzie. 2011. Bilberry (*Vaccinium myrtillus* L.). In *Herbal Medicine: Biomolecular and Clinical Aspects*, 77–94. USA: Taylor & Francis Group, LLC.

Cignarella, A., M. Nastasi, E. Cavalli, and L. Puglisi. 1996. Novel lipid-lowering properties of *Vaccinium myrtillus* L. leaves, a traditional antidiabetic treatment, in several models of rat dyslipidaemia: A comparison with ciprofibrate. *Thromb. Res.* 84 (5):311–322.

Crook, M. 2004. Type 2 diabetes mellitus: A disease of the innate immune system? An update. *Diabet. Med.* 21 (3):203–207.

Culpeper, N. Reprinted, 1981. *Culpeper's Complete Herbal and English Physician*. Manchester: J Gleave.

Dandona, P., A. Aljada, A. Chaudhuri, and P. Mohanty. 2004. Endothelial dysfunction, inflammation and diabetes. *Rev. Endocr. Metab. Disord.* 5 (3):189–197.

de Sales, P. M., P. M. de Souza, L. A. Simeoni, P. D. Magalhaes, and D. Silveira. 2012. Alpha-amylase inhibitors: A review of raw material and isolated compounds from plant source. *J. Pharm. Pharm. Sci.* 15 (1):141–183.

Donath, M. Y., and S. E. Shoelson. 2011. Type 2 diabetes as an inflammatory disease. *Nat. Rev. Immunol.* 11 (2):98–107.

Dos Santos, J. M., S. Tewari, and R. H. Mendes. 2019. The role of oxidative stress in the development of diabetes mellitus and its complications. *J. Diabetes Res.* 3.

Dregan, A., J. Charlton, P. Chowienczyk, and M. C. Gulliford. 2014. Chronic inflammatory disorders and risk of type 2 diabetes mellitus, coronary heart disease, and stroke a population-based cohort study. *Circulation.* 130 (10):837–844.

Duthie, S. J., A. M. Jenkinson, A. Crozier, W. Mullen, L. Pirie, J. Kyle, L. S. Yap, P. Christen, and G. G. Duthie. 2006. The effects of cranberry juice consumption on antioxidant status and biomarkers relating to heart disease and cancer in healthy human volunteers. *Eur. J. Nutr.* 45 (2):113–122.

Erlund, I., R. Koli, G. Alfthan, J. Marniemi, P. Puukka, P. Mustonen, P. Mattila, and A. Jula. 2008. Favorable effects of berry consumption on platelet function, blood pressure, and HDL cholesterol. *Am. J. Clin. Nutr.* 87 (2):323–331.

Ershad, M., M. K. Shigenaga, and B. Bandy. 2021. Differential protection by anthocyanin-rich bilberry extract and resveratrol against lipid micelle-induced oxidative stress and monolayer permeability in Caco-2 intestinal epithelial cells. *Food Funct.* 12 (7):2950–2961.

Fang, J. 2014. Bioavailability of anthocyanins. *Drug Metab. Rev.* 46 (4):508–520.

Felgines, C., S. Talavera, M. P. Gonthier, O. Texier, A. Scalbert, J. L. Lamaison, and C. Remesy. 2003. Strawberry anthocyanins are recovered in urine as glucuro- and sulfoconjugates in humans. *J. Nutr.* 133 (5):1296–1301.

Felgines, C., O. Texier, C. Besson, D. Fraisse, J. L. Lamaison, and C. Remesy. 2002. Blackberry anthocyanins are slightly bioavailable in rats. *J. Nutr.* 132 (6):1249–1253.

Fernandes, I., A. Faria, C. Calhau, V. de Freitas, and N. Mateus. 2014. Bioavailability of anthocyanins and derivatives. *J. Funct. Foods.* 7:54–66.

Freese, R., O. Vaarala, A. M. Turpeinen, and M. Mutanen. 2004. No difference in platelet activation or inflammation markers after diets rich or poor in vegetables, berries and apple in healthy subjects. *Eur. J. Nutr.* 43 (3):175–182.

Ginsberg, H. N., Y. L. Zhang, and A. Hernandez-Ono. 2006. Metabolic syndrome: Focus on dyslipidemia. *Obesity.* 14:41S–49S.

Giugliano, D., A. Ceriello, and G. Paolisso. 1996. Oxidative stress and diabetic vascular complications. *Diabetes Care.* 19 (3):257–267.

Grieve, M. 1994. *A Modern Herbal*, 3rd ed. London: Tiger Books Int.

Helmstädter, A., and N. Schuster. 2010. Vaccinium myrtillus as an antidiabetic medicinal plant – research through the ages. *Pharmazie.* 65 (5):315–321.

Heyman, L., U. Axling, N. Blanco, O. Sterner, C. Holm, and K. Berger. 2014. Evaluation of beneficial metabolic effects of berries in high-fat fed C57BL/6J mice. *J. Nutr. Metab.* 2014:403041.

Hoggard, N., M. Cruickshank, K. M. Moar, C. Bestwick, J. J. Holst, W. Russell, and G. Horgan. 2013. A single supplement of a standardised bilberry (*Vaccinium myrtillus* L.) extract (36 % wet weight anthocyanins) modifies glycaemic response in individuals with type 2 diabetes controlled by diet and lifestyle. *J. Nutr. Sci.* 2:e22.

Hurrle, S., and W. H. Hsu. 2017. The etiology of oxidative stress in insulin resistance. *Biomed. J.* 40 (5):257–262.

Ichiyanagi, T., Y. Shida, M. M. Rahman, Y. Hatano, and T. Konishi. 2006. Bioavailability and tissue distribution of anthocyanins in bilberry (*Vaccinium myrtillus* L.) extract in rats. *J. Agric. Food Chem.* 54 (18):6578–6587.

Johansen, J. S., A. K. Harris, D. J. Rychly, and A. Ergul. 2005. Oxidative stress and the use of antioxidants in diabetes: Linking basic science to clinical practice. *Cardiovasc. Diabetol.* 4 (1):5.

Judd, W. S., and G. A. Judd. 2017. *Flora of Middle-Earth: Plants of J.R.R. Tolkien's Legendarium.* Oxford: Oxford University Press.

Kalt, W., C. F. Forney, A. Martin, and R. L. Prior. 1999. Antioxidant capacity, vitamin C, phenolics, and anthocyanins after fresh storage of small fruits. *J. Agric. Food Chem.* 47 (11):4638–4644.

Karlsen, A., I. Paur, S. K. Bohn, A. K. Sakhi, G. I. Borge, M. Serafini, I. Erlund, P. Laake, S. Tonstad, and R. Blomhoff. 2010. Bilberry juice modulates plasma concentration of NF-kappa B related inflammatory markers in subjects at increased risk of CVD. *Eur. J. Nutr.* 49 (6):345–355.

Karlsen, A., L. Retterstol, P. Laake, I. Paur, S. Kjolsrud-Bohn, L. Sandvik, and R. Blomhoff. 2007. Anthocyanins inhibit nuclear factor-kappa B activation in monocytes and reduce plasma concentrations of pro-inflammatory mediators in healthy adults. *J. Nutr.* 137 (8):1951–1954.

Kim, J., C. S. Kim, Y. M. Lee, E. Sohn, K. Jo, and J. S. Kim. 2015. *Vaccinium myrtillus* extract prevents or delays the onset of diabetes-induced blood-retinal barrier breakdown. *Int. J. Food Sci. Nutr.* 66 (2):236–242.

Kolehmainen, M., O. Mykkänen, P. V. Kirjavainen, T. Leppanen, E. Moilanen, M. Adriaens, D. E. Laaksonen, M. Hallikainen, R. Puupponen-Pimia, L. Pulkkinen, H. Mykkänen, H. Gylling, K. Poutanen, and R. Torronen. 2012. Bilberries reduce low-grade inflammation in individuals with features of metabolic syndrome. *Mol. Nutr. Food Res.* 56 (10):1501–1510.

Kong, J. M., L. S. Chia, N. K. Goh, T. F. Chia, and R. Brouillard. 2003. Analysis and biological activities of anthocyanins. *Phytochemistry.* 64 (5):923–933.

Kopp, H. P., K. Krzyzanowska, M. Mohlig, J. Spranger, A.F.H. Pfeiffer, and G. Schernthaner. 2005. Effects of marked weight loss on plasma levels of adiponectin, markers of chronic subclinical inflammation and insulin resistance in morbidly obese women. *Int. J. Obes.* 29 (7):766–771.

Kowalczyk, E., P. Krzesinski, M. Kura, B. Szmigiel, and J. Blaszczyk. 2003. Anthocyanins in medicine. *Pol. J. Pharmacol.* 55 (5):699–702.

Larmo, P. S., A. J. Kangas, P. Soininen, H. M. Lehtonen, J. P. Suomela, B. R. Yang, J. Viikari, M. Ala-Korpela, and H. P. Kallio. 2013. Effects of sea buckthorn and bilberry on serum metabolites differ according to baseline metabolic profiles in overweight women: A randomized crossover trial. *Am. J. Clin. Nutr.* 98 (4):941–951.

Leopold, J. A., and J. Loscalzo. 2008. Oxidative mechanisms and atherothrombotic cardiovascular disease. *Drug Discov. Today Ther. Strateg.* 5 (1):5–13.

Manach, C., A. Scalbert, C. Morand, C. Remesy, and L. Jimenez. 2004. Polyphenols: Food sources and bioavailability. *Am. J. Clin. Nutr.* 79 (5):727–747.

Marczylo, T. H., D. Cooke, K. Brown, W. P. Steward, and A. J. Gescher. 2009. Pharmacokinetics and metabolism of the putative cancer chemopreventive agent cyanidin-3-glucoside in mice. *Cancer Chemother. Pharmacol.* 64 (6):1261–1268.

Marniemi, J., P. Hakala, J. Maki, and M. Ahotupa. 2000. Partial resistance of low density lipoprotein to oxidation in vivo after increased intake of berries. *Nutr. Metab. Cardiovasc. Dis.* 10 (6):331–337.

Martineau, L. C., A. Couture, D. Spoor, A. Benhaddou-Andaloussi, C. Harris, B. Meddah, C. Leduc, A. Burt, T. Vuong, P. M. Le, M. Prentki, S. A. Bennett, J. T. Arnason, and P. S. Haddad. 2006. Anti-diabetic properties of the Canadian lowbush blueberry *Vaccinium angustifolium* Ait. *Phytomedicine.* 13 (9–10):612–623.

Matuschek, M. C., W. H. Hendriks, T. K. McGhie, and G. W. Reynolds. 2006. The jejunum is the main site of absorption for anthocyanins in mice. *J. Nutr. Biochem.* 17 (1):31–36.

Mazza, G., C. D. Kay, T. Cottrell, and B. J. Holub. 2002. Absorption of anthocyanins from blueberries and serum antioxidant status in human subjects. *J. Agric. Food Chem.* 50 (26):7731–7737.

McDougall, G. J., N. N. Kulkarni, and D. Stewart. 2008. Current developments on the inhibitory effects of berry polyphenols on digestive enzymes. *Biofactors.* 34 (1):73–80.

Morazzoni, P., and E. Bombardelli. 1996. *Vaccinium myrtillus* L. *Fitoterapia*. 67 (1):3–29.

Nijhuis, J., S. S. Rensen, Y. Slaats, F. M. van Dielen, W. A. Buurman, and J. W. Greve. 2009. Neutrophil activation in morbid obesity, chronic activation of acute inflammation. *Obesity (Silver Spring)*. 17 (11):2014–2018.

Piberger, H., A. Oehme, C. Hofmann, A. Dreiseitel, P. G. Sand, F. Obermeier, J. Schoelmerich, P. Schreier, G. Krammer, and G. Rogler. 2011. Bilberries and their anthocyanins ameliorate experimental colitis. *Mol. Nutr. Food Res.* 55 (11):1724–1729.

Podsedek, A., I. Majewska, M. Redzynia, D. Sosnowska, and M. Koziolkiewicz. 2014. In vitro inhibitory effect on digestive enzymes and antioxidant potential of commonly consumed fruits. *J. Agric. Food Chem.* 62 (20):4610–4617.

Pojer, E., F. Mattivi, D. Johnson, and C. S. Stockley. 2013. The case for anthocyanin consumption to promote human health: A review. *Compr. Rev. Food. Sci. Food Saf.* 12 (5):483–508.

Pravenec, M., T. Kajiya, V. Zidek, V. Landa, P. Mlejnek, M. Simakova, J. Silhavy, H. Malinska, O. Oliyarnyk, L. Kazdova, J. L. Fan, J. M. Wang, and T. W. Kurtz. 2011. Effects of human c-reactive protein on pathogenesis of features of the metabolic syndrome. *Hypertension*. 57 (4):731–737.

Prior, R. L., G. H. Cao, A. Martin, E. Sofic, J. McEwen, C. O'Brien, N. Lischner, M. Ehlenfeldt, W. Kalt, G. Krewer, and C. M. Mainland. 1998. Antioxidant capacity as influenced by total phenolic and anthocyanin content, maturity, and variety of *Vaccinium* species. *J. Agric. Food Chem.* 46 (7):2686–2693.

Prior, R. L., and X. L. Wu. 2006. Anthocyanins: Structural characteristics that result in unique metabolic patterns and biological activities. *Free Radic. Res.* 40 (10):1014–1028.

Qin, Y., M. Xia, J. Ma, Y. T. Hao, J. Liu, H. Mou, L. Cao, and W. H. Ling. 2009. Anthocyanin supplementation improves serum LDL- and HDL-cholesterol concentrations associated with the inhibition of cholesteryl ester transfer protein in dyslipidemic subjects. *Am. J. Clin. Nutr.* 90 (3):485–492.

Sidorova, Y., V. Shipelin, V. Mazo, S. Zorin, N. Petrov, and A. Kochetkova. 2017. Hypoglycemic and hypolipidemic effect of *Vaccinium myrtillus* L. leaf and *Phaseolus vulgaris* L. seed coat extracts in diabetic rats. *Nutrition*. 41:107–112.

Sjostrom, C. D., L. Lissner, H. Wedel, and L. Sjostrom. 1999. Reduction in incidence of diabetes, hypertension and lipid disturbances after intentional weight loss induced by bariatric surgery: The SOS intervention study. *Obes. Res.* 7 (5):477–484.

Sone, H., S. Tanaka, S. Tanaka, S. Iimuro, K. Oida, Y. Yamasaki, S. Oikawa, S. Ishibashi, S. Katayama, Y. Ohashi, Y. Akanuma, N. Yamada, and Study Japan Diabet Complications. 2011. Serum level of triglycerides is a potent risk factor comparable to LDL cholesterol for coronary heart disease in Japanese patients with type 2 diabetes: Subanalysis of the Japan Diabetes Complications Study (JDCS). *J. Clin. Endocrinol. Metab.* 96 (11):3448–3456.

Stefanut, M. N., A. Cata, R. Pop, C. Tanasie, D. Boc, I. Ienascu, and V. Ordodi. 2013. Anti-hyperglycemic effect of bilberry, blackberry and mulberry ultrasonic extracts on diabetic rats. *Plant Foods Hum. Nutr.* 68 (4):378–384.

Suzuki, R., M. Tanaka, M. Takanashi, A. Hussain, B. Yuan, H. Toyoda, and M. Kuroda. 2011. Anthocyanidins-enriched bilberry extracts inhibit 3T3-L1 adipocyte differentiation via the insulin pathway. *Nutr. Metab. (Lond.).* 8:9.

Tajik, N., S. A. Keshavarz, F. Masoudkabir, M. Djalali, H. H. Sadrzadeh-Yeganeh, M. R. Eshraghian, M. Chamary, Z. Ahmadivand, T. Yazdani, and M. H. Javanbakht. 2013. Effect of diet-induced weight loss on inflammatory cytokines in obese women. *J. Endocrinol. Invest.* 36 (4):211–215.

Takikawa, M., S. Inoue, F. Horio, and T. Tsuda. 2010. Dietary anthocyanin-rich bilberry extract ameliorates hyperglycemia and insulin sensitivity via activation of AMP-activated protein kinase in diabetic mice. *J. Nutr.* 140 (3):527–533.

Triebel, S., H. L. Trieu, and E. Richling. 2012. Modulation of inflammatory gene expression by a bilberry (*Vaccinium myrtillus* L.) extract and single anthocyanins considering their limited stability under cell culture conditions. *J. Agric. Food Chem.* 60 (36):8902–8910.

Upton, Roy. 2001. *Bilberry Fruit Vaccinium Myrtillus L. Standards of Analysis, Quality Control, and Therapeutics*. Santa Cruz, CA: American Herbal Pharmacopoeia and Therapeutic Compendium.

Valentova, K., J. Ulrichova, L. Cvak, and V. Simanek. 2007. Cytoprotective effect of a bilberry extract against oxidative damage of rat hepatocytes. *Food Chem.* 101 (3):912–917.

Vanzo, A., U. Vrhovsek, F. Tramer, F. Mattivi, and S. Passamonti. 2011. Exceptionally fast uptake and metabolism of cyanidin 3-glucoside by rat kidneys and liver. *J. Nat. Prod.* 74 (5):1049–1054.

Veljkovic, M., D. R. Pavlovic, N. Stojiljkovic, S. Ilic, I. Jovanovic, N. P. Ulrih, V. Rakic, L. Velickovic, and D. Sokolovic. 2017. Bilberry: Chemical profiling, in vitro and in vivo antioxidant activity and nephroprotective effect against gentamicin toxicity in rats. *Phytother. Res.* 31 (1):115–123.

Wilson, P.W.F., J. B. Meigs, L. Sullivan, C. S. Fox, D. M. Nathan, and R. B. D'Agostino. 2007. Prediction of incident diabetes mellitus in middle-aged adults – The Framingham Offspring Study. *Arch. Intern. Med.* 167 (10):1068–1074.

Winefield, Chris, Kevin Davies, and Kevin Gould. 2009. *Anthocyanins: Biosynthesis, Functions, and Applications.* New York: Springer Science & Business Media.

Zhu, Y. N., X. W. Huang, Y. H. Zhang, Y. Wang, Y. Liu, R. F. Sun, and M. Xia. 2014. Anthocyanin supplementation improves HDL-associated paraoxonase 1 activity and enhances cholesterol efflux capacity in subjects with hypercholesterolemia. *J. Clin. Endocrinol. Metab.* 99 (2):561–569.

Zhu, Y. N., W. Ling, H. Guo, F. Song, Q. Ye, T. Zou, D. Li, Y. Zhang, G. Li, Y. Xiao, F. Liu, Z. Li, Z. Shi, and Y. Yang. 2013. Anti-inflammatory effect of purified dietary anthocyanin in adults with hypercholesterolemia: A randomized controlled trial. *Nutr. Metab. Carbiovasc. Dis.* 23 (9):843–849.

Zhu, Y. N., M. Xia, Y. Yang, F. Q. Liu, Z. X. Li, Y. T. Hao, M. T. Mi, T. R. Jin, and W. H. Ling. 2011. Purified anthocyanin supplementation improves endothelial function via NO-cGMP activation in hypercholesterolemic individuals. *Clin. Chem.* 57 (11):1524–1533.

Ziccardi, P., F. Nappo, G. Giugliano, K. Esposito, R. Marfella, M. Cioffi, F. D'Andrea, A. M. Molinari, and D. Giugliano. 2002. Reduction of inflammatory cytokine concentrations and improvement of endothelial functions in obese women after weight loss over one year. *Circulation.* 105 (7):804–809.

Zorenc, Z., R. Veberic, and M. Mikulic-Petkovsek. 2018. Are processed bilberry products a good source of phenolics? *J. Food Sci.* 83 (7):1856–1861.

10 Common Purslane (*Portulaca oleracea*) Use in Diabetes
Molecular, Cellular, and Metabolic Effects

Vafa Baradaran Rahimi and Vahid Reza Askari

CONTENTS

ABBREVIATIONS

ACh	acetylcholine
AI	atherogenic index
Akt1	protein kinase B
ALA	α-linolenic acid
ALT	alanine transaminase
AMPK	activation of 5′ AMP-activated protein kinase
AR	androgen receptor
AST	aspartate transaminase
BCAAs	branched-chain amino acid
CaMKKβ	calmodulin-dependent protein kinase kinase β
CRF	cardiac risk factor
ErbB2	Erb-b2 receptor tyrosine kinase 2
ET-1	endothelin-1

FBG	fasting of blood glucose
FINS	fasting serum insulin
FST	forced swimming test
GLP1	glucagon-like peptide–1
GLUT	glucose transporter
GSH	glutathione
GSK	glycogen synthase kinase
HbA$_{1c}$	hemoglobin A1C
HDL	high-density lipoprotein
HOMA-IR	homeostatic model of assessment of insulin resistance
ICAM-1	intercellular adhesion molecule-1
IFN-γ	interferon γ
IL-6	interleukin-6
IκBα	inhibitors of NF-κB
ISI	insulin sensitivity index
LDL	low-density lipoprotein cholesterol
MDA	malondialdehyde
MMP	matrix metalloproteinase
MWM	Morris water maze
NF-κB	nuclear factor κB
OGTT	oral glucose tolerance test
OVX	ovariectomized
PBG	postprandial blood glucose
PI3K	phosphatidylinositol-3 kinase
PO	*Portulaca oleracea* L.
PPAR	proliferator-activated receptor
QUICKI	quantitative insulin sensitivity check index
ROCK	rho-associated protein kinase
SNP	sodium nitroprusside
SOD	superoxide dismutase
STZ	streptozotocin
TAS	total antioxidant status
TC	total cholesterol
TG	triglycerides
TGF-β1	transforming growth factor-β1
TNF-α	tumor necrosis factor-a
TPS	tail pinch stressor
T2D	type 2 diabetes
VCAM-1	vascular cell adhesion molecule-1
VEGF	vascular endothelial growth factor
VGSC	voltage-gated Na$^+$ channel

10.1 INTRODUCTION

Portulaca oleracea L. (PO, Figure 10.1), commonly known as purslane, is a herbaceous annual plant belonging to the family Portulacaceae (Askari et al. 2016). PO is cultured in many parts of the world, including Central Europe, North America, Africa, Australia, Asia, and the Mediterranean (Baradaran Rahimi and Askari 2021). PO is known by several names in different countries, such as *khorfeh* in Persian, *purslane* in the United States and Australia, *ma chi xian* or *chang shou cai* in China, *rigla* in Egypt, *pourpier* in France, and *pigweed* in England. It has also been introduced as a global panacea (Kumar et al. 2022).

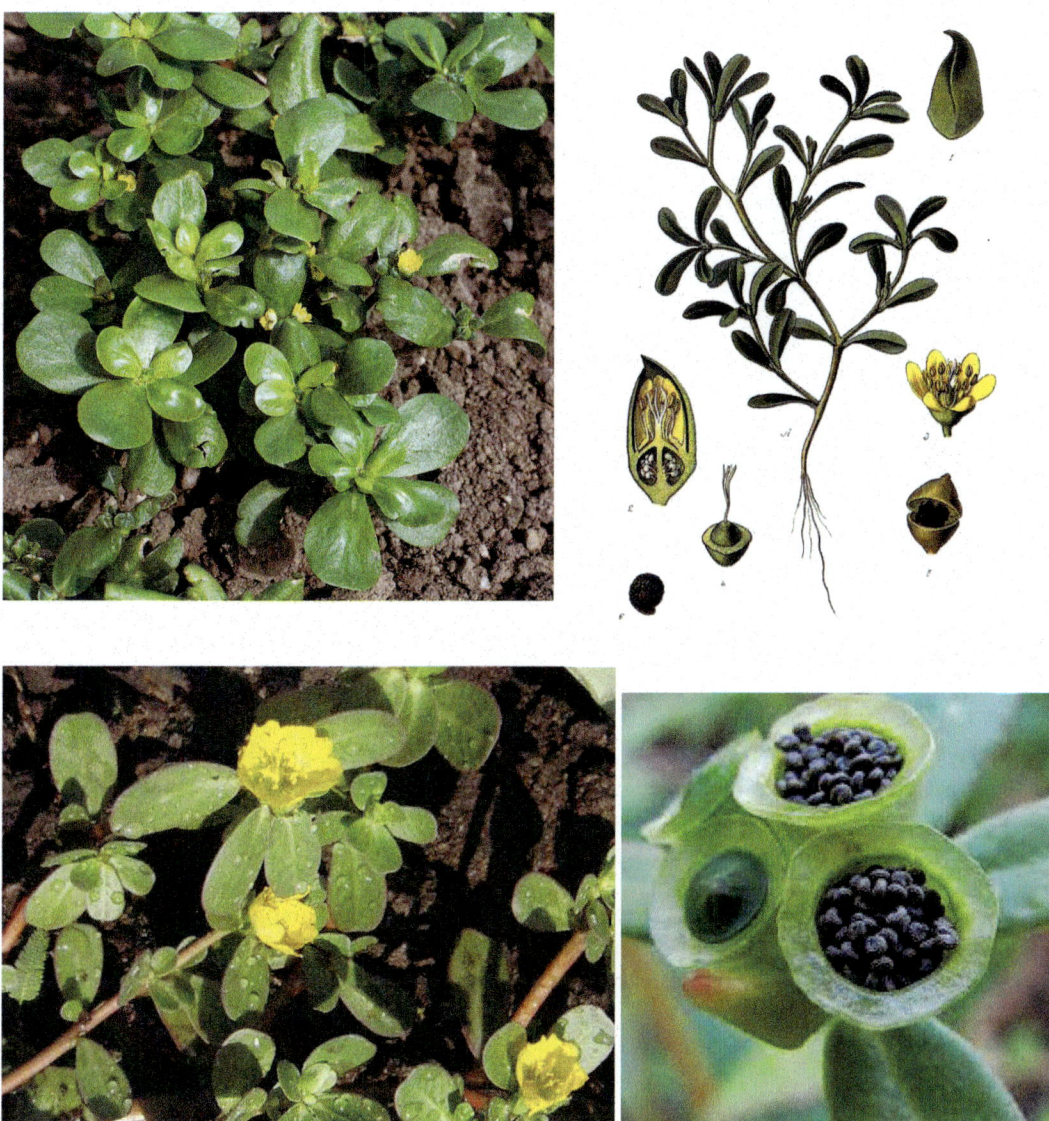

FIGURE 10.1   Different parts of *Portulaca oleracea* L.

PO stems are smooth, glabrous, green or red, up to 30 cm long and 2–3 mm in diameter, and scattered branched (Boskabady et al. 2016). Its leaves are green, thick, fleshy, succulent, smooth, alternative or subopposite, and stalkless or with very short stalks. PO has small yellow or white flowers with five petals and tiny black seeds 2–5 mm long (Uddin et al. 2014). The soft stem and succulent leaves of PO are edible and used raw or cooked in salads, soups, and other foods or as a pickle with a similar taste to spinach. In addition, the PO seeds are used in bread and juices. All parts of the PO plant, including roots, stems, leaves, and seeds, possess medicinal effects (Rahimi et al. 2019).

PO has multiple bioactive constituents, including flavonoids, alkaloids, terpenoids, vitamins, minerals, and fatty acids (Figure 10.2).

Flavonoids consists of portulacanones A–D, kaempferol, apigenin, luteolin, myricetin, quercetin, genistein, and genistin. Various alkaloids such as dopamine, DOPA, noradrenalin, oleraceins A–E, adenosine, and *N*-trans-feruloyltyramine have been derivated from PO. Furthermore, PO possesses

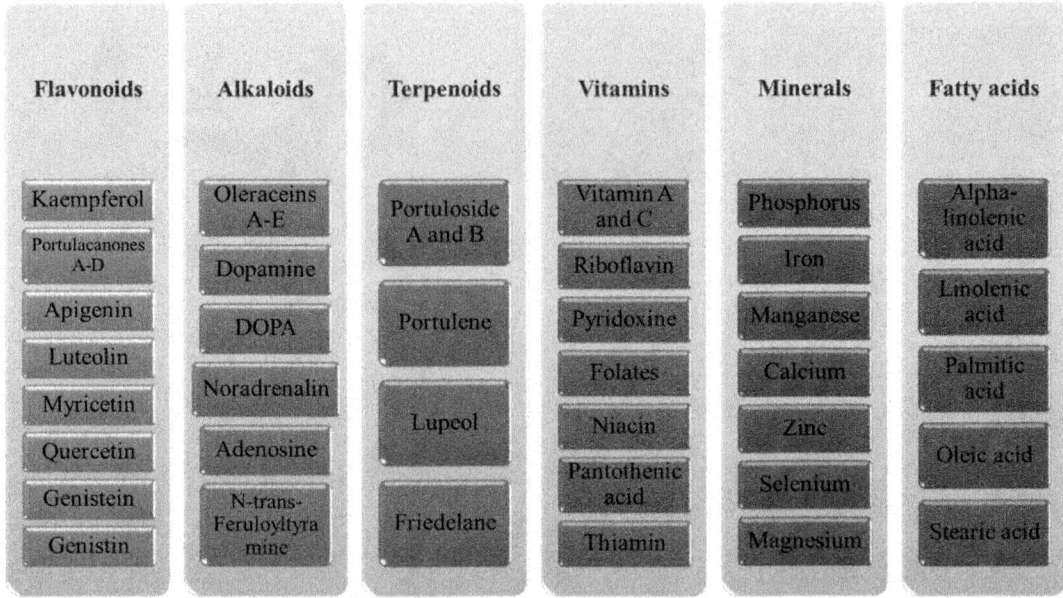

FIGURE 10.2 Active constituents of *Portulaca oleracea* L.

several terpenoids, including portuloside A and B, portulene, lupeol, and friedelane. Interestingly, it has been emphasized that PO contains numerous minerals such as phosphorus, iron, manganese, calcium, zinc, selenium, and magnesium, and vitamins including vitamin A and C, riboflavin, pyridoxine, folate, niacin, pantothenic acid, and thiamine (Zhou et al. 2015; Baradaran Rahimi, Mousavi, et al. 2019).

PO has been suggested as the richest source of omega-3 fatty acids among vegetables, especially α-linolenic acid (ALA). ALA is an essential omega-3 fatty acid that has a critical role in human growth, the immune system, and the prevention of various diseases such as cardiovascular disorders (Jaafari et al. 2021).

10.2 BACKGROUND

Different parts of PO have been widely used as folk medicine in several countries worldwide as a remedy for various disorders. It has been used to improve diarrhea, diabetes, obesity, throat infections, toothache, asthma, snake bites, ulcers, and jaundice (Baradaran Rahimi, Rakhshandeh, et al. 2019). In addition, it has been considered in several ancient texts from different parts of the world. In this regard, Dioscorides in the *Materia Medica* recommended PO as an astringent, febrifuge, and vermifuge, and for treatment of headache, burning of stomach, eye and other organ inflammation, and bladder diseases. Avicenna, a famous Iranian physician and philosopher, suggested PO for treating inflammation, pulsatile headaches, eye pain, gastritis, intestinal ulcers, liver pain and inflammation, and kidney and bladder pain and ulcers (Niazi et al. 2019; Petropoulos et al. 2016).

PO is known as a "vegetable for long life" in traditional Chinese medicine and is widely prescribed as medication for dysentery, swellings, uterine or hemorrhoid bleeding, sores, eczema, and snake and insect bite (Yang et al. 2016). Nowadays, its traditional applications are well investigated and documented by researchers worldwide.

The main anti-diabetic mechanisms and effects of PO are illustrated in Figure 10.3.

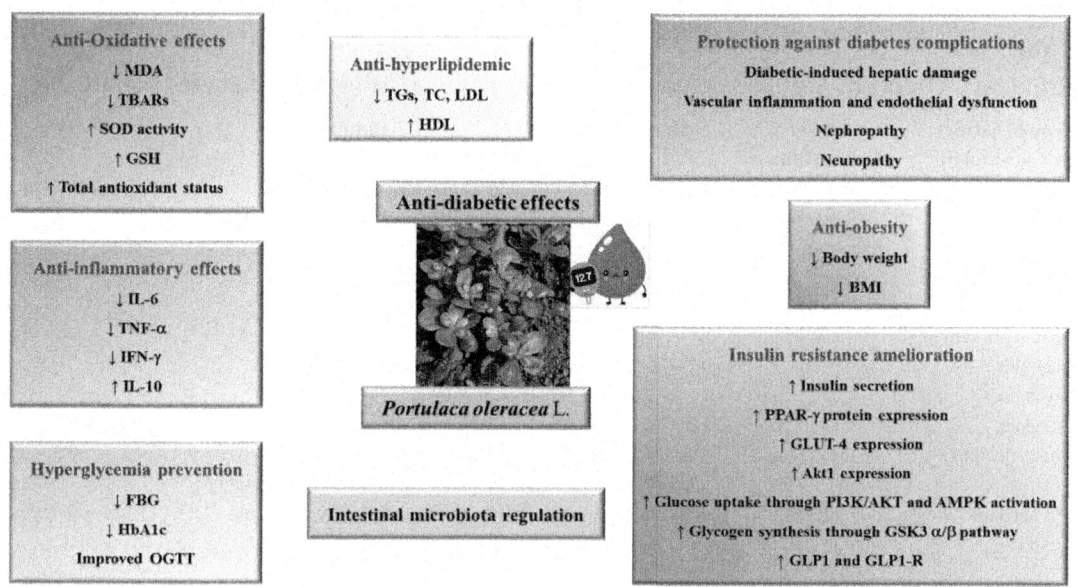

FIGURE 10.3 The anti-diabetic mechanisms of *Portulaca oleracea* L. Akt1, protein kinase B; AMPK, activation of 5′ AMP-activated protein kinase; FBG, fasting of blood glucose; GLP1, glucagon-like peptide 1; GLUT-4, glucose transporter 4; GSH, glutathione; GSK, glycogen synthase kinase; HbA$_{1c}$, hemoglobin A$_{1c}$; HDL, high-density lipoprotein cholesterol; IFN-γ, interferon γ; IL, interleukin; LDL, low-density lipoprotein cholesterol; MDA, malondialdehyde; OGTT, oral glucose tolerance test; PI3K, phosphatidylinositol-3 kinase; PPAR, proliferator-activated receptor; SOD, superoxide dismutase; TBARs, thiobarbituric acid reactive substances; TC, total cholesterol; TGs, triglycerides; TNF-α, tumor necrosis factor-α.

10.2.1 Animal Models of Diabetes Mellitus (DM)

The promising anti-diabetic effects of PO have been reported in different animal models of DM, including streptozotocin (STZ) and alloxan-induced DM (Table 10.1).

10.2.1.1 Protective Effects of *Portulaca oleracea* L. against STZ-Induced DM

Aqueous macerated extract of PO (200 and 400 mg/kg; orally) notably diminished fasting of blood glucose (FBG) and malondialdehyde (MDA) levels, improved oral glucose tolerance test (OGTT), and markedly elevated insulin secretion and superoxide dismutase (SOD) activity after 3 weeks in STZ-induced DM in C57BL/6J mice (Gu et al. 2015). Similarly, PO aqueous extract (100, 200, 400 mg/kg/day; IP) for 4 weeks meaningfully attenuated blood glucose, MDA, interleukin-6 (IL-6), and tumor necrosis factor-α (TNF-α) levels while propagating glutathione (GSH) and total antioxidant status (TAS) levels in STZ-induced DM in rats (Samarghandian, Borji, and Farkhondeh 2017). In addition, Hou et al. reported that PO seed (812.5, 1625, and 3250 mg/kg/day; orally) significantly reduced FBG, hemoglobin A$_{1c}$ (HbA$_{1c}$) levels, and protein kinase B (Akt1), vascular endothelial growth factor (VEGF), Erb-b2 receptor tyrosine kinase 2 (ErbB2), and androgen receptor (AR) mRNA expression levels in the pancreatic tissue after 4 weeks of treatment in STZ-induced DM in mice (Hou et al. 2020).

Similarly, a crude water-soluble polysaccharide isolated from PO (CPOP; 100, 200, and 400 mg/kg/day; orally) for 28 days remarkably elevated body weight, fasting serum insulin (FINS), insulin sensitivity index (ISI), and SOD activity in STZ-induced DM in the rat. Moreover, CPOP meaningfully mitigated the FBG, TNF-α, IL-6, and MDA levels and ameliorated the OGTT in diabetic rats.

TABLE 10.1

Protective Effects of *Portulaca oleracea* L. against Animal Models of Diabetes Mellitus

Type of Extract or Constituent	Dose/ Concentration	Study Model	Results	Reference
PO seed powder dissolved in normal saline containing 0.5% carboxymethyl cellulose sodium	812.5, 1625, and 3250 mg/kg/day; orally for 4 weeks	STZ-induced DM in mice	↓ FBG and HbA$_{1c}$ levels ↓ Akt1, VEGF, ErbB2, and AR mRNA expression levels in pancreatic tissue	(Hou et al. 2020)
Aqueous macerated PO extract	200 and 400 mg/kg; orally for 3 weeks	STZ-induced DM in C57BL/6J mice	↓ FBG, and MDA levels improved OGTT ↑ Insulin secretion and SOD activity	(Gu et al. 2015)
PO aqueous extract	100, 200, 400 mg/kg/day; IP for 4 weeks	STZ-induced DM in rats	↓ Blood glucose, MDA, IL-6, and TNF-α levels ↑ GSH, TAS levels	(Samarghandian, Borji, and Farkhondeh 2017)
Crude water soluble polysaccharide isolated from PO	100, 200, and 400 mg/kg/day; orally for 28 days	STZ-induced DM in rat	↑ Body weight, FINS, ISI, and SOD activity ↓ FBG, TNF-α, IL-6, and MDA level Ameliorated OGTT	(Bai et al. 2016)
P. oleracea polysaccharide fraction	25 and 50 mg/kg; orally for 3 weeks	STZ-induced DM in rat	↓ Blood glucose, and TBARs level ↑ Glutathione level, glutathione peroxidase, catalase, and SOD activities	(Sharma et al. 2012)
Mixture of aqueous extract of PO, *Spilanthes africana*, and *Sida rhombifolia*	50, 100, and 200 mg/kg; orally for 21 days	STZ-induced DM in rat	↓ Blood glucose, TG, LDL, ALT, AST, creatinine, and MDA levels ↑ HDL, glutathione, and TAS	(Moukette et al. 2017)
PO extract	50, 100, and 200 mg/kg; orally for 4 weeks	STZ-induced DM in C57BL/6J mice	↓ FBG, TNF-α, IL-6, and IFN-γ ↑ IL-10, glutamine Improved OGTT Modulates gut microbiota composition ↓ Firmicutes to Bacteroidetes ratio, *Blautia*, Ruminiclostridium_9, *Dubosiella*, and Lachnospiraceae_NK4A136_group abundancy ↑ *Bacteroides, Akkermansia*, and *Mucispirillum* genera ↓ BCAAs serum level, and bacterial biosynthesis of BCAAs ↑ expression of catabolic enzymes of BCAAs	(Bao et al. 2022)
PO aqueous extract	250 mg/kg/day; orally for 4 weeks	Alloxan-induced DM in mice	↓ HbA$_{1c}$, blood glucose, TNF-α, and IL-6 level ↑ C peptide and insulin levels Ameliorated pancreatic islet cell destruction	(Ramadan, Schaalan, and Tolba 2017)

Type of Extract or Constituent	Dose/ Concentration	Study Model	Results	Reference
Crude polysaccharide isolated from PO	200, 400 mg/kg/ day; orally for 28 days	Alloxan-induced DM in rat	↓ FBG, TG, and TC levels ↑ Body weight, HDL, and insulin levels	(Gong et al. 2009)

Abbreviations: Akt1, protein kinase B; ALT, alanine transaminase; AR, androgen receptor; AST, aspartate transaminase; DM, diabetes mellitus; ErbB2, Erb-b2 receptor tyrosine kinase 2; FBG, fasting of blood glucose; FINS, fasting serum insulin; GSH, glutathione; HbA_{1c}, hemoglobin A_{1c}; HDL, high-density lipoprotein cholesterol; IFN-γ, interferon γ; IL-6, interleukin-6; ISI, insulin sensitivity index; LDL, low-density lipoprotein cholesterol; MDA, malondialdehyde; OGTT, oral glucose tolerance test; SOD, superoxide dismutase; STZ, streptozotocin; TAS, total antioxidant status; TBARs, thiobarbituric acid reactive substances; TC, total cholesterol; TG, triglycerides; TNF-α, tumor necrosis factor-α; VEGF, vascular endothelial growth factor.

They supported that the antioxidant and anti-inflammatory effects of CPOP may be responsible for its anti-diabetic properties (Bai et al. 2016). Sharma et al. found that *P. oleracea* polysaccharide fraction (PPFt, 25 and 50 mg/kg; orally) for 3 weeks significantly decreased the blood glucose and thiobarbituric acid reactive substances level as an oxidative stress marker in STZ-induced DM in rats. In contrast, PPFt notably stimulated the antioxidant markers, including glutathione level, glutathione peroxidase, catalase, and SOD activities in diabetic rats (Sharma et al. 2012).

Another study evaluated the anti-diabetic effects of a mixture of aqueous extract of PO, *Spilanthes africana*, and *Sida rhombifolia* (MTPE) in STZ-induced DM in rats. MTPE (50, 100, and 200 mg/kg; orally) for 21 days considerably diminished blood glucose, triglycerides (TG), low-density lipoprotein cholesterol (LDL), alanine transaminase (ALT), aspartate transaminase (AST), creatinine, and MDA levels. Additionally, MTPE provided a significant increment in the level of high-density lipoprotein cholesterol (HDL), glutathione, and TAS in STZ-induced DM in rats (Moukette et al. 2017).

Recently, Bao et al. suggested that PO extract ameliorated type 2 diabetes (T2D) through regulating gut microbiota and metabolism of serum branched-chain amino acid (BCAAs). They found that PO extract (50, 100, and 200 mg/kg/day; orally) for 4 weeks markedly reduced FBG, serum level of inflammatory cytokines including TNF-α, IL-6, and interferon γ (IFN-γ) in STZ-induced T2D in C57BL/6J mice. PO extract also elevated the anti-inflammatory cytokine IL-10 and glutamine and improved OGTT in STZ-induced T2D mice. Additionally, PO extract modulates gut microbiota composition through decreasing Firmicutes to Bacteroidetes ratio, *Blautia*, Ruminiclostridium_9, *Dubosiella*, and Lachnospiraceae_NK4A136_group abundancy, while stimulating *Bacteroides, Akkermansia*, and *Mucispirillum* genera. Furthermore, PO extract attenuates BCAAs serum levels through decreasing bacterial biosynthesis of BCAAs while propagating the expression of catabolic enzymes of BCAAs (Bao et al. 2022).

10.2.1.2 Protective Effects of *Portulaca oleracea* L. against Alloxan-Induced DM

Ramadan et al. determined that aqueous extract of PO (250 mg/kg/day; orally) for 4 weeks notably diminished the HbA_{1c}, blood glucose, TNF-α, and IL-6 levels in alloxan-induced DM in the rat. In contrast, PO extract provided a significant increment in C-peptide and insulin levels in alloxan-induced DM in the rat. In addition, the histopathological evaluations of the pancreatic tissue revealed that treatment with PO extract firmly ameliorated the pancreatic islet cell destruction induced by alloxan (Ramadan, Schaalan, and Tolba 2017). Similarly, a crude polysaccharide isolated from PO (200, 400 mg/kg/day; orally) for 28 days strikingly alleviated FBG, TG, and total cholesterol (TC) levels in alloxan-induced DM in mice. Furthermore, the body weight, HDL, and insulin levels were significantly increased following treatment with crude polysaccharides isolated from PO in alloxan-induced DM in mice (Gong et al. 2009).

10.2.2 EFFECTS OF *PORTULACA OLERACEA* L. ON INSULIN RESISTANCE AND SECRETION

PO powder (5% and 10%, orally) for 12 weeks provided a significant decrement in the body weight gain, perirenal and epididymal fat contents, serum levels of LDL, TG, TG/LDL, atherogenic index (AI), cardiac risk factor (CRF), insulin, homeostatic model of assessment of insulin resistance (HOMA-IR), and ALT in HFD C57BL/6 mice. Interestingly, PO extract upregulated the protein expression of the proliferator-activated receptor (PPAR)-g, PPAR-a, and glucose transporter (GLUT) 4 while reducing the TNF-α protein expression in liver tissue. They emphasized that PO may regulate insulin resistance and possess anti-obesity and anti-diabetic properties (Jung et al. 2021).

The 80% hydroethanolic extract of PO (10–200 µg/ml) meaningfully stimulated insulin secretion in INS-1 pancreatic β cells. Surprisingly, this effect was propagated in the presence of insulin secretion stimulator agents, such as L-alanine, tolbutamide, and 3-isobutyl-1-methylxanthine. In contrast, it is inhibited in the presence of diazoxide (K^+_{ATP} channel opener) and verapamil (Ca^{2+} channel blocker). They concluded that PO extract increased insulin secretion in K^+_{ATP} channel-dependent manner (Park and Han 2018). In addition, Hu et al. emphasized that polysaccharides isolated from PO stimulated insulin secretion in INS-1 cells through the voltage-gated Na^+ channel (VGSC) mechanism (Hu et al. 2019).

Park et al. showed that an HM-chromanone (10 and 20 µM), a component isolated from PO, enhanced glycogen synthesis through the glycogen synthase kinase (GSK)3 a/β pathway and glucose uptake via phosphatidylinositol-3 kinase (PI3K)/AKT and calmodulin-dependent protein kinase kinase β (CaMKKβ) activation of 5′ AMP-activated protein kinase (AMPK) pathways activation in L6 skeletal muscle cells (Park, Seo, and Han 2021). Similarly, HM-chromanone (10 and 20 µM) propagated glucose uptake and translocation of GLUT4 to the plasma membrane through PI3K/AKT and AMPK activation in 3T3-L1 adipocytes (Park et al. 2019).

Lee and coworkers suggested that 80% ethanolic extract of PO (0.4%, w/w) significantly diminished the blood glucose, HbA_{1c}, and HOMA-IR while enhancing the quantitative insulin sensitivity check index (QUICKI) in C57BL/KsJ-db/db mice. Additionally, PO extract ameliorated insulin resistance in a PI3K/Akt and AMPK-dependent manner and stimulated the plasma membrane GLUT4 expression in the skeletal muscle of C57BL/KsJ-db/db mice (Lee, Park, and Han 2020).

10.2.3 PROTECTIVE EFFECTS OF *PORTULACA OLERACEA* L. AGAINST DIABETES COMPLICATIONS

DM is a complex chronic disorder that may cause plenty of chronic complications, including retinopathy, neuropathy, neuropathy, cardiovascular diseases, and hepatic failure. In this regard, DM is known as a silent killer (Cole and Florez 2020; Baradaran Rahimi et al. 2020). Interestingly, protective properties of PO against some DM complications have been reported (Table 10.2).

10.2.3.1 Diabetic-Induced Hepatic Damage

Zheng and coworkers investigated the effects of PO on hepatic injury in STZ-induced diabetic mice. They noticed that treatment with ethanolic extract of PO (100 and 200 mg/kg; orally) for 28 days strikingly alleviated food intake, serum glucose, ALT, AST, TG, TC, IL-6, IL-1b, and TNF-α levels. In contrast, PO extract markedly stimulated body weight and serum insulin level following STZ-induced liver injury in mice. In addition, it notably down-regulated the expression of Rho, Rho-associated protein kinase (ROCK)1, and ROCK2 and prevented the phosphorylation of nuclear factor κB (NF-κB) p65 and inhibitors of NF-κB (IκBα) in the liver tissue. PO extract also improved

TABLE 10.2

Protective Effects of *Portulaca oleracea* L. against Diabetes Mellitus Complications

Type of Extract or Constituent	Dose	Study Model	Results	Reference
Ethanolic extract of PO	100 and 200 mg/kg; orally for 28 days	STZ-induced hepatic damage	↓ Food intake, serum glucose, ALT, AST, TG, TC, IL-6, IL-1b, and TNF-α levels ↑ Body weight and serum insulin level Downregulated the expression of Rho, ROCK1, and ROCK2 Prevented the phosphorylation of NF-κBp65 and IκBα in liver tissue Improved pathologic liver changes	(Zheng et al. 2018)
Aqueous extract of PO	300 mg/kg/day; orally for 10 weeks	Diabetic male C57BL/KsJ-db/db mice–induced vascular inflammation and endothelial dysfunction	↓ Blood glucose, TG, LDL, and SBP ↑ HDL, insulin levels, and insulin immunoreactivity of the pancreatic islets Improved ACh and SNP-induced vascular relaxation of aortic rings impairment ↓ Over-expression of VCAM-1, ICAM-1, E-selectin, MMP-2, and ET-1 in aortic tissue	(Lee et al. 2012b)
Aqueous extract of PO	300 mg/kg; orally for 35 days	STZ-induced DM neuropathy in OVX female Wistar rats	↓ FBG level Improved spatial cognitive performance and total distance traveled at the probe trial in Morris water maze Improved non-functional masticatory activity in tail pinch stressor test No improve in the results of forced swimming test Showed anxiolytic effects in STZ-induced DM in OVX female Wistar rats	(Fatemi Tabatabaei et al. 2016)
Aqueous extract of PO	300 mg/kg; orally for 10 weeks	db/db diabetic mice-induced nephropathy	↓ Blood glucose, creatinine level, water intake, and urine volume ↓ Expression of TGF-β1, AGE, ICAM-1 ↓ Activation of NF-κB p65 in renal tissue	(Lee et al. 2012a)

Abbreviations: ACh, acetylcholine; AGE, advanced glycation end products; ALT, alanine transaminase; AST, aspartate transaminase; ET-1, endothelin-1; HDL, high-density lipoprotein cholesterol; ICAM-1, intercellular adhesion molecule-1; IL, interleukin; IκBα, inhibitors of NF-κB; LDL, low-density lipoprotein cholesterol; MMP, matrix metalloproteinase; NF-κB, nuclear factor κB; OVX, ovariectomized; ROCK, Rho-associated protein kinase; SBP, systolic blood pressure; SNP, sodium nitroprusside; STZ, streptozotocin; TC, total cholesterol; TG, triglycerides; TGF-β1, transforming growth factor-β1; TNF-α, tumor necrosis factor-α; VCAM-1, vascular cell adhesion molecule-1.

pathologic liver changes in STZ-induced liver injury mice. They emphasized that PO may possess protective effects against DM-induced hepatic damage through mitigating the Rho–NF-κB signaling pathway (Zheng et al. 2018).

Gu et al. showed that water macerated extract of PO (0.25, 0.5, and 1 mg/ml) provided a significant increment in extracellular glucose consumption while markedly attenuating insulin resistance in insulin-resistant HepG2 cells (Gu et al. 2015).

10.2.3.2 Diabetic Vascular Inflammation and Endothelial Dysfunction

It has been demonstrated that aqueous extract of PO (300 mg/kg/day; orally) for 10 weeks considerably attenuated blood glucose, TG, LDL, and systolic blood pressure (SBP) in diabetic male C57BL/KsJ-db/db mice. In contrast, the HDL and insulin levels and insulin immunoreactivity of the pancreatic islets were markedly enhanced following PO treatment. PO treatment also improved acetylcholine (ACh) and sodium nitroprusside (SNP)-induced vascular relaxation of aortic rings impairment in db/db mice. Additionally, PO extract remarkably inhibited the overexpression of vascular cell adhesion molecule-1 (VCAM-1), intercellular adhesion molecule-1 (ICAM-1), E-selectin, matrix metalloproteinase (MMP)-2, and endothelin-1 (ET-1) in aortic tissue of diabetic mice. They figured out that PO extract significantly mitigated diabetes-induced vascular inflammation and endothelial dysfunction and may be a potential agent for preventing diabetes vascular complications (Lee et al. 2012b).

10.2.3.3 Diabetic-Induced Neuropathy

Tabatabaei et al. measured the psychobiological effects of PO aqueous extract in STZ-induced DM in ovariectomized (OVX) female Wistar rats. They reported that PO extract (300 mg/kg; orally) for 35 days markedly reduced FBG level, improved spatial cognitive performance and total distance traveled at the probe trial in Morris water maze (MWM), and non-functional masticatory activity in tail pinch stressor (TPS) tests. However, it could not improve the forced swimming test (FST) results. PO extract also showed anxiolytic effects in STZ-induced DM in OVX female Wistar rats. They emphasized that PO extract may ameliorate stress, spatial cognitive performance, and locomotor deficit in STZ-induced DM in OVX female Wistar rats (Fatemi Tabatabaei et al. 2016).

10.2.3.4 Diabetic-Induced Nephropathy

Lee and coworkers evaluated the renoprotective properties of PO aqueous extract on db/db diabetic mice. PO extract (300 mg/kg/day; orally) for 10 weeks meaningfully diminished blood glucose, creatinine level, water intake, and urine volume in diabetic nephropathy mice. In addition, PO extract significantly suppressed the expression of transforming growth factor-β1 (TGF-β1), advanced glycation end products, ICAM-1, as well as NF-κB p65 activation in renal tissue of diabetic db/db mice. They supported that PO extract ameliorates diabetic nephropathy in mice through preventing inflammation and fibrosis in kidney tissue (Lee et al. 2012a).

10.2.4 CLINICAL INVESTIGATIONS

The ameliorating effects of PO on T2D have also been reported in clinical trial studies (Table 10.3). In this regard, El-Sayed conducted a double-blind controlled clinical trial on 30 T2D patients and assigned them to receive 5 g PO seed powder twice daily or 1500 mg metformin/day for 8 weeks in addition to usual care and exercise. He showed that PO seed consumption meaningfully alleviated TG, TC, LDL, FBG, postprandial blood glucose (PBG), insulin, ALT, AST, γ-glutamyl transferase, total and direct bilirubin, body weight and BMI following 8 weeks of treatment. In contrast, the HDL and albumin levels notably enhanced following 8 weeks of treatment with PO seed powder. Interestingly, the decreasing effect of PO seed on insulin, PBG, FBG, body weight, and BMI levels was significantly stronger than in the metformin group. He suggested that PO seed may ameliorate

TABLE 10.3

Clinical Studies of the Anti-Diabetic Effects of *Portulaca oleracea* L.

Extract Type or Plant Part	Study Design	Study Model	Results	Reference
PO seed powder	• 5 g twice daily • 1500 mg metformin/day for 8 weeks	Double-blind controlled clinical trial on T2D patients	↓ Levels of TG, TC, LDL, FBG, PBG, insulin, ALT, AST, GGT, total and direct bilirubin, body weight, and BMI ↑ HDL and albumin level	(El-Sayed 2011)
PO seed powder	• Placebo • Placebo and aerobic training • PO seed powder (2.5 g lunch and 5 g dinner) • PO seed powder along with aerobic training for 16 weeks	Double-blind, placebo-controlled clinical trial on atherosclerosis markers in women with T2D	↓ Glucose, LDL, TC, creatinine, urea, uric acid ↑ HDL level ↓ Protein and mRNA levels of NF-κB, TIMP-1, MMP2 and 9, CRP, CST3, and CTSS ↑ Protein and mRNA levels of GLP1 and GLP1-R	(Dehghan et al. 2016)
PO extract	• PO extract (60 mg) three times a day • Placebo	Double-blind, randomized, placebo-controlled clinical trial on T2D patients treated with a single oral hypoglycemic agent	↓ Systolic blood pressure and HbA_{1c}	(Wainstein et al. 2016)
PO seed powder	• PO seed powder (10 g/day) with 240 mL low-fat yogurt • Only 240 mL low-fat yogurt for 5 weeks • After a 2-week washout period, subjects were moved to the alternate arm for an additional 5 weeks	Crossover, randomized, controlled clinical trial on T2D patients	↓ Body weight, BMI, TG, TC, SBP, and DBP No significant changes in FBG, HOMA-IR, HDL, and LDL	(Esmaillzadeh et al. 2015)
PO seed powder	• PO seed powder (10 g/day) with 240 mL low-fat yogurt • Only 240 mL low-fat yogurt for 5 weeks • After a 2-week washout period, subjects were moved to the alternate arm for an additional 5 weeks	Crossover, randomized, controlled clinical trial on T2D patients	No significant changes in TAC, MDA, and Ox-LDL plasma levels	(Zakizadeh et al. 2015)
PO seed powder	• PO seed powder (2.5 g lunch and 5 g dinner) • Placebo	Randomized placebo-controlled clinical trial on T2D women	↑ GLP1 level No significant difference in the concentration of GLP1 receptor	(Heidarzadeh et al. 2013)

Abbreviations: ALT, liver alanine transaminase; AST, aspartate transaminase; CRP, C-reactive protein; CST3, cystatin C; CTSS, cathepsin S; DBP, diastolic blood pressure; FBG, fasting blood glucose; GGT, γ-glutamyl transferase; GLP1-R, glucagon-like peptide-1 receptor; GLP1, glucagon-like peptide−1; HbA_{1c}, hemoglobin A_{1c}; HDL, high-density lipoprotein cholesterol; HOMA-IR, homeostatic model of assessment of insulin resistance; LDL, low-density lipoprotein cholesterol; MDA, malondialdehyde; MMP, matrix metalloproteinase; NF-κB, nuclear factor κB; Ox-LDL, and oxidized–low-density lipoprotein; PBG, postprandial blood glucose; T2D, type 2 diabetes; TAC, total antioxidant capacity; TG, triglycerides; TC, total cholesterol; TIMP-1, metallopeptidase inhibitor 1.

T2D patients through its hypoglycemic, hypolipidemic and decreased insulin resistance properties (El-Sayed 2011).

Similarly, Dehghan et al. investigated the effects of PO seed powder and aerobic training on atherosclerosis markers in 196 women with T2D for 16 weeks. They divided patients into four groups: placebo; placebo and aerobic training; PO seed powder (2.5 g lunch and 5 g dinner); PO seed powder; and aerobic training. They revealed that PO, and PO along with aerobic training, markedly diminished glucose, LDL, TC, creatinine, urea, and uric acid levels but strikingly elevated HDL levels compared to the before-investigation levels or the placebo group. In addition, the PO and PO along with aerobic training groups considerably mitigated the protein and mRNA levels of NF-κB, metallopeptidase inhibitor 1, MMP2 and 9, C-reactive protein, cystatin C, and cathepsin S while notably promoting glucagon-like peptide-1 (GLP1) and GLP1 receptor compared to the before-investigation levels or the placebo group. Interestingly, the effect of PO along with aerobic exercise was remarkably greater than the PO group in all measured parameters. They supported that PO seed alone or along with exercise ameliorates atherosclerosis plaque biomarkers in women with T2D (Dehghan et al. 2016). Similarly, PO seed powder (2.5 g lunch and 5 g dinner) for 8 weeks markedly improved T2DM in women through elevating the GLP1 level (Heidarzadeh et al. 2013).

Additionally, Wainstein and coworkers conducted a randomized, placebo-controlled clinical trial on 63 T2D patients treated with a single oral hypoglycemic agent. They evaluated the effects of 12 months of treatment with PO extract or placebo. Patients received PO extract capsules (60 mg) three times a day, equal to 750 mg dried or 15 g fresh PO herb. They noticed that 12 months of treatment with PO extract provided a significant decrement in SBP and HbA$_{1c}$ levels than the placebo group (Wainstein et al. 2016).

Although promising results of PO in T2D patients, some studies reported no significant changes following PO treatment. Esmaillzadeh et al. evaluated the effect of 10 g/day PO seed powder with 240 mL low-fat yogurt on 48 T2D patients in a crossover, randomized controlled clinical trial. They demonstrated that PO seed markedly mitigated body weight, BMI, TG, TC, SBP, and diastolic blood pressure compared to the control group. However, they didn't find significant changes in FBG, insulin, HOMA-IR, HDL, and LDL levels between the two groups (Esmaillzadeh et al. 2015). In addition, Zakizadeh and coworkers determined the effect of 10 g/day PO seed powder with 240 mL low-fat yoghurt on oxidative stress markers in 40 T2D patients. They found no significant changes in total antioxidant capacity, MDA, and oxidized-LDL plasma levels following treatment with PO seed than in the control group. They suggested that PO seed powder could not improve oxidative stress in T2D patients (Zakizadeh et al. 2015).

10.3 OTHER FOODS, HERBS, SPICES, AND BOTANICALS USED IN DIABETES

Recently, herbal medicine has attracted a lot of attention, and many researchers reported the antidiabetic properties of several plants and their constituents (Baradaran Rahimi, Askari, and Mousavi 2019). In this regard, *Scutellaria baicalensis* and its two active components, baicalin and baicalein (Baradaran Rahimi, Askari, and Hosseinzadeh 2021); *Crocus sativus* L. and its major constituents crocin, safranal and crocetin (Razavi and Hosseinzadeh 2017); *Silybum marianum* (milk thistle) and its main constituent, silymarin (Tajmohammadi, Razavi, and Hosseinzadeh 2018); and *Capsicum annuum* L. and its component, capsaicin (Sanati, Razavi, and Hosseinzadeh 2018) have been suggested to have promising anti-diabetic effects. In addition, other plants such as *Crataegus pinnatifida* from Rosaceae (Dehghani, Mehri, and Hosseinzadeh 2019); *Cinnamomum verum* from Lauraceae (Mollazadeh and Hosseinzadeh 2016); *Allium sativum* from Alliaceae (Hosseini and Hosseinzadeh 2015); *Vitis vinifera* from Vitaceae (Akaberi and Hosseinzadeh 2016); and *Persea americana* (avocado) from Lauraceae (Tabeshpour, Razavi, and Hosseinzadeh 2017) ameliorated DM in several studies.

10.4 TOXICITY AND CAUTIONARY NOTES

In multiple *in-vitro* studies, PO showed no cytotoxic effects, and the IC_{50} of PO extract was reported to be more than 100 µg/mL in human hormone-dependent breast cancer MCF-7 cell, colon cancer HT-29, cervical cancer HeLa cell, and nasopharyngeal cancer CNE-1 cells (Yen, Chen, and Peng 2001; Tan et al. 2013). In addition, the IC_{50} of chloroform extract of PO was 1132.02 µg/ml and 767.60 µg/ml against human colon adenocarcinoma HCT-15 and Vero cell line, respectively (Mali 2015).

In animal studies, the LD_{50} for the methanolic extract of PO was 1853 mg/kg in Swiss albino mice (Musa Yusuf et al. 2007). Furthermore, Aljeboori et al. observed no toxic effects following treatment with ethanolic extract of PO up to 9500 mg/kg on Swiss albino balb/C mice (Aljeboori et al. 2014).

PO is well tolerated in patients, and almost all clinical trials have reported no adverse effects following treatment with PO (Zakizadeh et al. 2015). In one clinical trial study, constipation was reported as a side effect; however, it was not severe and was well resolved (Wainstein et al. 2016).

10.5 SUMMARY POINTS

- This chapter focuses on the anti-diabetic effects of *Portulaca oleracea* L. (PO), commonly known as purslane, a herbaceous annual plant belonging to Portulacaceae.
- Different parts of PO have been widely used as folk medicine in several countries as a remedy for various disorders.
- The promising anti-diabetic effects of PO have been reported in different animal models of DM, including streptozotocin (STZ) and alloxan-induced DM.
- PO increased insulin secretion and improved insulin resistance.
- PO possessed protective effects against diabetes complications, such as diabetic-induced hepatic damage, vascular inflammation and endothelial dysfunction, nephropathy, and neuropathy.
- The ameliorating effects of PO on T2D have also been reported in clinical trial studies.

REFERENCES

Akaberi, M., and H. Hosseinzadeh. 2016. "Grapes (Vitis vinifera) as a potential candidate for the therapy of the metabolic syndrome." *Phytother Res* 30 (4):540–556.

Aljeboori, Khalil H., O. H. Rubai, and O. H. Nahi. 2014. "Study of pathological, effects of crude extract of Portulaca olercea L. in the albino mice organs." *Int J Techn Res Yassen Appl* 2 (1):29–32.

Askari, V. R., S. A. Rezaee, K. Abnous, M. Iranshahi, and M. H. Boskabady. 2016. "The influence of hydro-ethanolic extract of Portulaca oleracea L. on Th(1)/Th(2) balance in isolated human lymphocytes." *J Ethnopharmacol* 194:1112–1121.

Bai, Y., X. Zang, J. Ma, and G. Xu. 2016. "Anti-diabetic effect of Portulaca oleracea L. polysaccharide and its mechanism in diabetic rats." *Int J Mol Sci* 17 (8).

Bao, M., K. Hou, C. Xin, D. Zeng, C. Cheng, H. Zhao, Z. Wang, and L. Wang. 2022. "Portulaca oleracea L. extract alleviated type 2 diabetes via modulating the gut microbiota and serum branched-chain amino acid metabolism." *Mol Nutr Food Res*:e2101030.

Baradaran Rahimi, Vafa, and Vahid Reza Askari. 2021. "Promising anti-melanogenic impacts of Portulaca oleracea on B16F1 murine melanoma cell line: An in-vitro vision." *South African Journal of Botany* 142:477–485.

Baradaran Rahimi, V., V. R. Askari, and H. Hosseinzadeh. 2021. "Promising influences of Scutellaria baicalensis and its two active constituents, baicalin, and baicalein, against metabolic syndrome: A review." *Phytother Res* 35 (7):3558–3574.

Baradaran Rahimi, V., V. R. Askari, and S. H. Mousavi. 2019. "Ellagic acid dose and time-dependently abrogates d-galactose-induced animal model of aging: Investigating the role of PPAR-γ." *Life Sci* 232:116595.

Baradaran Rahimi, V., S. H. Mousavi, S. Haghighi, S. Soheili-Far, and V. R. Askari. 2019. "Cytotoxicity and apoptogenic properties of the standardized extract of Portulaca oleracea on glioblastoma multiforme cancer cell line (U-87): A mechanistic study." *Excli J* 18:165–186.

Baradaran Rahimi, V., A. Rajabian, H. Rajabi, E. Mohammadi Vosough, H. R. Mirkarimi, M. Hasanpour, M. Iranshahi, H. Rakhshandeh, and V. R. Askari. 2020. "The effects of hydro-ethanolic extract of Capparis spinosa (C. spinosa) on lipopolysaccharide (LPS)-induced inflammation and cognitive impairment: Evidence from in vivo and in vitro studies." *J Ethnopharmacol* 256:112706.

Baradaran Rahimi, V., H. Rakhshandeh, F. Raucci, B. Buono, R. Shirazinia, A. Samzadeh Kermani, F. Maione, N. Mascolo, and V. R. Askari. 2019. "Anti-inflammatory and antioxidant activity of Portulaca oleracea extract on LPS-induced rat lung injury." *Molecules* 24 (1).

Boskabady, Mohammad Hossein, Milad Hashemzehi, Mohammad Reza Khazdair, and Vahid Reza Askari. 2016. "Hydro-ethanolic extract of Portulaca oleracea affects beta-adrenoceptors of guinea pig tracheal smooth muscle." *IJPR* 15 (4):867–874.

Cole, J. B., and J. C. Florez. 2020. "Genetics of diabetes mellitus and diabetes complications." *Nat Rev Nephrol* 16 (7):377–390.

Dehghan, F., R. Soori, K. Gholami, M. Abolmaesoomi, A. Yusof, S. Muniandy, S. Heidarzadeh, P. Farzanegi, and M. Ali Azarbayjani. 2016. "Purslane (Portulaca oleracea) seed consumption and aerobic training improves biomarkers associated with atherosclerosis in women with type 2 diabetes (T2D)." *Sci Rep* 6:37819.

Dehghani, S., S. Mehri, and H. Hosseinzadeh. 2019. "The effects of crataegus pinnatifida (Chinese hawthorn) on metabolic syndrome: A review." *Iran J Basic Med Sci* 22 (5):460–468.

El-Sayed, M. I. 2011. "Effects of Portulaca oleracea L. seeds in treatment of type-2 diabetes mellitus patients as adjunctive and alternative therapy." *J Ethnopharmacol* 137 (1):643–651.

Esmaillzadeh, A., E. Zakizadeh, E. Faghihimani, M. Gohari, and S. Jazayeri. 2015. "The effect of purslane seeds on glycemic status and lipid profiles of persons with type 2 diabetes: A randomized controlled cross-over clinical trial." *J Res Med Sci* 20 (1):47–53.

Fatemi Tabatabaei, S. R., M. Rashno, S. Ghaderi, and M. Askaripour. 2016. "The aqueous extract of Portulaca oleracea ameliorates neurobehavioral dysfunction and hyperglycemia related to streptozotocin-diabetes induced in ovariectomized rats." *Iran J Pharm Res* 15 (2):561–571.

Gong, F., F. Li, L. Zhang, J. Li, Z. Zhang, and G. Wang. 2009. "Hypoglycemic effects of crude polysaccharide from Purslane." *Int J Mol Sci* 10 (3):880–888.

Gu, J. F., Z. Y. Zheng, J. R. Yuan, B. J. Zhao, C. F. Wang, L. Zhang, Q. Y. Xu, G. W. Yin, L. Feng, and X. B. Jia. 2015. "Comparison on hypoglycemic and antioxidant activities of the fresh and dried Portulaca oleracea L. in insulin-resistant HepG2 cells and streptozotocin-induced C57BL/6J diabetic mice." *J Ethnopharmacol* 161:214–223.

Heidarzadeh, S., P. Farzanegi, M. A. Azarbayjani, and R. Daliri. 2013. "Purslane effect on GLP-1 and GLP-1 receptor in type 2 diabetes." *Electron Physician* 5 (1):582–587.

Hosseini, A., and H. Hosseinzadeh. 2015. "A review on the effects of Allium sativum (Garlic) in metabolic syndrome." *J Endocrinol Invest* 38 (11):1147–1157.

Hou, J., X. Zhou, P. Wang, C. Zhao, Y. Qin, F. Liu, L. Yu, and H. Xu. 2020. "An integrative pharmacology-based approach for evaluating the potential effects of purslane seed in diabetes mellitus treatment using UHPLC-LTQ-orbitrap and TCMIP V2.0." *Front Pharmacol* 11:593693.

Hu, Q., Q. Niu, H. Song, S. Wei, S. Wang, L. Yao, and Y. P. Li. 2019. "Polysaccharides from Portulaca oleracea L. regulated insulin secretion in INS-1 cells through voltage-gated Na(+) channel." *Biomed Pharmacother* 109:876–885.

Jaafari, Ali, Vafa Baradaran Rahimi, Nasser Vahdati-Mashhadian, Roghayeh Yahyazadeh, Alireza Ebrahimzadeh-Bideskan, Maede Hasanpour, Mehrdad Iranshahi, Sajjad Ehtiati, Hamed Rajabi, Mohammadreza Mahdinezhad, Hassan Rakhshandeh, and Vahid Reza Askari. 2021. "Evaluation of the therapeutic effects of the hydroethanolic extract of Portulaca oleracea on surgical-induced peritoneal adhesion." *Mediators Inflamm* 2021:8437753–8437753.

Jung, J. H., S. B. Hwang, H. J. Park, G. R. Jin, and B. H. Lee. 2021. "Antiobesity and antidiabetic effects of Portulaca oleracea powder intake in high-fat diet-induced obese C57BL/6 mice." *Evid Based Complement Alternat Med* 2021:5587848.

Kumar, A., S. Sreedharan, A. K. Kashyap, P. Singh, and N. Ramchiary. 2022. "A review on bioactive phytochemicals and ethnopharmacological potential of purslane (Portulaca oleracea L.)." *Heliyon* 8 (1): e08669.

Lee, A. S., Y. J. Lee, S. M. Lee, J. J. Yoon, J. S. Kim, D. G. Kang, and H. S. Lee. 2012a. "An aqueous extract of Portulaca oleracea ameliorates diabetic nephropathy through suppression of renal fibrosis and inflammation in diabetic db/db mice." *Am J Chin Med* 40 (3):495–510.

Lee, A. S., Y. J. Lee, S. M. Lee, J. J. Yoon, J. S. Kim, D. G. Kang, and H. S. Lee. 2012b. "Portulaca oleracea ameliorates diabetic vascular inflammation and endothelial dysfunction in db/db mice." *Evid Based Complement Alternat Med* 2012:741824.

Lee, J. H., J. E. Park, and J. S. Han. 2020. "Portulaca oleracea L. extract reduces hyperglycemia via PI3k/Akt and AMPK pathways in the skeletal muscles of C57BL/KsJ-db/db mice." *J Ethnopharmacol* 260:112973.

Mali, P. Y. 2015. "Assessment of cytotoxicity of Portulaca oleracea Linn. against human colon adenocarcinoma and vero cell line." *Ayu* 36 (4):432–436.

Mollazadeh, H., and H. Hosseinzadeh. 2016. "Cinnamon effects on metabolic syndrome: A review based on its mechanisms." *Iran J Basic Med Sci* 19 (12):1258–1270.

Moukette, B. M., V. J. Ama Moor, C. P. Biapa Nya, P. Nanfack, F. T. Nzufo, M. A. Kenfack, J. Y. Ngogang, and C. A. Pieme. 2017. "Antioxidant and synergistic anti-diabetic activities of a three-plant preparation used in cameroon folk medicine." *Int Sch Res Notices* 2017:9501675.

Musa Yusuf, Kabir, Ahmed Abubakar, G. Ibrahim, O. E. Ojonugwa, M. Bisalla, Hamidu Musa, and Habib Danmalam. 2007. "Toxicity studies on the methanolic extract of Portulaca oleracea L. (Fam. Portulacaceae)." *Journal of Biological Sciences* 7.

Niazi, A., S. Yousefzadeh, H. Rakhshandeh, H. Esmaily, and V. R. Askari. 2019. "Promising effects of purslane cream on the breast fissure in lactating women: A clinical trial." *Complement Ther Med* 43:300–305.

Park, J. E., and J. S. Han. 2018. "A Portulaca oleracea L. extract promotes insulin secretion via a K(+)(ATP) channel dependent pathway in INS-1 pancreatic β-cells." *Nutr Res Pract* 12 (3):183–190.

Park, J. E., J. Y. Park, Y. Seo, and J. S. Han. 2019. "A new chromanone isolated from Portulaca oleracea L. increases glucose uptake by stimulating GLUT4 translocation to the plasma membrane in 3T3-L1 adipocytes." *Int J Biol Macromol* 123:26–34.

Park, J. E., Y. Seo, and J. S. Han. 2021. "HM-chromanone, a component of Portulaca oleracea L., stimulates glucose uptake and glycogen synthesis in skeletal muscle cell." *Phytomedicine* 83:153473.

Petropoulos, Spyridon, Anestis Karkanis, Natalia Martins, and Isabel C.F.R. Ferreira. 2016. "Phytochemical composition and bioactive compounds of common purslane (Portulaca oleracea L.) as affected by crop management practices." *Trends Food Sci Technol* 55:1–10.

Rahimi, V. B., F. Ajam, H. Rakhshandeh, and V. R. Askari. 2019. "A pharmacological review on Portulaca oleracea L.: Focusing on anti-inflammatory, anti-oxidant, immuno-modulatory and antitumor activities." *J Pharmacopuncture* 22 (1):7–15.

Ramadan, B. K., M. F. Schaalan, and A. M. Tolba. 2017. "Hypoglycemic and pancreatic protective effects of Portulaca oleracea extract in alloxan induced diabetic rats." *BMC Complement Altern Med* 17 (1):37.

Razavi, B. M., and H. Hosseinzadeh. 2017. "Saffron: A promising natural medicine in the treatment of metabolic syndrome." *J Sci Food Agric* 97 (6):1679–1685.

Samarghandian, S., A. Borji, and T. Farkhondeh. 2017. "Attenuation of oxidative stress and inflammation by Portulaca oleracea in streptozotocin-induced diabetic rats." *J Evid Based Complementary Altern Med* 22 (4):562–566.

Sanati, S., B. M. Razavi, and H. Hosseinzadeh. 2018. "A review of the effects of capsicum annuum L. and its constituent, capsaicin, in metabolic syndrome." *Iran J Basic Med Sci* 21 (5):439–448.

Sharma, Alok, Gaurav Kaithwas, M. Vijayakumar, M. K. Unnikrishnan, and Ch. V. Rao. 2012. "Antihyperglycemic and antioxidant potential of polysaccharide fraction from portulaca oleracea seeds against streptozotocin-induced diabetes in rats." *J Food Biochem* 36 (3):378–382.

Tabeshpour, J., B. M. Razavi, and H. Hosseinzadeh. 2017. "Effects of avocado (Persea americana) on metabolic syndrome: A comprehensive systematic review." *Phytother Res* 31 (6):819–837.

Tajmohammadi, A., B. M. Razavi, and H. Hosseinzadeh. 2018. "Silybum marianum (milk thistle) and its main constituent, silymarin, as a potential therapeutic plant in metabolic syndrome: A review." *Phytother Res* 32 (10):1933–1949.

Tan, Gek, Kar Wong, Gui Pearle-Wong, Siau Yeo, Swee Keong Yeap, Beow Chin Yiap, and Megan Chong. 2013. "In vitro cytotoxic and antiproliferative effects of Portulaca oleracea methanol extract on breast, cervical, colon and nasopharyngeal cancerous cell lines." *Sains Malays* 42:927–935.

Uddin, M. K., A. S. Juraimi, M. S. Hossain, M. A. Nahar, M. E. Ali, and M. M. Rahman. 2014. "Purslane weed (Portulaca oleracea): A prospective plant source of nutrition, omega-3 fatty acid, and antioxidant attributes." *Sci World J* 2014:951019.

Wainstein, J., Z. Landau, Y. Bar Dayan, D. Jakubowicz, T. Grothe, T. Perrinjaquet-Moccetti, and M. Boaz. 2016. "Purslane extract and glucose homeostasis in adults with type 2 diabetes: A double-blind, placebo-controlled clinical trial of efficacy and safety." *J Med Food* 19 (2):133–140.

Yang, Xiaohang, Yongmei Yan, Jiankang Li, Zhishu Tang, Jing Sun, Huan Zhang, Siyang Hao, Aidong Wen, and Li Liu. 2016. "Protective effects of ethanol extract from Portulaca oleracea L on dextran sulphate sodium-induced mice ulcerative colitis involving anti-inflammatory and antioxidant." *Am J Transl Res* 8 (5):2138–2148.

Yen, G. C., H. Y. Chen, and H. H. Peng. 2001. "Evaluation of the cytotoxicity, mutagenicity and antimutagenicity of emerging edible plants." *Food and Chem Toxicol* 39 (11):1045–1053.

Zakizadeh, E., E. Faghihimani, P. Saneei, and A. Esmaillzadeh. 2015. "The effect of purslane seeds on biomarkers of oxidative stress in diabetic patients: A randomized controlled cross-over clinical trial." *Int J Prev Med* 6:95.

Zheng, G., F. Mo, C. Ling, H. Peng, W. Gu, M. Li, and Z. Chen. 2018. "Portulaca oleracea L. alleviates liver injury in streptozotocin-induced diabetic mice." *Drug Des Devel Ther* 12:47–55.

Zhou, Y. X., H. L. Xin, K. Rahman, S. J. Wang, C. Peng, and H. Zhang. 2015. "Portulaca oleracea L.: A review of phytochemistry and pharmacological effects." *Biomed Res Int* 2015:925631.

11 Corn Silk (*Stigma maydis*) Use in Diabetes
Molecular, Cellular, and Metabolic Effects

Ramesh Bhandari, Raushan Kumar Chaudhary,
Pukar Khanal and Madiwalayya S. Ganachari

CONTENTS

ABBREVIATIONS

ACC	acetyl-CoA carboxylase
AMPK	adenosine monophosphate-activated protein kinase
C/EBPs	CCAAT/enhancer-binding proteins
CAMKKB	calcium/calmodulin-dependent protein kinase kinase 2
CPT	carnitine palmitoyl transferase
EGFR	epidermal growth factor receptor
ERK	extracellular signal-regulated kinases
FAS	fatty acid synthase
GLP-1	glucagon-like peptide-1
GLUT4	glucose transporter type 4
HDL-C	high-density lipoprotein cholesterol
HMG-CoA	hydroxy methylglutaryl coenzyme A
HMGCR	3-hydroxy-3-methylglutaryl coenzyme A reductase
IFN-α	interferon-α
IKB	inhibitor of nuclear factor-κB (IκB)
IKK	inhibitor of nuclear factor-κB (IκB) kinase
IL-6	interleukin-6
IRS1	insulin receptor substrate 1
LPS	lipopolysaccharides

DOI: 10.1201/9781003220930-13

LXR α	liver X receptor α
MCP-1	monocyte chemoattractant protein-1
NF-κB	nuclear factor κ-light-chain-enhancer of activated B cells
NO	nitric oxide
PDGFR	platelet-derived growth factor receptor α
PDX-1	pancreatic and duodenal homeobox factor-1
PEPCK	phosphoenolpyruvate carboxykinase
PI3K	phosphoinositide 3-kinase
PKC	protein kinase C
PPAR-α	peroxisome proliferator-activated receptor-α
PPAR-γ	peroxisome proliferator-activated receptor-γ
PTP1B	protein tyrosine phosphatase 1B
ROS	reactive oxygen species
SREBP-1C	sterol regulatory element binding protein-1c
TNF-α	tumor necrosis factor α
VEGR-2	vasculotropin receptor 2
VLDL-C	very-low-density lipoprotein cholesterol

11.1 INTRODUCTION

Corn (*Zea mays* L.) belongs to the family Poaceae (or Gramineae) and is native to the Western Hemisphere. It originated from Mexico in the 12th century and later spread all over the American continent. The United States, China, Brazil, and India are the largest producers of corn worldwide (Nawaz H et al. 2018). The mature corn kernel consists of a radicle, four roots, and three seminal roots (Buzás I et al. 2006). The average height of a maize plant is 3 m (10 ft); however, some strains can reach 13 m (43 ft). The stem generally consists of 20 internodes, each 18 cm (7 in.) long. The leaves develop from the nodes and are arranged alternately on the stalk's opposite sides (Russell WA and Hallauer AR 1980; Goss JA 2008). Most of the corn is considered waste except for the corn seed. Corn seed is the edible part of corn served as a food in Asian countries. *Zea mays* are the only cultivable species, whereas others are wild grasses such as *Z. diploperennis*, *Z. luxurians*, *Z. nicaraguensis*, and *Z. perennis*. The corn plant emerges as a monoecious flowering plant from the bisexual during development (Nawaz H et al. 2018). Corn silk is a long, pigmented (yellowish to reddish) hair-like structure that covers the edible portion of corn and can be 30 cm or more in length.

11.2 BACKGROUND

Corn silk gets pollinated to produce one kernel of corn, but it has been harvested before pollination for medicinal uses (Sahib AS et al. 2012). Corn silk is nontoxic and safe and has traditionally been used to treat various diseases. It has been used to treat cystitis, edema, kidney stones, diuretic, prostate disorder, urinary infections, bedwetting, and obesity in Turkey, China, United States, and France. The medicinal value of corn silk is mainly due to bioactives such as phenols, polyphenols, phenolic acids, flavonoids, flavone glycosides, anthocyanins, carotenoids, terpenoids, alkaloids, steroids, luteins, tannins, saponins, volatile oils, vitamins, some sugars, and polysaccharides. Thus, it exerts various therapeutic effects like antioxidant, antihyperlipidemic, antidiabetic, anti-inflammatory, antifatigue, neuroprotective, diuresis, and kaliuresis (Chaudhary RK et al. 2022). Apart from this, it has been used as tea and in medical drinks in Asia, as additives in food, and as flavoring agents (Nawaz H et al. 2018). Polyphenols, including anthocyanins, quercetin, and phenolic acids in purple corn silk, have anti-obesity activity (Chaiittianan R et al. 2017). The purple waxy corn silk at the milky stage presents with the highest concentration of phenols, flavonoids, and anthocyanin.

In contrast, sweet and white corn presented these at the highest values in silking stage (Sarepoua E et al. 2015). Purple corn silk extract can also be used in cosmetic products as an anti–ultraviolet

B agent (Poorahong W et al. 2021). Despite having several therapeutic advantages, corn plants are linked to health risks. Mycotoxins, including ochratoxin A, zeralenone, fumonisins, and alfatoxins have caused fungal infections in humans (Widstrom NW 1996; Norred WP et al. 1998). Along with fungal infections, corn can also cause allergies as it contains lipid transfer protein, an indigestible protein that does not degrade even after cooking, which can result in asthma attacks, skin rashes, itching, swelling of mucous membranes, and rarely anaphylaxis. The prevalence of these allergies is unknown (Asero R et al. 2001). Another health risk connected to corn is pellagra, which was more common in non-native Americans but not in native Americans owing to niacin deficiency (Bollet AJ 1992). Corn silk has a subchronic toxic dose of 9.354 g/kg/day and 10.308 g/kg/day for male and female Wistar rats, respectively (Wang C et al. 2011). The corn earworm infestation, which causes damage to the corn ear, is a massive problem in the cultivation of maize. Still, Inbred T218 produces active levels of isoorientin, which inhibits the growth of corn earworm larvae (Widstrom NW and Snook ME 1998).

11.3 DIABETES

The glucose level in our body is regulated by the two crucial pancreatic hormones, glucagon and insulin. Whenever the glucose level goes up in the blood, it stimulates the release of insulin via the ATP-dependent inhibition of the potassium channel leading to depolarization of pancreatic β cells due to the influx of calcium which in turn promotes the exocytosis of insulin. This insulin acts on the extracellular domain of the insulin receptor in the cell, which activates the intracellular phosphorylation of insulin receptor substrate 1 (IRS1) by the intracellular domain of the insulin receptor. The phosphorylated IRS1 activates phosphoinositide 3-kinase (PI3K), which promotes the phosphorylation of AKT, leading to translocalization of glucose transporter type 4 (GLUT4), which is responsible for glucose uptake in the skeletal muscle. The insulin release also promotes glucose uptake and glycogen synthesis, reducing gluconeogenesis in the liver and skeletal muscle.

Further, it activates lipoprotein lipase, promotes adipogenesis, and decreases lipolysis (Al-Ishaq RK et al. 2019). Diabetes is a polygenic metabolic alteration generally characterized by altered insulin secretion and/or sensitization (Chaudhary RK et al. 2021). Various factors contribute to the development of diabetes, such as environment, genetics, obesity, and autoimmunity (Sun C et al. 2020). The cellular and molecular pathology of diabetes include the modulation of several pathways related to glucose uptake (e.g., SLC2 gene, IRS-1, PI3K), glucose metabolism by liver enzymes (glucose-6-phosphatase, hexokinase, PEPCK, fructose 1,6-bisphosphatase), programmed β cell death (pro-apoptotic proteins BCL2 family), lipid metabolism (e.g., PPAR-α, PPAR-γ), energy homeostasis (LKB1, CAMKKB, TAK-1), growth factor signaling (C-Abl, PDGFR, EGFR, VEGR-2), and survival of β cells (IKB, IKK, NF-κB). The modulation of the SLC2 gene, IRS-1, PI3K results in decreased GLUT translocation, glucose uptake, and insulin resistance. Similarly, the modulation of liver enzymes is responsible for the downregulation of insulin signaling and liver glycogen. In contrast, it upregulates gluconeogenesis, insulin resistance, endogenous glucose production, and lipid properties of the smooth endoplasmic reticulum. Likewise, downregulation of apoptotic regulatory genes and caspases, and upregulation of oxidative stress, mitochondrial dysfunction, and insulin resistance contribute toward the modulation of programmed β cell death. However, modulation of PPAR contributes to reduced lipid metabolism leading to hyperlipidemia, hyperinsulinemia, and hyperglycemia. Further, downregulation of AMPK and glucose homeostasis contributes to the modulation of energy homeostasis. Additionally, increased NF-κB expression, oxidative stress, and pro-inflammatory cytokines are responsible for modulation in the control of β cell survival (Al-Ishaq RK et al. 2019).

Corn silk has been reported as one of the nontoxic and potent medicinal herbs for the treatment of diabetes and its complications. The antidiabetic effect of corn silk is due to the potential druggable candidates such as the presence of flavonoids, phenolic acids, phytosterols, carotenoids, and tannins as reported by Chaudhary RK et al. 2022. The authors reported the higher affinity of flavones, β-carotene, gallotannins, 3-O-caffeoylquinic acid, and stigmasterol from corn silk toward

PTPN1B, GLUT1, DPP4, α-glucosidase, and α-amylase, respectively, using in silico molecular docking (Chaudhary RK et al. 2022).

11.4 FLAVONOIDS

The flavonoids are polyphenolic compounds made up of 15 carbon skeletons and two aromatic rings linking each other with the help of three carbon chains. The flavonoids, after ingestion, get converted from oligomeric to monomeric form in the stomach with the help of lactase. The liver further metabolizes this monomeric form once absorbed from the intestine via sulfonation, methylation, and glucuronidation, and the metabolites are excreted in bile and urine. In contrast, the unabsorbed flavonoids undergo hydrolysis in the large intestine and eventually get absorbed (Al-Ishaq RK et al. 2019). The corn silk contains druggable flavonoids such as quercetin, rutin, catechin, kaempferol, 3-O-caffeoylquinic acid, flavone, and formononetin (Chaudhary RK et al. 2022). These flavonoids are reported to act through various pathways to pose antidiabetic properties.

Quercetin has been reported to prevent glucose absorption from the intestine via the inhibition of GLUT2 transporter, α-glucosidase, and α-amylase (Al-Ishaq RK et al. 2019; Yi H et al. 2021; Sok Yen F et al. 2021). Further, it inhibits the insulin-dependent stimulation of PI3K and promotes glucose uptake via the activation of AMPK by translocation of GLUT4 (Al-Ishaq RK et al. 2019; Yi H et al. 2021). It regulates the IRS1/PI3K/PIP2/PIP3/PDK1/AKT/AS160/RABS/GLUT4 signaling pathway by reducing blood glucose (Al-Ishaq RK et al. 2019; Yi H et al. 2021; Sok Yen F et al. 2021). Similarly, AMPK activation by quercetin leads to suppression of glucose-6-phosphate (G6Pase) and phosphoenolpyruvate carboxylase (PEPCK) activity contributing to the antidiabetic effect. It also promotes hepatic glycogen synthesis by regulating glucokinase (GSK) expression mediated through the phosphorylation of Ser9 and Akt. Similarly, hexokinase activity is generally increased, and fructose-bisphosphatase (FBPase) activity is decreased in the presence of quercetin (Yi H et al. 2021). Quercetin can increase insulin secretion via three different pathways: promoting the expression of VERGF and VEGFR2 in the pancreas, which helps in β cell recovery, stimulating extracellular signal-regulated kinase (ERK1/2), and upregulated calcium signaling pathways. Likewise, quercetin also improves insulin resistance by reducing endoplasmic reticulum stress and oxidative stress in the pancreas, along with mitigating the inflammatory mediators and cell apoptosis. It blocks the TNF-α–mediated insulin resistance by inhibiting the IRS1 and PTP1B gene expression phosphorylation. It also improves insulin resistance by counteracting the hypothalamic insulin signaling pathway via the phosphorylation of insulin receptors and protein kinase B (AKT) (Yi H et al. 2021). Quercetin acts as an anti-inflammatory by inhibiting TNF-α/TNFR/IKK/IKB/NF-κB signaling pathways (Al-Ishaq RK et al. 2019; Yi H et al. 2021). It also acts as an antioxidant via upregulating the PPAR-γ activity and scavenges radicals via upregulating SIRT1 expression (Yi H et al. 2021). Quercetin decreases the pro-apoptotic markers such as caspases 3/9 and BAX, whereas it increases the anti-apoptotic markers like BCL2 proteins. It also diminishes the expression of autophagy via the downregulation of beclin-1 and LC-3B (Al-Ishaq RK et al. 2019; Yi H et al. 2021).

Rutin is another polyphenolic flavonoid compound reported to possess antidiabetic properties. The antidiabetic property of rutin is conferred to inhibition of α-glucosidase, α-amylase, glucose-6-phosphatase, PEPCK, glycogen phosphorylase, and fructose 1,6-bisphosphatase enzyme, whereas it activates hexokinase activity (Al-Ishaq RK et al. 2019; Sok Yen F et al. 2021; Ghorbani A 2017). Rutin also promotes glucose uptake in the tissue via the phosphoinositide 3-kinase (PI3K), protein kinase C, and mitogen-activated protein kinase (MAPK), similar to the insulin signaling pathway. In contrast, it decreases blood glucose levels and regulates the IRS1/PI3K/PIP2/PIP3/PDK1/AKT/AS160/RABS/GLUT4 signaling pathway (Al-Ishaq RK et al. 2019; Ghorbani A 2017). It promotes the uptake of glucose in muscle and adipocytes via the activation of PPAR-γ (Ghorbani A 2017). Rutin reduces β cell apoptosis via the inhibition of caspases 3/9 and activation of BCL2 family proteins (Al-Ishaq RK et al. 2019). It maintains the morphological structure of the islet of Langerhans and promotes calcium-dependent insulin exocytosis from the pancreatic β cell (Sok Yen F et al. 2021; Ghorbani A 2017).

Kaempferol inhibits α-glucosidase, regulates the IRS1/PI3K/PIP2/PIP3/PDK1/AKT/AS160/RABS/GLUT4 signaling pathway by reducing blood sugar, and activates the expression of AMPK and GLUT4 which is vital for antidiabetic property (Al-Ishaq RK et al. 2019; Sok Yen F et al. 2021). Like rutin, it also reduces β cell apoptosis (Al-Ishaq RK et al. 2019). It also suppresses the hexokinase activity in the liver and muscle (Alkhalidy H et al. 2018).

Catechin is a flavonoid compound that acts as an antidiabetic by inhibiting α-glucosidase, α-amylase, and sodium-dependent glucose transport (SGLT1) (Sun C et al. 2020; Pawar MR and Karthikeyan E 2020). It promotes the GLUT4 translocation via the PI3K and AMPK pathways. It also increases glycogen synthesis and glucose uptake but decreases lipogenesis in the hepatic cell. Further, it has a role in preventing insulin resistance by protecting the phosphorylation of insulin receptors and IRS on serine residue. Catechin acts as an antioxidant by scavenging the ROS, decreasing the JNK-activated pathway. Further, epigallocatechin also modulates the antioxidant and PTP1B gene expression via nuclear translocation of Nrf2 (Sun C et al. 2020).

Formononetin is an isoflavone found in the corn silk, which acts antidiabetically via the activation of the IRS1/PI3K/AKT/AMPK/P38/GLUT4 signaling pathways. It also inhibits the tubular reabsorption of glucose via the inhibition of SGLT2. It increases the expression of SIRT1 in pancreatic cells, which helps counteract insulin resistance. Further, it protects pancreatic β cells from necrosis and atrophy. Apart from antidiabetic action, it has a role in inflammation. It acts as an anti-inflammatory by inhibiting PKC/PARP/NF-κB signaling pathways in cardiac tissue. It also possesses antihyperlipidemic properties and can scavenge free radicals and exert antioxidant activity by inhibiting ROS formation.

11.5 PHENOLIC ACIDS

Corn silk has three different druggable phenolic acids: chlorogenic acid, protocatechuic acid, and 3-O-caffeoylquinic acid (Chaudhary RK et al. 2022).

Chlorogenic acid is phenolic acid that acts as antidiabetic by hindering glucose absorption via inhibition of α-glucosidase, α-amylase, and glucose-6-phosphatase translocase 1 and interrupting sodium-driven glucose transport (Meng S et al. 2013; Santana-Gálvez J et al. 2017). It activates the AMPK-mediated translocation of GLUT4 and stimulates GLP-1 secretion, which contributes to antidiabetic activity. Further, it reduces cholesterol synthesis and promotes fatty acid oxidation via inhibiting HMG-CoA enzymes and strengthening the activity of carnitine palmitoyl transferase (CPT). It also inhibits the activity of aldose reductase and hepatic pyruvate carboxylase and restores the activity of hexokinase in the liver and skeletal muscle (Meng S et al. 2013). Apart from glucose metabolism, it also has a role in lipid metabolism. Chlorogenic acid increases the expression of PPAR-α and PPAR-γ, which is responsible for the β-oxidation of fatty acids leading to improvements in insulin sensitivity. It also reduces the activity of LXR-α, which regulates fatty acid and triglyceride synthesis via the activation of genes encoding lipogenic enzymes, including FAS and ACC. Further, it decreases 3-hydroxy-3-methylglutaryl CoA reductase (HMGCR) and increases adiponectin and AMPK phosphorylation, leading to increased insulin sensitivity and glucose tolerance. It also scavenges ROS produced by a high-fat diet, suppressing inflammation and lowering fat storage, weight gain, and insulin resistance (Santana-Gálvez J et al. 2017).

Protocatechuic acid shows antidiabetic properties via activating the IRS1/PI3K/AKT/AMPK/P38/GLUT4 signaling pathway. It also acts as an antioxidant due to the inhibition of ROS. An increase in ROS generally occurs via the polyol and AGE pathway, which is responsible for forming inflammatory cytokines such as IL1β, IL6, IL12, and TNF-α. Further, it also exerts anti-inflammatory activity by inhibiting the PARP/PKC/NF-κB signaling cascade in myocardial tissue (Bhattacharjee N et al. 2017).

Caffeoylquinic acid is another phenolic acid reported to exert antidiabetic action by increasing the PDX-1 expression via IRS-2/Akt/PI3K signaling pathway and ERK1/2 expression (Marcelino G et al. 2020). It also shows antidiabetic activity by inhibiting human salivary and pancreatic α-amylase and hepatic glucose-6-phosphatase. It also promotes insulin secretion and insulin response (Sun C et al. 2020).

11.6 β-CAROTENE

The carotenoid is structurally composed of polyenes with 11 conjugated double bonds and a β-ionone ring on each end. β-Carotene has been reported to reduce insulin resistance. It suppresses the activity of PPAR-γ, leading to adipogenesis. Visceral fat, subcutaneous fat, triglycerides, VLDL-c levels, and the total-/HDL-c ratio are decreased by β-carotene. It also acts as an antioxidant by chelating with singlet oxygen and other free-radical species. It also possesses anti-inflammatory properties via the inhibition of nuclear factor κB (NF-κB) and inflammatory cytokines. Adiponectin is increased by the consumption of β-carotene, a critical factor for insulin sensitivity and glucose tolerance (Marcelino G et al. 2020).

11.7 PHYTOSTEROL

Phytosterol is the sterol that resembles human cholesterol concerning its structure and action. The phytosterol found in corn silk is stigmasterol and β-sitosterol. This phytosterol exerts antidiabetic activity via inhibiting glucose absorption from the intestine or decreasing glycogenolysis and gluconeogenesis. It are also responsible for reducing cholesterol absorption from the intestine and helpful in managing obesity and, thereby, insulin resistance. Further, phytosterol regulates the IR/IRS1/PI3K/AKT/AS160/GLUT4 pathway to possess antidiabetic activity. It also acts as anti-inflammatory via inhibiting IKK/NF-κB/JNK signaling pathway.

Further, phytosterol reduces pro-inflammatory cytokines such as leptin, resistin, TNF-α, and IL-6, whereas it increases anti-inflammatory properties such as adiponectin. It also stimulates the expression of PPAR-γ and decreases the sterol regulatory element binding protein-1c (SREBP-1C) expression. It protects against oxidative damage by increasing glucose-6-phosphate dehydrogenase, which has a role in pentose phosphate pathways (Prasad M et al. 2022).

11.8 GALLOTANNINS

Gallotannins are the polygalloyl ester of glucose molecules that undergo hydrolysis to give gallic acid. Gallotannins has been reported to pose antidiabetic, anti-inflammatory, and antioxidant properties (He HF 2022). Gallotannins show antidiabetic properties by inhibiting the α-glucosidase and α-amylase enzymes. It also phosphorylates IR, PI3K, and AKT, leading to the translocation of GLUT4. Further, it has a role in the translocation of GLUT4 via the activation of PPAR-γ and C/EBPs in adipocytes. Gallotannins also enhance insulin sensitivity via the activation of PPAR-γ, AKT, and AMPK. Gallic acid acts as an antioxidant by scavenging free radicals and forming metal chelation which counteracts the ROS. Further, it acts as an anti-inflammatory by impeding the activity of NO synthase and inducible NO synthase, which could hinder the induction of TNF-α, lipopolysaccharides (LPS), IL-6, and interferon-α (IFN-α) expression. It also inhibits p 65-NF-κB and IL-6/STAT3 pathways in adipose and reduces adipogenesis via the inhibition of monocyte chemoattractant protein-1 (MCP-1) expression and increasing that of adiponectin and PPAR-γ (He HF 2022; Xu Y et al. 2021).

The effect of druggable candidates from corn silk on cellular and molecular pathways involved in diabetes is represented in Figure 11.1.

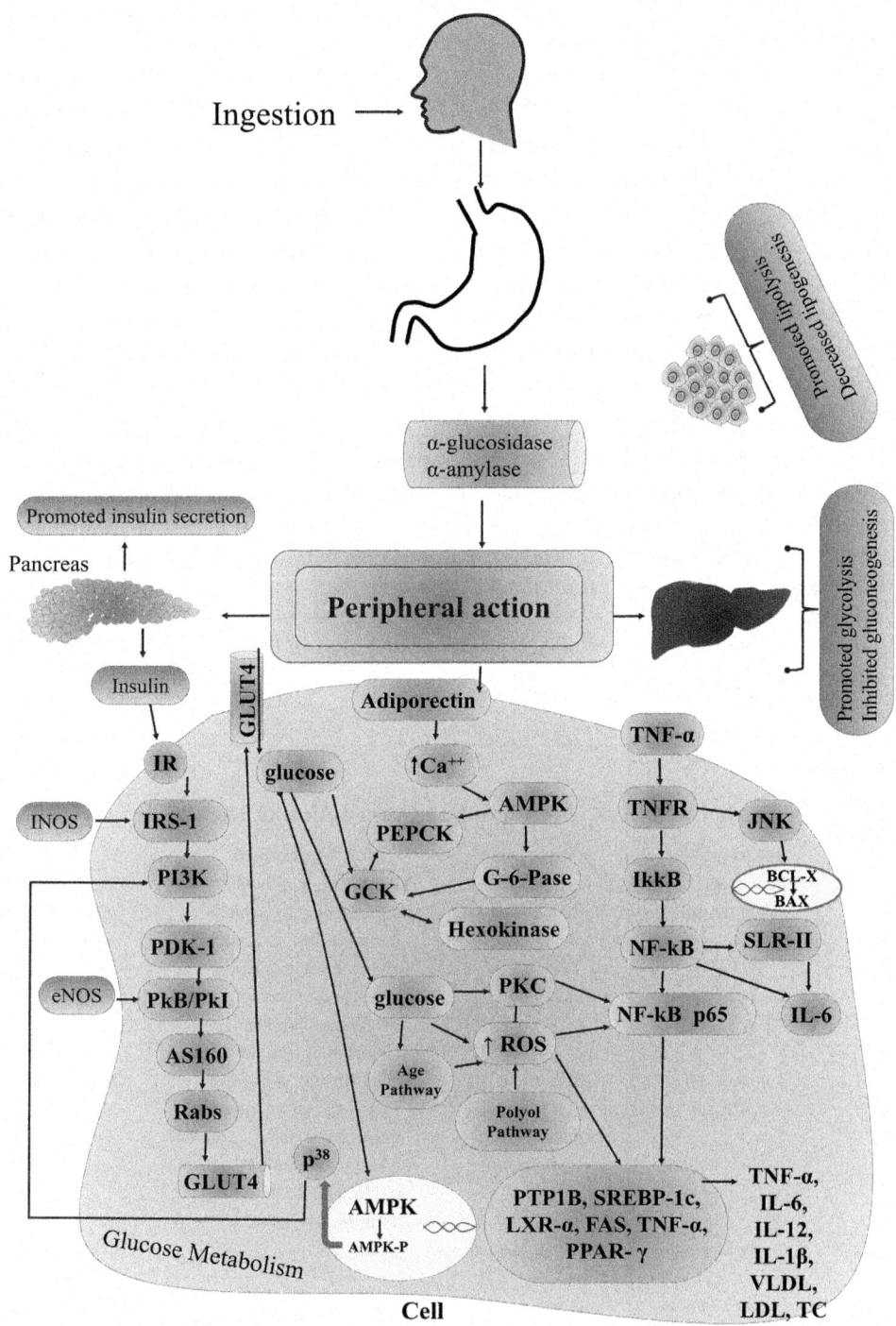

FIGURE 11.1 Cellular and molecular mechanism of bioactives from cornsilk. Arrow represents activation. AMPK, adenosine monophosphate-activated protein kinase; FAS, fatty acid synthase; GLUT4, glucose transporter type 4; IL-6, interleukin-6; IRS1, insulin receptor substrate 1; LXR-α, liver X receptors α; NF-κB, nuclear factor κ-light-chain-enhancer of activated B cells; PEPCK, phosphoenolpyruvate carboxykinase; PI3K, phosphoinositide 3-kinase; PPAR-γ, peroxisome proliferator-activated receptor-γ; PTP1B, protein tyrosine phosphatase 1B; ROS, reactive oxygen species; TNF-α, tumor necrosis factor α; VLDL-C, very-low-density lipoprotein cholesterol.

11.9 OTHER FOODS, HERBS, SPICES, AND BOTANICALS USED IN DIABETES

The presences of natural antioxidants are responsible for therapeutic effects in traditional herbs. Random screening, *in vitro*, *in vivo*, and clinical trials were employed to explore the mechanisms and effects of those compounds and extracts in preventing and treating diabetes. Isolated compounds and extracts from various plants were studied for their potential use in diabetes treatment. It is known that the extract of *Aphloia theiformis*, *Phyllanthus amarus*, the methanol extract of *Salvia acetabulosa*, *Terminalia arjuna*, *Aegle marmelos*, *Eugenia cumin*, and a mixture of oleanolic and ursolic acids extract possess significant α-amylase inhibition activity (Salehi B et al. 2019). Similarly, the extract of *Comarum palustre*, *Phoenix dactylifera*, hydroalcoholic extracts (Salehi B et al. 2019) of *Ludwigia octovalvis*, *Camellia sinensis*, *Iostephane heterophylla*, *Juniperus oxycedrus*, and a mixture of ursolic acid and oleanolic acids extract showed potent inhibition of α-glucosidase. Inhibiting carbohydrate hydrolyzing enzymes (both α-amylase and α-glucosidase) contributes to the reduction of glucose absorption in the human intestinal tract. *Moringa oleifera* and *Boerhavia diffusa* leaf extract and ginger (*Zingiber officinale*) extract are related to the increased plasma adiponectinin plasma and PPAR-α, PPAR-γ, and GLUT-2 expression in the liver, which improves the liver enzymes. *Ficus carica* leaves extract changes in carbohydrate metabolizing enzymes (glucose-6-phosphatase, fructose-1,6-bisphosphatase, and hexokinase). Aqueous and alcoholic extracts of *Tinospora cordifolia* and *Eugenia jambolana* kernels showed antihyperglycemic activity, whereas *Artemisia ludoviciana* organic extract showed dose-dependent reduction of blood glucose level (Jugran AK et al. 2021). Other plants used in treating and preventing diabetes are described in Table 11.1.

TABLE 11.1

Plants and Their Parts Used in the Treatment and Prevention of Diabetes

Plant Name	Botanical Name	Parts Used	Mechanism	Reference
Fenugreek	*Trigonella foenum-graecum*	Dried ripe seeds, leaves, and extract	Inhibits intestinal sodium-dependent glucose uptake, improves insulin resistance and β cell regeneration	Zhou J et al. 2012; Salehi B et al. 2019; Governa P et al. 2018
Aloe vera	*Aloe barbadensis miller*	Extract	α-Amylase inhibitor, improves insulin secretion and pancreatic β cell function	Salehi B et al. 2019
Tulsi	*Ocimum tenuiflorum*	Fresh or dried Leaves, aqueous extracts	Delays insulin resistance, improves fasting blood glucose and glucose tolerance	Governa P et al. 2018
Garlic	*Allium sativum*	Garlic bulb water extract	α-Amylase inhibitor, α-glucosidase inhibitor, antihyperglycemic	Salehi B et al. 2019
Turmeric	*Curcuma longa*	Rhizome, extracts	Antidiabetic	Pivari F et al. 2019; Salehi B et al. 2019
Cluster fig, red river fig	*Ficus racemosa*	Bark, leaves extract	Antihyperglycemic, hypoglycemic, α-glucosidase and α-amylase inhibitor	Salehi B et al. 2019
Bitter melon	*Momordica charantia*	Fresh or dried fruits, fruit pulp, seeds, and leaves	α-Amylase inhibitor, hypoglycemic, antihyperglycemic	Salehi B et al. 2019; Governa P et al. 2018
White mulberry	*Morus alba*	Leaves extract	Antidiabetic, hypoglycemic, α-glucosidase and α-amylase inhibitor	Salehi B et al. 2019

Plant Name	Botanical Name	Parts Used	Mechanism	Reference
Curry leaf tree	*Murraya koenigii*	Leaves	α-Amylase inhibitor, hypoglycemic effects, antihyperglycemic	Salehi B et al. 2019
Indian gooseberry	*Phyllanthus amarus*	Plant extract	α-Glucosidase inhibitor, hypoglycemic, α-amylase inhibitor	Salehi B et al. 2019
Guava	*Psidium guajava*	Leaf extract, juice	Psidium guajava	Salehi B et al. 2019
Black plum/ jamun	*Syzygium cumini*	Skeels, fruit, seed extract	α-Glucosidase and α-amylase inhibitor, antihyperglycemic	Salehi B et al. 2019
Chebulic myrobalan	*Terminalia chebula*	Seeds extract	α-Amylase inhibitor	Salehi B et al. 2019
Guduchi	*Tinospora cordifolia*	Leaf, stem, roots, and whole plant extract	α-Amylase inhibitor, hypoglycemic, antihyperglycemic	Salehi B et al. 2019
Petawali	*Tinospora crispa*	Stems extract, plant extract	Hypoglycemic, antihyperglycemic	Salehi B et al. 2019
Creat	*Andrographis paniculata*	Roots extract	Antihyperglycemic	Salehi B et al. 2019
Neem	*Azadirachta indica*	Dried leaves, ethanolic extract,	α-Glucosidase and α-amylase inhibitor, antihyperglycemic	Salehi B et al. 2019; Governa P et al. 2018
Madagascar periwinkle/ vinca rosea/ lochnera rosea	*Catharanthus roseus*	Fresh leaves, leaf juice, leaf powder, leaf extract	α-Amylase inhibitor, antihyperglycemic, hypoglycemic	Salehi B et al. 2019
Gotu kola	*Centella asiatica*	Leaf extract, Plant extract	Antidiabetic	Salehi B et al. 2019
Black cumin	*Nigella sativa*	Seed extract	Antidiabetic	Salehi B et al. 2019
Avocado	*Persea americana*	Fruit and Leaves extract	Antidiabetic	Salehi B et al. 2019
Onion	*Allium cepa*	Fresh or dried bulbs, extracts, juice, freeze-dried powder, essential oil	Reducing fasting blood glucose, reducing hyperglycemia, antihyperglycemic	Governa P et al. 2018

11.10 TOXICITY AND CAUTIONARY NOTES

Occurring naturally, users think the herbal medicines are safe and harmless, which is not always true. In a study, authors have shown that intake of 10 g/kg/day body weight of corn in the rat is safe irrespective of gender (Wang C et al. 2011). The corn silk extract (dose within 500 mg/kg body weight) is known to be safe in mice (Ha A. W. et al. 2018). The aqueous extract of corn silk did not exhibit any significant ($p > 0.05$) effect on hematological indices in Wistar rats at 24 hours after 1, 7, 14, 21, and 28 days upon administering 100, 200, and 400 mg/kg body weight (Saheed S et al. 2015). A study showed that polysaccharide-rich extract from corn silk is safe (7.5, 15, and 20 g/kg body weight) in mice (Zhao H. P. et al. 2017). Despite the enormous research on corn silk (*Stigma maydis*), there is a lack of information on its toxicity profile in human studies.

11.11 SUMMARY POINTS

- This chapter focuses on corn silk's cellular, molecular, and metabolic effects on diabetes.
- Other plants or their parts used in the diabetes treatment are summarized.
- Corn is cultivated in Asian countries; seeds are edible and the rest is considered waste.

- Flavonoids, phenolic acids, phytosterols, carotenoids, and tannins in corn silk are responsible for antidiabetic activity.
- The chapter discusses the effect of candidates from corn silk on cellular and molecular pathways involved in preventing and treating diabetes.

REFERENCES

Al-Ishaq, R. K., Abotaleb, M., Kubatka, P., Kajo, K., & Büsselberg, D. 2019. Flavonoids and Their Antidiabetic Effects: Cellular Mechanisms and Effects to Improve Blood Sugar Levels. *Biomolecules* 9(9): 430.

Alkhalidy, H., Moore, W., Wang, Y., Luo, J., McMillan, R., Zhen, W., Zhou, K., & Liu, D. 2018. The Flavonoid Kaempferol Ameliorates Streptozotocin-Induced Diabetes by Suppressing Hepatic Glucose Production. *Molecules* 23(9): 2338.

Asero, R., Mistrello, G., Roncarolo, D., Amato, S., & van Ree, R. 2001. A Case of Allergy to Beer Showing Cross-Reactivity Between Lipid Transfer Proteins. *Annals of Allergy, Asthma & Immunology: Official Publication of the American College of Allergy, Asthma, & Immunology* 87(1): 65–67.

Bhattacharjee, N., Dua, T. K., Khanra, R., Joardar, S., Nandy, A., Saha, A., De Feo, V., & Dewanjee, S. 2017. Protocatechuic Acid, a Phenolic from Sansevieria Roxburghiana Leaves, Suppresses Diabetic Cardiomyopathy via Stimulating Glucose Metabolism, Ameliorating Oxidative Stress, and Inhibiting Inflammation. *Frontiers in Pharmacology* 8: 251.

Bollet, A. J. 1992. Politics and Pellagra: The Epidemic of Pellagra in the U.S. in the Early Twentieth Century. *The Yale Journal of Biology and Medicine* 65(3): 211–221.

Buzás, I., Hoyk, E., Cserni, I., & Borsné, P. J. 2006. Evaluation of the Optimum Nitrogen Fertilizer Depending on the Nitrate Content of the Soil in Sweet Corn Plantation. *Cereal Research Communications* 34(1): 421–424.

Chaiittianan, R., Sutthanut, K., & Rattanathongkom, A. 2017. Purple Corn Silk: A Potential Anti-obesity Agent with Inhibition on Adipogenesis and Induction on Lipolysis and Apoptosis in Adipocytes. *Journal of Ethnopharmacology* 201: 9–16.

Chaudhary, R. K., Karoli, S. S., Dwivedi, P., & Bhandari, R. 2022. Antidiabetic Potential of Corn Silk (*Stigma maydis*): An *in-silico* Approach. *Journal of Diabetes and Metabolic Disorders* 21(1): 445–454.

Chaudhary, R. K., Philip, M. J., Santhosh, A., Karoli, S. S., Bhandari, R., & Ganachari, M. S. 2021. Health Economics and Effectiveness Analysis of Generic Antidiabetic Medication from Jan Aushadhi: An Ambispective Study in Community Pharmacy. *Diabetes & Metabolic Syndrome* 15(6): 102303.

Ghorbani, A. 2017. Mechanisms of Antidiabetic Effects of Flavonoid Rutin. *Biomedicine & Pharmacotherapy* 96: 305–312.

Goss, J. A. 2008. Development, Physiology, and Biochemistry of Corn and Wheat Pollen. *The Botanical Review* 34: 333–359.

Governa, P., Baini, G., Borgonetti, V., Cettolin, G., Giachetti, D., Magnano, A. R., Miraldi, E., & Biagi, M. 2018. Phytotherapy in the Management of Diabetes: A Review. *Molecules (Basel, Switzerland)* 23(1): 105.

Ha, A. W., Kang, H. J., Kim, S. L., Kim, M. H., & Kim, W. K. 2018. Acute and Subacute Toxicity Evaluation of Corn Silk Extract. *Preventive Nutrition and Food Science* 23(1): 70–76.

He, H. F. 2022. Recognition of Gallotannins and the Physiological Activities: From Chemical View. *Frontiers in Nutrition* 9: 888892.

Jugran, A. K., Rawat, S., Devkota, H. P., Bhatt, I. D., & Rawal, R. S. (2021). Diabetes and Plant-Derived Natural Products: From Ethnopharmacological Approaches to Their Potential for Modern Drug Discovery and Development. *Phytotherapy Research: PTR* 35(1): 223–245.

Marcelino, G., Machate, D. J., Freitas, K. C., Hiane, P. A., Maldonade, I. R., Pott, A., Asato, M. A., Candido, C. J., & Guimarães, R. 2020. β-Carotene: Preventive Role for Type 2 Diabetes Mellitus and Obesity: A Review. *Molecules (Basel, Switzerland)* 25(24): 5803.

Meng, S., Cao, J., Feng, Q., Peng, J., & Hu, Y. 2013. Roles of Chlorogenic Acid on Regulating Glucose and Lipids Metabolism: A Review. *Evidence-Based Complementary and Alternative Medicine* 2013: 801457.

Nawaz, H., Muzaffar, S., Aslam, M., & Ahmad, S. 2018. Phytochemical Composition: Antioxidant Potential and Biological Activities of Corn. *Corn-Production and Human Health in Changing Climate* 10: 49–68.

Norred, W. P., Voss, K. A., Riley, R. T., Meredith, F. I., & Bacon, C. W. 1998. Mycotoxins and Health Hazards: Toxicological Aspects and Mechanism of Action of Fumonisins. *The Journal of Toxicological Sciences* 23(Supplement I): 160–164.

Pawar, M. R., & Karthikeyan, E. 2020. Role of Catechins in Diabetes Mellitus. *European Journal of Molecular & Clinical Medicine* 7(11): 2515–2826.

Pivari, F., Mingione, A., Brasacchio, C., & Soldati, L. 2019. Curcumin and Type 2 Diabetes Mellitus: Prevention and Treatment. *Nutrients* 11(8): 1837.

Poorahong, W., Innalak, S., Ungsurungsie, M., & Watanapokasin, R. 2021. Protective Effect of Purple Corn Silk Extract Against Ultraviolet-B-Induced Cell Damage in Human Keratinocyte Cells. *Journal of Advanced Pharmaceutical Technology & Research* 12(2): 140–146.

Prasad, M., Jayaraman, S., Eladl, M. A., El-Sherbiny, M., Abdelrahman, M., Veeraraghavan, V. P., Vengadassalapathy, S., Umapathy, V. R., Jaffer Hussain, S. F., Krishnamoorthy, K., Sekar, D., Palanisamy, C. P., Mohan, S. K., & Rajagopal, P. 2022. A Comprehensive Review on Therapeutic Perspectives of Phytosterols in Insulin Resistance: A Mechanistic Approach. *Molecules (Basel, Switzerland)* 27(5): 1595.

Russell, W. A., & Hallauer, A. R. 1980. Corn. In *Hybridization of Crop Plants*, pp. 299–312. Madison, WI: American Society of Agronomy and Crop Science Society of America Publishers.

Saheed, S., Oladipipo, A. E., Abdulazeez, A. A., Olarewaju, S. A., Ismaila, N. O., Emmanuel, I. A., Fatimah, Q. D., & Aisha, A. Y. 2015. Toxicological Evaluations of Stigma Maydis (Corn Silk) Aqueous Extract on Hematological and Lipid Parameters in Wistar Rats. *Toxicology Reports* 2: 638–644.

Sahib, A. S., Mohammed, I. H., & Hamdan, S. J. 2012. Use of Aqueous Extract of Corn Silk in the Treatment of Urinary Tract Infection. *Journal of Complementary Medicine Research* 1(2): 93–96.

Salehi, B., Ata, A., Kumar, N.V.A., Sharopov, F., Ramírez-Alarcón, K., Ruiz-Ortega, A., Abdulmajid Ayatollahi, S., Tsouh Fokou, P. V., Kobarfard, F., Amiruddin Zakaria, Z., Iriti, M., Taheri, Y., Martorell, M., Sureda, A., Setzer, W. N., Durazzo, A., Lucarini, M., Santini, A., Capasso, R., Ostrander, E. A., Atta-ur-Rahman, Choudhary, M. I., Cho, W. C., & Sharifi-Rad, J. 2019. Antidiabetic Potential of Medicinal Plants and Their Active Components. *Biomolecules* 9(10): 551.

Santana-Gálvez, J., Cisneros-Zevallos, L., & Jacobo-Velázquez, D. A. 2017. Chlorogenic Acid: Recent Advances on Its Dual Role as a Food Additive and a Nutraceutical against Metabolic Syndrome. *Molecules (Basel, Switzerland)* 22(3): 358.

Sarepoua, E., Tangwongchai, R., Suriharn, B., & Lertrat, K. 2015. Influence of Variety and Harvest Maturity on Phytochemical Content in Corn Silk. *Food Chemistry* 169: 424–429.

Sok Yen, F., Shu Qin, C., Tan Shi Xuan, S., Jia Ying, P., Yi Le, H., Darmarajan, T., Gunasekaran, B., & Salvamani, S. 2021. Hypoglycemic Effects of Plant Flavonoids: A Review. *Evidence-Based Complementary and Alternative Medicine: eCAM*, 2021: 2057333.

Sun, C., Zhao, C., Guven, E. C., Paoli, P., Simal-Gandara, J., Ramkumar, K. M., Wang, S. P., Buleu, F., Pah, A., Turi, V., Damian, G., Dragan, S., Tomas, M., Khan, W., Wang, M. F., Delmas, D., Portillo, M., Dar, P., Chen, L., & Xiao, J. 2020. Dietary Polyphenols as Antidiabetic Agents: Advances and Opportunities. *Food Frontiers* 1(1): 18–44.

Wang, C., Zhang, T., Liu, J., Lu, S., Zhang, C., Wang, E., Wang, Z., Zhang, Y., & Liu, J. 2011. Subchronic Toxicity Study of Corn Silk with Rats. *Journal of Ethnopharmacology* 137(1): 36–43.

Widstrom, N. W. 1996. The Aflatoxin Problem with Corn Grain. *Advances in Agronomy* 12: 219–280.

Widstrom, N. W., & Snook, M. E. 1998. A Gene Controlling Biosynthesis of Isoorientin, a Compound in Corn Silks Antibiotic to the Corn Earworm. *Entomologia Experimentalis et Applicate* 89: 119–124.

Xu, Y., Tang, G., Zhang, C., Wang, N., & Feng, Y. 2021. Gallic Acid and Diabetes Mellitus: Its Association with Oxidative Stress. *Molecules (Basel, Switzerland)* 26(23): 7115.

Yi, H., Peng, H., Wu, X., Xu, X., Kuang, T., Zhang, J., Du, L., & Fan, G. 2021. The Therapeutic Effects and Mechanisms of Quercetin on Metabolic Diseases: Pharmacological Data and Clinical Evidence. *Oxidative Medicine and Cellular Longevity* 2021: 6678662.

Zhao, H. P., Zhang, Y., Liu, Z., Chen, J. Y., Zhang, S. Y., Yang, X. D., & Zhou, H. L. 2017. Acute Toxicity and Anti-Fatigue Activity of Polysaccharide-Rich Extract from Corn Silk. *Biomedicine & Pharmacotherapy* 90: 686–693.

Zhou, J., Chan, L., & Zhou, S. 2012. Trigonelline: A Plant Alkaloid with Therapeutic Potential for Diabetes and Central Nervous System Disease. *Current Medicinal Chemistry* 19(21): 3523–3531.

12 Egyptian Balsam (*Balanites aegyptiaca*) Use in Diabetes
Molecular, Cellular, and Metabolic Effects

Osama M. Ahmed, Asmaa S. Zaky and
Mohammed Abdel-Gabbar

CONTENTS

12.1 INTRODUCTION

Diabetes mellitus (DM), a chronic metabolic syndrome with several etiologies, is a common condition. Patients are badly affected and their risk of contracting further disorders is increased (He et al. 2019). It is characterized by aberrant catabolism and anabolism of carbohydrates, lipids, and proteins as a result of insulin resistance or hypoinsulinemia (Reach et al. 2017). According to recent data from the International Diabetes Federation (IDF), 700 million persons between the ages of 20 and 79 are predicted to have diabetes by 2045, up from the current estimate of 463 million adults, the majority of whom reside in underdeveloped and poor nations (International Diabetes Federation [IDF] 2019). Population expansion, urbanization, nutritional change, physical inactivity, and dietary change are only a few of the many factors that contribute to the rising prevalence of DM (Hirst 2013; Guariguata et al. 2014).

The synthetic anti-diabetic medications currently available offer many advantages, but they also come with a number of negative side effects (Osadebe et al. 2014). Alternative anti-diabetic medications are therefore required, ideally with fewer or no negative side effects (Osadebe et al. 2014; Abd El Mgeed et al. 2009; Ahmed et al. 2020). Recently, new active medications that are derived from plants have been developed that are more potent than oral chemical hypoglycemic medications used in proven therapies and have anti-diabetic activity. Pharmaceutical plants have a variety of bioactive substances with varied functions in insulin synthesis, insulin activity, or both (Chang et al. 2013).

For the treatment of DM, Eskander and Jun described a variety of Egyptian plant and herb prescriptions that come from different families (Eskander and Jun 1995). African nations have long employed the Zygophyllaceae family plant *Balanites aegyptiaca* L. Delile as an anthelmintic and to treat jaundice (Koko et al. 2000; Sarker et al. 2000). The fruit is sold by herbalists in the Egyptian market as an anti-diabetic drug and is used as an oral antihyperglycemic medication in Egyptian folkloric medicine (Kamel et al. 1991). But it is still quite challenging to keep the quality of these

DOI: 10.1201/9781003220930-14

herbal products high. In streptozotocin (STZ)-induced diabetic mice and rats, the mesocarp of the *B. aegyptiaca* fruit's aqueous extract has shown anti-diabetic properties (Kamel et al. 1991; Gad et al. 2006; Zaky et al. 2022), and various saponins were extracted from the mesocarp (Kamel et al. 1991; Hosny et al. 1992; Staerk et al. 2006). Additionally, the *B. aegyptiaca* seed kernel has a high protein and oil content that varies according on the source (Elfeel and Warrag 2011).

This chapter highlights the anti-diabetic effects of the *B. aegyptiaca* fruit and seed on the glycemic state and lipid profile as well as molecular, cellular, and metabolic effects to indicate their probable modes in DM.

12.2 DIABETES MELLITUS (DM)

DM is a prevalent metabolic disease condition that results in abnormally high blood sugar levels and diabetic complications in both developed and developing nations. It is characterized by defects in insulin secretion, insulin receptor, and/or postreceptor events, as well as disturbances in carbohydrate, protein, and lipid metabolism (Ahmed et al. 2012; Albarakat and Guzu 2019; Sarkar et al. 2019; World Health Organization [WHO] 2023).

One of the issues that doctors face the most frequently in the 21st century is DM (Chrysavgis et al. 2022). About 537 million people worldwide have DM, the majority living in low- and middle-income countries, and 1.5 million deaths are directly attributed to DM each year. Both the number of cases and the prevalence of DM have been steadily increasing over the past few decades; the total number of people living with DM is projected to rise to 643 million by 2030 and 783 million by 2045 (International Diabetes Federation [IDF] 2021; WHO 2023). The destructive effects of DM are expected to worsen as the prevalence as a result of population growth, an aging population, urbanization, decreased physical activity, and unfavorable dietary trends (Hu 2011; Hirst 2013; Guariguata et al. 2014; Zheng et al. 2018 Saeedi et al. 2019). About 9 million persons between the ages of 20 and 79 had DM in 2019 according to the International Diabetes Federation (IDF), which ranked Egypt among the top ten nations in the world with the highest prevalence of the disease. From roughly 4.5 million in 2007 to 7.5 million in 2013 and 13.1 million by 2035, the number of DM patients in Egypt has expanded quickly (Hegazi et al. 2015). Given this high prevalence, countries with low and moderate levels of income experience the highest rates of DM-related death (Shaw et al. 2010; Jagannathan et al. 2019).

DM patients have a doubled chance of getting Alzheimer disease (AD) compared to non-diabetics, according to some studies (Peila et al. 2002; Mushtaq et al. 2015).

12.2.1 *BALANITES AEGYPTIACA*

B. aegyptiaca (Figure 12.1) has a wide ecological distribution. It belongs to the family Balanitaceae and is also known as *Hegleg* or *Balah El-Abeed*. The date is dark brown in color, and the fleshy pulp of both unripe and ripe fruits is edible and eaten dried or fresh. It is known by various names: Arabic names include *heglig* (tree), *lalob* (fruit); trade names include Zaccone, Zachun, and Desert Date (dried fruit) (Yadav and Panghal 2010). Heglig is an extremely useful tree which has been utilized over thousands of years. All parts of the tree have medicinal uses including fruits, seeds, bark, and roots (Elfeel 2010). The most important parts are fruit pulp and kernel that contain saponin, which have wide industrial and medicinal values (Beit-Yannai 2010; Farid et al. 2002; FAO 1985). The bark and roots are used as laxatives or tranquilizers (for colic). The bark is used against stomachaches, sterility, mental diseases, epilepsy, yellow fever, syphilis, and as a vermifuge. Fruits and leaves, and especially the kernel oil, are applied for rheumatism and bark extracts for toothaches (Fregon 2015). Previous research indicates that the methanol leaf extracts of *B. aegyptiaca* has good antioxidant potential which indicates that this plant can have great scope of important antioxidant molecules which can be formulated to make antioxidant dosage forms (Najjaa et al. 2020). The debittered kernels are used as snacks (nuts) by humans. The extracted oil used for many uses, and

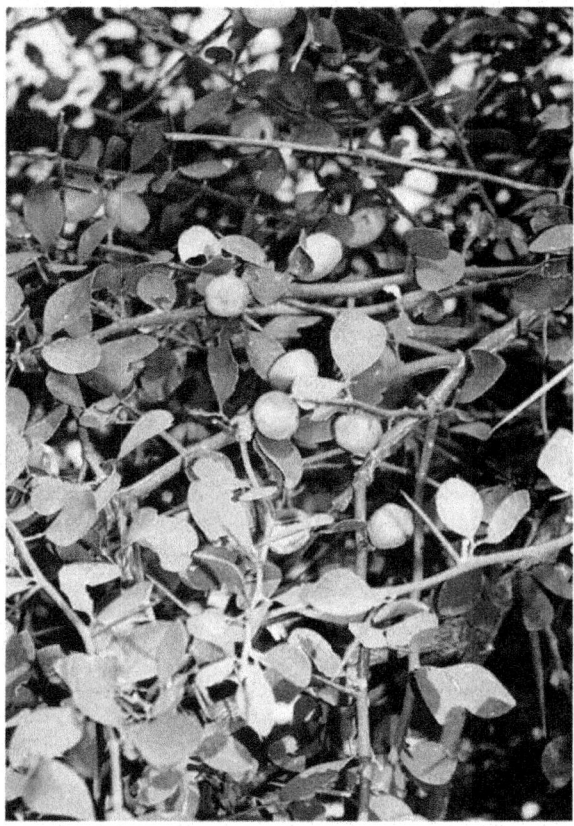

FIGURE 12.1   Tree with fruits of *Balanites aegyptiaca*.

Source: https://commons.wikimedia.org/wiki/File:Balanites_aegyptiaca_MS4917.JPG.

the remaining cake is used as fodder (Alkaltham et al. 2022). Both fruits and kernels were widely used in many countries during the dry season and drought periods.

B. *aegyptiaca* is known to be an all-purpose tree with various uses and values. The extracts of B. *aegyptiaca* have commonly been used in various traditional folk medicines, especially in Africa and southern Asia. Trigonelline identified and quantified in the crude extract of the peel and pulp of B. *aegyptiaca* fruit (mesocarp) is a well-characterized hypoglycemic alkaloid (Farag et al. 2015). The most studies dealing with the diverse biological activities in B. *aegyptiaca* extracts reported the active compounds to be steroidal saponins (Chapagain et al. 2008). B. *aegyptiaca* was used in Sudanese folk medicine for treatment of jaundice (Sarker et al. 2000). In Egyptian folk medicine, the fruits are commonly used as an oral anti-diabetic drug (Neuwinger 2004; Kamel 1998). The plant is used as a purgative to remove intestinal parasites with the root, branches, bark, fruit, and kernel extracts shown to be lethal to the miracidia and cercariae of *Shistosoma man-soni* and to *Fasciola gigantic* (Koko et al. 2005). Additionally, extracts of the tree display abortive and antiseptic properties (Koko et al. 2000). This plant may offer an opportunity for a new natural anthelmintic and an alternative source for the control of such infectious disease in sheep (Shalaby et al. 2020). The importance of B. *aegyptiaca* is due to the presence of a steroidal sapogenin compound named diosgenin which is useful in pharmaceutical industries as a natural source of steroidal hormones (Speroni et al. 2005). In addition, B. *aegyptiaca* protects the livers of treated mice against paracetamol hepatotoxicity as evidenced by a significant improvement of liver function tests (Zaahkouk et al. 2015). The aqueous extracts of whole fruit, mesocarp, endocarp, and seeds of *B. aegyptiaca* have molluscicidal and cercariacidal activities which were tested against Ethiopian *Biomphalaria pfeifferi, Lymnaea natalensis,* and *Schistosoma mansoni* cercariae (Molla et al. 2013).

12.3 CHEMICAL CONSTITUENTS OF *BALANITES AEGYPTIACA* AND ANTI-DIABETIC POTENCIES

B. aegyptiaca contains saponin, furanocoumarin, and flavonoid namely quercetin 3-glucoside, quercetin-3-rutinoside; 3-glucoside, 3-rutinoside, 3–7-diglucoside and 3-rhamnogalactoside of isorhamnetin Balanitoside (furostanol glycoside) and 6-methyldiosgenin, balanitin-3 (spirostanol glycoside), Balanitin-6 and -7: Diosgenyl saponins, two pregnane glycosides namely pregn-5-ene-3β,16β,20(R)-triol 3-O-(2,6-di-O-α-l-rhamnopyranosyl)-β-d glucopyranoside (balagyptin), and pregn-5-ene-3β,16β,20(R)-triol 3-O-β-d-glucopyranoside major sapogenin is yamogenin, two alkaloid namely, N-trans feruloyltyramine and N-cisferuloyltyramine, and three common metabolites, vanillic acid, syringic acid; and 3-hydroxy-1-(4-hydroxy-3-methoxyphenyl)-1-propanone, β-sitosterol, bergapten, marmesin, and β-sitosterol glucoside, balanitin-1,-2, and -3; 3 (Saboo et al. 2014).

In a randomized controlled clinical trial, the saponin and phenolic extract of this fruit was reported to be beneficial in controlling the blood glucose level and lipid profile in people with type 2 DM (Zeid et al. 2019). The pure saponin, extracted from the balamite fruit mesocarp, and water extract have been reported as hypoglycemic agent when tested on albino rats in different concentrations and Daonil (as a standard medication). It also reported that it inhibits *Escherichia coli* growth in rats (George et al. 2006). The aqueous extract of the mesocarp of fruits of *B. aegyptiaca* was reported to have anti-diabetic effect in STZ-induced diabetic mice (Mansour and Newairy 2000). It is reported that whole and extracted pulp of *B. aegyptiaca* fruits reported a hypocholesterolemic effect when tested on adult albino rats (Abdel-Rahim et al. 1986). The study showed that *B. aegyptiaca* and aqueous extracts have anti-diabetic and antioxidant effects on the diabetic rats. These extracts can be potentially used with insulin therapy to minimize its side effects and to improve the treatment of type 1 DM and probably other oxidative stress-associated diseases.

Treatment with the *B. aegyptiaca* fruit and seed aqueous extract produced a significant increase in the mRNA expression of insulin receptor β-subunit, reflecting the ability of this extract to reduce IR and enhance IS in the adipose tissues (Zaky et al. 2022). The treatment of diabetic rats with *B. aegyptiaca* extracts significantly decreased MDA, which is attributed to the increased levels of antioxidants that fight free radicals (Çelik et al. 2017) and markedly increased GSH level and SOD and GPx activities. Thus, it is worth noting that the improvement in glycemic state, lipid profile, and insulinotropic and insulin-sensitizing effects is associated with the suppression of oxidative stress and enhancement of the antioxidant defense system. This indicated that the decrease in oxidative stress and enhancement of the antioxidant defense system may have an important role in the improvement of the architecture and tissue IS of the pancreatic islets, which in turn result in the effective management of DM. Hassanin et al. (2018) indicated that *B. aegyptiaca* exerted hypoglycemic, hypolipidemic, and insulinotropic actions associated with the reduction in oxidative stress, enhancement in the antioxidant defense system, and reduced apoptosis in pancreatic β cells. Some hypotheses by which the pericarp of *B. aegyptiaca* fruits aqueous extract as explained by regenerated islet β cells and increased the size of pancreatic islets at the cellular can be explained by Abou Khalil et al. (2016). It is well known that β cell apoptosis is a common feature of type 1 DM (Roep et al. 2021). In fact, *B. aegyptiaca* (Maksoud and El Hadidi 1988), like many herbal extracts, is rich in flavonoids. The flavonoid genistein reduced β cell apoptosis in pancreatic islets, increased the number of insulin-positive β cells in the islets, promoted islet β cell survival, and preserved islet mass (Racine 2022). Previous study by Abdel-Mageed et al. (2019) proved that *B. aegyptiaca* methanolic extract protect pancreatic β cells of STZ-induced DM was at least partly due to the reduction of IL-1β and iNOS gene over the expression which can have a protective effect on β cell. In the treatment of diabetic animals with *B. aegyptiaca* aqueous extracts, a reduction in the amount of serum FFA levels that could be associated with the insulin-sensitizing activity of the extract was observed (Liu et al. 2022). Abd El-Rahman and Al-ahmari (2013) proved that *B. aegyptiaca* treatment improvement lipid profile, and that may be due to the presence of saponins in its extract, indicating antihypercholesterolemic and hypoglycemic activities. Moreover, diosgenin in *B. aegyptiaca* seed kernels plays an important role in the regulation of cholesterol metabolism (Zeid et al. 2019). The treatment with the *B. aegyptiaca* fruit and seed extracts significantly improved the lowered liver glycogen content and elevated hepatic glucose-6-phosphatase and glycogen phosphorylase activities. These ameliorations may be secondary to the increase in the insulin levels in the blood and the enhanced IS (Zaky et al. 2022). The administration of the *B. aegyptiaca* fruit and seed aqueous extracts produced a significant increase in serum insulin and C-peptide levels of diabetic rats, and this finding is consistent with that of Abou Khalil et al. (2016). In this regard, Abdel-Moneim (1998) hypothesized that the hypoglycemic action of the *B. aegyptiaca* aqueous extract stimulated the β cells of the pancreatic islets to secrete insulin, potentiate glucose-stimulated insulin secretion, and increase the number and sensitivity of insulin receptors and postreceptor effects in peripheral tissues.

Kamel et al. (1991) demonstrated the anti-diabetic effect of an aqueous extract of fruit in STZ-induced diabetic mice after oral administration. They also identified steroidal saponins, 26-O-β-D-glucopyranosyl-(25R)-furost-5-ene-3β,22,26-triol-3-O-[α-Lrhamnophyranosyl-(1→1)]-[β-D-xylopyranosyl-(1→3)]-[α-L-rhamnopyronosyl-(1→4)]-β-D-glucopyranoside and its 22-methyl ether in the extract and recognized two additional saponins, 26-O-β-D-glycopyranosyl-(25R)-furost-5-ene-3β,22,26,-triol-3-O-[2,4-di-O-α-L-rhamnopyranosyl)-β-D-glucopyranoside and its methyl ether. A combination of saponins exhibited greater anti-diabetic activity than individual saponins. Gad et al. (2006) administered fruit extracts (1.5 g/kg body weight) to STZ-induced diabetic rats and studied the glycogen content of liver and kidney and on some key enzymes of liver involved in carbohydrate metabolism. STZ (50 mg/kg body weight) caused a fivefold increase in blood glucose level, an 80% reduction in serum insulin level, a 58% decrease in liver glycogen, and a sevenfold increase in kidney glycogen content. A marked increment in the activity of glucose-6-phosphatase activity and decreased activity of glucose-6-phosphate dehydrogenase and phosphofructokinase were recorded. Treatment of rats with fruit extract reduced blood glucose levels by 24% and significantly decreased liver glucose-6-phosphatase activity. The authors also demonstrated that the extract inhibited α-amylase activity *in vitro*. The major component in the extract was diosgenin, based on high-performance thin-layer chromatography. Additionally, Al-Malki et al. (2015) showed that ethyl acetate extract containing β-sitosterol modulated oxidative stress induced by STZ. Hassanin et al. (2018) tested a crude ethanolic fruit extract and its butanolic and dichloromethane fractions on stress-activated protein kinase/c-Jun N-terminal kinase (SAPK-JNK) signaling in experimental diabetic rats. Six groups of male Wistar rats were used: normal control, diabetic, diabetic rats treated with crude, butanol or dichloromethane factions (50 mg/kg body weight), and diabetic rats were treated with gliclazide as a reference drug. Treatments continued for 1 month. Extract treatments produced a reduction in plasma glucose, hemoglobin A_{1c}, lactic acid, lipid profile, and malondialdehyde levels, which induced an increase in insulin and reduced glutathione (GSH) levels and catalase and superoxide dismutase activities. Moreover, the authors observed the downregulation of apoptosis signal-regulating kinase 1, c-Jun N-terminal kinase 1 and protein 53 and the upregulation of insulin receptor substrate 1 in rat pancreas. Glucose transporter 4 was upregulated in rat muscle. Liquid chromatography and high-resolution mass spectrometry (LC-HRMS) analysis identified balanitin-2, hexadecenoic acid, methyl protodioscin and 26-(O-β-D-glucopyranosyl)-3-β-[4-O-(β-D-glucopyranosyl)-2-O-(α-L-rhamnopyranosyl)-β-D-glucopyranosyloxy]-22,26-dihydroxyfurost-5-ene in crude extract and balanitin-1 and trigonelloside C in butanol and dichloromethane fractions of crude extract. Ezzat et al. (2017) isolated several compounds from pericarp, including stigmasterol-3-O-β-D-glucopyranoside (**a**), a pregnane glucoside: pregn-5-ene-3β,16β,20(R)-triol–3-O-β-D-glucopyranoside (**b**); a furostanol saponin: 26-(O-β-D-glucopyranosyl)-22-O-methylfurost-5-ene-3β,26-diol-3-O-β-D glucopyranosyl-(1→4)-[α-L-rhamnopyranosyl-(1→2)]-β-D glucopyranoside (**c**). The latter component possessed significant α-glucodidase (AG) and aldose reductase inhibitory activities in STZ-induced diabetic Wistar rats. Compound (**c**) also caused a significant increment in insulin and C-peptide levels.

In clinical trial, Rashad et al. (2017) found that the administration of the *B. aegyptiaca* capsules to type 2 DM patients resulted in significant improvements in the glycemic markers and the lipid profile, without adverse effects or hypoglycemia.

12.4 CONCLUSIONS

Balanites aegyptiaca fruits and seeds have potent anti-diabetic potentials in experimentally induced diabetic animals and in diabetic humans. The anti-diabetic effects may be mediated via improvements in the insulin secretory response, β cell function, and antioxidant defense system in addition to suppression of insulin resistance, oxidative stress, and inflammation.

12.5 SUMMARY POINTS

- The number of patients with diabetes mellitus (DM), which is one of the most common problems challenging the physicians in 21st century, has increased rapidly worldwide.
- The current treatments of type 2 DM include mainly oral anti-diabetic drugs, which have serious side effects. Therefore, search for alternative, safer, and more effective treatments for DM has been extended to natural plant-based remedies, which cause fewer adverse effects compared to modern synthetic drugs.
- The fruits of *Balanitis aegyptiaca*, belonging to Zygophyllaceae, is used traditionally in Egyptian folkloric medicine as oral anti-diabetic treatment. The extracts of various parts of *B. aegyptiaca* fruits including epicarp, mesocarp and seed kernel have been applied as treatments.
- *B. aegyptiaca* exerted antihyperglycemic, antihyperlipidemic, and insulinotropic actions associated with the reduction in oxidative stress, enhancement in the antioxidant defense system, and reduced apoptosis in pancreatic β cells. The treatment effects may be due to presence of saponins, flavonoids, and alkaloids.
- In conclusion, the present chapter provides scientific evidence for the probable use of *B. aegyptiaca* fruit and seed extracts as anti-diabetic agents in DM.

REFERENCES

Abd El Mgeed, A., Bstawi, M., Mohamed, U., Gabbar, M.A. 2009. Histopathological and biochemical effects of green tea and/or licorice aqueous extracts on thyroid functions in male albino rats intoxicated with dimethylnitrosamine. *Nutr. Metab.* 6: 2.

Abdel-Mageed, A.M., Osman, A.K., Awad, N.S., Abdein, M.A., 2019. Evaluation of antidiabetic potentiality of truffles and *Balanites aegyptiaca* among streptozotocin induced diabetic rats. *Int. J. Pharm. Res. Allied Sci.* 8(1): 36–44.

Abdel-Moneim, A. 1998. Effect of some medicinal plants and gliciazide on insulin release in vitro. *J. Egypt. German Soc. Zool.* 25: 423–445.

Abdel-Rahim, E.A., El-Saadany, S.S., Wasif, M.M. 1986. Biochemical dynamics of hypocholesterolemic action of *Balanites aegyptiaca* fruit. *Food Chem.* 20: 69–78.

Abd El-Rahman, S.N., Al-Ahmari, H.S. 2013. Evaluation of fertility potential of *Balanites aegyptiaca* sapogenin extract in male rats. *Inter. J. Sudan Res.* 3(1): 15–33.

Abou Khalil, N. S., Abou-Elhamd, A. S., Wasfy, S. I., El Mileegy, I. M., Hamed, M. Y., Ageely, H. M. 2016. Antidiabetic and antioxidant impacts of desert date (*Balanites aegyptiaca*) and parsley (*Petroselinum sativum*) aqueous extracts: Lessons from experimental rats. *J Diabetes Res.* 2016: 8408326.

Ahmed, O.M., Hassan, M.A., Saleh, A.S. 2020. Combinatory effect of hesperetin and mesenchymal stem cells on the deteriorated lipid profile, heart and kidney functions band antioxidant activity in STZ-induced diabetic rats. *Biocell*. 44: 27–29.

Ahmed, O.M., Mahmoud, A.M., Abdel-Moneim, A., Ashour, M.B. 2012. Antidiabetic effects of hesperidin and naringin in type 2 diabetes rats. *Diabet. Croat*. 41(2): 53–67.

Albarakat, M., Guzu, A. 2019. Prevalence of type 2 diabetes and their complications among home health care patients at Al-Kharj military industries corporation hospital. *J. Family Med. Prim. Care* 8(10): 3303–3312.

Alkaltham, M. S., Özcan, M. M., Uslu, N., Salamatullah, A. M., Hayat, K. 2022. Comparison of heglig (*Balanites aegyptiaca*) fruit parts in terms of bioactive properties, phenolic component, and mineral content. *J. Food Process. Preserv*. 46(2): e16254.

Al-Malki, A.L., Barbour, E.K., Abulnaja, K.O., Moselhy, S.S. 2015. Management of hyperglycaemia by ethyl acetate extract of *Balanites aegyptiaca* (desert date). *Molecules* 20: 14425–14434.

Beit-Yannai, E., Ben-Shabat, S., Gold, N., Chapagain, B.P., Wiesman, R.Z. 2010. Antiproliferative activity of steroidal saponins from Balanites aegyptiaca-An *in vitro* study. *Phytochem. Lett*. 4(1): 43–47.

Çelik, N., Vurmaz, A., Kahraman, A. 2017. Protective effect of quercetin on homocysteine-induced oxidative stress. *Nutrition*. 33: 291–296.

Chang, C.L., Lin, Y., Bartolome, A.P., Chen, Y.C., Chiu, S.C., Yang, W.C. 2013. Herbal therapies for type 2 diabetes mellitus: Chemistry, biology, and potential application of selected plants and compounds. *Evid. Based Complement. Altern. Med*. 2013: 378657.

Chapagain, B.P., Saharan, V., Wiesman, Z. 2008. Larvicidal activity of saponins from *Balanites aegyptiaca* callus against *Aedes aegypti* mosquito. *Bioresour. Technol*. 99: 1165–1168.

Chrysavgis, L., Giannakodimos, I., Diamantopoulou, P., Cholongitas, E. 2022. Non-alcoholic fatty liver disease and hepatocellular carcinoma: Clinical challenges of an intriguing link. *World J. Gastroenterol*. 28(3): 310.

Elfeel, A. A. 2010. Variability in *Balanites aegyptiaca* var. aegyptiaca seed kernel oil, protein and minerals contents between and within locations. *Agr. Biol. J. North Am*. 1: 170–174.

Elfeel, A.A., Warrag, E.I. 2011. Uses and conservation status of *Balanites aegyptiaca* (L.) del. (hegleig tree) in Sudan: Local people perspective. *Asian J. Agric. Sci*. 3: 286–290.

Eskander, E.F., Jun, H.W. 1995. Hypoglycaemic and hyperinsulinemic effects of some Egyptian herbs used for the treatment of diabetes mellitus (type II) in rats. *Egypt. J. Pharm. Sci*. 36: 331–342.

Ezzat, S.M., Motaal, A.A., Awdan, S.A.W.E., 2017. In vitro and in vivo antidiabetic potential of extracts and a furostanol saponin from *Balanites aegyptiaca*. *Pharm. Biol*. 55: 1931–1936.

FAO. 1985. An all purpose tree for Africa offers food and income. *Ceres*. 18: 6–7.

Farag, M.A., Porzel, A., Wessjohann, L.A. 2015. Unraveling the active hypoglycemic agent trigonelline in *Balanites aegyptiaca* date fruit using metabolite fingerprinting by NMR. *J. Pharm. Biomed. Anal*. 115: 383–387.

Farid, H., Haslinger, E., Kunert, O., Wegner, C., Hamburger, M. 2002. New steroidal glycosides from *Balanites aegyptiaca*. *Helv. Chim. Acta*. 88(4): 1019–1026.

Fregon, S.M.E. 2015. *Physicochemical properties of Balanites aegyptiaca (Laloub) seed oil* (Doctoral dissertation, Sudan University of Science and Technology).

Gad, M.Z., El-Sawalhi, M.M., Ismail, M.F., El-Tanbouly, N.D. 2006. Biochemical study of the anti-diabetic action of the Egyptian plants Fenugreek and Balanites. *Mol. Cell. Biochem*. 281: 173–183.

George, D.H., Ali, H.K., El Abbas, O.A. 2006. Evaluation of the biological activity of *Balanites aegyptiaca* Del Saponin in the control of type 11 diabetes mellitus on rats and the growth of *Escherichia coli*. *Ahfad J Women Change*. 23: 2. Available from: http://findarticles.com/ p/articles/mi_hb003/is_2_23/ai_n29364027.

Guariguata, L., Whiting, D.R., Hambleton, I., Beagley, J., Linnenkamp, U., Shaw, J.E. 2014. Global estimates of diabetes prevalence for 2013 and projections for 2035. *Diabetes Res. Clin. Pract*. 103: 137–149.

Hassanin, K.M., Mahmoud, M.O., Hassan, H.M., Abdel-Razik, A.R.H., Aziz, L.N., Rateb, M.E. 2018. *Balanites aegyptiaca* ameliorates insulin secretion and decreases pancreatic apoptosis in diabetic rats: Role of SAPK/JNK pathway. *Biomed. Pharmacoth*. 102: 1084–1091.

He, J.H., Chen, L.X., Li, H. 2019. Progress in the discovery of naturally occurring anti-diabetic drugs and in the identification of their molecular targets. *Fitoterapia* 134: 270–289.

Hegazi, R., El-Gamal, M., Abdel-Hady, N., Hamdy, O. 2015. Epidemiology of and risk factors for type 2 diabetes in Egypt. *Ann. Glob. Health* 81(6): 814–820.

Hirst, M. 2013. The new figures. *Diabetes Res. Clin. Pract*. 102: 265.

Hosny, M., Khalifa, T., Calig, I., Wright, A.D., Sticher, O. 1992. Balanitoside, a furostanol glycoside, and 6-methyldiosgenin from *Balanites aegyptiaca*. *Phytochemistry* 31: 3565–3569.

Hu, F.B. 2011. Globalization of diabetes: The role of diet, life style, and genes. *Diabetes Care* 34: 1249–1257.

International Diabetes Federation (IDF). 2019. *Diabetes Atlas*, 9th ed. International Diabetes Federation: Brussels, Belgium. Available online: www.diabetesatlas.org/en/ (accessed on 16 January 2019).

International Diabetes Federation (IDF). 2021. *Diabetes Facts & Figures*. Avenue Herrmann-Debroux 54 B-1160 Brussels, Belgium. Available online: https://idf.org/aboutdiabetes/what-is-diabetes/facts-figures. html

Jagannathan, R., Patel, S. A., Ali, M. K., Narayan, K. V. 2019. Global updates on cardiovascular disease mortality trends and attribution of traditional risk factors. *Curr. Diabetes Rep.* 19(7): 44.

Kamel, M.S. 1998. A furostanol saponin from fruits of *Balanites aegyptiaca*. *Phytochemistry*. 48: 755–757.

Kamel, M.S., Ohtani, K., Kurokawa, T., Assaf, M. H., El-Shanawany, M. A., Ali, A. A., Tanaka, O. 1991. Studies on Balanites aegyptiaca fruits, an antidiabetic Egyptian folk medicine. *Chem. Pharm. Bull.* 39(5): 1229–1233.

Koko, W.S., Abdalla, H.S., Galal, M., Khalid, H.S. 2005. Evaluation of oral therapy on Mansonial Shistosomiasis using single dose of Balanites aegyptiaca fruits and praziquantel. *Fitoterapia* 76: 30–34.

Koko, W.S., Galal, M., Khalid, H.S. 2000. Fasciolicidal efficacy of *Albizia anthelmintica* and *Balanites aegyptiaca* compared with albendazole. *J. Ethnopharmacol.* 71: 247–252.

Liu, Y., Wang, Q., Wu, K., Sun, Z., Tang, Z., Li, X., Zhang, B. 2022. Anthocyanins' effects on diabetes mellitus and islet transplantation. *Crit. Rev. Food Sci. Nutr.* 1–24. http://doi.org/10.1080/10408398.2022.2098464

Maksoud, S.A., El Hadidi, M.N. 1988. The flavonoids of *Balanites aegyptiaca* (*Balanitaceae*) from Egypt. *Plant Syst. Evol.* 160(3–4): 153–158.

Mansour, H.A., Newairy, A.A. 2000. Amelioration of impaired renalfunction associated with diabetes by Balanites aegyptiaca fruits in streptozotocin-induced diabetic rats. *J. Med. Res. Inst.* 21: 115–125.

Molla, E., Giday, M., Erko, B. 2013. Laboratory assessment of the molluscicidal and cercariacidal activities of *Balanites aegyptiaca*. *Asian Pac. J. Trop. Biomed.* 3(8): 657–662.

Mushtaq, G., Khan, J. A., Kumosani, T. A., Kamal, M. A. 2015. Alzheimer's disease and type 2 diabetes *via* chronic inflammatory mechanisms. *Saudi J Biol. Sci.* 22(1): 4–13.

Najjaa, H., Ben Arfa, A., Elfalleh, W., Zouari, N., Neffati, M. 2020. Jujube (*Zizyphus lotus* L.): Benefits and its effects on functional and sensory properties of sponge cake. *PloS ONE*, 15(2): e0227996.

Neuwinger, H.D. 2004. Plants used for poison fishing in tropical Africa. *Toxican* 44: 417–430.

Osadebe, P.O., Odoh, E.U., Uzor, P.F. 2014. Natural products as potential sources of antidiabetic drugs. *Br. J. Pharmaceut. Res.* 4: 2075–2095.

Peila, R., Rodriguez, B. L., Launer, L. J. 2002. Type 2 diabetes, APOE gene, and the risk for dementia and related pathologies: The Honolulu-Asia aging study. *Diabetes*. 51(4): 1256–1262.

Racine, K.C. 2022. *Protective effects of cocoa flavanols against obesity and type 2 diabetes are influenced by biological sex and host gut microbiome composition*. (North Carolina State University ProQuest Dissertations Publishing, 2022. 29228655). https://www.proquest.com/openview/dc835718630389556 c7347b8dbbc6fa4/1?pq-origsite=gscholar&cbl=18750&diss=y

Rashad, H., Metwally, F.M., Ezzat, S.M., Salama, M.M., Hasheesh, A., Abdel Motaal, A. 2017. Randomized double-blinded pilot clinical study of the antidiabetic activity of Balanites aegyptiaca and UPLC-ESI-MS/MS identification of its metabolites. *Pharmaceut. Biol.* 55(1): 1954–1961.

Reach, G., Pechtner, V., Gentilella, R., Corcos, A., Ceriello, A. 2017. Clinical inertia and its impact on treatment intensification in people with type 2 diabetes mellitus. *Diabetes Metab.* 43: 501–511.

Roep, B.O., Thomaidou, S., van Tienhoven, R., Zaldumbide, A. (2021). Type 1 diabetes mellitus as a disease of the β-cell (do not blame the immune system?). *Nat. Rev. Endocrinol.* 17(3): 150–161.

Saboo, S.S., Chavan, R.W., Tapadiya, G. G., Khadabadi, S.S. 2014. An important ethnomedicinal plant *Balanite Aegyptiaca* del. *Int. J. Phytopharm.* 4(3): 75–78.

Saeedi, P., Petersohn, I., Petersohn, I., Salpea, P., Malanda, B. 2019. Global and regional diabetes prevalence estimates for 2019 and projections for 2030 and 2045: Results from the international diabetes federation diabetes atlas, 9th edition. *Diabetes Res. Clin. Pract.* 157: 107843.

Sarkar, B.K., Akter, R., Das, J., Das, A., Modak, P., Halder, S., Sarkar, A.P., Kundu, S.K. 2019. Diabetes mellitus: A comprehensive review. *J. Pharmacogn. Phytochem.* 8(6): 2362–2371.

Sarker, S.D., Bartholomew, B., Nash, R.J. 2000. Alkaloids from *Balanites aegyptiaca*. *Fitoterapia*. 71(3): 328–330.

Shalaby, H.A., Hassan, N.M., Nasr, S.M., Korany, T., El Ezz, A., Mohamed Talaat, N. 2020. An anthelmintic assessment of balanites aegyptiaca fruits on some multiple drug resistant gastrointestinal helminthes affecting sheep. *Egypt. J. Vet. Sci.* 51(1): 93–103.

Shaw, J. E., Sicree, R. A., Zimmet, P. Z. 2010. Global estimates of the prevalence of diabetes for 2010 and 2030. *Diabetes Res. Clin. Pract.* 87: 4–14.

Speroni, E., Cervellati, R., 2005. Anti-inflammatory, anti-nociceptive and antioxidant activities of *Balanites aegyptiaca* (L.) Delile. *J. Ethnopharmacol.* 98: 117–125.

Staerk, D., Chapagain, B.P., Lindin, T., Wiesman, Z., Jaroszewski, J.W. 2006. Structural analysis of complex saponins of Balanites aegyptiaca by 800 MHz 1H NMR spectroscopy. *Magn. Reson. Chem.* 44: 923–928.

World Health Organization (WHO). 2023. *Diabetes.* Available online: https://www.who.int/health-topics/diabetes#tab=tab_1

Yadav, J., Panghal, M. 2010. *Balanites aegyptiaca* (L.) Del.(Hingot): A review of its traditional uses, phyto-chemistry and pharmacological properties. *Int. J. Green Pharm.* 4(3): 140.

Zaahkouk, S. A., Aboul-Ela, E. I., Ramadan, M. A., Bakry, S., Mhany, A. B. 2015. Anti carcinogenic activity of methanolic extract of Balanites aegyptiaca against breast, colon, and liver cancer cells. *Int. J. Adv. Res.* 3(6): 255–266.

Zaky, A.S., Kandeil, M., Abdel-Gabbar, M., Fahmy, E.M., Almehmadi, M.M., Ali, T.M., Ahmed, O.M. 2022. The antidiabetic effects and modes of action of the *Balanites aegyptiaca* fruit and seed aqueous extracts in NA/STZ-induced diabetic rats. *Pharmaceutics* 14: 263.

Zeid, I.M.A., Al-Thobaiti, S. A., Almalki, D. A., Ali, S. S., Umar, A. 2019. *Balanites aegyptiaca* modulates the lipid profile and testicular histopathology in streptozotocin-induced diabetic rats through an antioxidant mechanism. *Glob. J. Med. Plant Res.* 7(1): 1–6.

Zheng, Y., Ley, S. H., Hu, F. B. 2018. Global aetiology and epidemiology of type 2 diabetes mellitus and its complications. *Nat. Rev. Endocrinol.* 14(2): 88.

13 Fenugreek (*Trigonella foenum*) and Use in Diabetes
Molecular and Cellular Aspects

Vafa Baradaran Rahimi, Pouria Rahmanian-Devin
and Vahid Reza Askari

CONTENTS

ABBREVIATIONS

ALP	alkaline phosphatase
ALT	alanine transaminase
AST	alanine transaminase
BUN	blood urine nitrogen
CAT	catalase
DM	diabetes mellitus
FBG	fasting of blood glucose
G6PD	glucose-6-phosphate dehydrogenase
GLUT	glucose transporter
GPx	glutathione peroxidase
GSH	glutathione reduced
GST	glutathione S-transferase
HbA_{1c}	hemoglobin A_{1c}
HDL	high-density lipoprotein cholesterol

DOI: 10.1201/9781003220930-15

HOMA-IR	Homeostatic Model of Assessment of Insulin Resistance
IL	interleukin
LDH	lactate dehydrogenase
LDL	low-density lipoprotein cholesterol
MDA	malondialdehyde
NF-κB	nuclear factor κB
PKC	protein kinase C
PPAR-γ	peroxisome proliferator-activated receptor γ
SOD	superoxide dismutase
STZ	streptozotocin
T2D	type 2 diabetes
TC	total cholesterol
TG	triglycerides
TGF-β1	transforming growth factor-β1
TNF-α	tumor necrosis factor-α

13.1 INTRODUCTION

Trigonella foenum-graecum L. (Figure 13.1), commonly known as fenugreek, is an annual herbaceous plant belonging to the family Fabaceae. Fenugreek is widely cultivated in various parts of Asia, Africa, and Europe, including Spain, Italy, India, Algeria, China, Pakistan, Saudi Arabia, Egypt, Turkey, and Iran (Visuvanathan et al. 2022).

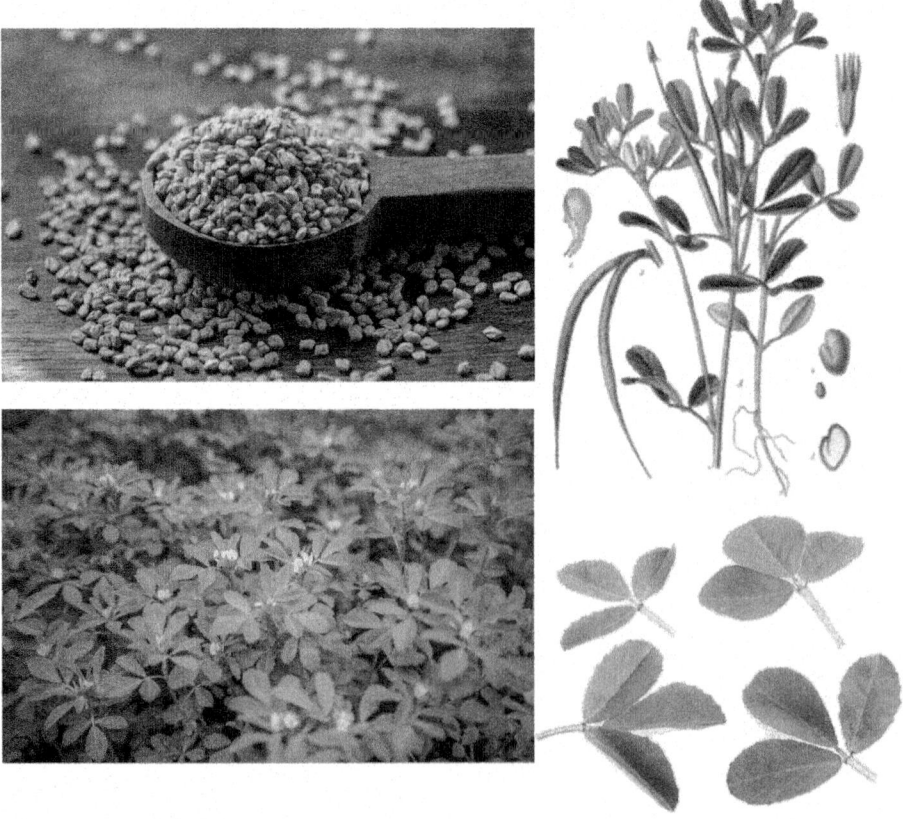

FIGURE 13.1 Different parts of fenugreek.

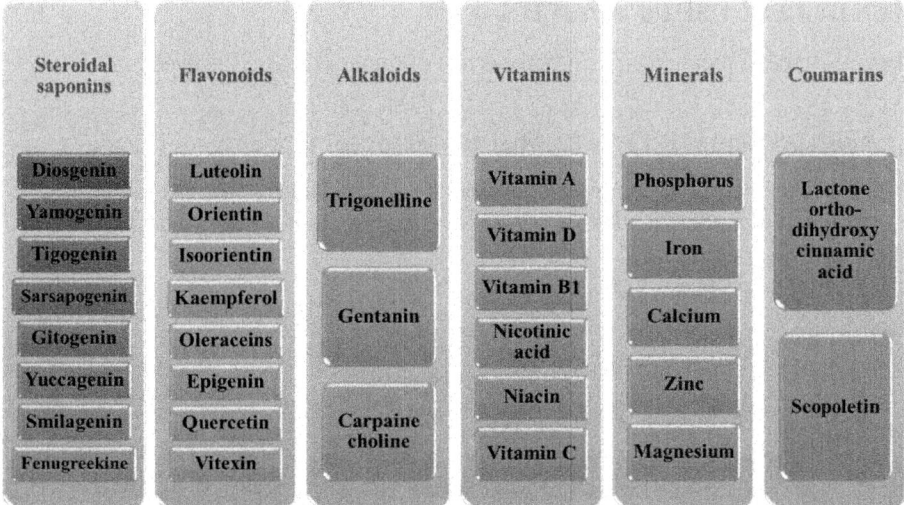

FIGURE 13.2 Active constituents of fenugreek.

Fenugreek stems are glabrous, green, and not branched, reaching up to 50 cm long. Leaves are green, oval, petiolate, serrated, and formed of three small obovate to oblong leaflets. The flowers are small, white to yellow in color, solitary or geminate, and covered with soft hairs. Its fruits are sickle-shaped pods, about 7 to 10 cm in length, and comprise 10 to 20 seeds. The seeds are angled-shaped, yellow in color, about 3 to 6 mm long, with a bitter, aromatic, and oily taste (Ruwali et al. 2022).

The edible parts of fenugreek are its green leaves and seeds, which have nutritional and medicinal value. In fact, fenugreek seeds are considered the most important and well-studied part of the plant. For centuries, fenugreek was used as a spice and herb in several foods in different countries. Fenugreek seeds were also used to make bread and pastes (Singh et al. 2022).

Fenugreek possesses plenty of bioactive constituents (Figure 13.2), such as steroidal saponins, alkaloids, oils, flavonoids, protein compounds, carbohydrates, aromatic compounds, and coumarins. Steroidal saponins consist of diosgenin, yamogenin, tigogenin, sarsapogenin, gitogenin, yuccagenin, smilagenin, and fenugreekine. In addition, several flavonoids, including luteolin, orientin, isoorientin, kaempferol, oleraceins, epigenin, vitexin, and quercetin, have been derived from fenugreek. Furthermore, fenugreek possesses various alkaloids, such as trigonelline, gentanin, carpaine choline, and coumarins, including lactone orthodihydroxy cinnamic acid and scopoletin. Interestingly, it has been supported that fenugreek contains numerous minerals, including iron, phosphate, calcium, and vitamins such as nicotinic acid, vitamin B1, D, A, and C (Nagulapalli Venkata et al. 2017).

13.2 BACKGROUND

Fenugreek has been extensively consumed as folk medicine in many countries worldwide. The leaves have been used to improve splenomegaly, hepatitis, cough, backache, loss of appetite, and gastrointestinal diseases. In addition, fenugreek seeds have been used as a local emollient, sedative, expectorant, and laxative, and to alleviate inflammation and arthralgia. In ancient Egypt, it was used to accelerate childbirth, stimulate breast milk, and decrease menstrual pain. It has been traditionally used in India as a tonic, to improve digestion, and lactation. Additionally, it was used to improve body weakness, gout, and leg edema in traditional Chinese medicine (Yadav and Baquer 2014). Avicenna, a well-known Iranian physician and philosopher, mentioned fenugreek for improving undesired mouth or body odor, skin disorders such as black spots, and sweating in the *Canon of Medicine*. In addition, Zakariya al-Razi, a famous Iranian philosopher, physician, and alchemist, suggested fenugreek to treat diabetes (Bahmani et al. 2016). Interestingly, its traditional usage is nowadays well evaluated and reported by researchers worldwide.

13.3 FENUGREEK USE IN DIABETES

The main anti-diabetic mechanisms and properties of fenugreek are illustrated in Figure 13.3.

13.3.1 ANIMAL MODELS OF DIABETES MELLITUS (DM)

The anti-diabetic properties of fenugreek have been investigated in various animal models of DM, including streptozotocin (STZ), alloxan, nitrate, and high-fat diet-induced DM (Table 13.1).

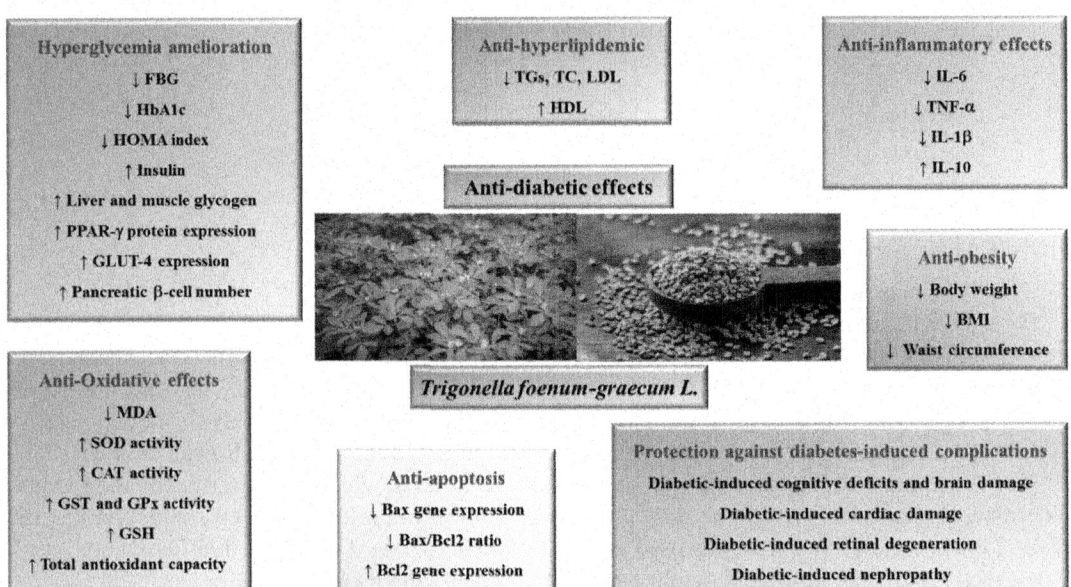

FIGURE 13.3 The anti-diabetic mechanisms of fenugreek. CAT, catalase; FBG, fasting blood glucose; GLUT4, glucose transporter-4; GPx, glutathione peroxidase; HbA_{1c}, hemoglobin A_{1c}; HDL, high-density lipoprotein cholesterol; HOMA, Homeostasis Model Assessment; IL, interleukin; LDL, low-density lipoprotein cholesterol; MDA, malondialdehyde; PPAR-γ, peroxisome proliferator-activated receptor γ; SOD, superoxide dismutase; TC, total cholesterol; TGs, triglycerides; TNF-α, tumor necrosis factor-α.

TABLE 13.1

Protective Effects of Fenugreek against Animal Models of DM

Type of Extract	Dose/Concentration	Study Model	Results	Reference
Fenugreek seed	1 g/kg; orally for 30 days	STZ-induced DM in rat	↓ Serum glucose, TGs, TC, AST, AST, ALP ↑ Insulin, liver and muscle glycogen, GSH levels ↑ GST and CAT activities	(Marzouk, Soliman, and Omar 2013)
Ethanolic extract of fenugreek seed	20 and 80 mg/kg; orally for 4 weeks	High-fat diet–fed and STZ-induced DM mice	↓ Blood glucose and MDA level ↑ SOD and CAT activities Improved histopathology of kidney, liver, and pancreas tissues	(Li et al. 2018)

Type of Extract	Dose/Concentration	Study Model	Results	Reference
Aqueous extract of fenugreek seed	200 mg/5 ml/kg/day; orally for 21 days	STZ-induced DM in rat	↑ Body weight, serum insulin, glycogen in the liver and skeletal muscle, and HDL levels ↓ FBG, HbA$_{1c}$, TC, TGs, LDL, ALT, and AST levels ↑ Hexokinase and glucose-6-phosphate dehydrogenase activities in liver tissue	(Bera et al. 2013)
Aqueous extract of fenugreek seed	0.87 and 1.74 g/kg; orally for 6 weeks	STZ-induced DM in rat	↓ Blood glucose level 4 Activities of SOD, CAT, and GPx in heart tissue	(Haghani, Bakhtiyari, and Doost Mohammadpour 2016)
Hydroethanolic extract of fenugreek seeds	100 mg/kg; orally for 4 weeks	STZ-induced DM in rat	↓ Blood glucose, insulin, HOMA index, TGs, TC, and LDL level ↑ HDL level	(Hosseini et al. 2020)
Fenugreek seed powder	10%; orally for 6 weeks	STZ-induced DM in rat	↑ Body weight and insulin ↓ Blood glucose, HOMA index, HbA$_{1c}$, urea, Cr, and advanced glycation end products Ameliorated pancreatic β cell islet area, number, and diameter	(Pradeep and Srinivasan 2017)
Ethanolic extracts of fenugreek seeds	100 mg/kg; orally for 21 days	Alloxan-induced DM in rats	↓ Blood glucose, TC, TGs, LDL, ALT, AST, urea, and creatinine levels ↑ Body weight and HDL levels	(Yella et al. 2019)
Aqueous extract of fenugreek leaves	0.5 and 1 g/kg/day; orally for 6 weeks	Alloxan-induced DM in rats	↓ Blood glucose ↓ MDA level in serum and liver ↑ Body weight ↑ GPx level and SOD activity in serum and liver	(Middha et al. 2011)
Hydroethanolic extract of fenugreek seeds	500, 1000, and 2000 mg/kg; orally for 30 days	Alloxan-induced DM in rats	↓ Blood glucose, HbA$_{1c}$, TNF-α and IL-6, α-amylase, lipase, and MDA levels ↑ Liver and muscle glycogen, GSH level, and SOD activity in liver and pancreas tissue	(Joshi, Patil, and Naik 2015)
Fenugreek seed powder	5%; orally for 21 days	Alloxan-induced DM in rats	↓ Blood glucose, level of MDA in heart, muscle, and brain tissues ↓ PKC-β2 levels in the heart membrane and skeletal muscle ↑ Body weight, serum insulin, SOD, CAT, GSH, glutathione reductase, pyruvate kinase, and LDH activities in heart, muscle, and brain	(Kumar, Taha, et al. 2012)

(Continued)

TABLE 13.1
(Continued)

Type of Extract	Dose/Concentration	Study Model	Results	Reference
Fenugreek seed	5% w/w; orally for 4 months	Nitrate-induced diabetes in young and adult male rats	↓ Serum glucose, HbA$_{1c}$, TGs, TC, phospholipids, LDL, ALT, AST, total bilirubin, urea, and creatinine levels ↑ Serum insulin, T3, T4, and HDL levels	(El-Wakf et al. 2015)
Hydroethanolic extract of fenugreek seed	2 g/kg/day; orally for 18 weeks	High-fat diet–induced diabetes in C57BL/6J mice	↓ Body weight, serum glucose, TGs, TC, and HOMA ↑ HDL level	(Hamza et al. 2012)
Petroleum ether fraction of fenugreek seed extract	50 mg/kg/day; orally for 12 weeks	High-fat–fed ovariectomized rats	↓ Blood glucose, TC, TGs, LDL, atherogenic index, cardiac risk index, ALT, AST, MDA, TNF-α, and leptin levels ↑ HDL and GSH levels ↑ Adiponectin and PPAR-γ mRNA expression in liver tissue	(Nagamma et al. 2022)
Hydroethanolic extract of fenugreek seed	100 and 200 mg/kg orally for 4 weeks	high-fructose–induced DM in rats	↓ FBG, TC, TGs, LDL, and MDA levels ↑ HDL, GPx, and TAC levels and CAT activity	(Mohammad-Sadeghipour et al. 2020)

Abbreviations: ALP, alkaline phosphatase; AST, alanine transaminase; AST, aspartate transaminase; CAT, catalase; DM, diabetes mellitus; FBG, fasting blood glucose; GPx, glutathione peroxidase; GSH, glutathione reduced; GST, glutathione S-transferase; HbA$_{1c}$, hemoglobin A1C; HDL, high-density lipoprotein cholesterol; HOMA, Homeostasis Model Assessment; LDH, lactate dehydrogenase; LDL, low-density lipoprotein cholesterol; MDA, malondialdehyde; PPAR-γ, peroxisome pro-liferator-activated receptor γ; SOD, superoxide dismutase; STZ, streptozotocin; T3, triiodothyronine; T4, thyroxin; TAC, total antioxidant capacity; TC, total cholesterol; TGs, triglycerides.

13.3.1.1 Protective Effects of Fenugreek against STZ-Induced DM

Marzouk et al. showed that fenugreek seed (1 g/kg; orally) meaningfully reduced serum glucose, triglycerides (TGs), total cholesterol (TC), alanine transaminase (AST), aspartate transaminase (AST), alkaline phosphatase (ALP), whereas it enhanced insulin, liver and muscle glycogen, and glutathione reduced (GSH) levels and glutathione S-transferase (GST) and catalase (CAT) activi-ties in STZ-induced diabetic rats (Marzouk et al. 2013). Similarly, ethanolic extract of fenugreek seed (20 and 80 mg/kg; orally) notably alleviated blood glucose and malondialdehyde (MDA) levels while markedly increased superoxide dismutase (SOD) and CAT activities in high-fat diet–fed and STZ-induced DM mice. In addition, fenugreek seed extract also improved the histopathology of kidney, liver, and mmuness tissues of diabetic mice (Li et al. 2018).

Bera and coworkers noticed that aqueous extract of fenugreek seed (200 mg/5 ml/kg/day) remarkably propagated body weight, serum insulin, glycogen in the liver and skeletal muscle, high-density lipoprotein cholesterol (HDL) while decreased fasting blood glucose (FBG), hemoglobin A$_{1c}$ (HbA$_{1c}$), TC, TGs, low-density lipoprotein cholesterol (LDL), ALT, AST, in STZ-induced dia-betic rats. Furthermore, fenugreek significantly stimulated hexokinase and glucose-6-phosphate dehydrogenase activities in the liver tissue of diabetic rats (Bera et al. 2013). Another similar study emphasized that aqueous extract of fenugreek (0.87 and 1.74 g/kg; orally) provided a significant decrement in blood glucose level while significantly increasing the activities of SOD, CAT, and glutathione peroxidase (GPx) in the heart tissue of STZ-induced diabetic rats (Haghani et al. 2016).

Hosseini et al. also revealed that hydroethanolic extract of fenugreek seeds (100 mg/kg; orally) considerably diminished the blood glucose, insulin, Homeostasis Model Assessment (HOMA) index, TGs, TC, and LDL levels, whereas it strikingly enhanced HDL levels in STZ-induced diabetic rats (Hosseini et al. 2020). Haritha et al. supported that fenugreek seed powder (1 g/kg; orally for 8 weeks) provided a significant decrement in MDA level while showing a significant increment in GSH, GST, glycogen levels, and glucose-6-phosphate dehydrogenase (G6PD), Na^+,K^+-ATPase activity, Mg^{2+}-ATPase, and cytochrome P450 activities in liver tissue of STZ-induced DM in rats (Haritha et al. 2013). Additionally, fenugreek seed powder (10%) significantly propagated body weight and insulin, while markedly diminished blood glucose, HOMA index, HbA_{1c}, urea, Cr, and advanced glycation end products in STZ-induced diabetic rats. Moreover, fenugreek notably ameliorated pancreatic β cell islet area, number, and diameter in diabetic rats (Pradeep and Srinivasan 2017).

13.3.1.2 Protective Effects of Fenugreek against Alloxan-Induced DM

Yella and coworkers revealed that ethanolic extracts of fenugreek seeds (100 mg/kg; orally) strikingly attenuated blood glucose, TC, TGs, LDL, ALT, AST, urea, and creatinine levels but elevated body weight and HDL levels in alloxan-induced DM in rats (Yella et al. 2019). Similarly, aqueous extract of fenugreek leaves (0.5 and 1 g/kg/day; orally) remarkably reduced blood glucose and MDA level in serum and liver but notably enhanced body weight, GPx level, and SOD activity in serum and liver of alloxan-induced DM in rats (Middha et al. 2011). In another study, hydroethanolic extract of fenugreek seeds (500, 1000, and 2000 mg/kg; orally) considerably diminished blood glucose, HbA_{1c}, inflammatory cytokines including tumor necrosis factor-α (TNF-α) and interleukin (IL)-6, pancreatic enzymes including α-amylase and lipase, and MDA levels in alloxan-induced DM in rats. On the other hand, fenugreek extract significantly propagated liver and muscle glycogen, GSH level, and SOD activity in the liver and pancreas tissue in diabetic rats (Joshi et al. 2015).

Kumar et al. emphasized that fenugreek seed powder (5%; orally for 21 days) meaningfully attenuated blood glucose, level of MDA in heart, muscle, and brain tissues, and protein kinase C (PKC)-β2 levels in the heart membrane and skeletal muscle in alloxan-induced DM in rats. In contrast, fenugreek remarkably promoted body weight, serum insulin, SOD, CAT, GSH, glutathione reductase, pyruvate kinase, and lactate dehydrogenase (LDH) activities in heart, muscle, and brain of diabetic rats (Kumar, Taha, et al. 2012). Mohamed and coworkers reported that aqueous extract of fenugreek seeds (100 mg/kg/day; orally for 4 weeks) notably mitigated blood glucose, TC, TGs, LDL, ALT, AST, and LDH levels and enhanced HDL and insulin levels in alloxan-induced DM rats. Additionally, fenugreek markedly elevated the pancreatic β cell number, while attenuating pancreatic β cell diameter and nuclear diameters in diabetic rats (Mohamed et al. 2015).

13.3.1.3 Protective Effects of Fenugreek against Nitrate-Induced DM

El-Wak et al. revealed that treatment with fenugreek seeds (5% w/w; orally) considerably mitigated the serum glucose, HbA_{1c}, TGs, TC, phospholipids, LDL, ALT, AST, total bilirubin, urea, and creatinine levels in nitrate-induced diabetes in young and adult male rats. In contrast, fenugreek seeds provided a significant increment in serum insulin, triiodothyronine, thyroxin, and HDL levels in nitrate-induced diabetes in young and adult male rats (El-Wakf et al. 2015).

13.3.1.4 Protective Effects of Fenugreek against High-Fat or High-Fructose Diet–Induced DM

Hamza and coworkers determined that hydroethanolic extract of fenugreek seed (2 g/kg/day; orally) attenuated the body weight, serum glucose, TGs, TC, and the HOMA as insulin resistance marker while remarkably elevating the HDL level in high-fat diet–induced diabetes in C57BL/6J mice

(Hamza et al. 2012). Additionally, petroleum ether fraction of fenugreek seed extract (50 mg/kg/day; orally for 12 weeks) strikingly mitigated blood glucose, TC, TGs, LDL, atherogenic index, cardiac risk index, ALT, AST, MDA, TNF-α, and leptin levels while notably enhancing HDL, GSH levels, and adiponectin and peroxisome proliferator-activated receptor γ (PPAR-γ) mRNA expression in liver tissue of high-fat–fed ovariectomized rats (Nagamma et al. 2022).

Sadeghipour et al. measured the effects of fenugreek against high-fructose–induced DM in rats. They found that hydroethanolic extract of fenugreek seed (100 and 200 mg/kg orally) strikingly diminished FBG, TC, TGs, LDL, and MDA levels, while markedly increasing the HDL, GPx, and total antioxidant capacity levels and CAT activity in high-fructose–induced diabetic rats (Mohammad-Sadeghipour et al. 2020).

13.3.2 PROTECTIVE EFFECTS OF FENUGREEK AGAINST DIABETES COMPLICATIONS

DM is a complex chronic disease that may give rise to several chronic complications, including cognitive deficits and brain damage, cardiovascular diseases, retinopathy, nephropathy, and hepatic failure. In this regard, DM is known as a silent killer (Cole and Florez 2020; Askari et al. 2020). In this regard, the protective effects of fenugreek against some DM complications have been investigated (Table 13.2).

TABLE 13.2
Protective Effects of Fenugreek against Diabetes Mellitus Complications

Type of Extract	Dose	Study Model	Results	Reference
Fenugreek seed extract	1 g/kg; orally for 6 weeks	STZ-induced cognitive deficits	↑ Learning, memory impairment, and performance in behavioral tasks ↑ Neuronal survival in the CA1 and CA3 regions of the hippocampus ↓ Blood glucose and MDA level ↑ GSH, GPx, SOD, and CAT	(Kodumuri et al. 2019)
Hydroethanolic fenugreek seed extract	50, 100, and 200 mg/ kg; orally for 6 weeks	STZ-induced cognitive deficits	Improved passive avoidance test ↓ MDA and NO metabolites ↑ GSH level, SOD, and CAT activities in the hippocampal and cortical tissues	(Bafadam et al. 2019)
Fenugreek seed powder	5%; orally for 21 days	Alloxan-induced diabetic brain injury in rat	↓ Serum glucose level ↓ Activity of MAO from synaptosomal and supernatant fractions, membrane fluidity, and neurolipofuscin content in brains ↑ GLUT4 protein levels and restored the distribution of GLUT4 to the neuronal membranes in the cerebral cortex	(Kumar, Kale, and Baquer 2012)
Fenugreek seed powder	5%, orally for 3 weeks	Alloxan-induced diabetic brain injury in rat	↓ Blood glucose, brain MDA level ↑ Body weight, insulin level, membrane Na$^+$,K$^+$-ATPase, Ca^{2+}ATPase, SOD, and GST activities in the brain Improved synaptosomal membrane fluidity, intrasynaptosomal calcium levels ↓ Deposition of lipofuscin in neurons	(Kumar, Kale, McLean, et al. 2012)

Type of Extract	Dose	Study Model	Results	Reference
Fenugreek seed powder	9 g/kg; orally for 12 weeks	STZ-induced diabetic nephropathy in rat	↓ Blood glucose, HbA$_{1c}$, BUN, creatinine levels, and kidney index Prevented extracellular matrix accumulation in glomeruli and glomerular morphological alterations ↑ SOD, CAT, and GSH-Px activities ↓ MDA level, mRNA, and protein expressions of TGF-β1 and CTGF	(Jin et al. 2014)
Fenugreek seed powder	10%; orally for 6 weeks	STZ-induced diabetic nephropathy in rat	↓ Kidney weight, creatinine clearance, TC, TG levels in serum ↓ ROS, MDA, and protein carbonyl levels in kidney ↓ Renal mRNA and protein expression of RAGE, NF-κB, TGF-β1, TNF-α, COX-2, Bax, and Bax/Bcl-2 ratio ↑ Renal activity of CAT and level of GSH	(Pradeep and Srinivasan 2018)
Fenugreek extract	100 and 200 mg/kg; orally for 24 weeks	STZ-induced diabetic retinal damage in rats	↑ GSH level and SOD and CAT activities in the retinal tissue ↓ Retinal levels of inflammatory cytokines including TNF-α and IL-1β and angiogenic markers including VEGF and PKC-β The retina showed no vascular leakage and vasodilation and had lower thickening of capillary basement membrane	(Gupta et al. 2014)
Hydroethanolic extract of fenugreek seed	50, 100, and 200 mg/kg; orally for 6 weeks	STZ-induced cardiac damage in rats	↓ FBG, TC, TG levels ↓ MDA level in heart tissue ↓ Gene expression of Bax and Bax/Bcl2 ratio in heart tissue ↑ GSH level, SOD, CAT activities, and gene expression of Bcl2 and ICAM-1 in heart tissue	(Bafadam et al. 2021)
Aqueous extract of fenugreek seed	0.87 and 1.74 g/kg; orally for 6 weeks	STZ-induced cardiac damage in rats	↑ Body weight, CAT, GPx, and SOD activities in the heart tissue ↓ Blood glucose level	(Arshadi et al. 2015)
Fenugreek seed	9 g/kg/day; orally for 30 days	Alloxan-induced DM in rats	↓ FBG, MDA level ↑ GSH level, SOD, CAT, GST activities in heart tissue	(Tripathi and Chandra 2009)

Abbreviations: BUN, blood urine nitrogen; CAT, catalase; COX-2, cyclooxygenase-2; CTGF, connective growth factor; DM, diabetes mellitus; FBG, fasting blood glucose; GLUT4, glucose transporter-4; GPx, glutathione peroxidase; GST, glutathione S-transferase; HbA$_{1c}$, hemoglobin A1C; ICAM1, intercellular adhesion molecule-1; IL-1β, interleukin-1β; MAO, monoamine oxidase; MDA, malondialdehyde; NF-κB, nuclear factor-κB; PKC, protein kinase C; RAGE, receptor for advanced glycation end products; SOD, superoxide dismutase; STZ, streptozotocin; TC, total cholesterol; TGF-β1, transforming growth factor-β1; TGs, triglycerides; TNF-α, tumor necrosis factor-α; VEGF, vascular endothelial growth factor.

13.3.2.1 Diabetic-Induced Cognitive Deficits and Brain Damage

Kodumuri and coworkers evaluated the effects of fenugreek on cognitive deficits in STZ-induced diabetic rats. They showed that fenugreek seed extract (1 g/kg; orally) significantly ameliorated learning, memory impairment, and performance in behavioral tasks and propagated neuronal survival in the CA1 and CA3 regions of the hippocampus in diabetic rats. In addition, fenugreek seed extract notably decreased the blood glucose and MDA level, while increasing GSH, GPx, SOD, and CAT levels in STZ-induced diabetic rats. They suggested that fenugreek seed extract improved diabetes-induced cognitive deficits through attenuating oxidative stress and elevating antioxidative markers and neuronal survival in the hippocampus (Kodumuri et al. 2019). Similarly, hydroethanolic fenugreek seed extract (50, 100, and 200 mg/kg; orally for 6 weeks) meaningfully improved passive avoidance test and prevented MDA and NO metabolites while providing a significant increment in GSH level, SOD, and CAT activities in the hippocampal and cortical tissues of STZ-induced DM in rats (Bafadam et al. 2019).

Kumar et al. investigated the effects of fenugreek seed powder in the alloxan-induced diabetic rat brain. They suggested that fenugreek seed (5%, orally) remarkably diminished serum glucose level, monoamine oxidase (MAO) activity from synaptosomal and supernatant fractions, membrane fluidity, and neurolipofuscin content in diabetic brains. Moreover, it stimulated the glucose transporter-4 (GLUT4) protein levels and restored the distribution of GLUT4 to the neuronal membranes in the cerebral cortex of alloxan-induced diabetic rats (Kumar, Kale, and Baquer 2012). In another study, fenugreek seed powder (5%, orally for 3 weeks) notably mitigated blood glucose and brain MDA level while promoting body weight, insulin level, membrane Na^+,K^+-ATPase, Ca^{2+}-ATPase, SOD, and GST activities in the brain of alloxan-induced DM in rats. Additionally, fenugreek significantly improved synaptosomal membrane fluidity, intrasynaptosomal calcium levels, and diminished lipofuscin deposition in neurons (Kumar, Kale, McLean, et al. 2012).

13.3.2.2 Diabetic-Induced Cardiac Damage

Bafadam et al. revealed the cardioprotective properties of fenugreek in STZ-induced diabetic rats. They reported that hydroethanolic extract of fenugreek seed (50, 100, and 200 mg/kg; orally) markedly alleviated FBG, TC, and TGs levels, MDA levels in heart tissue, and the gene expression of Bax, and Bax/Bcl2 ratio in heart tissue of STZ-induced diabetic rat. In contrast, fenugreek notably stimulated GSH level, SOD, CAT activities and gene expression of Bcl2 and intercellular adhesion molecule-1 in the heart tissue of diabetic rats (Bafadam et al. 2021). Similarly, aqueous extract of fenugreek seed (0.87 and 1.74 g/kg; orally) considerably enhanced body weight, CAT, GPx, and SOD activities in the heart tissue while firmly preventing blood glucose levels in STZ-induced diabetic rats (Arshadi et al. 2015). Tripathi and coworkers suggested that fenugreek seed (9 g/kg/day; orally for 30 days) significantly decreased FBG and MDA levels and remarkably propagated GSH level, SOD, CAT, GST activities in heart tissue of alloxan-induced DM in rats (Tripathi and Chandra 2009).

13.3.2.3 Diabetic-Induced Retinal Degeneration

Gupta et al. determined the effects of fenugreek on retinal damage in STZ-induced diabetic rats. They showed that fenugreek extract (100 and 200 mg/kg; orally) firmly stimulated the GSH level and SOD and CAT activities in the retinal tissue of diabetic rats. However, it meaningfully alleviated the retinal levels of inflammatory cytokines including TNF-α and IL-1β and angiogenic markers including vascular endothelial growth factor and PKC-β. In addition, the retinas of animals receiving fenugreek showed no vascular leakage and vasodilation and had lower thickening of capillary basement membrane than the diabetic groups (Gupta et al. 2014).

13.3.2.4 Diabetic-Induced Nephropathy

Jin and coworkers evaluated the effects of fenugreek on diabetic nephropathy in STZ-induced diabetic rats. They supported that fenugreek seed (9 g seed powder/kg; orally) significantly mitigated blood glucose, HbA_{1c}, blood urine nitrogen (BUN), creatinine levels, and kidney index following STZ-induced diabetic nephropathy in rats. Additionally, fenugreek considerably prevented extracellular matrix accumulation in glomeruli and glomerular morphological alterations of diabetic rats. Fenugreek also promoted SOD, CAT, and GSH-Px activities while decreasing MDA level, mRNA, and protein expressions of transforming growth factor-β1 (TGF-β1) and connective growth factor in kidney tissue of diabetic rats. They demonstrated that fenugreek seed improved diabetic nephropathy in STZ-induced diabetic rats (Jin et al. 2014). Similarly, fenugreek seed powder (10%; orally for 6 weeks) markedly alleviated kidney weight, creatinine clearance, TC, TGs levels in serum, ROS, MDA, and protein carbonyl levels in kidney, renal mRNA, and protein expression of the receptor for advanced glycation end products, nuclear factor κB (NF-κB), TGF-β1, TNF-α, cyclooxygenase-2, Bax, and Bax/Bcl-2 ratio in STZ-induced diabetic rats. However, fenugreek strikingly enhanced the renal activity of CAT and the level of GSH in diabetic rats (Pradeep and Srinivasan 2018).

13.3.3 Clinical Investigations

The promising anti-diabetic properties of fenugreek have also been supported in clinical trial studies (Table 13.3). In this regard, 12 weeks of treatment with fenugreek seed powder (2 g/day) significantly reduced FBG, HOMA index, HbA$_{1c}$, TC, TGs, and LDL while enhancing fasting insulin and

TABLE 13.3

Clinical Evaluations of the Anti-Diabetic Properties of Fenugreek

Extract Type or Plant Part	Study Design	Study Model	Results	Reference
Fenugreek seed powder	• 2 g/day	A randomized controlled clinical trial on T2D patients	↓ FBG, HOMA index, HbA$_{1c}$, TC, TGs, LDL ↑ Enhanced fasting insulin, and HDL level	(Najdi et al. 2019)
Fenugreek seed powder solution	• 25 g; orally twice a day for 1 month	A randomized controlled clinical trial on T2D patients	↓ TC, TGs, and LDL level ↑ HDL level compared to the baseline level and control group	(Geberemeskel, Debebe, and Nguse 2019)
Fenugreek seed powder	• 5 g, three times a day for 8 weeks	A parallel-group, randomized controlled clinical trial on T2D patients	↓ FBG, systolic blood pressure, BUN, GFR, irisin, ALT, and AST	(Hadi et al. 2020)
Fenfuro (novel fenugreek seed extract enriched in furostanolic saponins)	• 500 mg twice a day for 90 days	A multicenter randomized controlled clinical trial on T2D patients	↓ FBG, postprandial plasma glucose, HbA$_{1c}$, fasting, and postprandial C-peptide	(Verma et al. 2016)
Fenugreek seeds soaked in hot water	• 10 g/day for 6 months	A parallel-group, randomized controlled single-blind clinical trial on T2D patients	↓ FBG and HbA$_{1c}$ level	(Ranade and Mudgalkar 2017)
Fenugreek seed powder	• 5 g/day for 2 months	A randomized, double-blinded, placebo-controlled clinical trial on T2D patients	↓ FBG, HbA$_{1c}$, BMI, waist circumference, and diastolic blood pressure Improved quality of life	(Hassani et al. 2019)
Fenugreek seeds	• 10 g/day for 8 weeks	A randomized controlled clinical trial on T2D patients	↓ FBG, TGs, and LDL	(Kassaian et al. 2009)

Abbreviations: ALT, aspartate transaminase; AST, alanine transaminase; FBG, fasting blood glucose; HbA$_{1c}$, hemoglobin A$_{1c}$; HDL, high-density lipoprotein cholesterol; HOMA, Homeostasis Model Assessment; LDL, low-density lipoprotein cholesterol; T2D, type 2 diabetes mellitus; TC, total cholesterol; TGs, triglycerides.

HDL level in patients with type 2 DM (Najdi et al. 2019). Geberemeskel et al. also demonstrated that fenugreek seed powder solution (25 g; orally twice a day for 1 month) meaningfully diminished TC, TG, and LDL levels, while increasing HDL levels compared to the baseline level and control group in type 2 diabetic patients (Geberemeskel et al. 2019). Similarly, fenugreek seeds (10 g) soaked in hot water firmly alleviated the FBG and HbA_{1c} levels following 6 months of treatment in type 2 diabetic patients (Ranade and Mudgalkar 2017). In addition, fenugreek seed powder (10 g/day for 8 weeks) remarkably decreased FBG, TGs, and LDL in type 2 diabetic patients (Kassaian et al. 2009).

Hadi and coworkers determined that fenugreek seed powder (5 g, three times a day) remarkably mitigated FBG, systolic blood pressure, BUN, GFR, irisin, ALT, and AST following 8 weeks of treatment in type 2 diabetic patients (Hadi et al. 2020). Fenfuro, a novel fenugreek seed extract enriched in furostanolic saponins (500 mg twice daily for 90 days), considerably attenuated FBG, postprandial plasma glucose, HbA_{1c}, fasting, and postprandial C-peptide in type 2 diabetic patients (Verma et al. 2016). Hassani et al. revealed that 2 months of treatment with fenugreek seed powder (5 g) provided a significant decrement in FBG, HbA_{1c}, BMI, waist circumference, and diastolic blood pressure while notably improving the quality of life in type 2 diabetic patients (Hassani et al. 2019).

13.4   OTHER FOODS, HERBS, SPICES, AND BOTANICALS USED IN DIABETES

Nowadays, phytotherapy research has attracted a lot of attention, and the promising anti-diabetic effects of multiple medicinal plants have been reported worldwide (Baradaran Rahimi et al. 2019). In this regard, *Portulaca oleracea* L. (Rahimi et al. 2019); *Punica granatum* (pomegranate) and its constituent ellagic acid (Baradaran Rahimi et al. 2020); *Scutellaria baicalensis* and its two major active constituents, baicalin and baicalein (Baradaran Rahimi et al. 2021); *Silybum marianum* (milk thistle) and its major component, silymarin (Tajmohammadi et al. 2018); and *Crocus sativus* L. and its important constituents crocin, safranal, and crocetin (Razavi and Hosseinzadeh 2017) have been shown to possess anti-diabetic properties. Furthermore, many other plants ameliorated DM in cellular, animal, and clinical studies, including *Cinnamomum verum* from Lauraceae (Mollazadeh and Hosseinzadeh 2016); *Opuntia dillenii* from Cactaceae (Shirazinia et al. 2019); *Persea americana* (avocado) from Lauraceae (Tabeshpour et al. 2017); and *Allium sativum* from Alliaceae (Hosseini and Hosseinzadeh 2015).

13.5   TOXICITY AND CAUTIONARY NOTES

The ethanolic extract of fenugreek seeds (orally) showed no acute toxicity at the dose of 3 g/kg in Wister albino rats and Swiss albino mice (Mowla et al. 2009). Similarly, no mortality, gross toxicity, adverse pharmacological effects, or abnormal behavior was observed with fenugreek seed extract (Fenfuro; orally) at doses of 500, 1000, 2000, and 5,000 mg/kg in Sprague-Dawley rats or Swiss Albino mice. Interestingly, the LD_{50} of the Fenuro was stimulated as more than 5000 mg/kg (Swaroop et al. 2014). Middha and coworkers reported that the LD_{50} of the aqueous extract of fenugreek leaves was 8.4 g/kg body weight in mice (Middha et al. 2011).

Additionally, Najdi et al. reported no hepatic or renal adverse effects following 12 weeks of treatment with fenugreek seed powder (2 g/day) in patients with type 2 DM (Najdi et al. 2019).

13.6   SUMMARY POINTS

- This chapter focuses on the anti-diabetic properties of *Trigonella foenum-graecum* L. (fenugreek), a herbaceous annual plant belonging to the family Fabaceae.
- The edible parts of fenugreek are its green leaves and seeds, which have nutritional and medicinal value.
- The promising anti-diabetic effects of fenugreek have been supported in several animal models of DM, including STZ, alloxan, nitrate, and high-fat diet–induced DM.

- Fenugreek possessed antioxidative, anti-inflammatory, and antihyperlipidemia effects in different studies.
- Fenugreek significantly decreased blood glucose, HbA_{1c}, and HOMA index while increasing insulin levels in diabetic animal models.
- Fenugreek showed protective effects against diabetes-induced complications, such as diabetic-induced cognitive deficits and brain damage, cardiovascular diseases, retinopathy, nephropathy, and hepatic failure.
- The ameliorating effects of fenugreek on T2D have also been supported in clinical trial studies.

REFERENCES

Arshadi, S., S. Bakhtiyari, K. Haghani, and A. Valizadeh. 2015. "Effects of fenugreek seed extract and swimming endurance training on plasma glucose and cardiac antioxidant enzymes activity in streptozotocin-induced diabetic rats." *Osong Public Health Res Perspect* 6 (2):87–93.

Askari, V. R., V. B. Rahimi, R. Zargarani, R. Ghodsi, M. Boskabady, and M. H. Boskabady. 2020. "Antioxidant and anti-inflammatory effects of auraptene on phytohemagglutinin (PHA)-induced inflammation in human lymphocytes." *Pharmacol Rep* 73 (1):154–162.

Bafadam, S., F. Beheshti, T. Khodabakhshi, A. Asghari, B. Ebrahimi, H. R. Sadeghnia, M. Mahmoudabady, S. Niazmand, and M. Hosseini. 2019. "Trigonella foenum-graceum seed (Fenugreek) hydroalcoholic extract improved the oxidative stress status in a rat model of diabetes-induced memory impairment." *Horm Mol Biol Clin Investig* 39 (2).

Bafadam, S., M. Mahmoudabady, S. Niazmand, S. A. Rezaee, and M. Soukhtanloo. 2021. "Cardioprotective effects of fenugreek (Trigonella foenum-graceum) seed extract in streptozotocin induced diabetic rats." *J Cardiovasc Thorac Res* 13 (1):28–36.

Bahmani, M., H. Shirzad, M. Mirhosseini, A. Mesripour, and M. Rafieian-Kopaei. 2016. "A review on ethnobotanical and therapeutic uses of fenugreek (Trigonella foenum-graceum L.)." *J Evid Based Complementary Altern Med* 21 (1):53–62.

Baradaran Rahimi, V., V. R. Askari, and H. Hosseinzadeh. 2021. "Promising influences of Scutellaria baicalensis and its two active constituents, baicalin, and baicalein, against metabolic syndrome: A review." *Phytother Res* 35 (7):3558–3574.

Baradaran Rahimi, V., V. R. Askari, and S. H. Mousavi. 2019. "Ellagic acid dose and time-dependently abrogates d-galactose-induced animal model of aging: Investigating the role of PPAR-γ." *Life Sci* 232:116595.

Baradaran Rahimi, V., M. Ghadiri, M. Ramezani, and V. R. Askari. 2020. "Anti-inflammatory and anti-cancer activities of pomegranate and its constituent, ellagic acid: Evidence from cellular, animal, and clinical studies." *Phytother Res* 34 (4):685–720.

Bera, T. K., K. M. Ali, K. Jana, A. Ghosh, and D. Ghosh. 2013. "Protective effect of aqueous extract of seed of Psoralea corylifolia (Somraji) and seed of Trigonella foenum-graecum L. (Methi) in streptozotocin-induced diabetic rat: A comparative evaluation." *Pharmacognosy Res* 5 (4):277–285.

Cole, J. B., and J. C. Florez. 2020. "Genetics of diabetes mellitus and diabetes complications." *Nat Rev Nephrol* 16 (7):377–390.

El-Wakf, A. M., H. A. Hassan, A. Z. Mahmoud, and M. N. Habza. 2015. "Fenugreek potent activity against nitrate-induced diabetes in young and adult male rats." *Cytotechnology* 67 (3):437–447.

Geberemeskel, G. A., Y. G. Debebe, and N. A. Nguse. 2019. "Anti-diabetic effect of fenugreek seed powder solution (Trigonella foenum-graecum L.) on hyperlipidemia in diabetic patients." *J Diabetes Res* 2019:8507453.

Gupta, S. K., B. Kumar, T. C. Nag, B. P. Srinivasan, S. Srivastava, S. Gaur, and R. Saxena. 2014. "Effects of Trigonella foenum-graecum (L.) on retinal oxidative stress, and proinflammatory and angiogenic molecular biomarkers in streptozotocin-induced diabetic rats." *Mol Cell Biochem* 388 (1–2):1–9.

Hadi, A., A. Arab, H. Hajianfar, B. Talaei, M. Miraghajani, S. Babajafari, W. Marx, and R. Tavakoly. 2020. "The effect of fenugreek seed supplementation on serum irisin levels, blood pressure, and liver and kidney function in patients with type 2 diabetes mellitus: A parallel randomized clinical trial." *Complement Ther Med* 49:102315.

Haghani, K., S. Bakhtiyari, and J. Doost Mohammadpour. 2016. "Alterations in plasma glucose and cardiac antioxidant enzymes activity in streptozotocin-induced diabetic rats: Effects of Trigonella foenum-graecum extract and swimming training." *Can J Diabetes* 40 (2):135–142.

Hamza, N., B. Berke, C. Cheze, R. Le Garrec, A. Umar, A. N. Agli, R. Lassalle, J. Jové, H. Gin, and N. Moore. 2012. "Preventive and curative effect of Trigonella foenum-graecum L. seeds in C57BL/6J models of type 2 diabetes induced by high-fat diet." *J Ethnopharmacol* 142 (2):516–522.

Haritha, C., A. G. Reddy, Y. R. Reddy, Y. Anjaneyulu, T. M. Rao, B. A. Kumar, and M. U. Kumar. 2013. "Evaluation of protective action of fenugreek, insulin and glimepiride and their combination in diabetic Sprague Dawley rats." *J Nat Sci Biol Med* 4 (1):207–212.

Hassani, S. S., F. Fallahi Arezodar, S. S. Esmaeili, and M. Gholami-Fesharaki. 2019. "Effect of fenugreek use on fasting blood glucose, glycosylated hemoglobin, body mass index, waist circumference, blood pressure and quality of life in patients with type 2 diabetes mellitus: A randomized, double-blinded, placebo-controlled clinical trials." *Galen Med J* 8:e1432.

Hosseini, S. A., K. Hamzavi, H. Safarzadeh, and O. Salehi. 2020. "Interactive effect of swimming training and fenugreek (Trigonella foenum graecum L.) extract on glycemic indices and lipid profile in diabetic rats." *Arch Physiol Biochem*:1–5.

Hosseini, S. A., and H. Hosseinzadeh. 2015. "A review on the effects of Allium sativum (Garlic) in metabolic syndrome." *J Endocrinol Invest* 38 (11):1147–1157.

Jin, Y., Y. Shi, Y. Zou, C. Miao, B. Sun, and C. Li. 2014. "Fenugreek prevents the development of STZ-induced diabetic nephropathy in a rat model of diabetes." *Evid Based Complement Alternat Med* 2014:259368.

Joshi, D. V., R. R. Patil, and S. R. Naik. 2015. "Hydroalcohol extract of Trigonella foenum-graecum seed attenuates markers of inflammation and oxidative stress while improving exocrine function in diabetic rats." *Pharm Biol* 53 (2):201–211.

Kassaian, N., L. Azadbakht, B. Forghani, and M. Amini. 2009. "Effect of fenugreek seeds on blood glucose and lipid profiles in type 2 diabetic patients." *Int J Vitam Nutr Res* 79 (1):34–39.

Kodumuri, P. K., C. Thomas, R. Jetti, and A. K. Pandey. 2019. "Fenugreek seed extract ameliorates cognitive deficits in streptozotocin-induced diabetic rats." *J Basic Clin Physiol Pharmacol* 30 (4).

Kumar, P., R. K. Kale, and N. Z. Baquer. 2012. "Antihyperglycemic and protective effects of Trigonella foenum graecum seed powder on biochemical alterations in alloxan diabetic rats." *Eur Rev Med Pharmacol Sci* 16 (Suppl 3):18–27.

Kumar, P., R. K. Kale, P. McLean, and N. Z. Baquer. 2012. "Anti-diabetic and neuroprotective effects of Trigonella foenum-graecum seed powder in diabetic rat brain." *Prague Med Rep* 113 (1):33–43.

Kumar, P., A. Taha, R. K. Kale, P. McLean, and N. Z. Baquer. 2012. "Beneficial effects of Trigonella foenum graecum and sodium orthovanadate on metabolic parameters in experimental diabetes." *Cell Biochem Funct* 30 (6):464–473.

Li, X. Y., S. S. Lu, H. L. Wang, G. Li, Y. F. He, X. Y. Liu, R. Rong, J. Li, and X. C. Lu. 2018. "Effects of the fenugreek extracts on high-fat diet-fed and streptozotocin-induced type 2 diabetic mice." *Animal Model Exp Med* 1 (1):68–73.

Marzouk, M., A. M. Soliman, and T. Y. Omar. 2013. "Hypoglycemic and anti-oxidative effects of fenugreek and termis seeds powder in streptozotocin-diabetic rats." *Eur Rev Med Pharmacol Sci* 17 (4):559–565.

Middha, S. K., B. Bhattacharjee, D. Saini, M. S. Baliga, M. B. Nagaveni, and T. Usha. 2011. "Protective role of Trigonella foenum graceum extract against oxidative stress in hyperglycemic rats." *Eur Rev Med Pharmacol Sci* 15 (4):427–435.

Mohamed, Waleed S., Ashraf M. Mostafa, Khaled M. Mohamed, and Abdel Hamid Serwah. 2015. "Effects of fenugreek, Nigella, and termis seeds in nonalcoholic fatty liver in obese diabetic albino rats." *Arab Gastroenterol* 16 (1):1–9.

Mohammad-Sadeghipour, M., M. Afsharinasab, M. Mohamadi, M. Mahmoodi, S. K. Falahati-Pour, and M. R. Hajizadeh. 2020. "The effects of hydro-alcoholic extract of fenugreek seeds on the lipid profile and oxidative stress in fructose-fed rats." *J Obes Metab Syndr* 29 (3):198–207.

Mollazadeh, H., and H. Hosseinzadeh. 2016. "Cinnamon effects on metabolic syndrome: A review based on its mechanisms." *Iran J Basic Med Sci* 19 (12):1258–1270.

Mowla, A., M. Alauddin, M. A. Rahman, and K. Ahmed. 2009. "Antihyperglycemic effect of Trigonella foenum-graecum (fenugreek) seed extract in alloxan-induced diabetic rats and its use in diabetes mellitus: a brief qualitative phytochemical and acute toxicity test on the extract." *Afr J Tradit Complement Altern Med* 6 (3):255–261.

Nagamma, T., A. Konuri, K. M. Bhat, P. Udupa, G. Rao, and Y. Nayak. 2022. "Prophylactic effect of Trigonella foenum-graecum L. seed extract on inflammatory markers and histopathological changes in high-fat-fed ovariectomized rats." *J Tradit Complement Med* 12 (2):131–140.

Nagulapalli Venkata, K. C., A. Swaroop, D. Bagchi, and A. Bishayee. 2017. "A small plant with big benefits: Fenugreek (Trigonella foenum-graecum Linn.) for disease prevention and health promotion." *Mol Nutr Food Res* 61 (6).

Najdi, R. A., M. M. Hagras, F. O. Kamel, and R. M. Magadmi. 2019. "A randomized controlled clinical trial evaluating the effect of Trigonella foenum-graecum (fenugreek) versus glibenclamide in patients with diabetes." *Afr Health Sci* 19 (1):1594–1601.

Pradeep, S. R., and K. Srinivasan. 2017. "Amelioration of hyperglycemia and associated metabolic abnormalities by a combination of fenugreek (Trigonella foenum-graecum) seeds and onion (Allium cepa) in experimental diabetes." *J Basic Clin Physiol Pharmacol* 28 (5):493–505.

Pradeep, S. R., and K. Srinivasan. 2018. "Alleviation of oxidative stress-mediated nephropathy by dietary fenugreek (Trigonella foenum-graecum) seeds and onion (Allium cepa) in streptozotocin-induced diabetic rats." *Food Funct* 9 (1):134–148.

Rahimi, V. B., F. Ajam, H. Rakhshandeh, and V. R. Askari. 2019. "A pharmacological review on Portulaca oleracea L.: Focusing on anti-inflammatory, anti-oxidant, immune-modulatory and antitumor activities." *J Pharmacopuncture* 22 (1):7–15.

Ranade, M., and N. Mudgalkar. 2017. "A simple dietary addition of fenugreek seed leads to the reduction in blood glucose levels: A parallel group, randomized single-blind trial." *Ayu* 38 (1–2):24–27.

Razavi, B. M., and H. Hosseinzadeh. 2017. "Saffron: A promising natural medicine in the treatment of metabolic syndrome." *J Sci Food Agric* 97 (6):1679–1685.

Ruwali, Pushpa, Niharika Pandey, Khusboo Jindal, and Rahul Vikram Singh. 2022. "Fenugreek (Trigonella foenum-graecum): Nutraceutical values, phytochemical, ethnomedicinal and pharmacological overview." *S Afr J Bot* 151 (B):423-431.

Shirazinia, R., V. B. Rahimi, A. R. Kehkhaie, A. Sahebkar, H. Rakhshandeh, and V. R. Askari. 2019. "Opuntia dillenii: A forgotten plant with promising pharmacological properties." *J Pharmacopuncture* 22 (1):16–27.

Singh, Neetu, Surender Singh Yadav, Sanjiv Kumar, and Balasubramaniam Narashiman. 2022. "Ethnopharmacological, phytochemical and clinical studies on Fenugreek (Trigonella foenum-graecum L.)." *Food Bioscience* 46:101546.

Swaroop, A., M. Bagchi, P. Kumar, H. G. Preuss, K. Tiwari, P. A. Marone, and D. Bagchi. 2014. "Safety, efficacy and toxicological evaluation of a novel, patented anti-diabetic extract of Trigonella Foenum-Graecum seed extract (Fenfuro)." *Toxicol Mech Methods* 24 (7):495–503.

Tabeshpour, J., B. M. Razavi, and H. Hosseinzadeh. 2017. "Effects of avocado (Persea americana) on metabolic syndrome: A comprehensive systematic review." *Phytother Res* 31 (6):819–837.

Tajmohammadi, A., B. M. Razavi, and H. Hosseinzadeh. 2018. "Silybum marianum (milk thistle) and its main constituent, silymarin, as a potential therapeutic plant in metabolic syndrome: A review." *Phytother Res* 32 (10):1933–1949.

Tripathi, U. N., and D. Chandra. 2009. "The plant extracts of Momordica charantia and Trigonella foenum-graecum have anti-oxidant and anti-hyperglycemic properties for cardiac tissue during diabetes mellitus." *Oxid Med Cell Longev* 2 (5):290–296.

Verma, N., K. Usman, N. Patel, A. Jain, S. Dhakre, A. Swaroop, M. Bagchi, P. Kumar, H. G. Preuss, and D. Bagchi. 2016. "A multicenter clinical study to determine the efficacy of a novel fenugreek seed (Trigonella foenum-graecum) extract (Fenfuro™) in patients with type 2 diabetes." *Food Nutr Res* 60:32382.

Visuvanathan, T., L.T.L. Than, J. Stanslas, S. Y. Chew, and S. Vellasamy. 2022. "Revisiting Trigonella foenum-graecum L.: Pharmacology and therapeutic potentialities." *Plants (Basel)* 11 (11).

Yadav, U. C., and N. Z. Baquer. 2014. "Pharmacological effects of Trigonella foenum-graecum L. in health and disease." *Pharm Biol* 52 (2):243–254.

Yella, S.S.T., R. N. Kumar, C. Ayyanna, A. M. Varghese, P. Amaravathi, and Y. Vangoori. 2019. "The combined effect of Trigonella foenum seeds and Coriandrum sativum leaf extracts in alloxan-induced diabetes mellitus wistar albino rats." *Bioinformation* 15 (10):716–722.

14 Foxtail Orchid (*Rhynchostylis retusa*)
Anti-Diabetic Properties, Biodiversity, and Propagation

Pema Lhamo, Abinash Kumar, Biswanath
Mahanty and Bula Choudhury

CONTENTS

ABBREVIATIONS

6-BA	6-benzylaminopurine
AC	activated charcoal
CITES	Convention on International Trade in Endangered Species of Wild Fauna and Flora
IAA	indoleacetic acid
KT	kinetin
MS	Murashige and Skoog
MTAQ	2-methyl-1,3,6-trihydroxy-9,10-anthraquinone
NAA	α-naphthaleneacetic acid
PLB	protocorm-like bodies
PPARγ	peroxisome proliferator-activated receptor γ
TDZ	thidiazuron
VW	Vacin and Went

DOI: 10.1201/9781003220930-16

14.1   INTRODUCTION

The orchid family (Orchidaceae) is one of the most widespread flowering plants with 31,000 species (Hinsley et al. 2018). These species are absent only from polar and desert regions and are particularly abundant in the wet tropics worldwide (Zhang et al. 2018). The flowers of Orchidaceae exhibit diverse speciation, with wide variations in floral features such as morphology, color, size, and fragrance for the attraction of pollinators. Orchids are traded for a wide range of purposes and at many different scales, from large-scale commercial trades through minimal use such as medicines, materials for weaving, ornaments, food, and dyes (C. Li et al. 2021). There are also other, emerging commercial uses of orchids, such as in perfumes and cosmetic products (Lubinsky et al. 2008).

Among the various species *Rhynchostylis retusa* (L.) (*R. retusa*) Blume has been identified as an endangered species with a robust stem and dense pendulous inflorescences with long, attractive flowers (Sinha and Jahan 2012). The plant is reported to grow in Sri Lanka, India, and Bangladesh up to the Philippines (Fonseka 2020). Apart from its beauty, it has been consumed as a nutraceutical since ancient times. Its therapeutic benefits have been realized and utilized in traditional medicine in China and India (Tsering et al. 2017). Orchids are known for their medicinal value from the Vedic period. References to orchids as medicinal plants are available in Sanskrit literature, namely *Nighantus* and *Amarakosha* by Sushruta and Vagbhata, respectively (250–300 BC). In Sanskrit, *R. retusa* is known as *Seetha Pushpa* and *Kapou Phul* in Assam. The plants are erect and leafy, producing densely flowered decurved inflorescences which are 40–50 cm long. The flowering period is April to June (Hegde 1984). *R. retusa* has been used to treat conditions like paralysis, rheumatism, allergies, abnormal menstruation, and malaria fever in traditional medicine (Akhter et al. 2017).

Diabetes mellitus is a metabolic disorder caused by insufficient insulin secretion, action, or a combination of the two. Destruction of pancreatic β cells leads to type 1 or insulin-dependent diabetes, whereas insulin resistance compensated by β cell insulin hypersecretion leads to type-2 or insulin-independent diabetes (Teoh and Das 2018). The condition can be controlled by preventing the breakdown of complex carbohydrates or the diffusion of glucose through the intestinal membrane (Chakrabarti and Rajagopalan 2002). Phytochemicals from various plant species have been identified to have α-amylase inhibitory properties and are used for controlling diabetes (Nyambe-Silavwe et al. 2015). The *R. retusa* plant contains various phytochemical compounds which have been reported for antibacterial, antifungal, anti-inflammatory, and antioxidant properties which could be used to treat diabetes (Abinash Kumar et al. 2021).

This chapter highlights the anti-diabetic properties of phytochemical compounds found in the *R. retusa* plant while discussing its biodiversity, ethnomedicinal uses, and micropropagation techniques.

14.2   BIODIVERSITY

Countries with the most orchids are India, Myanmar, China, Philippines, Sri Lanka, Thailand, Malaysia, Australia, and New Guinea. *R. retusa* grows in most of these countries, as well as in Bangladesh, Bhutan, Nepal, Vietnam, Laos, and Cambodia (Adhikari, Jentsch, and Kunwar 2021). In India, orchids are among the largest flowering plant, accounting for 9% of total flora. India has 1256 species of orchid, with the highest in the North East, followed by the Western Ghats, Deccan Plateau, and the Andaman and Nicobar Islands (Sundararaju 2020). Arunachal Pradesh in the North East has the most, with 577 species in 147 genera, followed by Sikkim with 561 species in 144 genera, Meghalaya with 380 species in 113 genera, Nagaland with 387 species in 107 genera, Manipur with 314 species in 93 genera, Mizoram with 253 species in 86 genera, Assam with 231 species in 82 genera, and Tripura with 39 species in 29 genera (Ninawe and Swapna 2017). *R. retusa* grows predominately in Arunachal Pradesh, Assam, and Andhra Pradesh. Other states with its distribution include Chhattisgarh, Odisha, West Bengal, Sikkim, Meghalaya, Madhya Pradesh, Uttarakhand, Kerala, Tamil Nadu, Karnataka, Telangana, and the Andaman and Nicobar Islands (Figure 14.1) (Saxena 2020). Over the years, *R. retusa* has greatly declined in number and

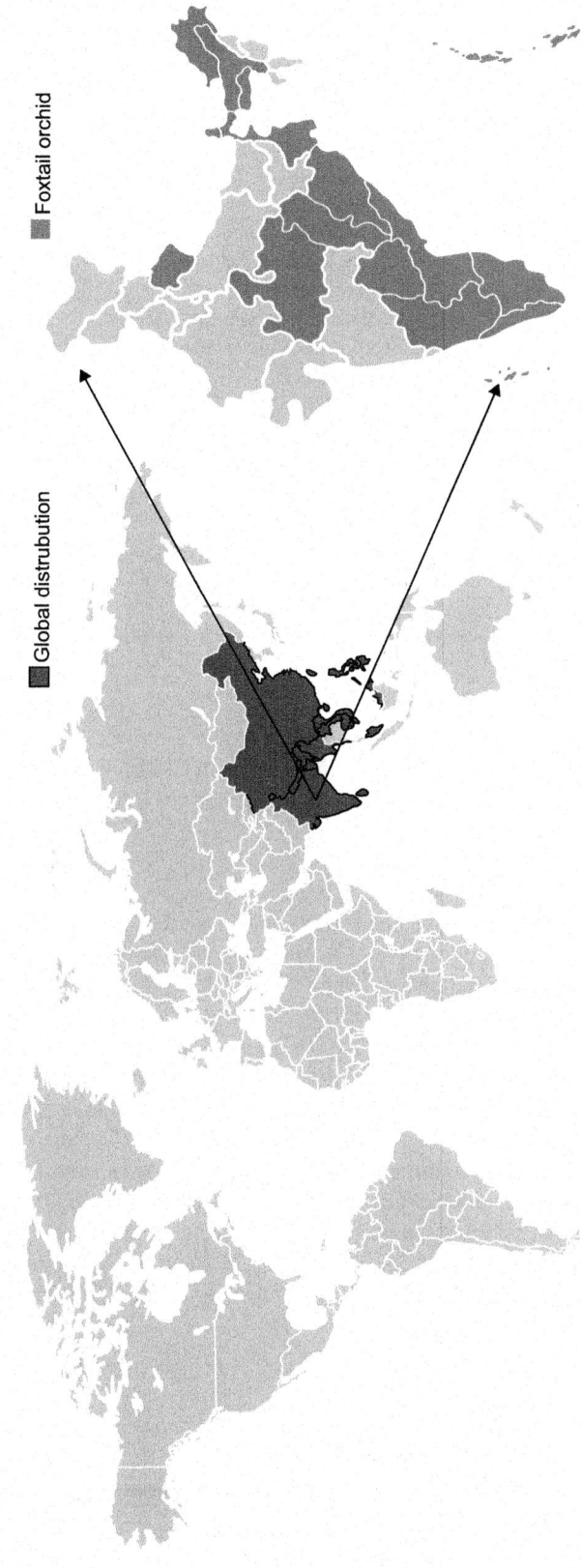

FIGURE 14.1 Distribution of foxtail orchid (*R. retusa*) globally and in different states of India.

TABLE 14.1

Ethnomedicinal Uses of *R. retusa* in Different Countries and Indian States of India

Plant Part Used	State/Country	Traditional Uses	Reference
Root	Nepal	Roots are used as an emollient for treating asthma, tuberculosis, nervous twitching, cramps, rheumatism, kidney stones, and menstrual irregularities.	(Acharya and Rokaya 1970)
	Nagaland, India	Root paste mixed with *Pisum sativum* is used to cure blood dysentery.	(Nongdam 2014)
	Arunachal Pradesh, India	Root juice is used for treating cuts, wounds, menstrual pain.	(Tsering et al. 2017)
Leaf	Uttarakhand and Arunachal Pradesh, India	Paste of leaves is used to treat rheumatism, wounds, paralysis.	(Tsering et al. 2017; Jalal, Kumar, and Pangtey 2008)
	Bangladesh	The paste is used to treat rheumatism.	(Shanavaskhan et al. 2012)
Flower	Arunachal Pradesh, India	Dried flowers are used as an emetic.	(Tsering et al. 2017)

has been listed as "Endangered" by the Government of India in CITES (Convention on International Trade in Endangered Species of Wild Fauna and Flora) Appendix II (Das et al. 2013).

14.3   ETHNOMEDICINAL USES

Different parts of the *R. retusa* plant have been traditionally used as medicines for a very long time (Table 14.1). Roots are used to treat cuts, wounds, rheumatism, menstrual troubles, kidney stones, asthma, vertigo, tuberculosis, and malaria fever. In Nepal, the root has been used as an emollient for treating asthma, tuberculosis, nervous twitching, cramps, rheumatism, kidney stones, and menstrual irregularities (Acharya and Rokaya 1970). In Nagaland, the root is mostly used as herbal medicine in a paste form by mixing it with *Pisum sativum* and consuming it twice a day to cure blood dysentery (Nongdam 2014). The locals of Arunachal Pradesh also use root juice for treating cuts, wounds, menstrual pain; dried flower is also used as an emetic (Tsering et al. 2017).

Paste of leaves is used to treat rheumatism in Uttarakhand and Arunachal Pradesh (Tsering et al. 2017). Leaf paste is also used as an emollient to treat wounds (Nongdam 2014). Leaves have also been used to cure paralysis by rubbing a paste made by mixing its leaves and ghee or with *Datura metel* roots and *Piper nigrum* fruits (Rohani et al. 2018). In Bangladesh, *R. retusa* plant leaves are used to treat rheumatism. The entire plant is also used as an emollient to treat throat inflammation (Shanavaskhan et al. 2012).

14.4   PROPAGATION TECHNIQUES

14.4.1   MICROPROPAGATION OR *IN VITRO* PROPAGATION

Division propagation and seed propagation are traditional breeding methods of *R. retusa* (Xi, Zeng, and Huang 2021). Division propagation can preserve parent traits but has a low efficiency making it unsuitable for factory production, whereas the lack of cotyledon and endosperm in seeds result in incomplete embryo development (Islam and Bhattacharjee 2015). Tissue culture has emerged as a potential method that is not limited by season, region, or climate and can overcome problems such as distant incompatibility and stunted development of hybrid embryos (Thomas and Michael 2007). Orchids are propagated through protocorm-like bodies (PLB) explants in a different culture medium which is then followed by shoot and root formation leading to well-developed plantlets (Figure 14.2) (Chugh, Guha, and Rao 2009). Leaves, stem tips, and root tips have been used as explants for *R. retusa* propagation; a study revealed that the regenerative potential of the various explants differed with shoot showing maximum growth and the least found in the root (Devi and Neelashree 2018). The study also reported Vacin and Went (VW) medium to be better for growth compared to Nitsch and Knudson media where the formation of PLB took place when the explant was still green in color and calli formation from Went turned brown. Naing et al. (2010) reported the successful formation of shoot and root among the micropropagation of seedling culture, thin root section, and thin leaf section on half-strength Murashige and Skoog (MS) medium with thidiazuron (TDZ) α-naphthaleneacetic acid (NAA) and activated charcoal (AC). Other explants such as callus and protocorm mixtures have shown optimum growth in half-strength MS medium with banana puree, NAA, 6-benzylaminopurine (6-BA), and kinetin (KT) (Xi, Zeng, and Huang 2021).

Plantlets from micro shoots have been also attempted which showed effective regeneration eliminating the need for callus induction (Sinha and Jahan 2012). The rapid increase in micro shoots was reported to be due to the supplement of L-glutamine and coconut water. Asymbiotic seed germination has been one of the most used strategies for orchid maintenance and propagation (Yeung 2017). Regeneration protocol of *R. retusa* plant from immature seeds has been developed using callus and PLB (Parab and Krishnan 2012). For callus formation, VW medium supplemented with coconut water was effective, whereas, in terms of PLB formation, MS medium showed maximum growth.

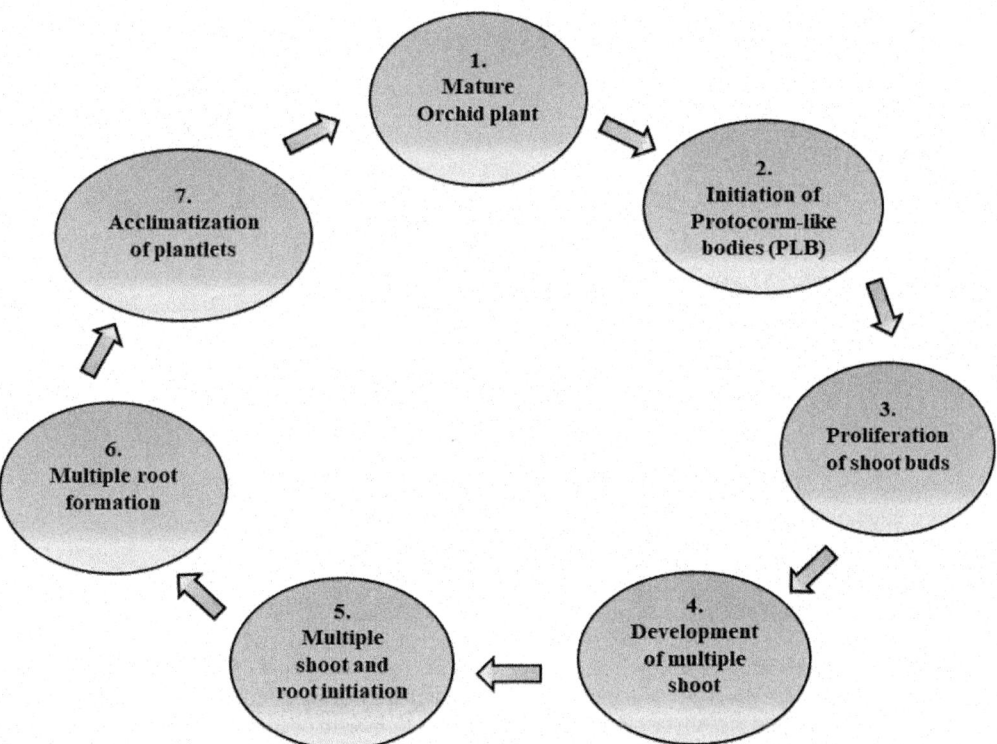

FIGURE 14.2 Micropropagation technique of orchids from protocorm-like bodies (PLB) explant.

R. retusa has been also successfully mass propagated using embryo culture where the correct maturity stage for *R. retusa* was 6 months after pollination, and *in-vitro* seed germination took 20 days for 6-month-old pods (Fonseka 2020).

14.4.2 Effect of Culture Media on Germination

Culture media is important for micropropagation to be successful as it contains essential macroelements, microelements, iron chelate, and supplements such as plant growth regulators, vitamins, complex additives, darkening agents, and a solidifier (Chugh, Guha, and Rao 2009). Plant growth regulators (BA and NAA) and growth additives (coconut water, yeast extract, and peptone) have been tested for seed germination, proliferation, and plantlet development (Lal et al. 2019). MS medium supplemented with coconut water was reported as optimum for germination and PLB formation. Coconut water has a positive effect on explants as it boosts cell proliferation while avoiding mutations, and therefore it is often used with various media (Yam and Arditti 2018).

Different mediums (half-strength MS, MS, Gamborg B5), cytokinins, and auxins have been tested for germination and development of PLBs, where half-strength MS medium supplemented with 6-BA, sucrose, and indoleacetic acid (IAA) was reported to be the best (Bhattacharjee 2015). The study also reported the importance of 6-BA and kinetin for somatic embryogenesis from root and leaf explants. Basal medium with 6-BA showed a high multiplication rate of PLB from green pods (Anil Kumar et al. 2002). Effect of phytagel, sucrose, and photosynthetically active radiation was examined which showed elevated growth compared to their absence in the medium with up to 70% of plantlets surviving when acclimatized.

Different strengths (full, half, and quarter) of MS medium and full-strength MS medium supplemented with 6-BA, NAA, and coconut water were tested for *in vitro* seed germination from immature seeds of *R. retusa* (Figure 14.3) (Oliya et al. 2021). Half and quarter-strength

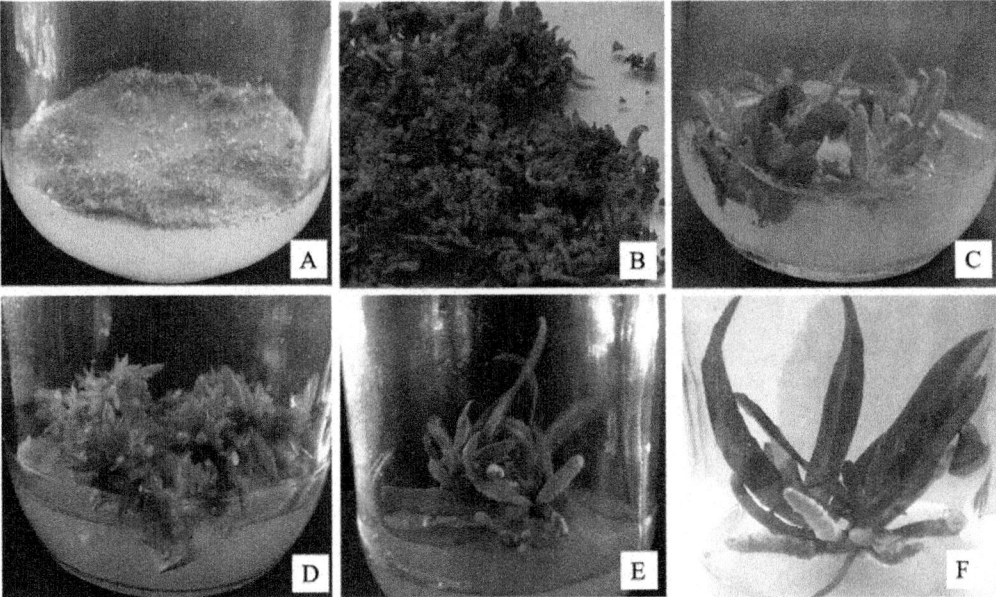

FIGURE 14.3 Germination and development of protocorm, root, and shoot in different strengths of MS medium supplemented with growth regulators. (A, B) Half-strength MS medium; I full-strength MS medium supplemented with 6-BA and NAA; (D, E) full-strength MS medium with coconut water; (F) full-strength MS medium with fungal elicitor.

Source: From (Oliya et al. 2021) with permission (licence no. 5250220314577).

medium were reported to be best for germination and protocorm development showing low nutrient medium to be more effective.

14.5 PHYTOCHEMICAL COMPOUNDS AND THEIR ANTI-DIABETIC PROPERTIES

R. retusa contains a wide range of phytochemical compounds such as phenols, flavonoids, tannins, alkaloids, saponins, and phytosterol with antioxidant, antibacterial, anti-inflammatory, and antiseptic properties (Table 14.2) (Abinash Kumar et al. 2021). Phytocompounds including fucoidan, phenols, tannins, and sterols including a few marine algae are reported to have blood glucose–lowering activities (Zhao et al. 2018). Flavonoids such as naringin, hesperidin, myricetin, rutin, and especially quercetin are found to have inhibition of intestinal glucose absorption, glucose homeostasis, utilization in peripheral tissues, and increased insulin sensitivity (AL-Ishaq et al. 2019).

14.5.1 PHENOLIC COMPOUNDS

Phenolic compounds such as curcumin, ellagic acid, gallic acid, chlorogenic acid, and resveratrol are known for their anti-diabetic, anti-inflammatory, and antioxidation properties and help in maintaining pancreatic β cells and insulin activity (Szkudelski and Szkudelska 2015). Studies reveal that resveratrol enhances enzymatic and clinical limitations for type 1 and type 2 animal models of diabetic nephropathy (Bastianetto, Ménard, and Quirion 2015), type 1 diabetes mellitus–induced cerebrovascular dysfunction and diabetes-induced liver injury (El-Maksoud, Hussein, and Abd El-Maksoud 2013).

TABLE 14.2
Pharmacological Activities of Different Phytochemical Compounds Found in *R. retusa*

Name of Compound	Reported Activity	Reference
Resveratrol	Anti-diabetic	(Szkudelski and Szkudelska 2015)
Curcumin	Anti-diabetic, antiproliferative	(Nishiyama et al. 2005; Chattopadhyay et al. 2004)
Cyclohexene	Anti-inflammatory, antibacterial	(Vuuren and Viljoen 2007)
Hydroxytyrosol	Anti-inflammatory, anti-diabetic, antioxidant, antithrombotic	(Hamden et al. 2009)
Ellagic acid	Antimutagen, antioxidative, anticarcinogenic, anti-diabetic, anti-inflammatory	(Malini, Kanchana, and Rajadurai 2011; Muthenna, Akileshwari, and Reddy 2012)
Steroid alkaloids	Hypoglycemic effect	(Ullah Jan et al. 2018)
Saponins	Anti-diabetic	(Gong et al. 2020)
Terpenoids	Anti-diabetic	(Hadjzadeh et al. 2017)
Damnacanthol-3-O-β-D-primeveroside and lucidin-3-O-β-D-primeveroside	Anti-diabetic	(Kamiya et al. 2008)
1-O-methyl chrysophanol	Anti-diabetic, antihyperglycemic activity	(Chandrasekhar et al. 2021)
Cardiac glycosides	Anti-diabetic	(Tofighi et al. 2017)
3-methoxy-hexane-1,6-diol	Antioxidant, antimicrobial	(Kumar et al. 2021)
1-methylene-2b-hydroxymethyl-3,3-dimethyl-4b-(3-methylbut-2-enyl)-cyclohexane	Antioxidant	(Kumar et al. 2021)
Butyl 9,12,15-octa-decatrienoate	Anti-inflammatory	(Kumar et al. 2021)

Curcumin has been observed for anti-inflammatory, antioxidant, and anti-diabetic activities where it has exhibited hypoglycemic effect for type 2 diabetic KK-Ay in mice due to activation of peroxisome proliferator-activated receptor γ (PPARγ) (Nishiyama et al. 2005). Very low doses of curcumin can inhibit the formation of a galactose-induced cataract, reducing insulin resistance and improving β cell functions (Chuengsamarn et al. 2012).

Ellagic acid has pharmaceutical properties such as antioxidative, anti-diabetic, and anti-inflammatory (Muthenna, Akileshwari, and Reddy 2012). Diabetic rats showed improvement in hyperglycemia, dyslipidemia, liver, and kidney function markers after treatment with ellagic acid, pioglitazone, or their combinations. The treatment of diabetic rats with the same combination significantly increased the expression levels of GLUT4, PPAR-γ, and adiponectin in skeletal muscle (Nankar and Doble 2017).

14.5.2 ALKALOIDS

Alkaloids such as atropine, nicotine, morphine, caffeine, and berberine have been used in the treatment for their inflammatory activities (Habtemariam 2020). Steroid alkaloids isolated from *Sarcococca saligna* were reported to possess hypoglycemic effects and improve diabetes-associated complications (Ullah Jan et al. 2018). Alkaloids of benzylisoquinoline such as palmatine and berberine found in the roots and rhizomes of the Berberidaceae plant family show anti-diabetic activities. Scequinadoline D can be used as a insulin sensitizer that targets adipocytes used in the treatment of type 2 diabetes mellitus. Study have reported isolation of fumiquinazoline alkaloids from the marine fungus *Scedosporium apiospermum* F41–1, which was later evaluated for its anti-diabetic potential by determining its triglyceride-promoting activity using 3T3-L1 adipocytes (C.-J. Li et al. 2020).

Steroids are known for their immunomodulatory antimicrobial, anti-inflammatory, and anti-fungal activities which can be useful in cardiovascular diseases, inflammatory bowel diseases, and type 1 diabetes mellitus (Marahatha et al. 2021). γ-Oryzanol and β-sitosterol are found extensively in rice milk and have anti-diabetic, antioxidative, and anti-inflammatory effects (Biswas et al. 2011).

Saponins can inhibit α-glucosidase, α-amylase, and aldose reductase that are responsible for diabetes mellitus, and they lower the absorption of carbohydrates in the colon and small intestine (Gong et al. 2020). Saponins of *Momordica charantia* L. can regulate the levels of triglycerides and low- and high-density lipoprotein cholesterol, and exhibit significant antihyperlipidemic effects mitigating diabetic complications (Q. Wang et al. 2019). *M. charantia* saponins have an anti-diabetic effect by improving the lipid metabolism disorder, reducing oxidative stress level, and regulating the insulin signaling pathway (Jiang et al. 2020).

14.5.3 TERPENOIDS

Terpenoids are isoprene molecules possessing antifungal, antibacterial, anti-inflammatory, and anti-diabetic activity. Terpenoids are reported to have potential uses for the treatment of anti-diabetic activities by targeting the tyrosine phosphatase, α-amylase, and α-glucosidase enzymes (Kjaerulff et al. 2020). *In vivo* studies report that terpenoids improve the metabolism of glucose by maintaining the glucose and insulin levels and also by preventing the development of insulin resistance (Nazaruk and Borzym-Kluczyk 2015). Terpenoids can activate AMPK, reduce obesity-induced metabolic disorders, such as hyperlipidemia, type 2 diabetes, and insulin resistance (Smitha Grace, Chandran, and Chauhan 2019). *Annona diversifolia* Safford and acyclic terpenoids have antihyperglycemic activity for the treatment of diabetes mellitus where the hydrolysis of complex disaccharides is inhibited and absorption of simple monosaccharides through inhibition of α-glucosidase and selective SGLT-1 inhibition in the small intestine (Valdés et al. 2020).

14.5.4 Quinones

Quinone derivatives such as quinoxalinones, phtalazine, isoquinolones, quinolinones, quinazolines, quinolines, quinazolones, quinazolinone, quinoxalines, N-hydroxypyridones, and phenylhydrazones have been used in the treatment of antihypercholesterolemic, antihyperlipidemic activities, and type 1 diabetes mellitus (Lourenço et al. 2014). Quinones act as antioxidants and protect the cells against oxidative damage and reactive oxygen species (ROS); however, some of the quinone-mediated ROS cause cellular damage due to alkylation against proteins, DNA, and lipids. Anthraquinone has shown potential inhibitory effects against aldose reductase, which is an essential strategy for the attenuation and prevention of diabetic complications (Demir et al. 2019). Aglycon anthraquinones such as rhein, catenarin, aloe-emodin, chrysophanol, and emodin have been reported to have inhibitory activities against α-glucosidase and α-amylase enzymes (Mohammed et al. 2020). Anthraquinones compounds such as damnacanthol-3-O-β-D-primeveroside and lucidin-3-O-β-D- primeveroside, isolated from *Morinda citrifolia* L. roots, are reported to have potent anti-diabetic activities on STZ-induced diabetic mice (Kamiya et al. 2008). A hydroxyanthraquinone (1-O-methyl chrysophanol [OMC]) derived from *Amycolatopsis thermoflava* strain SFMA-103 was found to exhibit moderate antihyperglycemic activity in both *in vitro* and *in vivo* models. This anti-diabetic property of OMC was further confirmed based on in silico molecular interactions with α-amylase and α-glucosidase enzymes (Chandrasekhar et al. 2021).

14.5.5 Cardiac Glycosides

The cardiac glycosides have various medicinal properties and are found in different plant species and mammal tissues. It improves the cardiac output force by increasing the heart rate that enhances the Na^+, K^+-ATPase pump (Patel 2016); moreover, it is used in treatment for various cardiovascular-related aligned diseases and treatment of diabetes. Some of the widely used cardiac glycosides include digitoxin, bufalin, ouabain, digoxin, oleandrin, marinobufagenin, telocinobufagin, and aerobufagenin (Botelho et al. 2019). The cardiac glycosides are steroid compounds that improve myocardial contractility and have cardiotonic biological activity. Various *in vitro* and *in vivo* studies confirmed that the cardiac glycosides present in different plant species possess anti-diabetic activity (Tofighi et al. 2017).

14.6 CONCLUSION

Since ancient times, many plants have been discovered and used as medicines which have eventually led to the production of several plant-based pharmaceuticals. Tribal communities of India have used *R. retusa* to treat wounds, fever, rheumatism, paralysis, and other conditions. Its medicinal and ornamental use has led the species to overexploitation and endangered plant status. Emphasis on the need for micropropagation for ecological restoration of the species is needed as there have not many reported studies on this species to date. The species contains many phytochemicals with antimicrobial, antifungal, anti-diabetic properties. There is a lack of information on the pharmacological activities of the plant, which restricts the development of a pharmaceutical product from *R. retusa*. Much more work on its effect on different diseases is needed.

14.7 OTHER FOODS, HERBS, SPICES, AND BOTANICALS USED IN DIABETES

A variety of herbs and functional foods have been suggested to be effective in glycemic control and improved management of diabetic conditions. Recently, Venkatakrishnan et al. (2019) comprehensively reviewed such functional foods and herbs used by traditional medicinal practitioners in Asia, especially China, Taiwan, and India. Leaves and bark of *Ginkgo biloba* from the family

Ginkgoaceae containing flavonoid glycosides, terpene lactones, and ginkgolic acid show antioxidant and anti-inflammatory properties. Ginkgo biloba extract can inhibit the α-glucosidase synthesis, increasing uptake of peripheral glucose while regulating the AMPK signaling pathway (Aziz et al. 2018). Positive regulation of PPAR-α/γ induces lipoprotein lipase expression and hence lowers TGs level, enhances β oxidation and insulin sensitivity (Rhee et al. 2015). Use of ginkgo biloba alone or supplementation with standard hypoglycemic drugs can have better glycemic control (lowering fasting blood glucose, glycosylated hemoglobin) than placebo in clinical trials with type 2 diabetic patients (Lasaite et al. 2014; Aziz et al. 2018).

Ginseng, a slow-growing perennial herb with fleshy roots is reported to show hypoglycemic activity with ginsenoside Rb1/2/c/d/e/f and g1, panaxadiol, and protopanaxadiol (Nuri et al. 2016). Ginseng effectively inhibits PTP1B and positively regulates various insulin signaling pathways, increasing glycogen synthesis, inhibiting gluconeogenesis, impairing intestinal glucose absorption, and acting as a potent antioxidant and anti-inflammatory, reversing impaired glucose tolerance or insulin resistance (Wang, Wang, and Chan 2013). Data from different clinical trials suggest ginseng supplementation (0.96–13.6 g/day) for 4–20 weeks can significantly lower fasting blood glucose and postprandial insulin in type 2 diabetes patients (Gui et al. 2016).

Leaves of *Gymnema sylvestre*, a perennial woody vine rich in phytocomponents like gymnemic acid, gurmarin, and triterpenoid saponins, possesses potent antioxidant, anti-inflammatory, anti-diabetic properties. Animal and *in vivo* studies suggest lowered intestinal glucose absorption (inhibiting α-amylase and glucosidase), improved glycolysis and glycogenesis, and suppression of gluconeogenesis with *G. sylvestre* (Pothuraju et al. 2014). Supplementation of leaf extract in type 2 diabetes patients showed a significant decrease in blood glucose level and increase in the levels of insulin to maintain glucose homeostasis.

Apart from phytochemicals various functional foods can be adopted in the management regime of type 2 diabetes (Alkhatib et al. 2017). Gel from leaves of *Aloe vera*, a succulent plant of tropical and subtropical region is particularly rich in carbohydrates, protein, sterols, lignins, saponins. Phytoconstituents such as aloresin A, lophenol, cycloartenol, and emodin are responsible for hypoglycemic properties (Kaur, Fernandez, and Sim 2017). Active constituents regulate various insulin signaling pathways, lower glucose output, increase glucose input (uptake), inhibit glucose absorption (α-glucosidase), and delay gastric emptying (Pothuraju et al. 2016). Reduced fasting blood glucose, HbA$_{1c}$ was observed among type 2 diabetes patient participants in randomized, double-blind clinical trial following supplemental intake of *A. vera* (capsule, 600 mg/day) for 2 months (Huseini et al. 2012).

Fruits of bitter melon (*Momordica charantia*) containing an array of phytoactive compounds, including sterols and triterpenes like charantin, vicine, and cucurbitane show an insulinomimetic property, inhibiting glucose absorption in the gut (potent α-glucosidase), preserving β cells (insulin secretagogue), and impeding gluconeogenesis and glycogenolysis (Governa et al. 2018). Consumption of bitter melon juice has been shown to lower mean blood glucose level in type 2 diabetes patients in clinical trials (Selvakumar et al. 2017).

Flavored spice from the inner bark of *Cinnamonum cassia* (Chinese), *C. verum*, or *C. zeylanicum* contains cinnamaldehyde, cinnamic acid, and tannins and is known for effective regulation of glucose homeostasis by increasing insulin secretion and glucose uptake and inhibiting intestinal and pancreatic amylase and glucosidase enzymes (Governa et al. 2018). Cinnamon administration with a standard hypoglycemic drug can substantially lower FBG and HbA$_{1c}$ levels improving glycemic control in type 2 diabetes patients (Lu et al. 2012). *Fenugreek*, used as a spice, primarily contains 4-hydroxyisleucine, trigonelline, saponins and can improve sensitivity of insulin receptors, inhibit α-amylase, sucrase, and α-glycosidase, and delay gastric emptying (K. Kumar et al. 2015). Other spices such as garlic (*Allium sativum* L.), ginger (*Zingiber officinale*), and turmeric (*Curcuma longa*) are well documented for their anti-diabetic properties.

Though this list is far from being an exhaustive representation, it definitely indicates the vast phytochemical reserve potentially available or to be explored for diabetic management. A few exhaustive reviews published in recent years may be consulted for further information (Jayaraman et al. 2021; Willcox et al. 2021; Tripathy, Sahoo, and Sahoo 2021).

14.8 TOXICITY AND CAUTIONARY NOTES

No rigorously controlled clinical trial studies have been conducted on *R. retusa* extract. Most studies are based on *in vitro* assays, and a few suggest pharmacological activities in animal studies. Al-Amin et al. studied analgesic activity of *R. retusa* extract on acetic acid–induced writhing and carrageenan- and formaldehyde-induced paw edema in mice models (Al-Amin, Sultana, and Hossain 2011). The authors observed 35.81% inhibition of acetic acid–induced writhing and 14.32% mean inhibition of carrageenan-induced paw edema at doses of 400 mg/kg. Methanolic extract *R. retusa* leaves screened for toxicity against brine shrimp had LC_{50} values less than 100 μg/ml (Radhika, Murthy, and Grace 2013). Chloroform extract *R. retusa* has been shown to be effective against *Bacillus subtilis* and *Vibrio cholerae*, while chloroform extract (10 mg/ml) exhibited antifungal activity against *Penicillium* sp., *Rhizopus* sp., and *Aspergillus niger* (Saxena 2020). Diethyl ether fraction of the roots of *R. retusa* has been shown to have promising leishmanicidal activity with IC_{50} values of 56.04 and 18.4 μg/mL against promastigotes and intracellular amastigotes, respectively (Bhatnagar et al. 2017). The author observed negligible cytotoxic effect from active fractions of extract against normal J774G8 murine macrophages in MTT assay, though parasitic cells were largely affected at those concentrations (100.7 ± 1.7 μg/mL). Though potential medicinal application of *R. retusa* is widely implicated, detailed *in vivo* and clinical trials studies need to be conducted.

14.9 SUMMARY POINTS

- This chapter focuses on the anti-diabetic properties of the foxtail orchid.
- Foxtail orchids are mainly found in the North East region of India.
- The species has been used to treat cuts, wounds, rheumatism, and menstrual troubles, among other conditions.
- The plant has been listed as "Endangered" by the Government of India in CITES Appendix II.
- Phytochemical compounds such as alkaloids, quinones, terpenoids, and cardiac glycosides from *R. retusa* show anti-diabetic properties.

REFERENCES

Acharya, K.P., and M.B. Rokaya. 1970. "Medicinal Orchids of Nepal: Are They Well Protected?" *Our Nature* 8 (1): 82–91. https://doi.org/10.3126/on.v8i1.4315.

Adhikari, Yagya P., Anke Jentsch, and Ripu M. Kunwar. 2021. "*Rhynchostylis Retusa* (L.) Blume Orchidaceae." In Kunwar, R.M., Sher, H., Bussmann, R.W. (eds) *Ethnobotany of the Himalayas. Ethnobotany of Mountain Regions*, 1–6. Cham: Springer. https://doi.org/10.1007/978-3-030-45597-2_264-1.

Akhter, M., M. Hoque, M. Rahman, and M. K. Huda. 2017. "Ethnobotanical Investigation of Some Orchids Used by Five Communities of Cox's Bazar and Chittagong Hill Tracts Districts of Bangladesh." *Journal of Medicinal Plants Studies* 5 (3): 265–268.

Al-Amin, M., G.N.N. Sultana, and C.F. Hossain. 2011. "Analgesic and Anti-Inflammatory Activities of Rhynchostylis Retusa." *Biology and Medicine* 3 (5): 55–59.

AL-Ishaq, R.K., M. Abotaleb, P. Kubatka, K. Kajo, and D. Büsselberg. 2019. "Flavonoids and Their Anti-Diabetic Effects: Cellular Mechanisms and Effects to Improve Blood Sugar Levels." *Biomolecules* 9 (9): 430. https://doi.org/10.3390/biom9090430.

Alkhatib, Ahmad, Catherine Tsang, Ali Tiss, Theeshan Bahorun, Hossein Arefanian, Roula Barake, Abdelkrim Khadir, and Jaakko Tuomilehto. 2017. "Functional Foods and Lifestyle Approaches for Diabetes Prevention and Management." *Nutrients* 9 (12): 1310. https://doi.org/10.3390/nu9121310.

Aziz, Tavga, Saad Hussain, Taha Mahwi, Zheen Aorahman Ahmed, Heshu Rahman, and Abdullah Rasedee. 2018. "The Efficacy and Safety of Ginkgo Biloba Extract as an Adjuvant in Type 2 Diabetes Mellitus Patients Ineffectively Managed with Metformin: A Double-Blind, Randomized, Placebo-Controlled Trial." *Drug Design, Development and Therapy* 12 (April): 735–742. https://doi.org/10.2147/DDDT.S157113.

Bastianetto, Stéphane, Caroline Ménard, and Rémi Quirion. 2015. "Neuroprotective Action of Resveratrol." *Biochimica et Biophysica Acta (BBA) – Molecular Basis of Disease* 1852 (6): 1195–1201. https://doi.org/10.1016/j.bbadis.2014.09.011.

Bhatnagar, Manisha, Nandan Sarkar, Nigam Gandharv, Ona Apang, Sarman Singh, and Sabari Ghosal. 2017. "Evaluation of Antimycobacterial, Leishmanicidal and Antibacterial Activity of Three Medicinal Orchids of Arunachal Pradesh, India." *BMC Complementary and Alternative Medicine* 17 (1): 379. https://doi.org/10.1186/s12906-017-1884-z.

Bhattacharjee, Bakul, S.M. Shahinul Islam. 2015. "The Effect of PGRs on in Vitro Development of Protocorms, Regeneration and Mass Multiplication Derived from Immature Seeds of *Rhynchostylis Retusa* (L.) Blume." *Global Journal of Bio-Science and Biotechnology* 4 (1): 121–127.

Biswas, Sinchan, Debabrata Sircar, Adinpunya Mitra, and Bratati De. 2011. "Phenolic Constituents and Antioxidant Properties of Some Varieties of Indian Rice." *Nutrition & Food Science* 41 (2): 123–135. https://doi.org/10.1108/00346651111117391.

Botelho, Ana Flávia M., Felipe Pierezan, Benito Soto-Blanco, and Marília Martins Melo. 2019. "A Review of Cardiac Glycosides: Structure, Toxicokinetics, Clinical Signs, Diagnosis and Antineoplastic Potential." *Toxicon* 158 (February): 63–68. https://doi.org/10.1016/j.toxicon.2018.11.429.

Chakrabarti, Ranjan, and Ramanujam Rajagopalan. 2002. "Diabetes and Insulin Resistance Associated Disorders: Disease and the Therapy." *Current Science* 83 (12): 1533–1538.

Chandrasekhar, Cheemalamarri, Hemshikha Rajpurohit, Kalpana Javaji, Madhusudana Kuncha, Aravind Setti, A. Zehra Ali, Ashok K. Tiwari, Sunil Misra, and C. Ganesh Kumar. 2021. "Anti-Hyperglycemic and Genotoxic Studies of 1-O-Methyl Chrysophanol, a New Anthraquinone Isolated from Amycolatopsis Thermoflava Strain SFMA-103." *Drug and Chemical Toxicology* 44 (2): 148–160. https://doi.org/10.1080/01480545.2018.1551406.

Chattopadhyay, Ishita, Kaushik Biswas, Uday Bandyopadhyay, and Ranajit K. Banerjee. 2004. "Turmeric and Curcumin: Biological Actions and Medicinal Applications." *Current Science*, 87 (1): 44–53.

Chuengsamarn, Somlak, Suthee Rattanamongkolgul, Rataya Luechapudiporn, Chada Phisalaphong, and Siwanon Jirawatnotai. 2012. "Curcumin Extract for Prevention of Type 2 Diabetes." *Diabetes Care* 35 (11): 2121–2127. https://doi.org/10.2337/dc12-0116.

Chugh, Samira, Satyakam Guha, and I. Usha Rao. 2009. "Micropropagation of Orchids: A Review on the Potential of Different Explants." *Scientia Horticulturae* 122 (4): 507–520. https://doi.org/10.1016/j.scienta.2009.07.016.

Das, Amar Jyoti, Mohammad Athar, Manoj Kumar, and Rajesh Kumar. 2013. "FTIR Analysis for Screening Variation in Antimicrobial Activity of Fresh and Dried Leaf Extract of Rhynchostylis Retusa: A Threatened Orchid Species of Assam, North East India." *International Research Journal of Pharmacy* 4 (7): 187–189. https://doi.org/10.7897/2230-8407.04741.

Demir, Yeliz, Muhammet Serhat Özaslan, Hatice Esra Duran, Ömer İrfan Küfrevioğlu, and Şükrü Beydemir. 2019. "Inhibition Effects of Quinones on Aldose Reductase: Antidiabetic Properties." *Environmental Toxicology and Pharmacology* 70 (August): 103195. https://doi.org/10.1016/j.etap.2019.103195.

Devi, Sunitabala Y., and N. Neelashree. 2018. "Micropropagation of the Monopodial Orchid, Rhynchostylis Retusa (L.)." *International Journal of Life Sciences International* 6 (1): 181–186.

El-Maksoud, Hussein, Mohammed A. Hussein, and Hussein Abd El-Maksoud. 2013. "Biochemical Effects of Resveratrol and Curcumin Combination on Obese Diabetic Rats." *Molecular & Clinical Pharmacology* 2013 (1): 1–10.

Fonseka, Kumari. 2020. "Asymbiotic Seed Germination, Mass Propagation and Conservation of Fox-Tail Orchid, Rhynchostylis Retusa L. Blume: An Endangered Orchid." *Asian Journal of Conservation Biology* 9 (2): 275–279.

Gong, Xue, Xue Li, Agula Bo, Ru-Yu Shi, Qin-Yu Li, Lu-Jing Lei, Lei Zhang, and Min-Hui Li. 2020. "The Interactions between Gut Microbiota and Bioactive Ingredients of Traditional Chinese Medicines: A Review." *Pharmacological Research* 157 (July): 104824. https://doi.org/10.1016/j.phrs.2020.104824.

Governa, Paolo, Giulia Baini, Vittoria Borgonetti, Giulia Cettolin, Daniela Giachetti, Anna Magnano, Elisabetta Miraldi, and Marco Biagi. 2018. "Phytotherapy in the Management of Diabetes: A Review." *Molecules* 23 (1): 105. https://doi.org/10.3390/molecules23010105.

Gui, Qi-feng, Zhe-rong Xu, Ke-ying Xu, and Yun-mei Yang. 2016. "The Efficacy of Ginseng-Related Therapies in Type 2 Diabetes Mellitus." *Medicine* 95 (6): e2584. https://doi.org/10.1097/MD. 0000000000002584.

Habtemariam, Solomon. 2020. "Berberine Pharmacology and the Gut Microbiota: A Hidden Therapeutic Link." *Pharmacological Research* 155 (May): 104722. https://doi.org/10.1016/j.phrs.2020.104722.

Hadjzadeh, Mousa-Al-Reza, Ziba Rajaei, Esmaeil Khodaei, Maryam Malek, and Habib Ghanbari. 2017. "Rheum Turkestanicum Rhizomes Possess Anti-Hypertriglyceridemic, but Not Hypoglycemic or Hepatoprotective Effect in Experimental Diabetes." *Avicenna Journal of Phytomedicine* 7 (1): 1–9.

Hamden, Khaled, Noureddine Allouche, Mohamed Damak, and Abdelfattah Elfeki. 2009. "Hypoglycemic and Antioxidant Effects of Phenolic Extracts and Purified Hydroxytyrosol from Olive Mill Waste in Vitro and in Rats." *Chemico-Biological Interactions* 180 (3): 421–432. https://doi.org/10.1016/j.cbi.2009.04.002.

Hegde, S. N. (Sadanand N.). 1984. *Orchids of Arunāchal Pradesh*. Itanagar, India: Forest Dept., Arunachal Pradesh.

Hinsley, Amy, Hugo J. de Boer, Michael F. Fay, Stephan W. Gale, Lauren M. Gardiner, Rajasinghe S. Gunasekara, Pankaj Kumar, et al. 2018. "A Review of the Trade in Orchids and Its Implications for Conservation." *Botanical Journal of the Linnean Society* 186 (4): 435–455. https://doi.org/10.1093/botlinnean/box083.

Huseini, Hasan, Saeed Kianbakht, Reza Hajiaghaee, and Fataneh Dabaghian. 2012. "Anti-Hyperglycemic and Anti-Hypercholesterolemic Effects of Aloe Vera Leaf Gel in Hyperlipidemic Type 2 Diabetic Patients: A Randomized Double-Blind Placebo-Controlled Clinical Trial." *Planta Medica* 78 (4): 311–316. https://doi.org/10.1055/s-0031-1280474.

Islam, S.M. Shahinul, and Bakul Bhattacharjee. 2015. "Plant Regeneration through Somatic Embryogenesis from Leaf and Root Explants of Rhynchostylis Retusa (L.) Blume." *Applied Biological Research* 17 (2): 158. https://doi.org/10.5958/0974-4517.2015.00025.7.

Jalal, Jeewan, Pankaj Kumar, and Y. Pangtey. 2008. "Ethnomedicinal Orchids of Uttarakhand, Western Himalaya." *Ethnobotanical Leaflets* 12: 1227–1230.

Jayaraman, Selvaraj, Anitha Roy, Srinivasan Vengadassalapathy, Ramya Sekar, Vishnu Priya Veeraraghavan, Ponnulakshmi Rajagopal, Gayathri Rengasamy, Raktim Mukherjee, Durairaj Sekar, and Reji Manjunathan. 2021. "An Overview on the Therapeutic Function of Foods Enriched with Plant Sterols in Diabetes Management." *Antioxidants* 10 (12): 1903. https://doi.org/10.3390/antiox10121903.

Jiang, Shuang, Lei Xu, Yan Xu, Yushan Guo, Lin Wei, Xueting Li, and Wu Song. 2020. "Antidiabetic Effect of Momordica Charantia Saponins in Rats Induced by High-Fat Diet Combined with STZ." *Electronic Journal of Biotechnology* 43 (January): 41–47. https://doi.org/10.1016/j.ejbt.2019.12.001.

Kamiya, Kohei, Wakako Hamabe, Sachiko Harada, Rie Murakami, Shogo Tokuyama, and Toshiko Satake. 2008. "Chemical Constituents of Morinda Citrifolia Roots Exhibit Hypoglycemic Effects in Streptozotocin-Induced Diabetic Mice." *Biological and Pharmaceutical Bulletin* 31 (5): 935–938. https://doi.org/10.1248/bpb.31.935.

Kaur, Narabjit, Ritin Fernandez, and Jenny Sim. 2017. "Effect of Aloe Vera on Glycemic Outcomes in Patients with Diabetes Mellitus." *JBI Database of Systematic Reviews and Implementation Reports* 15 (9): 2300–2306. https://doi.org/10.11124/JBISRIR-2016-002958.

Kjaerulff, Louise, Alexander Baekager Just Jensen, Chi Ndi, Susan Semple, Birger Lindberg Møller, and Dan Staerk. 2020. "Isolation, Structure Elucidation and PTP1B Inhibitory Activity of Serrulatane Diterpenoids from the Roots of Myoporum Insulare." *Phytochemistry Letters* 39 (October): 49–56. https://doi.org/10.1016/j.phytol.2020.07.001.

Kumar, Abinash, Biswanath Mahanty, Rajiv Chandra Dev Goswami, Prajjalendra Kumar Barooah, and Bula Choudhury. 2021. "In Vitro Antidiabetic, Antioxidant Activities and GC-MS Analysis of Rhynchostylis Retusa and Euphorbia Neriifolia Leaf Extracts." *3 Biotech* 11 (7): 315. https://doi.org/10.1007/s13205-021-02869-7.

Kumar, Anil, S. K. Nandi, N. Bag, and L.M.S. Palni. 2002. "Tissue Culture Studies in Two Important Orchid Taxa : *Rhynchostylis Retusa* (L.) Bl. and *Cymbidium Elegans* Lindl." In Nandi, S.K., Palni, L.M.S., Kumar, A. (eds) *Role of Plant Tissue Culture in Biodiversity Conservation and Economic Development*, 124, 113–124. Nainital, India: Gyanodaya Prakashan.

Kumar, Kamakhya, Shiv Kumar, Arunima Datta, and Arup Bandyopadhyay. 2015. "Effect of Fenugreek Seeds on Glycemia and Dyslipidemia in Patients with Type 2 Diabetes Mellitus." *International Journal of Medical Science and Public Health* 4 (7): 997. https://doi.org/10.5455/ijmsph.2015.11032015202.

Lal, Ankita, Manu Pant, A. Datta, and L.M.S. Palni. 2019. "In Vitro Propagation of Rhynchostylis Retusa (L.) Blume through Immature Seed Culture." *Ecology, Environment and Conservation* 26: 46–51.

Lasaite, Lina, Asta Spadiene, Nijole Savickiene, Andrejs Skesters, and Alise Silova. 2014. "The Effect of Ginkgo Biloba and Camellia Sinensis Extracts on Psychological State and Glycemic Control in Patients with Type 2 Diabetes Mellitus." *Natural Product Communications* 9 (9): 1934578X1400900. https://doi.org/10.1177/1934578X1400900931.

Li, Chan-Juan, Pei-Nan Chen, Hou-Jin Li, Taifo Mahmud, Dong-Lan Wu, Jun Xu, and Wen-Jian Lan. 2020. "Potential Antidiabetic Fumiquinazoline Alkaloids from the Marine-Derived Fungus Scedosporium Apiospermum F41–1." *Journal of Natural Products* 83 (4): 1082–1091. https://doi.org/10.1021/acs.jnatprod.9b01096.

Li, Chengru, Na Dong, Yamei Zhao, Shasha Wu, Zhongjian Liu, and Junwen Zhai. 2021. "A Review for the Breeding of Orchids: Current Achievements and Prospects." *Horticultural Plant Journal* 7 (5): 380–392. https://doi.org/10.1016/j.hpj.2021.02.006.

Lourenço, Elaine V., Maida Wong, Bevra H. Hahn, M. Fernando Palma-Diaz, and Brian J. Skaggs. 2014. "Laquinimod Delays and Suppresses Nephritis in Lupus-Prone Mice and Affects Both Myeloid and Lymphoid Immune Cells." *Arthritis & Rheumatology* 66 (3): 674–685. https://doi.org/10.1002/art.38259.

Lu, Ting, Hongguang Sheng, Johnna Wu, Yuan Cheng, Jianming Zhu, and Yan Chen. 2012. "Cinnamon Extract Improves Fasting Blood Glucose and Glycosylated Hemoglobin Level in Chinese Patients with Type 2 Diabetes." *Nutrition Research* 32 (6): 408–412. https://doi.org/10.1016/j.nutres.2012.05.003.

Lubinsky, Pesach, Séverine Bory, Juan Hernández Hernández, Seung-Chul Kim, and Arturo Gómez-Pompa. 2008. "Origins and Dispersal of Cultivated Vanilla (Vanilla Planifolia Jacks. [Orchidaceae])." *Economic Botany* 62 (2): 127–138. https://doi.org/10.1007/s12231-008-9014-y.

Malini, Palanisamy, Ganesan Kanchana, and Murugan Rajadurai. 2011. "Antibiabetic Efficacy of Ellagic Acid in Streptozotocin-Induced Diabetes Mellitus in Albino Wistar Rats." *Asian Journal of Pharmaceutical and Clinical Research* 4 (3): 127–128.

Marahatha, Rishab, Kabita Gyawali, Kabita Sharma, Narayan Gyawali, Parbati Tandan, Ashma Adhikari, Grishma Timilsina, et al. 2021. "Pharmacologic Activities of Phytosteroids in Inflammatory Diseases: Mechanism of Action and Therapeutic Potentials." *Phytotherapy Research* 35 (9): 5103–5124. https://doi.org/10.1002/ptr.7138.

Mohammed, Aminu, Mohammed Auwal Ibrahim, Nasir Tajuddeen, Abubakar Babando Aliyu, and Murtala Bindawa Isah. 2020. "Antidiabetic Potential of Anthraquinones: A Review." *Phytotherapy Research* 34 (3): 486–504. https://doi.org/10.1002/ptr.6544.

Muthenna, Puppala, Chandrasekhar Akileshwari, and G. Bhanuprakash Reddy. 2012. "Ellagic Acid, a New Antiglycating Agent: Its Inhibition of N ε-(Carboxymethyl)Lysine." *Biochemical Journal* 442 (1): 221–230. https://doi.org/10.1042/BJ20110846.

Naing, A. H., I. Park, Y. Hwang, Jae-Dong Chung, and K. Lim. 2010. "In Vitro Micropropagation and Conservation of Rhynchostylis Retusa BL." *Horticulture Environment and Biotechnology* 51 (5): 440–444.

Nankar, Rakesh P., and Mukesh Doble. 2017. "Hybrid Drug Combination: Anti-Diabetic Treatment of Type 2 Diabetic Wistar Rats with Combination of Ellagic Acid and Pioglitazone." *Phytomedicine* 37 (December): 4–9. https://doi.org/10.1016/j.phymed.2017.10.014.

Nazaruk, J., and M. Borzym-Kluczyk. 2015. "The Role of Triterpenes in the Management of Diabetes Mellitus and Its Complications." *Phytochemistry Reviews* 14 (4): 675–690. https://doi.org/10.1007/S11101-014-9369-X/FIGURES/7.

Ninawe, A. S., and T. S. Swapna. 2017. "Orchid Diversity of Northeast India – Traditional Knowledge and Strategic Plant for Conservation." *The Journal of The Orchid Society of India* 31: 41–56.

Nishiyama, Tozo, Tatsumasa Mae, Hideyuki Kishida, Misuzu Tsukagawa, Yoshihiro Mimaki, Minpei Kuroda, Yutaka Sashida, et al. 2005. "Curcuminoids and Sesquiterpenoids in Turmeric (Curcuma Longa L.) Suppress an Increase in Blood Glucose Level in Type 2 Diabetic KK-A y Mice." *Journal of Agricultural and Food Chemistry* 53 (4): 959–963. https://doi.org/10.1021/jf0483873.

Nongdam, P. 2014. "Ethno-Medicinal Uses of Some Orchids of Nagaland, North-East India." *Research Journal of Medicinal Plant* 8 (3): 126–139. https://doi.org/10.3923/rjmp.2014.126.139.

Nuri, Thimarul Huda Mat, June Choon Wai Yee, Manish Gupta, Muhammad Anwar Nawab Khan, and Long Chiau Ming. 2016. "A Review of Panax Ginseng as an Herbal Medicine." *Archives of Pharmacy Practice* 7 (5): 61. https://doi.org/10.4103/2045-080X.183030.

Nyambe-Silavwe, Hilda, Jose A. Villa-Rodriguez, Idolo Ifie, Melvin Holmes, Ebru Aydin, Jane Møller Jensen, and Gary Williamson. 2015. "Inhibition of Human α-Amylase by Dietary Polyphenols." *Journal of Functional Foods* 19 (December): 723–732. https://doi.org/10.1016/j.jff.2015.10.003.

Oliya, Bal Kumari, Krishna Chand, Laxmi Sen Thakuri, Manju Kanu Baniya, Anil Kumar Sah, and Bijaya Pant. 2021. "Assessment of Genetic Stability of Micropropagated Plants of Rhynchostylis Retusa (L.) Using RAPD Markers." *Scientia Horticulturae* 281 (April): 110008. https://doi.org/10.1016/j.scienta.2021.110008.

Parab, G. V., and S. Krishnan. 2012. "Rapid in Vitro Mass Multiplication of Orchids Aerides Maculosa Lindl. and Rhynchostylis Retusa (L.) Bl. from Immature Seeds." *Indian Journal of Biotechnology* 11: 288–294.

Patel, Seema. 2016. "Plant-Derived Cardiac Glycosides: Role in Heart Ailments and Cancer Management." *Biomedicine & Pharmacotherapy* 84 (December): 1036–1041. https://doi.org/10.1016/j.biopha.2016.10.030.

Pothuraju, Ramesh, Raj Kumar Sharma, Jayasimha Chagalamarri, Surender Jangra, and Praveen Kumar Kavadi. 2014. "A Systematic Review of Gymnema Sylvestre in Obesity and Diabetes Management." *Journal of the Science of Food and Agriculture* 94 (5): 834–840. https://doi.org/10.1002/jsfa.6458.

Pothuraju, Ramesh, Raj Kumar Sharma, Suneel Kumar Onteru, Satvinder Singh, and Shaik Abdul Hussain. 2016. "Hypoglycemic and Hypolipidemic Effects of Aloe Vera Extract Preparations: A Review." *Phytotherapy Research* 30 (2): 200–207. https://doi.org/10.1002/ptr.5532.

Radhika, B., Jvvsn Murthy, and D. Nirmala Grace. 2013. "Antifungal and Cytotoxic Activities of Medicinal Important Orchid Rhynchostylis Retusa Blume." *International Journal of Advanced Research* 1 (7): 31–35.

Rhee, Ki-Jong, Chang Gun Lee, Sung Woo Kim, Dong-Hyeon Gim, Hyun-Cheol Kim, and Bae Dong Jung. 2015. "Extract of Ginkgo Biloba Ameliorates Streptozotocin-Induced Type 1 Diabetes Mellitus and High-Fat Diet-Induced Type 2 Diabetes Mellitus in Mice." *International Journal of Medical Sciences* 12 (12): 987–994. https://doi.org/10.7150/ijms.13339.

Rohani, Shahanoor, Md Salahuddin Sarder, Moutushi Khan Tuti, Khoshnur Jannat, Mohammed Rahmatullah, and Tarana Afrooz. 2018. "Rhynchostylis Retusa (L.) Blume: A Potential Plant to Cure Paralysis." *Journal of Medicinal Plants Studies* 6 (4): 20–21.

Saxena, Shaiphali. 2020. "The Current Research Status of Endangered Rhynchostylis Retusa (L.) Blume: A Review." *Asian Journal of Research in Botany* 4 (2): 16–25.

Selvakumar, G., G. Shathirapathiy, R. Jainraj, and P. Yuvaraj Paul. 2017. "Immediate Effect of Bitter Gourd, Ash Gourd, Knol-Khol Juices on Blood Sugar Levels of Patients with Type 2 Diabetes Mellitus: A Pilot Study." *Journal of Traditional and Complementary Medicine* 7 (4): 526–531. https://doi.org/10.1016/j.jtcme.2017.01.009.

Shanavaskhan, A.E., M. Sivadasan, Ahmed H. Alfarhan, and Jacob Thomas. 2012. "Ethnomedicinal Aspects of Angiospermic Epiphytes and Parasites of Kerala, India." *Indian Journal of Traditional Knowledge* 11 (2): 250–258.

Sinha, Pinaki, and Miskat Ara Akhter Jahan. 2012. "Clonal Propagation of Rhynchostylis Retusa (Lin.) Blume through in Vitro Culture and Their Establishment in the Nursery." *Plant Tissue Culture and Biotechnology* 22 (1): 1–11. https://doi.org/10.3329/ptcb.v22i1.11242.

Smitha Grace, S. R., Girish Chandran, and Jyoti Bala Chauhan. 2019. "Terpenoids: An Activator of 'Fuel-Sensing Enzyme AMPK' with Special Emphasis on Antidiabetic Activity." In *Plant and Human Health, Volume 2*, 227–244. Cham: Springer International Publishing. https://doi.org/10.1007/978-3-030-03344-6_9.

Sundararaju, V. 2020. "India Must Conserve Its Orchid Wealth." *DownToEarth*, August 17, 2020.

Szkudelski, Tomasz, and Katarzyna Szkudelska. 2015. "Resveratrol and Diabetes: From Animal to Human Studies." *Biochimica et Biophysica Acta (BBA) – Molecular Basis of Disease* 1852 (6): 1145–1154. https://doi.org/10.1016/j.bbadis.2014.10.013.

Teoh, Seong Lin, and Srijit Das. 2018. "Phytochemicals and Their Effective Role in the Treatment of Diabetes Mellitus: A Short Review." *Phytochemistry Reviews* 17 (5): 1111–1128. https://doi.org/10.1007/s11101-018-9575-z.

Thomas, T. Dennis, and Alwin Michael. 2007. "High-Frequency Plantlet Regeneration and Multiple Shoot Induction from Cultured Immature Seeds of Rhynchostylis Retusa Blume., an Exquisite Orchid." *Plant Biotechnology Reports* 1 (4): 243–249. https://doi.org/10.1007/s11816-007-0038-z.

Tofighi, Zahra, Fahimeh Moradi-Afrapoli, Samad Nejad Ebrahimi, Saied Goodarzi, Abbas Hadjiakhoondi, Markus Neuburger, Matthias Hamburger, Mohammad Abdollahi, and Narguess Yassa. 2017. "Securigenin Glycosides as Hypoglycemic Principles of Securigera Securidaca Seeds." *Journal of Natural Medicines* 71 (1): 272–280. https://doi.org/10.1007/s11418-016-1060-7.

Tripathy, Bichitrananda, Nityananda Sahoo, and Sudhir Kumar Sahoo. 2021. "Trends in Diabetes Care with Special Emphasis to Medicinal Plants: Advancement and Treatment." *Biocatalysis and Agricultural Biotechnology* 33 (May): 102014. https://doi.org/10.1016/j.bcab.2021.102014.

Tsering, Jambey, Ngilyang Tam, Hui Tag, Baikuntha Jyoti Gogoi, and Ona Apang. 2017. "Medicinal Orchids of Arunachal Pradesh: A Review." *Bulletin of Arunachal Forest Research* 32 (1 & 2): 1–16.

Ullah Jan, Naeem, Amjad Ali, Bashir Ahmad, Naveed Iqbal, Achyut Adhikari, Inayat-ur-Rehman, Abid Ali, et al. 2018. "Evaluation of Antidiabetic Potential of Steroidal Alkaloid of Sarcococca Saligna." *Biomedicine & Pharmacotherapy* 100 (April): 461–466. https://doi.org/10.1016/j.biopha.2018.01.008.

Valdés, Miguel, Fernando Calzada, Jessica Elena Mendieta-Wejebe, Verenice Merlín-Lucas, Claudia Velázquez, and Elizabeth Barbosa. 2020. "Antihyperglycemic Effects of Annona Diversifolia Safford and Its Acyclic Terpenoids: α-Glucosidase and Selective SGLT1 Inhibitors." *Molecules* 25 (15): 3361. https://doi.org/10.3390/molecules25153361.

Venkatakrishnan, Kamesh, Hui-Fang Chiu, and Chin-Kun Wang. 2019. "Popular Functional Foods and Herbs for the Management of Type-2-Diabetes Mellitus: A Comprehensive Review with Special Reference to Clinical Trials and Its Proposed Mechanism." *Journal of Functional Foods* 57 (June): 425–438. https://doi.org/10.1016/j.jff.2019.04.039.

Vuuren, S. F. van, and A. M. Viljoen. 2007. "Antimicrobial Activity of Limonene Enantiomers and 1,8-Cineole Alone and in Combination." *Flavour and Fragrance Journal* 22 (6): 540–544. https://doi.org/10.1002/ffj.1843.

Wang, Qi, Xueyan Wu, Fulin Shi, and Yang Liu. 2019. "Comparison of Antidiabetic Effects of Saponins and Polysaccharides from Momordica Charantia L. in STZ-Induced Type 2 Diabetic Mice." *Biomedicine & Pharmacotherapy* 109 (January): 744–750. https://doi.org/10.1016/j.biopha.2018.09.098.

Wang, Zhijun, Jeffrey Wang, and Patrick Chan. 2013. "Treating Type 2 Diabetes Mellitus with Traditional Chinese and Indian Medicinal Herbs." *Evidence-Based Complementary and Alternative Medicine* 2013: 1–17. https://doi.org/10.1155/2013/343594.

Willcox, Merlin L., Christina Elugbaju, Marwah Al-Anbaki, Mark Lown, and Bertrand Graz. 2021. "Effectiveness of Medicinal Plants for Glycaemic Control in Type 2 Diabetes: An Overview of Meta-Analyses of Clinical Trials." *Frontiers in Pharmacology* 12 (November). https://doi.org/10.3389/fphar.2021.777561.

Xi, Yinkai, Biao Zeng, and Hengyu Huang. 2021. "Rapid Propagation of Rhynchostylis Retusa in Vitro." *Phyton* 90 (3): 987–1001. https://doi.org/10.32604/phyton.2021.014218.

Yam, Tim W., and J. Arditti. 2018. "Orchid Micropropagation: An Overview of Approaches and Methodologies." In Lee, Y.I., Yeung, E.T. (eds) *Orchid Propagation: From Laboratories to Greenhouses – Methods and Protocols*, 151–178. New York: Springer Protocols Handbooks, Humana Press. https://doi.org/10.1007/978-1-4939-7771-0_7.

Yeung, Edward C. 2017. "A Perspective on Orchid Seed and Protocorm Development." *Botanical Studies* 58 (1): 33. https://doi.org/10.1186/s40529-017-0188-4.

Zhang, Shibao, Yingjie Yang, Jiawei Li, Jiao Qin, Wei Zhang, Wei Huang, and Hong Hu. 2018. "Physiological Diversity of Orchids." *Plant Diversity* 40 (4): 196–208. https://doi.org/10.1016/j.pld.2018.06.003.

Zhao, Chao, Chengfeng Yang, Bin Liu, Luan Lin, Satyajit D. Sarker, Lutfun Nahar, Hua Yu, Hui Cao, and Jianbo Xiao. 2018. "Bioactive Compounds from Marine Macroalgae and Their Hypoglycemic Benefits." *Trends in Food Science & Technology* 72 (February): 1–12. https://doi.org/10.1016/j.tifs.2017.12.001.

15 Indian Ginseng (*Withania somnifera*) in the Management of Diabetes Mellitus
An Evidence-Based Narrative Review

Sharanbasappa Durg, Neelima Satrasala and Shivsharan Dhadde

CONTENTS

ABBREVIATIONS

A:G ratio	albumin:globulin ratio
ALP	alkaline phosphatase
ALT	alanine aminotransferase
AM	alloxan monohydrate
AST	aspartate aminotransferase
AUC	area under curve
BID	two times daily
BMI	body mass index
BP	blood pressure
CAT	catalase
CI	confidence interval
CK	creatinine kinase
DM	diabetes mellitus

DOI: 10.1201/9781003220930-17

DPP-IV	dipeptidyl peptidase-IV
FBG	fasting blood glucose
FBS	fasting blood sugar
GP_X	glutathione peroxidase
GR	glutathione reductase
GSH	reduced glutathione
GST	glutathione S-transferase
HbA_{1c}	glycosylated hemoglobin
HDL	high-density lipoprotein
HOMA-IR	Homeostasis Model Assessment of Insulin Resistance
i.p.	intraperitoneal
IV	inverse variance
LDH	lactate dehydrogenase
LDL	low-density lipoprotein
LPO	lipid peroxidation
MD	mean difference
MDA	malondialdehyde
MLD	multiple low dose
NIDDM	non–insulin dependent diabetes mellitus
NO	nitric oxide
PC	protein carbonyl
RCT	randomized controlled trial
RI	reflection index
SMD	standardized mean difference
SOD	superoxide dismutase
STZ	streptozotocin
TBARS	thiobarbituric acid reactive substances
TC	total cholesterol
TG	triglyceride
TID	three times daily
VLDL	very low-density lipoprotein

15.1   INTRODUCTION

Withania somnifera (L.) Dunal (family Solanaceae), commonly known as Indian ginseng, winter cherry, *ajagandha*, and *ashwagandha*, is widely used in Ayurveda – the traditional Indian system of medicine (Weiner and Weiner 1994; Durg et al. 2015). In Sanskrit (Hayagandhā/Vājigandhā), *ashwa* meaning "horse" and "*gandha* meaning "smell," which generally explains *WS* as "smell and strength of horse," thus supporting its claim in vigor and strength (Kaul and Wadhwa 2017; Department of AYUSH 1989). *Somnifera*, the species name, means "sleep-inducing" in Latin, which indicates its traditional Ayurvedic use in sleep disorders (Langade et al. 2021).

In Ayurveda, for more than 2500 years, *WS* has been used as *Rasayana* (rejuvenating tonic) that promotes longevity, happiness, and vitality (Weiner and Weiner 1994; Durg et al. 2015). *Rasayana* is an herbal or metallic preparation in Ayurveda that promotes the mental and physical state of health by halting the aging process, boosting defense against disease, revitalizing the body in debilitated conditions, raising an individual's ability to resist adverse environmental effects, and establishing a sense of mental well-being (Weiner and Weiner 1994; Durg et al. 2015; Durg, Shivaram, and Bavage 2018).

Generally, dried mature roots of *WS* are most widely used, besides the leaves, for their medicinal properties (Kulkarni and Dhir 2008; Weiner and Weiner 1994; Durg et al. 2015). *WS* is reported to possess immunomodulatory, antioxidant, antistress, hemopoietic, and rejuvenating properties and has been in use for insomnia, rheumatism, infertility, and diabetes mellitus (DM) (Kulkarni and Dhir 2008; Durg et al. 2015; Durg, Shivaram, and Bavage 2018; Kaul and Wadhwa 2017). In the form of tea, *WS* is known to improve immunity, cardiovascular system, and stimulate detoxification that in turn aids in maintaining well-being (Bhat et al. 2010; Reuland et al. 2013). The major chemical constituents of *WS* are steroidal lactones, which include withaferin A, withanone, withanolides, sitoindosides, and withanolide C, and all of these have antioxidant activity (Kulkarni and Dhir 2008; Durg et al. 2015).

This review documents the scientific evidence of *WS*, from both experimental and clinical studies, for its anti-diabetic activity. To assess its role in managing DM, *WS* has undergone various levels of securitization in both preclinical and clinical studies. The first experimental (preclinical) study reported the hypoglycemic activity of *WS* in an Ayurvedic formulation, Trasina, where *WS* is one of the active constituents, and the observed effect was attributed to its antioxidant property (Bhattacharya, Satyan, and Chakrabarti 1997). Following this, a clinical study was conducted to evaluate the hypoglycemic, diuretic, and hypocholesterolemic properties of *WS* in patients with type 2 DM and mild hypercholesterolemia (Andallu and Radhika 2000). Post this, many experimental and clinical studies evaluated the efficacy/effectiveness and safety of *WS* and its isolated markers in DM. Building on these, this review collates and highlights the inclusive scientific evidence to assess the overall efficacy/effectiveness, safety, and tolerability of *WS* in managing DM.

15.2 *WITHANIA SOMNIFERA* IN MANAGING DIABETES MELLITUS: EVIDENCE FROM EXPERIMENTAL AND CLINICAL STUDIES

Fourteen preclinical studies (mice model, $n = 3$; rat model, $n = 10$; dog model, $n = 1$) evaluating the anti-diabetic activity of *WS* (root/leaf) extracts and/or its active constitutes are included in this review: mice model (Parihar et al. 2004; Tekula et al. 2018; Thakur et al. 2015); rat model (Anwer et al. 2008, 2012, 2017; Jain et al. 2006; Kiasalari, Khalili, and Aghaei 2009; Kyathanahalli, Manjunath, and Muralidhara 2014; Parihar et al. 2016; Sarangi et al. 2013; Udayakumar et al. 2009, 2010); and one study performed in dogs (Gopinath et al. 2021). Of these 14 experimental studies, seven did not mention diabetes type (Gopinath et al. 2021; Kyathanahalli, Manjunath, and Muralidhara 2014; Parihar et al. 2004, 2016; Udayakumar et al. 2009, 2010; Sarangi et al. 2013). However, by virtue of diabetes inducing agent(s)/diagnostic observation, the diabetic animals in these studies partly mimicked either type 1 DM or type 2 DM, or both (Durg et al. 2017). Further details of these experimental studies are summarized in Table 15.1. In case of clinical evidence, five clinical studies accessed the efficacy/effectiveness and safety of *WS* in ($N = 194$) patients with type 2 DM (Andallu and Radhika 2000; Agnihotri et al. 2013; Nayak et al. 2015; Usharani, Fatima, et al. 2014; Usharani, Kishan, et al. 2014). Additional information of clinical studies is depicted in Table 15.2. Besides these, a case report of *WS* root extract use (400 mg BID for 3 months) in older women with prediabetes (Simon et al. 2018) is also part of this narrative review.

To review and summarize commonly reported outcomes, in both experimental (comparison: *WS* vs. diabetes control) and clinical studies (post-/pre-comparison; or patients taking *WS* vs. control patients not taking *WS*), meta-analysis was performed, where possible, in Review Manager (RevMan; Computer program, version 5.3.5, Copenhagen: Nordic Cochrane Centre, Cochrane Collaboration, 2014). For analysis of continuous outcomes, the data are presented in mean difference (MD: inverse variance [IV] method) and 95% confidence intervals (CIs). If studies reported the same continuous outcome in different units, then the results are measured in standardized MD (SMD) and 95% CI. The random-effects model is used to perform meta-analysis, considering the differences across studies, as experimental studies varied in *WS* extract/dose and treatment duration, and population as well in case of clinical studies (Borenstein et al. 2009). A p-value < 0.05 (two-tailed test) is considered statistically significant in the analysis.

TABLE 15.1

Details of Experimental (Preclinical) Studies

Study	Induction of Diabetes	Diabetes Type	WS Extract	Treatment Duration	Grouping and Dosage
Anwer et al. 2008	STZ (100 mg/kg, i.p.)	Type 2	Standardized powdered, aqueous root extract of WS (Batch No. WS/05002; withanolides, 3.9% w/w) was gifted by Natural Remedies, Bengaluru, India	5 weeks	Albino Wistar rats ($N = 30$); five groups (each containing six rats) Group 1: normal control (citrate buffer 0.1 ml/10 g, i.p.). Group 2: diabetic control (single dose of STZ). Group 3: single dose of STZ + WS (200 mg/kg). Group 4: single dose of STZ + WS (400 mg/kg). Group 5: only WS (400 mg/kg)
Anwer et al. 2012	STZ (100 mg/kg, i.p.)	Type 2	Same as Anwer et al. 2008	5 weeks	Albino Wistar rats ($N = 24$); four groups (each containing six rats) Group 1: normal control (citrate buffer). Group 2: diabetic control (single dose of STZ). Group 3: single dose of STZ + WS (200 mg/kg). Group 4: single dose of STZ + WS (400 mg/kg)
Anwer et al. 2017	STZ (100 mg/kg, i.p.)	Type 2	Same as Anwer et al. 2008	5 weeks	Albino Wistar rats ($N = 30$); five groups (each containing six rats) Group 1: normal control (citrate buffer, 0.1 ml/kg, i.p.). Group 2: diabetic control (single dose of STZ). Group 3: only WS (400 mg/kg). Group 4: single dose of STZ + WS (200 mg/kg). Group 5: single dose of STZ + WS (400 mg/kg)
Gopinath et al. 2021	Subclinically diabetic dogs (based on preliminary screening of random blood glucose, fasting blood glucose and Benedict's test for the presence of sugar in urine)	Not reported*	WS extract was prepared as per published literature	30 days	Subclinically diabetic dogs ($N = 30$); five groups (each containing six dogs) Group 1: positive control (no treatment). Group 2: *Terminalia chebula* extract (100 mg/kg). Group 3: WS (100 mg/kg). Group 4: *Terminalia chebula* extract + WS (100 mg/kg each). Group 5: standard antioxidant *N*-acetyl cysteine (10 mg/kg). Additionally, Group 6 ($N = 6$); negative control (healthy dogs; no treatment)

Study	Induction of Diabetes	Diabetes Type	*WS* Extract	Treatment Duration	Grouping and Dosage
Jain et al. 2006	STZ (60 mg/kg, i.p.)	Type 1	Alcoholic root extract of *WS* (1.5% withanolides) procured from Sanat Products, New Delhi, India	3 weeks	Sprague-Dawley rats (150–200 g) of either sex ($N = 36$); seven groups (each containing six rats) Group 1: diabetic control. Group 2: *WS* (20 mg/kg). Group 3: *Allium sativum* (100 mg/kg). Group 4: *Gymnema sylvestre* (100 mg/kg). Group 5: *Ferula foetida* (100 or 200 mg/kg). Group 6: *Murraya koenigii* (200 mg/kg). Group 7: insulin (5 u/kg subcutaneously daily)
Kiasalari, Khalili, and Aghaei 2009	STZ (60 mg/kg, i.p.)	Type 1	*WS* root was procured from the local market, then powdered and mixed in pelleted food at ratio of 6.25%	4 weeks	Adult male (195–220 g) Wistar rats ($N = 39$); four groups Group 1 ($n = 8$); normal control (*WS* [powdered root–mixed pelleted food at ratio of 6.25%], 4 weeks). Group 2 ($n = 11$): sham. Group 3 ($n = 9$): diabetic control. Group 4 ($n = 11$): single dose of STZ + *WS*
Kyathanahalli, Manjunath, and Muralidhara 2014	STZ (90 mg/kg, i.p.)	Not reported*	Standard root extract of *WS* powder (batch number: C81015; anolides, 2.57%; aferin A, 2.38%) was procured from M/s Sami Labs Ltd., Bengaluru, India	15 days	Four-week-old prepubertal male (40 ± 5 g) CFT-Wistar rats ($N = 18$); three groups (each containing six rats) Group 1: normal control. Group 2: diabetic control (single dose of STZ). Group 3: single dose of STZ + *WS* (500 mg/kg)
Parihar et al. 2004	STZ (60 mg/kg, i.p.)	Not reported*	Methanolic fraction of *WS* root extract was prepared according to the published research study	30 days	Female (25 g) Swiss albino mice ($N = 40$); five groups (each containing eight mice) Group 1: normal control. Group 2: diabetic control (single dose of STZ). Group 3: single dose of STZ + *WS* (20 mg/kg). Group 4: single dose of STZ + *Aloe vera* (32 mg/kg). Group 5: single dose of STZ + combination of *WS* and *Aloe vera*
Parihar et al. 2016	STZ (60 mg/kg, i.p.)	Not reported*	Same as Parihar et al. 2004	30 days	Adult (250–300 g) male Wistar rats ($N = 40$); four groups (each containing ten rats) Group 1: normal control. Group 2: *WS* (35 mg/kg). Group 3: diabetic control (single dose of STZ). Group 4: single dose of STZ + *WS* (35 mg/kg)

(Continued)

TABLE 15.1
(Continued)

Study	Induction of Diabetes	Diabetes Type	WS Extract	Treatment Duration	Grouping and Dosage
Sarangi et al. 2013	STZ (150 mg/kg, i.p.)	Not reported*	Root and leaf extract of WS were prepared according to the published research study	8 weeks	Adult (150–180 g) male albino Wistar rats ($N = 24$); four groups (each containing six rats) Group 1: normal control (distilled water). Group 2: diabetic control (single dose of STZ). Group 3: single dose of STZ + WS root extract (200 mg/kg). Group 4: single dose of STZ + WS leaf extract (200 mg/kg)
Tekula et al. 2018	STZ (40 mg/kg, i.p.)	Type 1	Withaferin A (>98% pure) was purchased from Aptus Therapeutics, Hyderabad, India (characterized by nuclear magnetic resonance and Fourier-transform infrared spectroscopy for integrity)	4 weeks	Male Swiss albino mice ($N = 40$); five groups (each containing eight mice) Group 1: normal control. Group 2: diabetic control (multiple low dose of STZ) + vehicle. Group 3: drug control (withaferin A per se) which were treated with 10 mg/kg withaferin A alone. Group 4: MLD-STZ + withaferin A (2 mg/kg). Group 5: MLD-STZ + withaferin A (10 mg/kg)
Thakur et al. 2015	STZ (65 mg/kg, i.p.)	Type 2	Methanolic extract prepared from root of WS according to the published research study	10 days	Adult male (25 ± 5 g) albino mice ($N = 30$); five groups (each containing six mice) Group 1: normal control. Group 2: diabetic control (single dose of STZ + vehicle only). Group 3: single dose of STZ + WS (25 mg/kg). Group 4: single dose of STZ + WS (50 mg/kg). Group 5: single dose of STZ + WS (100 mg/kg)
Udayakumar et al. 2009	Alloxan (150 mg/kg, i.p.)	Not reported*	Root and leaf extract of WS were prepared according to the published research study	8 weeks	Male (150–180 g) albino Wistar rats ($N = 42$) seven groups (each containing six rats) Group 1: normal control (distilled water). Group 2: diabetic control (single dose of alloxan). Group 3: single dose of alloxan + WS root extract (100 mg/kg). Group 4: single dose of alloxan + WS root extract (200 mg/kg). Group 5: single dose of alloxan + WS leaf extract (100 mg/kg). Group 6: single dose of alloxan + WS leaf extract (200 mg/kg). Group 7: single dose of alloxan + glibenclamide (0.6 mg/kg)

Study	Induction of Diabetes	Diabetes Type	WS Extract	Treatment Duration	Grouping and Dosage
Udayakumar et al. 2010	Alloxan (150 mg/kg, i.p.)	Not reported*	Same as Udayakumar et al. 2009	8 weeks	Male (150–180 g) albino Wistar rats (*N* = 42); seven groups (each containing six rats) Group 1: normal control (distilled water). Group 2: diabetic control (single dose of alloxan). Group 3: single dose of alloxan + *WS* root extract (100 mg/kg). Group 4: single dose of alloxan + *WS* root extract (200 mg/kg). Group 5: single dose of alloxan + *WS* leaf extract (100 mg/kg). Group 6: single dose of alloxan + *WS* leaf extract (200 mg/kg). Group 7: single dose of alloxan + glibenclamide (0.6 mg/kg)

* By virtue of diabetes inducing agent(s)/diagnostic observation, these studies partly mimicked either type 1 DM or type 2 DM, or both.

Abbreviations: N, total number of animals in the study; *n*, total number of animals in a group.

15.3   BODY WEIGHT

Unexplained weight loss is a common symptom in both type 1 and type 2 DM. Overweight or obesity can be one of the risk factors in type 2 DM but is not seen usually with type 1 DM. Experimental studies evaluated the effect of *WS* on body weight in diabetic animals. Kyathanahalli and colleagues reported decrease in body weight in prepubertal rats when injected with streptozotocin (STZ; 90 mg/kg single i.p. injection). Oral supplementation of *WS* root extract (500 mg/kg) for 15 days improved the weight loss (vs. baseline) by 35.90% in prepubertal diabetic rats (Kyathanahalli, Manjunath, and Muralidhara 2014). Alloxan monohydrate (AM; 150 mg/kg, i.p.), a diabetes-inducing agent, also produced continuous loss of weight in diabetic rats. Treatment with *WS* root and leaf extracts (200 mg/kg) for 8 weeks, respectively, increased body weight by 25.53% and 25.10% in diabetic rats (Udayakumar et al. 2009). Likewise, in type 2 diabetic mice, i.p. injection of STZ (65 mg/kg) and nicotinamide (120 mg/kg, 15 minutes after STZ) reduced body weight which was increased (19.90%) by *WS* (100 mg/kg for 10 days) root extract (Thakur et al. 2015). Tekula and team, using type 1 diabetes mice (STZ, 40 mg/kg, i.p.), evaluated the effect of withaferin A on body weight (Tekula et al. 2018). Withaferin A, a steroidal lactone, is one of the active constituents of *WS* and reported to possess antioxidant activity (Durg et al. 2015). There was insignificant decrease in body weight in diabetic mice and supplementation of withaferin A (2 and 10 mg/kg for 4 weeks) showed a trend in improving body weight (Tekula et al. 2018). A case report by Simon and coworkers described the use of *WS* root (400 mg BID for 3 months) in an older woman with prediabetes (class III obesity, BMI; 49.4 kg/m^2) and noted a reduction in body weight from 135 to 131.8 kg with no further changes in lifestyle (Simon et al. 2018).

TABLE 15.2

Details of Clinical Studies

Study (Study Design)	Population	Sex (Male %)	Age (Years)	BMI (Mean or Range, kg/m²)	Intervention (N /dose)	Control (N /dose)	Co-Interventions
Andallu and Radhika 2000 (observational study)	Mild hyperglycemic (NIDDM) and hypercholesterolemic	NR	40–60	NR	N = 12 (six each, NIDDM and hypercholesterolemic) WS: 500 mg capsule (six capsules/day, two after every meal) for 30 days	N = 12 (six each, NIDDM and hypercholesterolemic) Oral hypoglycemic drug (Daonil) for 30 days	Subjects undergoing any treatment before the study period was terminated after consultation with the physician
Agnihotri et al. 2013 (RCT)	Schizophrenia patients, suffering from metabolic syndrome, on second-generation antipsychotics for 6 months or more, with FBG level >100 mg/dL, serum TGs >150 mg/dL, HDL-C <40 mg/dL in men and <50 mg/dL in women	NR	>18	NR	N = 12 WS extract: 400 mg per capsule, one capsule TID for 1 month	N = 13 Placebo: one capsule TID for 1 month	Second-generation antipsychotics
Nayak et al. 2015 (RCT)	Type 2 DM patients treated with fixed oral anti-diabetic drugs, FBS ≥126 and ≤180 mg/dL, postprandial blood sugar ≤240 mg/dL, HbA$_{1c}$ ≥7%, and mean total diabetes distress scale scoring ≥3	Reported as "dominated by males"	41–50	NR	N = 28 WS: Capsule of 300 mg root extract in groundnut oil base, one capsule BID with a cup of lukewarm milk for 6 weeks, followed by another 6 weeks of follow-up	N = 27 Control group: soft gelatin capsule of only groundnut oil, one capsule BID with a cup of lukewarm milk for 6 weeks, followed by another 6 weeks of follow-up	Metformin 500 mg + glimepride 1 mg, 1 tablet BID

Study	Population				Intervention	Comparator
Usharani, Fatima, et al. 2014 (RCT)	Type 2 DM patients with FBG between 110–126 mg/dL, HbA$_{1c}$ between 6.5% and 8.0%, on oral hypoglycemic agents for last 8 weeks prior to screening visit, endothelial dysfunction defined as ≤6% change in RI post salbutamol challenge test	WS 250 mg: 70% WS 500 mg: 65% Placebo: 60%	WS 250 mg: 55.40 ± 8.07 WS 500 mg: 57.30 ± 9.40 Placebo: 57.45 ± 8.85	WS 250 mg: 24.89 ± 2.03 WS 500 mg: 25.01 ± 2.92 Placebo: 24.82 ± 1.86	N = 20 WS 250 mg: capsule of 250 mg root extract BID for 12 weeks N = 20 WS 500 mg: capsule of 500 mg root extract BID for 12 weeks	N = 20 Placebo: identical matching capsule to WS BID for 12 weeks — Metformin 1500–2500 mg/day
Usharani, Kishan, et al. 2014 (RCT)	Type 2 DM patients with FBG ≥110 mg/dL, HbA$_{1c}$ between 6.5% and 8.0%, on oral hypoglycemic agents for last 8 weeks prior to screening visit, endothelial dysfunction defined as ≤6% change in RI postsalbutamol challenge test	WS 250 mg: 90% *Phyllanthus emblica* 250 mg: 80% Combination of *P. emblica* + WS: 90%	WS 250 mg: 60.10 ± 6.47 *P. emblica* 250 mg: 58.60 ± 10.54 Combination of *P. emblica* + WS: 57.30 ± 9.23	WS 250 mg: 24.83 ± 2.20 WS 500 mg: 25.65 ± 3.517 Placebo: 24.97 ± 2.65	N = 10 WS: capsule of 250 mg root extract BID for 12 weeks N = 10 Combination of *P. emblica* + WS: capsule of 250 mg + 250 mg BID for 12 weeks	N = 10 *P. emblica*: capsule of 500 mg BID for 12 weeks — Metformin 1500–2500 mg/day

15.4 BLOOD GLUCOSE AND GLYCOSYLATED HEMOGLOBIN (HbA1c)

Induction of diabetes in experimental rats, via inducing agents such as AM/STZ, significantly increased blood glucose and HbA_{1c} levels. Eight and three studies, respectively, assessed the effect of *WS* root and leaf extract on blood glucose in diabetic rats. The overall effect of *WS* root (MD −183.64, 95% CI [−226.49, −140.79], $p < 0.00001$) and leaf (MD −211.18, 95% CI [−272.08, −150.28], $p < 0.00001$) extract in diabetic rats, as evident in meta-analysis, showed significant reduction in blood glucose level (Table 15.3). Similarly, Parihar and team in two different studies investigated the nutritional effect of *WS* on blood glucose in STZ-induced diabetic mice and rats. *WS* treatment (vs. diabetic control) reported significant (43.44%, $p < 0.05$) (Parihar et al. 2004) and numerical (31.70%) (Parihar et al. 2016) improvement in blood glucose levels. In another study, three different doses (25/50/100 mg/kg) of *WS* root extract were evaluated in diabetic mice, and all the doses showed significant ($p < 0.05$) decrease (27.32%/44.76%/55.81%) in plasma glucose levels (Thakur et al. 2015). The active constituents of *WS*, such as withaferin A (both 2 and 10 mg/kg in 3 and 4 weeks, respectively), also reported significant ($p < 0.001$ vs. diabetic control) reduction in the elevated blood glucose levels in type 1 diabetes mice (Tekula et al. 2018). In a study by Gopinath et al., *WS* root extract (100 mg/kg for 30 days) showed insignificant reduction in random and fasting blood glucose in subclinically diabetic dogs (Gopinath et al. 2021) (Table 15.3). *WS* (root/leaf extract) treatment also significantly ($p < 0.00001$) restored elevated HbA_{1c} levels to near normal in diabetic rats (Table 15.3).

The effect of *WS* root extract was also examined in clinical studies. A total of 40 patients with either metabolic syndrome in schizophrenia or type 2 DM were given 400 mg TID (1 month) or 300 mg BID (6 weeks) of *WS* root extract (Agnihotri et al. 2013; Nayak et al. 2015). In both groups of patients, *WS* treatment significantly reduced fasting blood glucose ($p = 0.001$; Table 15.3). Additionally, Nayak and coworkers also noted significant reduction in postprandial blood glucose and HbA_{1c} levels in patients with type 2 DM taking oral hypoglycemic agents (metformin, 500 mg + glimepride, 1 mg) with or without *WS*. However, the improvement was better (PPBS, 29.66% vs. 25.51%; HbA_{1c}, 13.73% vs. 9.31%) in patients receiving a combination of oral hypoglycemic agents and *WS* (Nayak et al. 2015). Further, in an elderly woman with prediabetes (class III obesity, BMI; 49.4 kg/m^2), *WS* root extract (400 mg BID) reduced HbA_{1c} (6.4% from baseline to 5.9% after 3 months) (Simon et al. 2018).

15.5 INSULIN LEVEL/SENSITIVITY AND HOMEOSTASIS MODEL ASSESSMENT OF INSULIN RESISTANCE (HOMA-IR)

The effect of *WS* on insulin and HOMA-IR (an index of hepatic insulin resistance) was assessed in animal studies. STZ-induced type 2 diabetic rats had hyperinsulinemia and *WS* (200 and 400 mg/kg, 5 weeks) treatment significantly ($p < 0.001$) decreased (17.71% and 30.21%) the elevated insulin levels (Anwer et al. 2008). However, Thakur and team noted statistically lower levels of insulin in type 2 diabetic mice when given STZ (65 mg/kg) and nicotinamide (120 mg/kg, 15 minutes after STZ). Treating these diabetic mice with *WS* (50 and 100 mg/kg, 10 days) increased ($p < 0.05$; 32.99% and 52.57%) plasma insulin levels, respectively, in a dose-dependent manner (Thakur et al. 2015). In type 1 diabetic mice (STZ, 40 mg/kg/day for 5 consecutive days), plasma and tissue insulin levels were significantly ($p < 0.001$) lower compared to healthy controls, and withaferin A intervention (4 weeks) significantly improved ($p < 0.001$) plasma (2 and 10 mg/kg) and tissue (10 mg/kg) insulin levels to near normal (Tekula et al. 2018). Anwer and team reported significant improvement in HOMA-IR ($p < 0.001$; 61.37% and 73.87%) and K_{ITT} (an index of peripheral insulin resistance, $p < 0.001$; 33.34% and 75.56%) in diabetic rats when treated with *WS* (200 and 400 mg/kg, 5 weeks) (Anwer et al. 2008).

TABLE 15.3
Summary of Meta-Analysis Outcomes

Outcome	Studies	Species (*WS* extract)	*N* (Total; *WS* / control)	Effect measure (95% CI)	I^2% (*p* value)
Blood glucose	Anwer et al. 2008 Anwer et al. 2017 Jain et al. 2006 Kiasalari, Khalili, and Aghaei 2009 Kyathanahalli, Manjunath, and Muralidhara 2014 Sarangi et al. 2013 Udayakumar et al. 2009 Udayakumar et al. 2010	Rat (Root extract)	53/51	MD −183.64 (−226.49, −140.79)	97 (< 0.00001)
	Sarangi et al. 2013 Udayakumar et al. 2009 Udayakumar et al. 2010	Rat (Leaf extract)	18/18	MD −211.18 (−272.08, −150.28)	99 (< 0.00001)
	Gopinath et al. 2021 (Random glucose)	Dog (Root extract)	6/6	MD −7.50 (−33.74, 18.74)	NA (= 0.58)
FBG	Gopinath et al. 2021	Dog (Root extract)	6/6	MD −6.75 (−27.97, 14.47)	NA (= 0.53)
	Agnihotri et al. 2013 Nayak et al. 2015	Human (Root extract)	40/40	MD −8.67 (−14.02, −3.32)	0 (= 0.001)
HbA_{1c}	Anwer et al. 2008 Udayakumar et al. 2009	Rat (Root extract)	12/12	SMD −7.61 (−10.37, −4.85)	0 (< 0.00001)
	Udayakumar et al. 2009	Rat (Leaf extract)	6/6	MD −2.38 (−2.73, −2.03)	NA (< 0.00001)
Lipid profile					
TC	Anwer et al. 2017 Kiasalari, Khalili, and Aghaei 2009 Sarangi et al. 2013 Udayakumar et al. 2009	Rat (Root extract)	29/27	MD −62.75 (−98.40, −27.11)	98 (= 0.0006)
	Sarangi et al. 2013 Udayakumar et al. 2009	Rat (Leaf extract)	12/12	MD −67.14 (−77.63, −56.64)	33 (< 0.00001)
TG	Anwer et al. 2017 Kiasalari, Khalili, and Aghaei 2009 Sarangi et al. 2013 Udayakumar et al. 2009	Rat (Root extract)	29/27	MD −35.34 (−60.50, −10.18)	96 (= 0.008)
	Sarangi et al. 2013 Udayakumar et al. 2009	Rat (Leaf extract)	12/12	MD −12.40 (−34.73, 9.93)	91 (= 0.28)
LDL	Anwer et al. 2017 Sarangi et al. 2013 Udayakumar et al. 2009	Rat (Root extract)	18/18	MD −43.23 (−63.28, −23.19)	98 (< 0.00001)
	Sarangi et al. 2013 Udayakumar et al. 2009	Rat (Leaf extract)	12/12	MD −25.28 (−28.93, −21.62)	0 (< 0.00001)
VLDL	Anwer et al. 2017 Udayakumar et al. 2009	Rat (Root extract)	18/18	MD −8.85 (−15.20, −2.50)	93 (= 0.0006)
	Udayakumar et al. 2009	Rat (Leaf extract)	6/6	MD −4.79 (−6.86, −2.72)	NA (< 0.00001)

(Continued)

TABLE 15.3
(Continued)

Outcome	Studies	Species (*WS* extract)	*N* (Total; *WS* / control)	Effect measure (95% CI)	I²% (*p* value)
HDL	Anwer et al. 2017 Sarangi et al. 2013 Udayakumar et al. 2009	Rat (Root extract)	18/18	MD 5.23 (3.72, 6.74)	53 (< 0.00001)
	Sarangi et al. 2013 Udayakumar et al. 2009	Rat (Leaf extract)	12/12	MD 3.67 (2.26, 5.07)	0 (< 0.00001)
Serum markers					
AST	Sarangi et al. 2013 Udayakumar et al. 2009	Rat (Root extract)	12/12	MD −73.47 (−77.97, −68.97)	0 (< 0.00001)
	Sarangi et al. 2013 Udayakumar et al. 2009	Rat (Leaf extract)	12/12	MD −62.80 (−68.23, −57.36)	15 (< 0.00001)
ALT	Sarangi et al. 2013 Udayakumar et al. 2009	Rat (Root extract)	12/12	MD −56.68 (−61.08, −52.27)	0 (< 0.00001)
	Sarangi et al. 2013 Udayakumar et al. 2009	Rat (Leaf extract)	12/12	MD −55.92 (−73.71, −38.13)	94 (< 0.00001)
ALP	Sarangi et al. 2013 Udayakumar et al. 2009	Rat (Root extract)	12/12	MD −3.39 (−5.02, −1.77)	0 (< 0.00001)
	Sarangi et al. 2013 Udayakumar et al. 2009	Rat (Leaf extract)	12/12	MD −2.61 (−4.23, −0.98)	0 (< 0.0002)
Total protein	Sarangi et al. 2013 Udayakumar et al. 2009	Rat (Root extract)	12/12	MD 1.41 (1.05, 1.77)	0 (< 0.00001)
	Sarangi et al. 2013 Udayakumar et al. 2009	Rat (Leaf extract)	12/12	MD 1.92 (1.13, 2.71)	73 (< 0.00001)
Albumin	Sarangi et al. 2013 Udayakumar et al. 2009	Rat (Root extract)	12/12	MD 1.48 (1.28, 1.68)	0 (< 0.00001)
	Sarangi et al. 2013 Udayakumar et al. 2009	Rat (Leaf extract)	12/12	MD 1.47 (1.10, 1.83)	0 (< 0.00001)
A:G ratio	Sarangi et al. 2013 Udayakumar et al. 2009	Rat (Root extract)	12/12	MD 0.79 (0.68, 0.90)	0 (< 0.00001)
	Sarangi et al. 2013 Udayakumar et al. 2009	Rat (Leaf extract)	12/12	MD 0.60 (0.46, 0.75)	21 (< 0.00001)
Liver glycogen	Udayakumar et al. 2009 Udayakumar et al. 2010	Rat (Root extract)	12/12	MD 8.36 (6.37, 10.35)	0 (< 0.00001)
	Udayakumar et al. 2009 Udayakumar et al. 2010	Rat (Leaf extract)	12/12	MD 9.47 (3.99, 14.94)	68 (= 0.0007)

15.6 LIPID PROFILE

Induction of diabetes in experimental rats exhibited elevation in lipid profile, such as total cholesterol (TC), triglyceride (TG), low-density lipoprotein (LDL) and very-low-density lipoprotein (VLDL), and decrease in high-density lipoprotein (HDL) levels. Treatment of diabetic rats with *WS* (root/ leaf) extract significantly restored altered lipid profile to near normal (Table 15.3). Alloxan-induced diabetic rats were also observed with elevated levels of TC, TG, and phospholipids in heart, liver, and kidney which were restored to near normal following *WS* supplementation (Udayakumar et al. 2009). In clinical studies, patients with type 2 DM also showed significant improvement in lipid profile when treated with *WS* (Andallu and Radhika 2000; Nayak et al. 2015; Usharani, Kishan, et al. 2014; Usharani, Fatima, et al. 2014).

15.7 SERUM MARKERS

Diabetes and hyperlipidemia can cause cell damage following disturbance in the cell membrane architecture leading to impaired liver function (Harris 2005; Salmela et al. 1984; Udayakumar et al. 2009). In experimental animals, AM/STZ-induced diabetes can cause elevation in aspartate aminotransferase (AST), alanine aminotransferase (ALT), creatinine kinase (CK), and alkaline phosphatase (ALP) levels. Additionally, diabetes can also decrease physiological levels of total protein, albumin and albumin:globulin (A:G) ratio, possibly due to albuminuria and microproteinuria and/ or increased protein catabolism (Almdal and Vilstrup 1988).

WS treatment reduced the elevated levels of AST, ALT, and ALP in diabetic rats to near normal (Table 15.3), and likewise, a significant decrease in the raised levels of acid phosphatase following *WS* root (28.93%)/leaf (31.53%) extract supplementation (Udayakumar et al. 2009). Diabetic rats were additionally observed with significant reduction in serum total protein, albumin, A:G ratio, and liver glycogen, and administration of *WS* root/leaf extract statistically restored these altered concentrations (Table 15.3). *WS* root extract also reduced elevated levels of CK in STZ-induced diabetic rats (Anwer et al. 2017). Induction of diabetes increased liver glucose-6-phosphatase (220%), which was significantly restored ($p < 0.05$) near to baseline following *WS* extract (root, 55%; leaf, 52%) supplementation (Udayakumar et al. 2009). Further, *WS* statistically ($p < 0.05$) improved the altered activities of glucose-6-phosphate dehydrogenase and β-hydroxysteroid dehydrogenase close to normal (Kyathanahalli, Manjunath, and Muralidhara 2014).

15.8 OXIDATIVE STRESS MARKERS

AM/STZ injection in experimental rats showed significant reduction in endogenous antioxidant levels including superoxide dismutase (SOD), catalase (CAT), reduced glutathione (GSH), glutathione peroxidase (GPx), glutathione S-transferase (GST), and glutathione reductase (GR) in myocardial, hepatic, and kidney as well as pancreatic (only GPx, GST, and GR) tissues. Treatment of these diabetic rats with *WS* (root/leaf) extract improved antioxidant levels to near normal. Additionally, elevated lipid peroxidation (LPO)/TBARS (n mole malondialdehyde [MDA]/mg protein) level in the myocardial, hepatic, pancreatic, and kidney tissues of diabetic rats decreased significantly following *WS* treatment (Anwer et al. 2017; Udayakumar et al. 2010).

Kyathanahalli and team, in prepubertal diabetic rats, observed significant elevation of reactive oxygen species generation (120%; in both testis cytosol and mitochondria), membrane LPO (66%; in both testis cytosol and mitochondria), GSH (cytosol, less altered; mitochondria, 22%), SOD (cytosol, less altered; mitochondria, 53%), GST and GR (in both testis cytosol and mitochondria). Further, decrease in total thiol concentration (cytosol, 43%; mitochondria, 16%) and CAT were noted. Administering *WS* for 15 days in these prepubertal diabetic rats significantly re-established diabetes-induced testicular oxidative impairments, besides improving the altered activity of lactate dehydrogenase (LDH) (Kyathanahalli, Manjunath, and Muralidhara 2014). In two separate studies, administration of *WS* (root/leaf) extract also significantly decreased elevated LDH levels (Anwer et al. 2017; Sarangi et al. 2013). Parihar and coworkers reported significant ($p < 0.05$) increase in LPO and protein carbonyl (PC) in hippocampus/hypothalamus and cerebral cortex brain regions of diabetic mice/rat (Parihar et al. 2004; Parihar et al. 2016). *WS* treatment in these diabetic mice/ rat significantly ($p < 0.05$) reduced LPO and PC in the analyzed brain regions. Also, *WS* significantly ($p < 0.05$) stabilized GSH and GPx levels to near normal in the hypothalamus (Parihar et al. 2016). In another study, type 1 diabetic mice also reported increased MDA and nitrosative stress levels (Tekula et al. 2018). Withaferin A administration reduced MDA levels by 3-fold and 4.1-fold at doses of 2 and 10 mg/kg, respectively. Both doses (2 mg/kg, $p < 0.001$; 10 mg/kg, $p < 0.01$) also lowered the elevated tissue nitrosative stress.

In two different randomized controlled trials (RCTs), *WS* root extract (250 and 500 mg) in patients with type 2 DM significantly ($p \leq 0.05$) increased GSH and nitric oxide (NO) levels and decreased

MDA and high-sensitivity C-reactive protein (an inflammatory biomarker) levels (Usharani, Kishan, et al. 2014; Usharani, Fatima, et al. 2014).

15.9   MECHANISM OF ACTION

The proposed mechanism(s) of action(s) of *WS* for its anti-diabetic activity is illustrated in Figure 15.1 (Durg, Bavage, and Shivaram 2020 – reproduced with permission). The antihyperglycemic profile of *WS* can be recognized from β cell protection (preserve the size and number of β cells) from oxidative stress (Anwer et al. 2012), and rejuvenation as well as activation of pancreatic β cells leading to insulin release (Udayakumar et al. 2010). It also acts by inhibiting α-glucosidase, α-amylase, and DPP-IV enzymes (Huerta et al. 2010; Khan, Khan, and Ali 2014; Singh, Joshi, and Jatwa 2013). *WS* also accelerates transport of glucose into cells by stimulating glucose transports (Nirupama et al. 2014). Further, withanolides are reported to increase glucose uptake in myotubes and adipocytes (Jonathan et al. 2015). The glucose-lowering activity of *WS* is noted via insulinotropic effects, improving insulin sensitivity by reducing hyperinsulinemia and insulin resistance in addition to improving glucose tolerance (Anwer et al. 2008). Aliper and colleagues via in silico

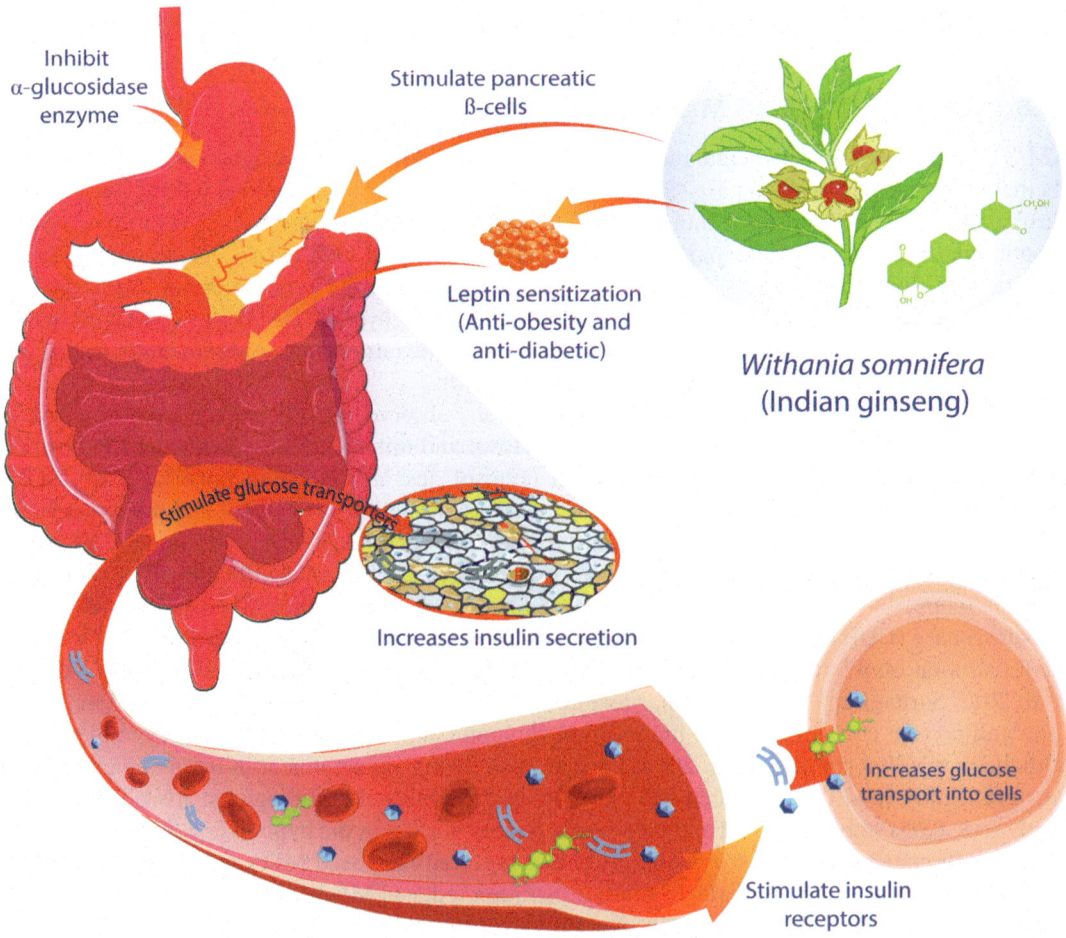

FIGURE 15.1   Mechanism of action of *Withania somnifera*.

Source: Reproduced with permission from Durg, Bavage, and Shivaram (2020).

screening showed that withaferin A mimics anti-aging properties of mammalian target of rapamycin inhibitors, i.e., metformin and rapamycin (Aliper et al. 2017), which tops the list of drugs mimicking caloric restriction (Ingram et al. 2004). Further, Lee and team from Harvard Medical School reported withaferin A as a potential leptin sensitizer with great anti-diabetic effects in mice (Lee et al. 2016).

15.10   OTHER FOODS, HERBS, SPICES, AND BOTANICALS USED IN DIABETES MELLITUS

There are many foodstuffs, spices, and herbs that have ethnic reference for their use in managing DM and are part of our daily diet. Table 15.4 lists clinical studies of some of the widely used foods, such as bitter gourd (*Momordica charantia*) (Kim et al. 2020; Cortez-Navarrete et al. 2018)

TABLE 15.4

RCTs Evaluating Anti-Diabetic Activity of Other Foods/Herbs/Spices/Botanicals in Type 2 DM

Study	Intervention (*N* /dose)	Control (*N* /dose)	Co-Intervention	Results	PMID
Allium sativum (garlic)					
Ashraf, Khan, and Ashraf 2011	Garlic (KWAI) 300 mg TID for 24 weeks (*n* = 30)	Placebo for 24 weeks (*n* = 30)	Metformin 500 mg BID	Supplementation of garlic showed decrease in FBS at 24 weeks ($p \leq 0.005$) Treatment with garlic improved serum lipid profile ($p \leq 0.005$), i.e., decrease in TC, LDL-C, TC, increase in HDL	21959822
Sobenin et al. 2008	Garlic powder tablet, i.e., Allicor for 4 weeks (*n* = 30)	Placebo for 4 weeks (*n* = 30)	Patients were additionally on dietary treatment/ sulfonylurea derivatives	Treatment with Allicor showed improved metabolic control by decreasing FBG, serum fructosamine, and serum TG levels	17823766
Momordica charantia (bitter gourd/bitter melon)					
Kim et al. 2020	Bitter melon extract for 12 weeks (*n* = 62)	Placebo for 12 weeks (*n* = 28)	Oral hypoglycemic agents	Supplementation of bitter melon extract for 12 weeks showed no change in HbA_{1c} in both groups Average FBG level was decreased in bitter melon group ($p = 0.014$)	32951763
Cortez-Navarrete et al. 2018	*M. charantia* (2000 mg/day) for 3 months (*n* = 12)	Placebo for 3 months (*n* = 12)	Not reported	*M. charantia* group significantly increased insulin AUC ($p = 0.043$), in total insulin secretion ($p = 0.028$), and during first phase of insulin secretion ($p = 0.043$) Significant decrease in weight, fat percentage, BMI, waist circumference, HbA_{1c}, 2-hour glucose in oral glucose tolerance test, glucose AUC	29431598

(*Continued*)

TABLE 15.4
(Continued)

Study	Intervention (*N* /dose)	Control (*N* /dose)	Co-Intervention	Results	PMID
Curcuma longa (turmeric)					
Neta et al. 2021	*C. longa* (500 mg/ day on empty stomach) with piperine 5 mg for 120 days (*n* = 38)	Placebo for 120 days (*n* = 38)	Not reported	Significant decrease in the levels of glycemia ($p = 0.013$), HbA$_{1c}$ ($p = 0.015$), HOMA-index ($p = 0.037$), TGs ($p = 0.002$) in *Curcuma* group	33586583
Adibian et al. 2019	Curcumin (1500 mg/day) for 10 weeks (*n* = 22)	Placebo for 10 weeks (*n* = 22)	Not reported	Curcumin, significantly decreased C-protein ($p < 0.05$) and increased levels of adiponectin ($p < 0.05$)	30864188
Zingiber officinale (ginger)					
Carvalho et al. 2020	600 mg of ginger/ capsule BID; one 30 minutes before breakfast and the other 30 minutes before lunch for 90 days (*n* = 47)	Placebo for 90 days (*n* = 56)	Not reported	Ginger supplementation reduced FBG, HbA$_{1c}$, TC, LDL, and elevated levels of HDL	33053078
Zarezadeh et al. 2018	Ginger powder (2 g/day) for 10 weeks (*n* = 23)	Placebo (2 g wheat flour) for 10 weeks (*n* = 22)	Not reported	Ginger supplementation diminished asymmetric dimethylarginine serum levels significantly ($p = 0.002$) and intercellular adhesion molecule-1 levels marginally ($p = 0.097$)	30099412
Trigonella foenum-graecum (fenugreek)					
Hadi et al. 2020	Fenugreek seed powder (5 g TID) for 8 weeks (*n* = 25)	Placebo for 8 weeks (*n* = 25)	Anti-diabetic agents	Supplementation of fenugreek significantly decreased FPG ($p = 0.024$), ALT ($p = 0.02$), ALP ($p = 0.001$), AST ($p = 0.014$), systolic BP ($p = 0.001$), irisin ($p = 0.001$) with no significant changes in diastolic BP and blood urea nitrogen	32147060
Geberemeskel, Debebe, and Nguse 2019	Fenugreek seed powder solution (25 g BID) for 1 month (*n* = 57)	Metformin for 1 month (*n* = 57)	Not reported	Significant reduction in TC ($p < 0.001$), TG ($p < 0.001$), LDL ($p < 0.001$) and increase in HDL ($p < 0.001$) in fenugreek group	31583253

and fenugreek (*Trigonella foenum* graecum) (Hadi et al. 2020; Geberemeskel, Debebe, and Nguse 2019); herbs like garlic (*Allium sativum*) (Ashraf, Khan, and Ashraf 2011; Sobenin et al. 2008); spices, for example turmeric (*Curcuma longa*) (Neta et al. 2021; Adibian et al. 2019) and ginger (*Zingiber officinale*) (Carvalho et al. 2020; Zarezadeh et al. 2018). Most of these foods, spices, and herbs are used as an adjuvant with main treatment in controlling, majorly, blood glucose level and lipid profile in DM. Further, *WS* being considered as food is also used in combination with other herbs in managing DM (Mutalik et al. 2005; Upadhyay, Kumar, and Mishra 2009), as a combination of herbal preparations can show greater synergistic activity over monocomponent preparations.

15.11 TOXICITY AND CAUTIONARY NOTES

WS, an age-old herb, has been in use since ancient times for treating and managing various ailments including DM, and has a long history of safe use (Narayana and Durg 2019). It is recognized as a food or food ingredient by the European Commission, and its access to the market is not subjected to the Novel Food Regulation (EC) No. 258/97 (http://ec.europa.eu/food/safety/novel_food/catalogue/search/public/index.cfm: Product Name – *Withania somnifera*). Further, as per the Dietary Supplement Health and Education Act (1994), it is freely available in the United States as a dietary supplement but is not given "generally recognized as safe" status (Mills, Simon Mills, and Bone 2004).

Three clinical studies evaluated the safety and tolerability of *WS* in patients with type 2 DM and noted no safety concerns when assessed from hematological, renal, and hepatic laboratory parameters (Nayak et al. 2015; Usharani, Fatima, et al. 2014; Usharani, Kishan, et al. 2014). Further, *WS* supplementation (300 mg BID) for 8 weeks in healthy participants ($N = 80$) reported no safety concerns and was well tolerated. The physical, hematological, and biochemical parameters (including hepatotoxicity assessment and thyroid function parameters) were found to be within limits in both male and female healthy participants (Verma et al. 2021). Likewise, *WS* administration in healthy young adults ($N = 40$; 500 mg/day) and aging overweight males (placebo to ashwagandha, $N = 29$; ashwagandha to placebo, $N = 28$: two tablets daily, each tablet containing 10.5 mg of withanolide glycosides) for 8 weeks reported to be safe and well tolerated (Sandhu et al. 2010; Lopresti, Drummond, and Smith 2019). Further, a prospective observational study evaluated the safety and tolerability of *WS* in healthy volunteers ($N = 18$), and reported significant reduction in cholesterol and LDL levels with decreasing trend in triglyceride as well as increase in muscle strength activity (Raut et al. 2012). The organ function tests were normal following *WS* intervention, and escalated doses (750–1250 mg/day) were well tolerated.

15.12 SUMMARY POINTS

- *WS* (*ashwagandha*: *ashwa* meaning "horse" and *gandha* meaning "smell" in Sanskrit) known as "smell and strength of horse," thus supporting its claim in vigor and strength.
- *WS*, being considered as *Rasayana* (rejuvenating tonic), is reported to have steroidal lactones including withaferin A, withanone, withanolides, sitoindosides, and withanolide C as active constituents.
- Fourteen experimental (preclinical) studies and six clinical trials/case reports assessing the efficacy/effectiveness and safety of *WS* in DM are discussed in this review.
- *WS* treatment, in general, significantly improved elevated blood glucose and HbA_{1c} levels in experimental and clinical studies.
- *WS* also significantly restored the altered lipid profile, insulin level, and serum and oxidative stress markers with no safety concerns.
- Protection of pancreatic β cells from oxidative stress is one of the main mechanisms of *WS* leading to insulin release.
- *WS* also acts by inhibiting α-glucosidase, α-amylase, and DPP-IV enzymes, thus accelerating the transport of glucose into cells.

REFERENCES

Adibian, Mahsa, Homa Hodaei, Omid Nikpayam, Golbon Sohrab, Azita Hekmatdoost, and Mehdi Hedayati. 2019. "The Effects of Curcumin Supplementation on High-Sensitivity C-Reactive Protein, Serum

Adiponectin, and Lipid Profile in Patients with Type 2 Diabetes: A Randomized, Double-Blind, Placebo-Controlled Trial." *Phytotherapy Research : PTR* 33 (5): 1374–1383. http://doi.org/10.1002/ptr.6328.

Agnihotri, Akshay P, Smita D Sontakke, Vijay R Thawani, Anand Saoji, and Vaidya Shishir S Goswami. 2013. "Effects of Withania Somnifera in Patients of Schizophrenia: A Randomized, Double Blind, Placebo Controlled Pilot Trial Study." *Indian Journal of Pharmacology* 45 (4): 417–18. doi:10.4103/0253-7613.115012.

Aliper, Alexander, Leslie Jellen, Franco Cortese, Artem Artemov, Darla Karpinsky-Semper, Alexey Moskalev, Andrew G. Swick, and Alex Zhavoronkov. 2017. "Towards Natural Mimetics of Metformin and Rapamycin." *Aging* 9 (11): 2245–68. doi:10.18632/aging.101319.

Almdal, T. P., and H Vilstrup. 1988. "Strict Insulin Therapy Normalises Organ Nitrogen Contents and the Capacity of Urea Nitrogen Synthesis in Experimental Diabetes in Rats." *Diabetologia* 31 (2): 114–118. http://doi.org/10.1007/BF00395558.

Andallu, B, and B Radhika. 2000. "Hypoglycemic, Diuretic and Hypocholesterolemic Effect of Winter Cherry (Withania Somnifera, Dunal) Root." *Indian Journal of Experimental Biology* 38 (6): 607–609.

Anwer, Tarique, Manju Sharma, Gyas Khan, Mohammad Firoz Alam, Nawazish Alam, Md Sajid Ali, and Md Sarfaraz Alam. 2017. "Preventive Role of Withania Somnifera on Hyperlipidemia and Cardiac Oxidative Stress in Streptozotocin Induced Type 2 Diabetic Rats." *Tropical Journal of Pharmaceutical Research* 16 (1): 119. http://doi.org/10.4314/tjpr.v16i1.15.

Anwer, Tarique, Manju Sharma, Krishna Kolappa Pillai, and Muzaffar Iqbal. 2008. "Effect of Withania Somnifera on Insulin Sensitivity in Non-Insulin-Dependent Diabetes Mellitus Rats." *Basic & Clinical Pharmacology & Toxicology* 102 (6): 498–503. http://doi.org/10.1111/j.1742-7843.2008.00223.x.

Anwer, Tarique, Manju Sharma, Krishna Kolappa Pillai, and Gyas Khan. 2012. "Protective Effect of Withania Somnifera against Oxidative Stress and Pancreatic Beta-Cell Damage in Type 2 Diabetic Rats." *Acta Poloniae Pharmaceutica* 69 (6): 1095–1101.

Ashraf, Rizwan, Rafeeq Alam Khan, and Imran Ashraf. 2011. "Garlic (*Allium Sativum*) Supplementation with Standard Antidiabetic Agent Provides Better Diabetic Control in Type 2 Diabetes Patients." *Pakistan Journal of Pharmaceutical Sciences* 24 (4): 565–570. http://www.ncbi.nlm.nih.gov/pubmed/21959822.

Bhat, Jyoti, Aparna Damle, Pankaj P. Vaishnav, Ruud Albers, Manoj Joshi, and Gautam Banerjee. 2010. "In Vivo Enhancement of Natural Killer Cell Activity through Tea Fortified with Ayurvedic Herbs." *Phytotherapy Research* 24 (1): 129–135. http://doi.org/10.1002/ptr.2889.

Bhattacharya, S K, K S Satyan, and A Chakrabarti. 1997. "Effect of Trasina, an Ayurvedic Herbal Formulation, on Pancreatic Islet Superoxide Dismutase Activity in Hyperglycaemic Rats." *Indian Journal of Experimental Biology* 35 (3): 297–299. www.ncbi.nlm.nih.gov/pubmed/9332177.

Borenstein, Michael, Larry V Hedges, Julian P. T. Higgins, and Hannah R Rothstein. 2009. *Introduction to Meta-Analysis.* Chichester: John Wiley & Sons, Ltd. http://doi.org/10.1002/9780470743386.

Carvalho, Gerdane Celene Nunes, José Claudio Garcia Lira-Neto, Márcio Flávio Moura de Araújo, Roberto Wagner Júnior Freire de Freitas, Maria Lúcia Zanetti, and Marta Maria Coelho Damasceno. 2020. "Effectiveness of Ginger in Reducing Metabolic Levels in People with Diabetes: A Randomized Clinical Trial." *Revista Latino-Americana de Enfermagem* 28: e3369. http://doi.org/10.1590/1518-8345.3870.3369.

Cortez-Navarrete, Marisol, Esperanza Martínez-Abundis, Karina G Pérez-Rubio, Manuel González-Ortiz, and Miriam Méndez-Del Villar. 2018. "Momordica Charantia Administration Improves Insulin Secretion in Type 2 Diabetes Mellitus." *Journal of Medicinal Food* 21 (7): 672–677. http://doi.org/doi:10.1089/jmf.2017.0114.

Department of AYUSH. 1989. *The Ayurvedic Pharmacopoeia, Part-I, Volume-I.* Vol. 1. Ministry of Health and Family Welfare: Government of India.

Durg, Sharanbasappa, Sachin Bavage, and Shivakumar B. Shivaram. 2020. "*Withania somnifera* (Indian Ginseng) in Diabetes Mellitus: A Systematic Review and Meta-analysis of Scientific Evidence from Experimental Research to Clinical Application." Phytotherapy Research 34 (5): 1041–1059. https://doi.org/10.1002/ptr.6589.

Durg, Sharanbasappa, Shivsharan B Dhadde, Ravichandra Vandal, Badamaranahalli S Shivakumar, and Chabbanahalli S Charan. 2015. "Withania Somnifera (Ashwagandha) in Neurobehavioural Disorders Induced by Brain Oxidative Stress in Rodents: A Systematic Review and Meta-Analysis." *Journal of Pharmacy and Pharmacology* 67 (7): 879–899. http://doi.org/10.1111/jphp.12398.

Durg, Sharanbasappa, Shivakumar Badamaranahalli Shivaram, and Sachin Bavage. 2018. "Withania Somnifera (Indian Ginseng) in Male Infertility: An Evidence-Based Systematic Review and Meta-Analysis." *Phytomedicine : International Journal of Phytotherapy and Phytopharmacology* 50 (November): 247–256. http://doi.org/10.1016/j.phymed.2017.11.011.

Durg, Sharanbasappa, Veeresh P Veerapur, Satrasala Neelima, and Shivsharan B Dhadde. 2017. "Antidiabetic Activity of Embelia Ribes, Embelin and Its Derivatives: A Systematic Review and Meta-Analysis."

Biomedicine and Pharmacotherapy 86. Elsevier Masson SAS: 195–204. http://doi.org/10.1016/j.biopha.2016.12.001.

Geberemeskel, Genet Alem, Yared Godefa Debebe, and Nigisty Abraha Nguse. 2019. "Antidiabetic Effect of Fenugreek Seed Powder Solution (*Trigonella Foenum-Graecum L.*) on Hyperlipidemia in Diabetic Patients." *Journal of Diabetes Research* 2019: 8507453. http://doi.org/10.1155/2019/8507453.

Gopinath, Devi, Umesh Dimri, Y Ajith, P. M. Deepa, M. I. Yatoo, A Gopalakrishnan, and E Madhesh. 2021. "The Anti-Oxidant and the Anti-Diabetic Effects of Terminalia Chebula and Withania Somnifera in Subclinically Diabetic Dogs." *Indian Journal of Animal Research* 55 (April): 1–9. Agricultural Research Communication Center. http://doi.org/10.18805/IJAR.B-4355.

Hadi, Amir, Arman Arab, Hossein Hajianfar, Behrouz Talaei, Maryam Miraghajani, Siavash Babajafari, Wolfgang Marx, and Rahele Tavakoly. 2020. "The Effect of Fenugreek Seed Supplementation on Serum Irisin Levels, Blood Pressure, and Liver and Kidney Function in Patients with Type 2 Diabetes Mellitus: A Parallel Randomized Clinical Trial." *Complementary Therapies in Medicine* 49 (March): 102315. http://doi.org/10.1016/j.ctim.2020.102315.

Harris, Elizabeth H. 2005. "Elevated Liver Function Tests in Type 2 Diabetes." *Clinical Diabetes* 23 (3): 115–119. http://doi.org/10.2337/diaclin.23.3.115.

Huerta, V, K Mihalik, K Becket, V Maitin, and D Vattem. 2010. "Anti-Diabetic and Anti-Energy Harvesting Properties of Common Traditional Herbs, Spices and Medicinal Plants from India." *Journal of Natural Remedies* 10 (2): 123–135. http://doi.org/10.18311/jnr/2010/253.

Ingram, Donald K, R Michael Anson, Rafael De Cabo, Jacek Mamczarz, Min Zhu, Julie Mattison, Mark A Lane, and George S Roth. 2004. "Development of Calorie Restriction Mimetics as a Prolongevity Strategy." *Annals of the New York Academy of Sciences* 1019: 412–423. http://doi.org/10.1196/annals.1297.074.

Jain, S, P Pandhi, A P Singh, and S Malhotra. 2006. "Efficacy of Standardised Herbal Extracts in Type 1 Diabetes-an Experimental Study." *African Journal of Traditional, Complementary and Alternative Medicines* 3 (4): 23–33.

Jonathan, Gorelick, Rosenberg Rivka, Smotrich Avinoam, Hanuš Lumír, and Bernstein Nirit. 2015. "Hypoglycemic Activity of Withanolides and Elicitated Withania Somnifera." *Phytochemistry* 116 (1): 283–289. http://doi.org/10.1016/j.phytochem.2015.02.029.

Kaul, Sunil C, and Renu Wadhwa. 2017. *Science of Ashwagandha: Preventive and Therapeutic Potentials.* Edited by Sunil C. Kaul and Renu Wadhwa. Cham: Springer International Publishing. http://doi.org/10.1007/978-3-319-59192-6.

Khan, Murad Ali, Haroon Khan, and Tahir Ali. 2014. "Withanolides Isolated from Withania Somnifera with α-Glucosidase Inhibition." *Medicinal Chemistry Research* 23 (5): 2386–2390. http://doi.org/10.1007/s00044-013-0838-3.

Kiasalari, Z, M Khalili, and M Aghaei. 2009. "Effect of Withania Somniferaon Levels of Sex Hormonesin the Diabetic Male Rats." *Iranian Journal of Reproductive Medicine* 7 (4): 163–168.

Kim, Soo Kyoung, Jaehoon Jung, Jung Hwa Jung, NalAe Yoon, Sang Soo Kang, Gu Seob Roh, and Jong Ryeal Hahm. 2020. "Hypoglycemic Efficacy and Safety of Momordica Charantia (Bitter Melon) in Patients with Type 2 Diabetes Mellitus." *Complementary Therapies in Medicine* 52 (August): 102524. http://doi.org/10.1016/j.ctim.2020.102524.

Kulkarni, S. K., and Ashish Dhir. 2008. "Withania Somnifera: An Indian Ginseng." *Progress in Neuro-Psychopharmacology and Biological Psychiatry* 32 (5): 1093–1105. http://doi.org/10.1016/j.pnpbp.2007.09.011.

Kyathanahalli, Chandrashekara Nagaraj, Mallayya Jayawanth Manjunath, and Muralidhara. 2014. "Oral Supplementation of Standardized Extract of Withania Somnifera Protects against Diabetes-Induced Testicular Oxidative Impairments in Prepubertal Rats." *Protoplasma* 251 (5): 1021–1029. http://doi.org/10.1007/s00709-014-0612-5.

Langade, Deepak, Vaishali Thakare, Subodh Kanchi, and Sunil Kelgane. 2021. "Clinical Evaluation of the Pharmacological Impact of Ashwagandha Root Extract on Sleep in Healthy Volunteers and Insomnia Patients: A Double-Blind, Randomized, Parallel-Group, Placebo-Controlled Study." *Journal of Ethnopharmacology* 264 (January): 113276. http://doi.org/10.1016/j.jep.2020.113276.

Lee, Jaemin, Junli Liu, Xudong Feng, Mario Andrés Salazar Hernández, Patrick Mucka, Dorina Ibi, Jae Won Choi, and Umut Ozcan. 2016. "Withaferin a Is a Leptin Sensitizer with Strong Antidiabetic Properties in Mice." *Nature Medicine* 22 (9): 1023–1032. http://doi.org/10.1038/nm.4145.

Lopresti, Adrian L, Peter D Drummond, and Stephen J Smith. 2019. "A Randomized, Double-Blind, Placebo-Controlled, Crossover Study Examining the Hormonal and Vitality Effects of Ashwagandha (Withania

Somnifera) in Aging, Overweight Males." *American Journal of Men's Health* 13 (2): 1–15. http://doi.org/10.1177/1557988319835985.

Mills, S Y, M.F.M.A. Simon Mills, and K Bone. 2004. *The Essential Guide to Herbal Safety*. Missouri: Elsevier Health Sciences.

Mutalik, S, M Chetana, B Sulochana, P Uma Devi, and N Udupa. 2005. "Effect of Dianex, a Herbal Formulation on Experimentally Induced Diabetes Mellitus." *Phytotherapy Research: PTR* 19 (5): 409–415. http://doi.org/10.1002/ptr.1570.

Narayana, D. B. Anantha, and Sharanbasappa Durg. 2019. "Approaches to Safety Evaluation of Botanicals and Processed Botanicals Known in Traditional Knowledge." In *Natural Medicines*, 187–214. Boca Raton: Taylor & Francis: CRC Press. http://doi.org/10.1201/9781315187853-10.

Nayak, S, S Nayak, B K Panda, and S Das. 2015. "A Clinical Study on Management of Stress in Type-2 Diabetes Mellitus (Madhumeha) with Ashwagandha (Withania Somnifera)." *Ayushdhara* 2 (6): 413–417.

Neta, Joana Furtado de Figueiredo, Vivian Saraiva Veras, Danilo Ferreira de Sousa, Maria da Conceição Dos Santos Oliveira Cunha, Maria Veraci Oliveira Queiroz, José Claudio Garcia Lira Neto, Marta Maria Coelho Damasceno, Márcio Flávio Moura de Araújo, and Roberto Wagner Júnior Freire de Freitas. 2021. "Effectiveness of the Piperine-Supplemented *Curcuma Longa* L. in Metabolic Control of Patients with Type 2 Diabetes: A Randomised Double-Blind Placebo-Controlled Clinical Trial." *International Journal of Food Sciences and Nutrition* 72 (7): 968–977. http://doi.org/10.1080/09637486.2021.1885015.

Nirupama, R, M Devaki, M Nirupama, and H N Yajurvedi. 2014. "In Vitro and in Vivo Studies on the Hypoglycaemic Potential of Ashwagandha (Withania Somnifera) Root." *Pharma Science Monitor* 5 (3): 45–58.

Parihar, Mordhwaj S, Madhulika Chaudhary, Rajani Shetty, and Taruna Hemnani. 2004. "Susceptibility of Hippocampus and Cerebral Cortex to Oxidative Damage in Streptozotocin Treated Mice: Prevention by Extracts of Withania Somnifera and Aloe Vera." *Journal of Clinical Neuroscience* 11 (4): 397–402. http://doi.org/10.1016/j.jocn.2003.09.008.

Parihar, Priyanka, R Shetty, P Ghafourifar, and Mordhwaj S Parihar. 2016. "Increase in Oxidative Stress and Mitochondrial Impairment in Hypothalamus of Streptozotocin Treated Diabetic Rat: Antioxidative Effect of Withania Somnifera." *Cellular and Molecular Biology* 62 (1): 73–83. http://doi.org/10.14715/cmb/2016.62.1.15.

Raut, Ashwinikumar, Nirmala N Rege, Sudatta G Shirolkar, Shefali N Pandey, Firoz M Tadvi, Punita V Solanki, Rama A Vaidya, Ashok B Vaidya, and Kirti R Kene. 2012. "Exploratory Study to Evaluate Tolerability, Safety, and Activity of Ashwagandha (Withania Somnifera) in Healthy Volunteers." *Journal of Ayurveda and Integrative Medicine* 3 (3): 111. http://doi.org/10.4103/0975–9476.100168.

Reuland, Danielle J., Shadi Khademi, Christopher J. Castle, David C. Irwin, Joe M. McCord, Benjamin F. Miller, and Karyn L. Hamilton. 2013. "Upregulation of Phase II Enzymes through Phytochemical Activation of Nrf2 Protects Cardiomyocytes against Oxidant Stress." *Free Radical Biology and Medicine* 56 (March): 102–111. http://doi.org/10.1016/j.freeradbiomed.2012.11.016.

Salmela, P I, E A Sotaniemi, M Niemi, and O Mäentausta. 1984. "Liver Function Tests in Diabetic Patients." *Diabetes Care* 7 (3): 248–254. http://doi.org/10.2337/diacare.7.3.248.

Sandhu, Jaspal Singh, Biren Shah, Shweta Shenoy, Suresh Chauhan, G S Lavekar, and M M Padhi. 2010. "Effects of Withania Somnifera (Ashwagandha) and Terminalia Arjuna (Arjuna) on Physical Performance and Cardiorespiratory Endurance in Healthy Young Adults." *International Journal of Ayurveda Research* 1 (3): 144–149. http://doi.org/10.4103/0974-7788.72485.

Sarangi, A, S Jena, A K Sarangi, and B Swain. 2013. "Anti-Diabetic Effects of Withania Somnifera Root and Leaf Extracts on Streptozotocin Induced Diabetic Rats." *Journal of Cell and Tissue Research* 13 (1): 3597–3601.

Simon, K, T Inoue, G Fenteany, G Bahtiyar, and A Sacerdote. 2018. "Ashwagandha Root in the Treatment of Prediabetes." *Endocrine Reviews* 39 (2): Supplement 1. www.abstractsonline.com/pp8/#!/4482/presentation/7233.

Singh, Anand Krishna, Jaya Joshi, and Rameshwar Jatwa. 2013. "Dipeptidyl Peptidase IV (CD26/DPP-IV) Inhibitory and Free Radical Scavenging Potential of W Somnifera and T Foenum-Graecum Extract." *International Journal of Phytomedicine* 5 (4): 503–509. http://doi.org/10.5138/ijpm.v5i4.1212.

Sobenin, Igor A, Lyudmila V Nedosugova, Lyudmila V Filatova, Mikhail I Balabolkin, Tatiana V Gorchakova, and Alexander N Orekhov. 2008. "Metabolic Effects of Time-Released Garlic Powder Tablets in Type 2 Diabetes Mellitus: The Results of Double-Blinded Placebo-Controlled Study." *Acta Diabetologica* 45 (1): 1–6. http://doi.org/10.1007/s00592-007-0011-x.

Tekula, Sravani, Amit Khurana, Pratibha Anchi, and Chandraiah Godugu. 2018. "Withaferin-A Attenuates Multiple Low Doses of Streptozotocin (MLD-STZ) Induced Type 1 Diabetes." *Biomedicine & Pharmacotherapy = Biomedecine & Pharmacotherapie* 106 (October): 1428–1440. http://doi.org/10.1016/j.biopha.2018.07.090.

Thakur, Ajit, Amitabha Dey, Shyam S Chatterjee, and Vikas Kumar. 2015. "Reverse Ayurvedic Pharmacology of Ashwagandha as an Adaptogenic Anti-Diabetic Plant: A Pilot Study." *Current Traditional Medicine* 1 (1): 51–61. http://doi.org/10.2174/2215083801999150527115205.

Udayakumar, Rajangam, Sampath Kasthurirengan, Thankaraj Salammal Mariashibu, Manoharan Rajesh, Vasudevan Ramesh Anbazhagan, Sei Chang Kim, Andy Ganapathi, and Chang Won Choi. 2009. "Hypoglycaemic and Hypolipidaemic Effects of Withania Somnifera Root and Leaf Extracts on Alloxan-Induced Diabetic Rats." *International Journal of Molecular Sciences* 10 (5): 2367–2382. http://doi.org/10.3390/ijms10052367.

Udayakumar, Rajangam, Sampath Kasthurirengan, Ayyappan Vasudevan, Thankaraj Salammal Mariashibu, Jesudass Joseph Sahaya Rayan, Chang Won Choi, Andy Ganapathi, and Sei Chang Kim. 2010. "Antioxidant Effect of Dietary Supplement Withania Somnifera L. Reduce Blood Glucose Levels in Alloxan-Induced Diabetic Rats." *Plant Foods for Human Nutrition* 65 (2): 91–98. http://doi.org/10.1007/s11130-009-0146-8.

Upadhyay, A K, K Kumar, and H Mishra. 2009. "Effects of Combination of Shilajit Extract and Ashwagandha (Withania Somnifera) on Fasting Blood Sugar and Lipid Profile." *Journal of Pharmacy Research* 2 (5): 897–899.

Usharani, P, N Fatima, C U Kumar, and P V Kishan. 2014. "Evaluation of a Highly Standardized Withania Somnifera Extract on Endothelial Dysfunction and Biomarkers of Oxidative Stress in Patients with Type 2 Diabetes Mellitus: A Randomized, Double Blind, Placebo Controlled Study." *International Journal of Ayurveda and Pharma Research* 2 (3): 22–32.

Usharani, P, P V Kishan, N Fatima, and C U Kumar. 2014. "A Comparative Study to Evaluate the Effect of Highly Standardised Aqueous Extracts of Phyllanthus Emblica, Withania Somnifera and Their Combination on Endothelial Dysfunction and Biomarkers in Patients with Type II Diabetes Mellitus." *International Journal of Pharmaceutical Sciences and Research* 5 (7): 2687–2697. http://doi.org/10.13040/IJPSR.0975-8232.5(6).2687-97.

Verma, Narsing, Sandeep Kumar Gupta, Shashank Tiwari, and Ashok Kumar Mishra. 2021. "Safety of Ashwagandha Root Extract: A Randomized, Placebo-Controlled, Study in Healthy Volunteers." *Complementary Therapies in Medicine* 57 (March): 102642. http://doi.org/10.1016/j.ctim.2020.102642.

Weiner, M A, and J Weiner. 1994. "Ashwagandha (India Ginseng)." In *Herbs That Heal*, edited by M A Weiner and J Weiner, 70–72. Mill Valley, CA: Quantum Books.

Zarezadeh, Meysam, Ahmad Saedisomeolia, Masoud Khorshidi, Hamed Kord Varkane, Motahareh Makhdoomi Arzati, Mina Abdollahi, Mir Saeed Yekaninejad, Rezvan Hashemi, Mohammad Effatpanah, and Niyaz Mohammadzadeh Honarvar. 2018. "Asymmetric Dimethylarginine and Soluble Inter-Cellular Adhesion Molecule-1 Serum Levels Alteration Following Ginger Supplementation in Patients with Type 2 Diabetes: A Randomized Double-Blind, Placebo-Controlled Clinical Trial." *Journal of Complementary & Integrative Medicine* 16 (2). http://doi.org/10.1515/jcim-2018-0019.

16 Medicinal Herbs and Spices in the Management of Diabetes

Debarupa Hajra and Santanu Paul

CONTENTS

16.1 INTRODUCTION

Diabetes mellitus is characterized by an imbalance of glucose level in the blood. It is mostly of 3 types: type 1, type 2, and gestational diabetes. The onset of type 1 diabetes mellitus is mostly observed at quite a young age. It is characterized by the absence of the formation of insulin in the β cells of the islet of Langerhans in the pancreas. The general treatment includes the external supply of insulin into the body. Type 2 diabetes mellitus (T2DM) is generally considered to be related to diet and lifestyle by a greater degree. In the case of T2DM, there can be a number of underlying reasons or processes. These include reduced production of insulin, insensitive insulin receptor, and disrupted PkB/Akt pathway. Gestational diabetes is a type of diabetes that develops in pregnant women leading to glucose imbalance.

T2DM is such a metabolic disease that can be considered to be a pandemic itself. It is of global concern now considering that many lives are affected by this deadly disease. Current lifestyles and the accompanying stress in daily life is a major contributor to this current scenario. It is multifactorial in nature. The management of this pathological condition requires lifelong drug therapy and definitely involves a complete overhaul of the lifestyle of the affected individual.

In recent decades, there have been several advances in the treatment and prevention of diabetes and in glycemic management. But the existence of cardiovascular complications remains an important issue of concern associated with T2DM (Pirola et al., 2010). The prevalent management strategy for T2DM treatment involves using antidiabetes drugs, monitoring of lipid profile and arterial pressure, and lifestyle intervention including regular physical activity and proper nutrition. As per recent research, there is growing knowledge and evidence of the efficacy of medicinal plants

DOI: 10.1201/9781003220930-18

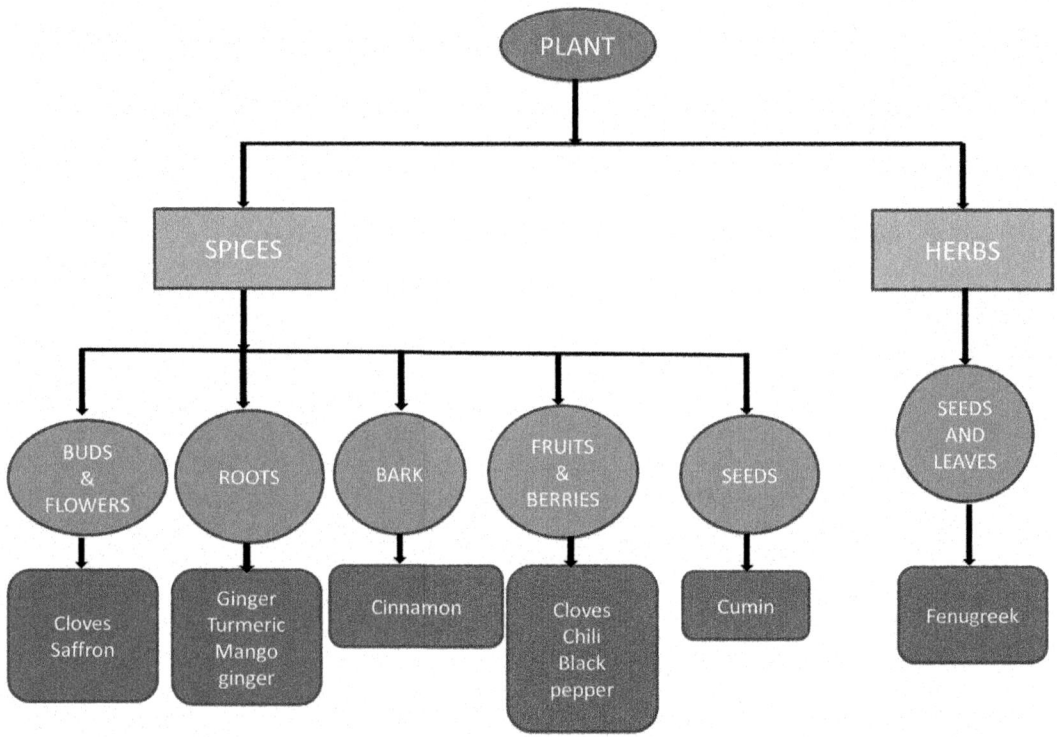

FIGURE 16.1   Various types of spices and herbs with the plant parts that are commonly consumed.

as supplements for T2DM prevention and subsequent management (Standards of Medical Care in Diabetes, 2019). There is evidence of the evolution of the use of medicinal plant supplements for T2DM management (Demmers et al., 2017; Poolsup et al., 2019; Suksomboon et al., 2011).

Several studies have shown that in developing countries, a 69% increase in incidence of diabetes has been observed. In developed countries, between 2010 and 2030 a nearly 20% increase is expected (Neelakantan et al., 2014). T2DM is a metabolic disease that can be controlled and mediated by diet and lifestyle. In Asia the incorporation of several spices and herbs in daily life has led to better health conditions as compared to the West, though Asia, too, is now becoming adversely affected by these lifestyle diseases such as cardiovascular diseases, obesity, and diabetes with the higher intake of processed and fast foods. Spices such as curcumin, black pepper, star anise, cinnamon, ginger, ginseng, fenugreek, and yellow and black mustard are a part of cuisines all over the world, mostly Asia. These spices were much sought after since ancient times, which was a major reason that eventually led to colonization by the European countries. It is said that the spices and condiments that Vasco da Gama had taken back on his return to Europe, had yielded him 60 times the total expenditure of the voyage! The various types of spices and herbs and the parts they are derived from are shown in Figure 16.1.

16.2   SPICES IN THE MANAGEMENT OF DIABETES

16.2.1   FENUGREEK (*TRIGONELLA FOENUM-GRAECUM*)

Fenugreek is a herb that belongs to the Fabaceae family (Hajra et al., 2018). Its scientific name is *Trigonella folium*. Fenugreek possesses a number of properties such as anti-inflammatory, anti-oxidant, antifungal, antibacterial, antilipidemic, hypocholesterolemic, anticarcinogenic, and also antidiabetic activities. Fenugreek contains soluble dietary fiber that enhances glycemic control by inhibiting lipid-hydrolyzing and carbohydrate-hydrolyzing enzymes in the digestive system. Flavonoids present in plants contribute to the color of fruits and flowers. They are polyphenolic compounds. These possess antioxidant, antitumor, and antibacterial activities. They are known to be present in fenugreek as well. Fenugreek seeds are reported to lower blood glucose levels in diabetic patients and also reduces fasting blood glucose levels. It also enhances glucose tolerance as revealed in clinical studies on human subjects (Neelakantan et al., 2014).

16.2.2 TURMERIC (*CURCUMA LONGA*)

Curcumin is a known bioactive molecule that is present in the rhizome of the *C. longa* plant (turmeric) and several other spices belonging to the genus *Curcuma*. It has a varied range of pathological and biological effects such as cardioprotective, nephroprotective, antineoplastic, hepatoprotective, anti-inflammatory, hypoglycemic, antioxidant, immunomodulatory, antimicrobial, and antirheumatic effects (Derosa et al., 2016; Mirzaei et al., 2017). An *in vivo* model study has shown that diabetes development is delayed by application of curcumin extracts. It also showed enhanced β cell functions, prevents β cell death and reduced insulin resistance (Pivari et al., 2019). *In vitro* studies with curcumin and its analogs have shown a mechanism of action quite close to that of thiazolidinedione. It is an antidiabetic drug that helps to manage diabetes through peroxisome proliferator-activated receptor-γ (PPAR-γ) activation (Nishiyama et al., 2005). Thus, curcumin may prove to be especially effective in the regulation and control of lipidemia and glycemia. Both these factors play crucial roles in T2DM treatment. Several randomized controlled trials (RCTs) have attested to the above findings (Rahmani et al., 2016).

16.2.3 AMADA (*CURCUMA AMADA*)

C. amada, or mango ginger, belongs to the Zingiberaceae family. It is a rhizome and is popular for its characteristic aroma. It is cultivated throughout India, Sri Lanka, Bangladesh, and in many Southeast Asian countries. It is not only valued for its culinary utilities but also for its inherent medicinal value. The fresh-cut rhizomes have the characteristic flavor, aroma, and color of mango. The herb generally attains a height of 60–90 cm. The leaves of mango ginger are long, petiolate, and oblong-lanceolate. They taper at both the ends and are green in color on both sides. The flowers of the plant are white or pale yellow. There are spikes that occur in the center of the leaves; the lip is semi-elliptic, yellow, three-lobed, the middle lobe emarginate. Studies have revealed that the ethanol extract of the mango ginger rhizome has hydroxyl, carbonyl, ester, and olefin functional groups and also methyl, methylene, methionine proteins, and olefinic proteins. According to a study by Dipanwita Mitra et al. on streptozotocin-induced diabetic rats orally administered with hydromethanolic extract of *C. amada* for 28 days, a significant antidiabetic and antioxidative effect of the extract in a dose-dependent manner was observed. Comparative studies of extract treated and untreated diabetic groups revealed recovery of fasting blood glucose level, serum insulin, activity of carbohydrate metabolic enzymes, and antioxidative enzymes. The treatment improved the size of pancreatic islet and cell population densities.

16.2.4 BLACK PEPPER (*PIPER NIGRUM*)

Black pepper is considered to be one of the most highly prized species globally. It is popularly known as "the king of spices" and "black gold" (Wei et al., 2019). It is of two types, one being black pepper, which is derived from the unripe and green berry of the plant *P. nigrum* L., and white pepper is derived from the white inside (Chithra et al., 2011). Pepper is known to possess several bioactive compounds such as alkaloids (piperine), polyphenols, amides, lignans, and flavonoids (Jin et al., 2013; Rathod et al., 2014; Wang et al., 2018). It has been found that black pepper contains a higher polyphenol proportion than white pepper (Agbor et al., 2006). Black pepper is also known to contain a major proportion of essential oil (Wei et al., 2019), with characteristic aroma and flavor. This is also known to exhibit DPPH and ABTS free radical inhibition potential and hence strong antioxidant potential.

16.2.5 CINNAMON (*CINNAMOMUM ZEYLANICUM*)

Nearly 300 species of the genus *Cinnamomum* are known to us. Out of these, Ceylon cinnamon (*C. zeylanicum*) are widely available and used for obtaining the spice cinnamon (Jayaprakasha et al., 2011). There are many well-known health effects of cinnamon such as antimicrobial, combating cardiovascular disease, reducing risk of onset of colon cancer, inflammatory properties, and management of blood glucose level. An *in vitro* study by Ranasinghe et al. (2012) showed *C. zeylanicum* exhibited reduced postprandial intestinal glucose absorption. This occurred due to inhibition of pancreatic α-amylase and α-glucosidase. It was also found to stimulate cellular glucose uptake by membrane translocation of glucose transporter-4, enhancing glucose metabolism and glycogen synthesis. Also, it was found to inhibit gluconeogenesis and stimulate insulin release and potentiating insulin receptor activity.

16.2.6 GINGER (*ZINGIBER OFFICINALE*)

Ginger (*Z. officinale* Roscoe) belongs to the Zingiberaceae family and is a herbaceous perennial plant. Ginger is quite popular for both its culinary utilities and its medicinal value. It has a characteristic pungent taste and aroma (Bi et al., 2017). Ginger has been well-known for centuries as a potent medicinal plant in the Indian Ayurvedic system of medicine.

16.2.7 CUMIN (*CUMINUM CYMINUM*)

Cumin (*C. cyminum* L.) seeds (green cumin) is a herbaceous plant that belongs to the Apiaceae family. Cumin is indigenous to the Mediterranean region, central Asia, and southwestern Asia and is popularly used as a spice (Mohamed, 2018). Cumin is very widely used in Indian cuisine. Previous studies suggested that cumin possesses a broad range of pharmacological activities such as antibacterial, antioxidant, hypoglycemic, and anticarcinogenic (El-Ghorab et al., 2010). Cumin seeds contain 5% volatile oil, 22% fat, 10% protein, and 11% fiber. The major volatile components known to be present in cumin are cuminaldehyde, cymene, and terpenoids. A specific study (Mohamed, 2018) found that crude ethanol extract of cumin seeds possesses antioxidant and antidiabetic effects. The extract showed complete safety. Ethanol fraction of cumin seeds may be used as an alternative treatment for diabetes mellitus.

16.2.8 ANISE (*PIMPINELLA ANISUM*)

An aromatic plant, widely used in traditional Iranian medicine, *P. anisum* of the Umbelliferae family is commonly known as anise, or star anise. It is an annual herb that grows up to a height of 50 cm and is characterized by white flowers and greenish yellow seeds. It is known to contain a substantial amount of essential oil which is used to relieve gastrointestinal pain and digestive issues. It is also used for its flavoring properties in food industries and is known to be beneficial for lactating mothers (Shojaii et al., 2012). Anise seeds are also known to show antioxidant properties, as attested by Vecchio et al. (2016). In a study by Gulcin, the antioxidant properties of aqueous and ethanolic extract of anise seeds were studied. They showed strong antioxidative properties when compared to standards such as butylated hydroxytoluene (BHT), α-tocopherol. The anise seeds exhibit strong superoxide anion scavenging power as well as enhanced DPPH radical scavenging potential. It is also a potent metal chelating properties as well as hydrogen peroxide scavenging properties. A study was conducted in 2000 (Faried and El-Mehi, 2020) to evaluate the effect of aqueous anise extract on the pancreatic damage in the streptozotocin (STZ)-induced diabetic rat model. The study concluded that there was a significant decrease in body weight and simultaneous increase in blood glucose and serum amylase levels. Marked degenerative changes were observed that resulted in significant decrease in islet perimeter size, vacuolated cytoplasm, pyknotic nuclei, depletion of zymogen granules, dilated congested blood vessels, and degenerated organelles affecting both β cells and acinar cells of the pancreas in the were reported. Hyperglycemia-induced oxidative stress with subsequent upregulation of caspase 3 and beclin 1 immunoreactivity was suggested to be implicated in diabetes mellitus pathogenesis. Anise extract thus shows potent hypoglycemic and antioxidant properties by subsequently downregulating apoptosis and autophagy.

16.2.9 ONION (*ALLIUM CEPA*)

A. cepa, commonly known as onion, belongs to the family of Liliaceae. This is a common part of the human diet in almost every cuisine. It is characterized by a strong pungent smell mostly attributed to its sulfur containing compounds. The sulfur-containing compounds such as S-methylcysteine, quercetin, and many others are the source for its antidiabetic property. Onion helps to combat T2DM through its regulation of hypoglycemic activity. These compounds help to lower blood glucose levels, lipid peroxidation, serum lipids, and oxidative stress. In several studies it has proved to enhance insulin secretion. *A. cepa* extracts regulate hypoglycemic and hypolipidemic activity through normalizing the activities of liver hexokinase, glucose-6-phosphatase, and HMG coenzyme-A reductase.

Of the above-mentioned spices and herbs, turmeric, black pepper, and fenugreek are quite frequently consumed by Asians, and mostly in India. Since time immemorial these have been considered part of both cuisine and traditional medicine. Even the West has come to acknowledge the benefits of these spices. Thus, these are extensively studied and the bioactive compounds present in these have also been subject of intensive studies. The bioactive compounds present in fenugreek, turmeric, and black pepper are listed in Tables 16.1–16.3, respectively, along with their 3D structures.

16.2.10 INSULIN PLANT (*COSTUS IGNEUS*)

C. igneus is popularly known as "insulin plant" due to its reported potent antidiabetic property. It belongs to the family Costaceae. It is known to contain tannins, saponins, alkaloids, triterpenois, ascorbic acid, β-carotene, flavonoids, and α-tocopherol. *C. igneus* possesses triterpenoids (Corosolic acid), which is responsible for imparting glucose uptake activity. Steroid diosgenin present in this plant is known to have hypoglycemic properties. It also contains β-sitosterol which increases plasma insulin level and also increases glucose uptake activity. Flavonoids such as quercetin are also a major component of this plant that increases insulin mediated glucose uptake and activity of antioxidant enzymes. Catechin, a phenol having α glucosidase inhibitory activity and antioxidant activity, is found in good proportions in *C. igneus* (Laha and Paul, 2018).

16.3 TOXICITY AND CAUTIONARY NOTES

The above mentioned spices are a part of the daily cuisine. They have been consumed over thousands of years, hence they are tried and tested years over. There are several studies conducted on these spices that show that that when consumed in limited quantity, they do not cause harm to the human body.

TABLE 16.1

Detailed Properties of Compounds Present in *Trigonella foenum-graecum* (Fenugreek)

Phytochemical Name	IMPPAT/PubMed	Molecular Structure (G/Ml)	Molecular Formula	Class and Subclass	3D Structure	Reference
Spirostan-3-ol, (3β,5β)-	CID:12304444	416.6	$C_{27}H_{44}O_3$	Prenol lipids; triterpenoids		(Pang et al., 2012)
2,3-Butanedione	CID:650	86.09	$C_4H_6O_2$	Organooxygen compounds; carbonyl compounds		(Guerra et al., 2011)
2,3-Dimethylaniline	CID:6893	121.18	$C_8H_{11}N$	Benzene and substituted derivatives; xylenes		(Kang et al., 2013; Swaroop et al., 2014)
3-Amino-4,5-dimethyl-2(5H)-furanone	CID:6421106	127.14	$C_6H_9NO_2$	Carboxylic acids and derivatives; amino acids, peptides, and analogues		(Guerra et al., 2011)
4,5-Dimethyl-3-hydroxy-25h-furanones	CID:62835	128.13	$C_6H_8O_3$	Dihydrofurans; furanones		(Korman et al., 2001)

Name	CID	Molecular Weight	Molecular Formula	Class	Structure	Reference
Apigenin	CID:5280443	270.24	$C_{15}H_{10}O_5$	Flavonoids; flavones		(Rayyan et al., 2010)
Biochanin A	CID:5280373	284.26	$C_{16}H_{12}O_5$	Isoflavonoids; O-methylated isoflavonoids		(Wang et al., 2010)
Calycosin	CID:5280448	284.26	$C_{16}H_{12}O_5$	Isoflavonoids; O-methylated isoflavonoids		(Wang et al., 2010)
Creatine	CID:586	131.13	$C_4H_9N_3O_2$	Carboxylic acids and derivatives; amino acids, peptides, and analogues		(Genet et al., 1999)
D-galactose	CID:6036	180.16	$C_6H_{12}O_6$	Organooxygen compounds; carbohydrates and carbohydrate conjugates		(Zambou et al., 1990)
D-raffinose	CID:10542	504.4	$C_{18}H_{32}O_{16}$	Organooxygen compounds; carbohydrates and carbohydrate conjugates		(Reid, 1971)
Diosgenin	CID:99474	414.6	$C_{27}H_{42}O_3$	—		(Taylor et al., 2000; Lu et al., 2005 Kaufmann et al.,2007; Li et al., 2010; Chaudhary et al., 2015)

(Continued)

TABLE 16.1
(Continued)

Phytochemical Name	IMPPAT/PubMed	Molecular Structure (G/Ml)	Molecular Formula	Class and Subclass	3D Structure	Reference
Eupatin	CASID:19587–65–6	360.32	$C_{18}H_{16}O_8$	Flavonoids; flavones		(Mandegary et al., 2012)
Falcarindiol	CID:5281148	260.399	$C_{17}H_{24}O_2$	Fatty acyls; fatty alcohols		(Yamazoe et al., 2007)
Formononetin	CID:5280378	268.26	$C_{16}H_{12}O_4$	Isoflavonoids; O-methylated isoflavonoids		(Wang et al., 2010)
Galactomannan	CID:439336	504.4	$C_{18}H_{32}O_{16}$	Organooxygen compounds; carbohydrates and carbohydrate conjugates		(Edwards et al., 1989; Wang et al., 2013)
Gitogenin	CID:441887	432.6	$C_{27}H_{44}O_4$	Prenol lipids; triterpenoids		(Shim et al., 2008)
Irilone	CID:5281779	298.25	$C_{16}H_{10}O_6$	Isoflavonoids; isoflav-2-enes		(Wang et al., 2010)

Kaempferol	CID:5280863	286.24	$C_{15}H_{10}O_6$	Flavonoids; flavones	(Han et al., 2001)
Mimosine	CID:3862	198.18	$C_8H_{10}N_2O_4$	Carboxylic acids and derivatives; amino acids, peptides, and analogues	(Sreekala et al., 1999; Sreekala and Lalitha, 2001a; Sreekala and Lalitha, 2001b)
Tolbutamide	CID:5505	270.35	$C_{12}H_{18}N_2O_3S$	Benzene and substituted derivatives; benzenesulfonamides	(Moorthy et al., 2010)
Trigonelline	CID:5570	137.14	$C_7H_7NO_2$	Alkaloids and derivatives	(Moorthy et al., 2010; Morani et al., 2012; Shailajan et al., 2011; Radwan et al., 1980)

TABLE 16.2

Detailed Properties of Compounds Present in *Curcuma longa* (Turmeric)

Phytochemical Name	IMPPAT/PubMed	Molecular Structure (G/Ml)	Molecular Formula	Class and Subclass	3D Structure	Reference
(+)-α-Phellandrene	CID:443160	136.23	$C_{10}H_{16}$	Prenol lipids; monoterpenoids		(Yang et al., 2007)
(+)-Sabinene	CID:10887971	136.230	$C_{10}H_{16}$	Prenol lipids; monoterpenoids		(Yang et al., 2007)
(1E,6E)-1-(4-Hydroxy-3-methoxyphenyl)-7-(4-hydroxyphenyl) hepta-1,6-diene-3,5-dione	CASID:24939–17–1	338.35	$C_{20}H_{18}O_5$	Diarylheptanoids; linear diarylheptanoids		(Rungphanichkul et al., 2011)
1,7-bis(4-Hydroxy-3-methoxyphenyl)-1,6-heptadiene-3,5,dione	CHEMSPIDER:9079552	370.4	$C_{21}H_{22}O_6$	Diarylheptanoids; linear diarylheptanoids		(Guglielmo et al., 2017)
2-Methylisoborneol	CID:16913	168.28	$C_{11}H_{20}O$	Prenol lipids; monoterpenoids		(Maehara et al., 2011)
2,6-Di-tert-butyl-4-methylphenol	CID:31404	220.35	$C_{15}H_{24}O$	Benzene and substituted derivatives;		(Zhao et al., 2019)
Ar-turmerone	CID:160512	216.32	$C_{15}H_{20}O$	Prenol lipids; sesquiterpenoids		(Chang and Chen, 2015)

Name	CID	MW	Formula	Class	Structure	Reference
Bisdemethoxy curcumin	CID:5315472	308.3	$C_{19}H_{16}O_4$	Diarylheptanoids; linear diarylheptanoids		(Neyrinck et al., 2013)
Butylhydroxy anisole	CID:24667	360.5	$C_{22}H_{32}O_4$	Phenols; methoxyphenols		(Valizadeh et al., 2016)
Curlone	CID:196216	218.33	$C_{15}H_{22}O$	Prenol lipids; sesquiterpenoids		(Nishiyama et al., 2005)
Demethoxy curcumin	CID:5469424	338.4	$C_{20}H_{18}O_5$	Diarylheptanoids; linear diarylheptanoids		(Guglielmo et al., 2017)
Dihydrocurcumin	CID:10429233	370.4	$C_{21}H_{22}O_6$	Diarylheptanoids; linear diarylheptanoids		(Akbar et al., 2016)
Eucalyptol	CID:2758	154.25	$C_{10}H_{18}O$	Organoheterocyclic compounds; oxanes		(Hu et al., 1998)
Go-Y022	CID:6474893	326.3	$C_{19}H_{18}O_5$	Cinnamic acids and derivatives; hydroxycinnamic acids and derivatives		(Zheng et al., 2016)
L-ascorbic acid	CID:54670067	176.12	$C_6H_8O_6$	Dihydrofurans; furanones		(Hossain et al., 2013)
Piperine	CID:638024	285.34	$C_{17}H_{19}NO_3$	Alkaloids and derivatives		(Zheng et al., 2016)
Tetrahydrobisde methoxycurcumin	CID:9796792	312.4	$C_{19}H_{20}O_4$	Diarylheptanoids; linear diarylheptanoids		(Zheng et al., 2016)

TABLE 16.3

Detailed Properties of Compounds Present in *Piper nigrum* (Black Pepper)

Phytochemical Name	IMPPAT/ PubMed	Molecular Structure (G/Ml)	Molecular Formula	Class and Subclass	3D Structure	Reference
(−)-Linalool	CID:443158	154.25	$C_{10}H_{18}O$	Prenol lipids; monoterpenoids		(Jhong et al., 2015)
(+)-α-Phellandrene	CID:443160	136.23	$C_{10}H_{16}$	Prenol lipids; monoterpenoids		(Jirovetz et al., 2002; Musenga et al., 2007)
2,6-Di-tert-butyl-4-methylphenol	CID:31404	220.35	$C_{15}H_{24}O$	Benzene and substituted derivatives; phenylpropanes		(Nakatani et al., 1986)
3-Carene	CID:26049	136.23	$C_{10}H_{16}$	Prenol lipids; monoterpenoids		(Jirovetz et al., 2002; Orav et al., 2004)
7-Epi-.α.-eudesmol	CID:6428428	222.37	$C_{15}H_{26}O$	Prenol lipids; sesquiterpenoids		(Orav et al., 2004)
α-Humulene	CID:5281520	204.35	$C_{15}H_{24}$	Prenol lipids; sesquiterpenoids		(Jirovetz et al., 2002)

Phytochemical Name	IMPPAT/ PubMed	Molecular Structure (G/MI)	Molecular Formula	Class and Subclass	3D Structure	Reference
β-Pinene	CID:14896	136.23	$C_{10}H_{16}$	Prenol lipids; monoterpenoids		(Musenga et al., 2007)
Bicyclogermacrene	CID:44583886	204.35	$C_{15}H_{24}$	Prenol lipids; sesquiterpenoids		(Jirovetz et al., 2002)
Butylhydroxyanisole	CID:24667	360.5	$C_{22}H_{32}O_4$	Phenols; methoxyphenols		(Nakatani et al., 1986)
Capsaicin	CID:1548943	305.4	$C_{18}H_{27}NO_3$	Phenols; methoxyphenols		(Suresh et al., 2010)
Eucalyptol	CID:2758	154.25	$C_{10}H_{18}O$	Organoheterocyclic compounds; oxanes		(Wrba et al., 1992)
Eugenol	CID:3314	164.2	$C_{10}H_{12}O_2$	Benzenoids; phenols		(Musenga et al., 2007)
Guineensine	CID:6442405	383.5	$C_{24}H_{33}NO_3$	Organoheterocyclic compounds; benzodioxoles		(Teoh and Das, 2018)

(Continued)

TABLE 16.3
(Continued)

Phytochemical Name	IMPPAT/ PubMed	Molecular Structure (G/Ml)	Molecular Formula	Class and Subclass	3D Structure	Reference
Hedycaryol	CID:6432240	222.37	$C_{15}H_{26}O$	Prenol lipids; sesquiterpenoids		(Orav et al., 2004)
Isobutyramide	CID:68424	87.12	C_4H_9NO	Organoheterocyclic compounds; benzodioxoles		(Park, 2012)
Kakoul	CID:596894	194.18	$C_{10}H_{10}O_4$	Organoheterocyclic compounds; benzodioxoles		(Siddiqui et al., 2008)
Moupinamide	CID:5280537	313.3	$C_{18}H_{19}NO_4$	Phenols; methoxyphenols		(Lin et al., 2007)
Oxirane	CID:6354	44.05	C_2H_4O	Organoheterocyclic compounds; epoxides		(Muraz and Chaigneau, 1985)
p-Anisidine	CID:7732	123.15	C_7H_9NO	Phenol ethers; aminophenyl ethers		(Kapoor et al., 2009)
Paroxetine	CID:43815	329.4	$C_{19}H_{20}FNO_3$	Piperidines; phenylpiperidines		(Subehan et al., 2006)

Phytochemical Name	IMPPAT/ PubMed	Molecular Structure (G/Ml)	Molecular Formula	Class and Subclass	3D Structure	Reference
Piperidine	CID:8082	85.15	$C_5H_{11}N$	Organoheterocyclic compounds; piperidines		(Khajuria et al., 1998; Mujumdar et al., 1990)
Piperine	CID: 638024	285.34	$C_{17}H_{19}NO_3$	Alkaloids and derivatives		(Lin et al., 1999; Hiwale et al., 2002; Pradeep and Kuttan, 2002; Vijayakumar and Nalini, 2006)
Pipernonaline	CID:9974595	341.4	$C_{21}H_{27}NO_3$	Organoheterocyclic compounds; benzodioxoles		(Lee et al., 2006, 2008)
Piperonal	CID:8438	150.13	$C_8H_6O_3$	Organoheterocyclic compounds; benzodioxoles		(EE et al., 2009)
Pyrocatechol	CID:289	110.11	$C_6H_6O_2$	Phenols; benzenediols		(Singh et al., 2008)
Retrofractamide A	CID:11012859	327.4	$C_{20}H_{25}NO_3$	Organoheterocyclic compounds; benzodioxoles		(Park et al., 2002)
Trichostachine	CID:636537	271.31	$C_{16}H_{17}NO_3$	Organoheterocyclic compounds; benzodioxoles		(Orav et al., 2004; Park et al., 2002)
Wisanine	CID:6441085	315.4	$C_{18}N_{21}NO_4$	Alkaloids and derivatives		(Siddiqui et al., 2004)

16.4 CONCLUSION

Since ancient times, it has been believed that the key to the solutions to various ailments is to be found in nature itself. Asia is home to a great many varieties of spices that form part of daily culinary practices in India and Asia. These spices have contributed to the better health of the people and resistance to several diseases. These spices were also subject to several studies leading to the discovery of several bioactive compounds that are today known to be antidiabetic in nature.

16.5 SUMMARY

- Herbs and spices are part of cuisine.
- They are responsible for protection against various ailments.
- Fenugreek, pepper, and turmeric possesses antidiabetic properties.
- Bioactive compounds present in herbs and spices are responsible for their activity against various diseases.

REFERENCES

Agbor GA, Vinson JA, Oben JE, Ngogang JY. Comparative analysis of the in vitro antioxidant activity of white and black pepper. *Nutr Res* [Internet]. 2006;26(12):659–663. Available from: www.sciencedirect.com/science/article/pii/S0271531706002351

Akbar A, Kuanar A, Joshi RK, Sandeep IS, Mohanty S, Naik PK, et al. Development of prediction model and experimental validation in predicting the curcumin content of turmeric (Curcuma longa L.). *Front Plant Sci.* 2016;7:1507.

Association AD. Standards of medical care in diabetes-2019 abridged for primary care providers. *Clin Diabetes* [Internet]. 2019;37(1):11–34. Available from: https://pubmed.ncbi.nlm.nih.gov/30705493

Bi X, Lim J, Henry CJ. Spices in the management of diabetes mellitus. *Food Chem* [Internet]. 2017;217:281–293. Available from: www.sciencedirect.com/science/article/pii/S0308814616313516

Chang H-B, Chen B-H. Inhibition of lung cancer cells A549 and H460 by curcuminoid extracts and nanoemulsions prepared from Curcuma longa Linnaeus. *Int J Nanomedicine.* 2015;10:5059–5080.

Chaudhary S, Chikara SK, Sharma MC, Chaudhary A, Alam Syed B, Chaudhary PS, et al. Elicitation of diosgenin production in Trigonella foenum-graecum (Fenugreek) seedlings by Methyl Jasmonate. *Int J Mol Sci.* 2015;16(12):29889–29899.

Chithra G, Mathew SM, Deepthi C. Performance evaluation of a power operated decorticator for producing white pepper from black pepper. *J Food Process Eng.* 2011;34(1):1–10.

Demmers A, Korthout H, van Etten-Jamaludin FS, Kortekaas F, Maaskant JM. Effects of medicinal food plants on impaired glucose tolerance: A systematic review of randomized controlled trials. *Diabetes Res Clin Pract.* 2017;131:91–106.

Derosa G, Maffioli P, Simental-Mendía LE, Bo S, Sahebkar A. Effect of curcumin on circulating interleukin-6 concentrations: A systematic review and meta-analysis of randomized controlled trials. *Pharmacol Res* [Internet]. 2016;111:394–404. Available from: www.sciencedirect.com/science/article/pii/S1043661816303929

Edwards M, Bulpin PV, Dea IC, Reid JS. Biosynthesis of legume-seed galactomannans in vitro: Cooperative interactions of a guanosine 5′-diphosphate-mannose-linked (1→4)-β-D-manno-syltransferase and a uridine 5′-diphosphate-galactose-linked α-D-galactosyltransferase in particulate enzyme preparations from developing endosperms of fenugreek (*Trigonella foenum-graecum* L.) and guar (*Cyamopsis tetragonoloba* [L.] Taub.). *Planta.* 1989;178(1):41–51.

Ee GCL, Lim CM, Lim CK, Rahmani M, Shaari K, Bong CFJ. Alkaloids from Piper sarmentosum and Piper nigrum. *Nat Prod Res.* 2009;23(15):1416–1423.

El-Ghorab A, Nauman M, Anjum F, Hussain S, Nadeem M. A comparative study on chemical composition and antioxidant activity of ginger (Zingiber officinale) and cumin (Cuminum cyminum). *J Agric Food Chem.* 2010;58:8231–8237.

Faried MA, El-Mehi AES. Aqueous anise extract alleviated the pancreatic changes in streptozotocin-induced diabetic rat model via modulation of hyperglycaemia, oxidative stress, apoptosis and autophagy: A biochemical, histological and immunohistochemical study. *Folia Morphol (Warsz).* 2020;79(3):489–502.

Genet S, Kale RK, Baquer NZ. Effects of vanadate, insulin and fenugreek (Trigonella foenum graecum) on creatine kinase levels in tissues of diabetic rat. *Indian J Exp Biol*. 1999;37(2):200–202.

Guerra PV, Yaylayan VA. Thermal generation of 3-amino-4,5-dimethylfuran-2(5H)-one, the postulated precursor of sotolone, from amino acid model systems containing glyoxylic and pyruvic acids. *J Agric Food Chem*. 2011;59(9):4699–4704.

Guglielmo A, Sabra A, Elbery M, Cerveira MM, Ghenov F, Sunasee R, et al. A mechanistic insight into curcumin modulation of the IL-1β secretion and NLRP3 S-glutathionylation induced by needle-like cationic cellulose nanocrystals in myeloid cells. *Chem Biol Interact*. 2017;274:1–12.

Hajra D, Paul S. Study of glucose uptake enhancing potential of fenugreek (Trigonella foenum graecum) leaves extract on 3T3 L1 cells line and evaluation of its antioxidant potential debarupa. *Pharmacognosy Res*. 2018;10(October):347–353.

Han Y, Nishibe S, Noguchi Y, Jin Z. Flavonol glycosides from the stems of Trigonella foenum-graecum. *Phytochemistry*. 2001;58(4):577–580.

Hiwale AR, Dhuley JN, Naik SR. Effect of co-administration of piperine on pharmacokinetics of beta-lactam antibiotics in rats. *Indian J Exp Biol*. 2002;40(3):277–281.

Hossain M, Ibnul Hasan Even ASM, Ahsanul Akbar M, Ganguly A, Abdur Rahman SM. Evaluation of analgesic activity of Sterculia villosa roxb. (Sterculiaceae) bark in Swiss-Albino mice. *Dhaka Univ J Pharm Sci*. 2013;12(2):167–171.

Hu Y, Du Q, Tang Q. [Determination of chemical constituents of the volatile oil from Curcuma longa by gas chromatography-mass spectrometry]. *Se pu = Chinese J Chromatogr*. 1998;16(6):528–529.

Jayaprakasha GK, Rao LJM. Chemistry, biogenesis, and biological activities of cinnamomum zeylanicum. *Crit Rev Food Sci Nutr*. 2011;51(6):547–562.

Jhong CH, Riyaphan J, Lin SH, Chia YC, Weng CF. Screening alpha-glucosidase and alpha-amylase inhibitors from natural compounds by molecular docking in silico. *Biofactors*. 2015;41(4):242–251.

Jin Y, Qian D, Du Q. Preparation of bioactive amide compounds from black pepper by countercurrent chromatography and preparative HPLC. *Ind Crops Prod* [Internet]. 2013;44:258–262. Available from: www.sciencedirect.com/science/article/pii/S0926669012006085

Jirovetz L, Buchbauer G, Ngassoum MB, Geissler M. Aroma compound analysis of Piper nigrum and Piper guineense essential oils from Cameroon using solid-phase microextraction-gas chromatography, solid-phase microextraction-gas chromatography-mass spectrometry and olfactometry. *J Chromatogr A*. 2002;976(1–2):265–275.

Kang L-P, Zhao Y, Pang X, Yu H-S, Xiong C-Q, Zhang J, et al. Characterization and identification of steroidal saponins from the seeds of Trigonella foenum-graecum by ultra-high-performance liquid chromatography and hybrid time-of-flight mass spectrometry. *J Pharm Biomed Anal*. 2013;74:257–267.

Kapoor IPS, Singh B, Singh G, De Heluani CS, De Lampasona MP, Catalan CAN. Chemistry and in vitro antioxidant activity of volatile oil and oleoresins of black pepper (Piper nigrum). *J Agric Food Chem*. 2009;57(12):5358–5364.

Kaufmann B, Rudaz S, Cherkaoui S, Veuthey J-L, Christen P. Influence of plant matrix on microwave-assisted extraction process. The case of diosgenin extracted from fenugreek (Trigonella foenum-graecum L.). *Phytochem Anal*. 2007;18(1):70–76.

Khajuria A, Zutshi U, Bedi KL. Permeability characteristics of piperine on oral absorption–an active alkaloid from peppers and a bioavailability enhancer. *Indian J Exp Biol*. 1998;36(1):46–50.

Korman SH, Cohen E, Preminger A. Pseudo-maple syrup urine disease due to maternal prenatal ingestion of fenugreek. *J Paediatr Child Health*. 2001;37(4):403–404.

Laha S, Paul S. Costus igneus – A therapeutic anti-diabetic herb with active phytoconstitutents. *IJPSR*. 2018;18(1):1–23.

Lee SW, Kim YK, Kim K, Lee HS, Choi JH, Lee WS, et al. Alkamides from the fruits of Piper longum and Piper nigrum displaying potent cell adhesion inhibition. *Bio Org Med Chem Lett*. 2008;18(16):4544–4546.

Lee SW, Rho M-C, Park HR, Choi J-H, Kang JY, Lee JW, et al. Inhibition of diacylglycerol acyltransferase by alkamides isolated from the fruits of Piper longum and Piper nigrum. *J Agric Food Chem*. 2006;54(26):9759–9763.

Li F, Fernandez PP, Rajendran P, Hui KM, Sethi G. Diosgenin, a steroidal saponin, inhibits STAT3 signaling pathway leading to suppression of proliferation and chemosensitization of human hepatocellular carcinoma cells. *Cancer Lett*. 2010;292(2):197–207.

Lin Z, Hoult JR, Bennett DC, Raman A. Stimulation of mouse melanocyte proliferation by Piper nigrum fruit extract and its main alkaloid, piperine. *Planta Med*. 1999;65(7):600–603.

Lin Z, Liao Y, Venkatasamy R, Hider RC, Soumyanath A. Amides from Piper nigrum L. with dissimilar effects on melanocyte proliferation in-vitro. *J Pharm Pharmacol*. 2007;59(4):529–536.

Lu X, Zhao H, Zhang C, Tang S. [Separation and identification of diosgenin in Trigonella foenum-graecum L. and its compound preparation by gradient thin-layer chromatography]. *Se pu = Chinese J Chromatogr*. 2005;23(2):216.

Maehara S, Ikeda M, Haraguchi H, Kitamura C, Nagoe T, Ohashi K, et al. Microbial conversion of curcumin into colorless hydroderivatives by the endophytic fungus Diaporthe sp. associated with Curcuma longa. *Chem Pharm Bull (Tokyo)*. 2011;59(8):1042–1044.

Mandegary A, Pournamdari M, Sharififar F, Pournourmohammadi S, Fardiar R, Shooli S. Alkaloid and flavonoid rich fractions of fenugreek seeds (Trigonella foenum-graecum L.) with antinociceptive and anti-inflammatory effects. *Food Chem Toxicol an Int J Publ Br Ind Biol Res Assoc*. 2012;50(7):2503–2507.

Mirzaei H, Shakeri A, Rashidi B, Jalili A, Banikazemi Z, Sahebkar A. Phytosomal curcumin: A review of pharmacokinetic, experimental and clinical studies. *Biomed Pharmacother* [Internet]. 2017;85:102–112. Available from: www.sciencedirect.com/science/article/pii/S0753332216320741

Mohamed D. Antioxidant and anti-diabetic effects of cumin seeds crude ethanol extract. *J Biol Sci*. 2018;18.

Moorthy R, Prabhu KM, Murthy PS. Anti-hyperglycemic compound (GII) from fenugreek (Trigonella foenum-graecum Linn.) seeds, its purification and effect in diabetes mellitus. *Indian J Exp Biol*. 2010;48(11):1111–1118.

Morani AS, Bodhankar SL, Mohan V, Thakurdesai PA. Ameliorative effects of standardized extract from Trigonella foenum-graecum L. seeds on painful peripheral neuropathy in rats. *Asian Pac J Trop Med*. 2012;5(5):385–390.

Mujumdar AM, Dhuley JN, Deshmukh VK, Raman PH, Naik SR. Anti-inflammatory activity of piperine. *Jpn J Med Sci Biol*. 1990;43(3):95–100.

Muraz B, Chaigneau M. [Decontamination of spices by ethylene oxide. The case of cloves (Eugenia caryophyllus Spreng.) and white pepper (Piper nigrum L.)]. *Ann Pharm Fr*. 1985;43(1):15–21.

Musenga A, Mandrioli R, Ferranti A, D'Orazio G, Fanali S, Raggi MA. Analysis of aromatic and terpenic constituents of pepper extracts by capillary electrochromatography. *J Sep Sci*. 2007;30(4):612–619.

Nakatani N, Inatani R, Ohta H, Nishioka A. Chemical constituents of peppers (Piper spp.) and application to food preservation: Naturally occurring antioxidative compounds. *Environ Health Perspect*. 1986;67:135–142.

Neelakantan N, Narayanan M, de Souza RJ, van Dam RM. Effect of fenugreek (Trigonella foenum-graecum L.) intake on glycemia: A meta-analysis of clinical trials. *Nutr J* [Internet]. 2014;13(1):7. https://doi.org/10.1186/1475-2891-13-7

Neyrinck AM, Alligier M, Memvanga PB, Névraumont E, Larondelle Y, Préat V, et al. Curcuma longa extract associated with white pepper lessens high fat diet-induced inflammation in subcutaneous adipose tissue. *PLoS ONE*. 2013;8(11):e81252.

Nishiyama T, Mae T, Kishida H, Tsukagawa M, Mimaki Y, Kuroda M, et al. Curcuminoids and sesquiterpenoids in turmeric (Curcuma longa L.) suppress an increase in blood glucose level in type 2 diabetic KK-Ay mice. *J Agric Food Chem*. 2005;53(4):959–963.

Orav A, Stulova I, Kailas T, Müürisepp M. Effect of storage on the essential oil composition of Piper nigrum L. fruits of different ripening states. *J Agric Food Chem*. 2004;52(9):2582–2586.

Pang X, Cong Y, Yu H-S, Kang L-P, Feng B, Han B-X, et al. Spirostanol saponins derivated from the seeds of Trigonella foenum-graecum by β-glucosidase hydrolysis and their inhibitory effects on rat platelet aggregation. *Planta Med*. 2012;78(3):276–285.

Park I-K. Insecticidal activity of isobutylamides derived from Piper nigrum against adult of two mosquito species, Culex pipiens pallens and Aedes aegypti. *Nat Prod Res*. 2012;26(22):2129–2131.

Park I-K, Lee S-G, Shin S-C, Park J-D, Ahn Y-J. Larvicidal activity of isobutylamides identified in Piper nigrum fruits against three mosquito species. *J Agric Food Chem*. 2002;50(7):1866–1870.

Pirola L, Balcerczyk A, Okabe J, El-Osta A. Epigenetic phenomena linked to diabetic complications. *Nat Rev Endocrinol* [Internet]. 2010;6(12):665–675. https://doi.org/10.1038/nrendo.2010.188

Pivari F, Mingione A, Soldati CB and L. Curcumin and type 2 diabetes mellitus: Prevention and treatment. *J R Soc Promot Health*. 2019;11:204–208.

Poolsup N, Suksomboon N, Kurnianta PDM, Deawjaroen K. Effects of curcumin on glycemic control and lipid profile in prediabetes and type 2 diabetes mellitus: A systematic review and meta-analysis. *PLoS ONE*. 2019;14(4):e0215840–e0215840.

Pradeep CR, Kuttan G. Effect of piperine on the inhibition of lung metastasis induced B16F-10 melanoma cells in mice. *Clin Exp Metastasis*. 2002;19(8):703–708.

Radwan SS, Kokate CK. Production of higher levels of trigonelline by cell cultures of Trigonella foenum-graecum than by the differentiated plant. *Planta*. 1980;147(4):340–344.

Rahmani S, Asgary S, Askari G, Keshvari M, Hatamipour M, Feizi A, et al. Treatment of non-alcoholic fatty liver disease with curcumin: A randomized placebo-controlled trial. *Phytother Res*. 2016;30(9):1540–1548.

Ranasinghe P, Jayawardana R, Galappaththy P, Constantine GR, de Vas Gunawardana N, Katulanda P. Efficacy and safety of "true" cinnamon (Cinnamomum zeylanicum) as a pharmaceutical agent in diabetes: A systematic review and meta-analysis. *Diabet Med*. 2012;29(12):1480–1492.

Rathod SS, Rathod VK. Extraction of piperine from Piper longum using ultrasound. *Ind Crops Prod* [Internet]. 2014;58:259–264. www.sciencedirect.com/science/article/pii/S0926669014001885

Rayyan S, Fossen T, Andersen ØM. Flavone C-glycosides from seeds of fenugreek, Trigonella foenum-graecum L. *J Agric Food Chem*. 2010;58(12):7211–7217.

Reid JS. Reserve carbohydrate metabolism in germinating seeds of Trigonella foenum-graecum L. (Leguminosae). *Planta*. 1971;100(2):131–142.

Rungphanichkul N, Nimmannit U, Muangsiri W, Rojsitthisak P. Preparation of curcuminoid niosomes for enhancement of skin permeation. *Pharmazie*. 2011;66(8):570–575.

Shailajan S, Menon S, Singh A, Mhatre M, Sayed N. A validated RP-HPLC method for quantitation of trigonelline from herbal formulations containing Trigonella foenum-graecum (L.) seeds. *Pharm Methods*. 2011;2(3):157–160.

Shim SH, Lee EJ, Kim JS, Kang SS, Ha H, Lee HY, et al. Rat growth-hormone release stimulators from fenugreek seeds. *Chem Biodivers*. 2008;5(9):1753–1761.

Shojaii A, Abdollahi Fard M. Review of pharmacological properties and chemical constituents of pimpinella anisum. *ISRN Pharm*. 2012;2012:1–8.

Siddiqui BS, Gulzar T, Begum S, Afshan F. Piptigrine, a new insecticidal amide from Piper nigrum Linn. *Nat Prod Res*. 2004;18(5):473–477.

Siddiqui BS, Gulzar T, Begum S, Afshan F, Sultana R. A new natural product and insecticidal amides from seeds of Piper nigrum Linn. *Nat Prod Res*. 2008;22(13):1107–1111.

Singh R, Singh N, Saini BS, Rao HS. In vitro antioxidant activity of pet ether extract of black pepper. *Indian J Pharmacol*. 2008;40(4):147–151.

Sreekala M, Lalitha K. Kinetic analyses of mitochondrial 75selenium uptake in Trigonella foenum-graecum seedlings exposed to selenium and mimosine. *Biol Trace Elem Res*. 2001a;79(3):271–285.

Sreekala M, Lalitha K. Uptake of 45Ca by mitochondria of Trigonella foenum-graecum as influenced by selenium and mimosine–detailed kinetic analyses. *Biol Trace Elem Res*. 2001b;82(1–3):217–229.

Sreekala M, Santosh TR, Lalitha K. Oxidative stress during selenium deficiency in seedlings of Trigonella foenum-graecum and mitigation by mimosine. Part I. Hydroperoxide metabolism. *Biol Trace Elem Res*. 1999;70(3):193–207.

Subehan, Usia T, Kadota S, Tezuka Y. Mechanism-based inhibition of human liver microsomal cytochrome P450 2D6 (CYP2D6) by alkamides of Piper nigrum. *Planta Med*. 2006;72(6):527–532.

Suksomboon N, Poolsup N, Boonkaew S, Suthisisang CC. Meta-analysis of the effect of herbal supplement on glycemic control in type 2 diabetes. *J Ethnopharmacol*. 2011;137(3):1328–1333.

Suresh D, Srinivasan K. Tissue distribution & elimination of capsaicin, piperine & curcumin following oral intake in rats. *Indian J Med Res*. 2010;131:682–691.

Swaroop A, Bagchi M, Kumar P, Preuss HG, Tiwari K, Marone PA, et al. Safety, efficacy and toxicological evaluation of a novel, patented anti-diabetic extract of Trigonella Foenum-Graecum seed extract (Fenfuro). *Toxicol Mech Methods*. 2014;24(7):495–503.

Taylor WG, Elder JL, Chang PR, Richards KW. Microdetermination of diosgenin from fenugreek (Trigonella foenum-graecum) seeds. *J Agric Food Chem*. 2000;48(11):5206–5210.

Teoh SL, Das S. Phytochemicals and their effective role in the treatment of diabetes mellitus: A short review. *Phytochem Rev* [Internet]. 2018;17(5):1111–1128. https://doi.org/10.1007/s11101-018-9575-z

Valizadeh Kiamahalleh M, Najafpour-Darzi G, Rahimnejad M, Moghadamnia AA, Valizadeh Kiamahalleh M. High performance curcumin subcritical water extraction from turmeric (Curcuma longa L.). *J Chromatogr B, Anal Technol Biomed Life Sci*. 2016;1022:191–198.

Vecchio MG, Gulati A, Minto C, Lorenzoni G. Pimpinella anisum and illicium verum: The multifaceted role of anise plants. *Open Agric J*. 2016;10(1):81–86.

Vijayakumar RS, Nalini N. Efficacy of piperine, an alkaloidal constituent from Piper nigrum on erythrocyte antioxidant status in high fat diet and antithyroid drug induced hyperlipidemic rats. *Cell Biochem Funct*. 2006;24(6):491–498.

Wang G-R, Tang W-Z, Yao Q-Q, Zhong H, Liu Y-J. New flavonoids with 2BS cell proliferation promoting effect from the seeds of Trigonella foenum-graecum L. *J Nat Med*. 2010;64(3):358–361.

Wang Y, Li R, Jiang Z-T, Tan J, Tang S-H, Li T-T, et al. Green and solvent-free simultaneous ultrasonic-microwave assisted extraction of essential oil from white and black peppers. *Ind Crops Prod* [Internet]. 2018;114:164–172. Available from: www.sciencedirect.com/science/article/pii/S0926669018300980

Wang Y, Mortimer JC, Davis J, Dupree P, Keegstra K. Identification of an additional protein involved in mannan biosynthesis. *Plant J*. 2013;73(1):105–117.

Wei X, Lau SK, Stratton J, Irmak S, Subbiah J. Radiofrequency pasteurization process for inactivation of Salmonella spp. and Enterococcus faecium NRRL B-2354 on ground black pepper. *Food Microbiol* [Internet]. 2019;82:388–397. Available from: www.sciencedirect.com/science/article/pii/S0740002018309729

Wrba H, el-Mofty MM, Schwaireb MH, Dutter A. Carcinogenicity testing of some constituents of black pepper (Piper nigrum). *Exp Toxicol Pathol Off J Gesellschaft fur Toxikologische Pathol*. 1992;44(2):61–65.

Yamazoe S, Hasegawa K, Shigemori H. Growth inhibitory indole acetic acid polyacetylenic ester from Japanese ivy (Hedera rhombea Bean). *Phytochemistry*. 2007;68(12):1706–1711.

Yang K-Y, Lin L-C, Tseng T-Y, Wang S-C, Tsai T-H. Oral bioavailability of curcumin in rat and the herbal analysis from Curcuma longa by LC-MS/MS. *J Chromatogr B, Anal Technol Biomed life Sci*. 2007;853(1–2):183–189.

Zambou K, Spyropoulos CG. d-Galactose uptake by fenugreek cotyledons: Effect of water stress. *Plant Physiol*. 1990;93(4):1417–1421.

Zhao X, Chen M, Zhao Y, Zha L, Yang H, Wu Y. GC-MS-based nontargeted and targeted metabolic profiling identifies changes in the Lentinula edodes mycelial metabolome under high-temperature stress. *Int J Mol Sci*. 2019;20(9).

Zheng J, Zhou Y, Li Y, Xu D-P, Li S, Li H-B. Spices for prevention and treatment of cancers. *Nutrients*. 2016;8(8).

17 Kola Nut (*Cola nitida* (Vent.) Schott & Endl.) Use in Diabetes
Molecular, Cellular, and Metabolic Effects

Almahi I. Mohamed, Ochuko L. Erukainure and Md. Shahidul Islam

CONTENTS

ABBREVIATIONS

ALT   alanine transaminase
AST   aspartate transaminase

DOI: 10.1201/9781003220930-19

CAT	catalase
DPPH	2,2′-diphenyl-1-picrylhydrazyl
$FeCl_3$	iron(III) chloride
FRAP	ferric-reducing antioxidant power
GCMS	gas chromatography/mass spectroscopy
GDM	gestational diabetes mellitus
GSH	reduced glutathione
GST	glutathione S-transferase
H_2O_2	hydrogen peroxide
HDL	high-density lipoprotein
HPLC	high-performance liquid chromatography
LD_{50}	50% of lethal dose
MDA	malondialdehyde
NAD^+	nicotinamide adenine dinucleotide (oxidized)
NADH	nicotinamide adenine dinucleotide (reduced)
O_2	superoxide anion
OH^*	hydroxyl radical
$ONOO^-$	peroxynitrite
SOD	superoxide dismutase
T1D	type 1 diabetes
T2D	type 2 diabetes
VLDL	very-low-density lipoprotein

17.0 SUMMARY POINTS

- *Cola nitida* is a commonly used medicinal plant in many African countries.
- Different types of bioactive compounds, such as alkaloid, flavonoids, phenols, tannins, saponins, are isolated from different parts of this plant.
- This chapter focuses on the effects of *C. nitida* on oxidative stress, hyperglycemia, and diabetes with molecular mechanisms.
- Based on the results presented in this chapter, *C. nitida* can be used a potential nutraceutical in the treatment of diabetes and its associated complications.

17.1 INTRODUCTION

Diabetes affects more than 1 out of 10 adults worldwide. Furthermore, there is an expanding list of nations where one-fifth or more of the adult population has diabetes. Diabetes has more than quadrupled among individuals aged 20–79 years since 2000, from an estimated 151 million (4.6% of the world population at the time) to 537 million (10.5%) now. However. without adequate effort, the cases will reach 643 million by 2030 (11.3% of the population globally). If the current trends continue, the figure will increase to 783 million individuals (12.2% of the population) by 2045 (IDF, 2021).

Several pharmacological medications have been developed to control diabetes, including metformin, biguanides, and thiazolidinediones. Despite their comprehensive therapeutic benefits, these pharmacological medicines have many disadvantages, including inaccessibility, high price, and a multitude of intrinsic adverse side effects (Kenny et al., 2019).

Due to the expenditure and restricted availability of current therapies for many individuals in developing nations, alternatives to modern pharmacotherapy for diabetes are continually needed (Pereira et al., 2016). Plants are extensively used throughout the African countries, with up to 90% of the community in certain places depend only on plant-based medicines to cure different conditions such as diabetes. One of these medicinal plants is *Cola nitida*, which has been utilized in folk medicine to manage diabetes mellitus from time immemorial (Erukainure et al., 2017).

17.2 BOTANICAL DESCRIPTIONS OF *COLA NITIDA*

C. nitida is an evergreen tree belonging to the family of Malvaceae, genus of *Cola*. It is around 20 m high, has ovoid leaves, and is pointed at both ends, having a leathery surface. The trees produce cream flowers with purplish-brown striations, as well as star-shaped fruits that are usually composed of five follicles each. Around a hundred prismatic seeds develop within each follicle, protected by a white seed shell. The fruits are shaped like an oval-ellipsoid and are 13 cm × 7 cm in size. They are green, with a glossy surface and a smooth texture (Quiroz et al., 2001).

17.2.1 ECOLOGICAL AND GEOGRAPHICAL DISTRIBUTION OF *COLA NITIDA*

The plant is indigenous to West Africa particularly, Nigeria, Ghana, Cote d'Ivoire, Liberia, and Sierra Leone. The plant grows typically in a tropical rainforest climate and requires a hot, humid environment to grow. However, it can tolerate dry season in areas where groundwater is accessible. The tree usually flowers for 3 months, from May to July, and produces fruit for 3 months, from October to December (Komlaga et al., 2019).

17.3 COMMON TRADITIONAL USES OF *COLA NITIDA*

In many West African nations, *C. nitida* seeds are chewed in personal and public ceremonies, such as when given to leaders or visitors. The plant is often used as a flavoring agent in sodas in the Western world. It is regularly utilized as an ingredient in energy drinks and performance boosters. It is being used as an extract or powder (Savi et al., 2019). Moreover, various ailments were treated in traditional medicine using *C. nitida* products, including diarrhea, dysentery, female sterility, early menopause, painful menstruation, difficult birth, diabetes, high blood pressure, charm, urinary infection, and hernia. It is thought to have a number of therapeutic pharmacological properties, including antioxidant, antibacterial, antifungal, antiviral, and anti-inflammatory properties. Additionally, *C. nitida* bark has been historically utilized as an antibacterial and antifungal agent. The seeds of the plant are renowned for their anti-inflammatory qualities. In Uganda, the plant's leaves and seeds are used to treat sexual and erectile dysfunction. The plant's seeds have been traditionally used in Nigeria to cure emesis and migraine headaches using a methanol extract. *C. nitida*'s bitter twigs have also been applied to clean teeth and gums. In Nigeria, *C. nitida* is also one of the herbal fruits utilized by pregnant women. Despite all of the research on *C. nitida*, there is still a paucity of knowledge concerning its effects on the developing brain. The plant is consumed before meals to improve digestion and has been shown to benefit the digestive system, particularly the liver. It has also been utilized as an antidepressant as reported in a number of previous studies (Durand et al., 2015; Nwobodo et al., 2017; Adesanwo et al., 2017).

17.4 PHYTOCHEMICAL CONSTITUENT SCREENING RESULTS OF *COLA NITIDA*

The phytochemical screening of *C. nitida* confirm the presence of alkaloids, phenols, flavonoids, saponins, and tannins, which are described in Table 17.1.

17.4.1 ALKALOIDS

Alkaloids (see Figure 17.1) are secondary metabolites found in plants. They are well-known natural nitrogen-containing bioactive chemicals. Alkaloids are the subject of cutting-edge research to discover innovative treatment techniques. According to the literature, alkaloids provide various biological functions, and certain alkaloids also change into active metabolites. It has been observed in many studies that alkaloids are the main constituents of *Cola nitida* (Erukainure et al., 2017).

TABLE 17.1

Bioactive Compounds Identified in the Different Extracts of *Cola nitida*

Phytochemicals	Compounds	Solvent for Extraction	Biological Effects	References
Alkaloids	Caffeine, spilanthol, cinchonine, cryptopine, and 9-octadecenamide	Methanol, hot water infusion	Antioxidant properties Antidiabetes properties Neuroprotective properties Antimicrobial activities	Erukainure et al. (2017) Erukainure et al. (2019a) Erukainure et al. (2019b) Oboh et al. (2019)
Phenols	Catechin, epicatechin, apigenin, and narigenin	Chloroform, methanol, aqueous, ethanol	Antioxidant properties Antidiabetes properties	Oboh et al. (2014)
Flavonoids	Quercetin and rutin	Chloroform, methanol, aqueous	Anti-inflammatory agent	Adamu et al. (2020)
Saponins	Saponin	Chloroform, aqueous	Antimicrobial activities	Muhammad et al. (2014)
Tannins	Gallotannin	Chloroform, Methanol, Aqueous, Ethanol	Anticarcinogenic properties Antidiabetes properties Antimicrobial activities	Boege (2005) Chung et al. (1998)

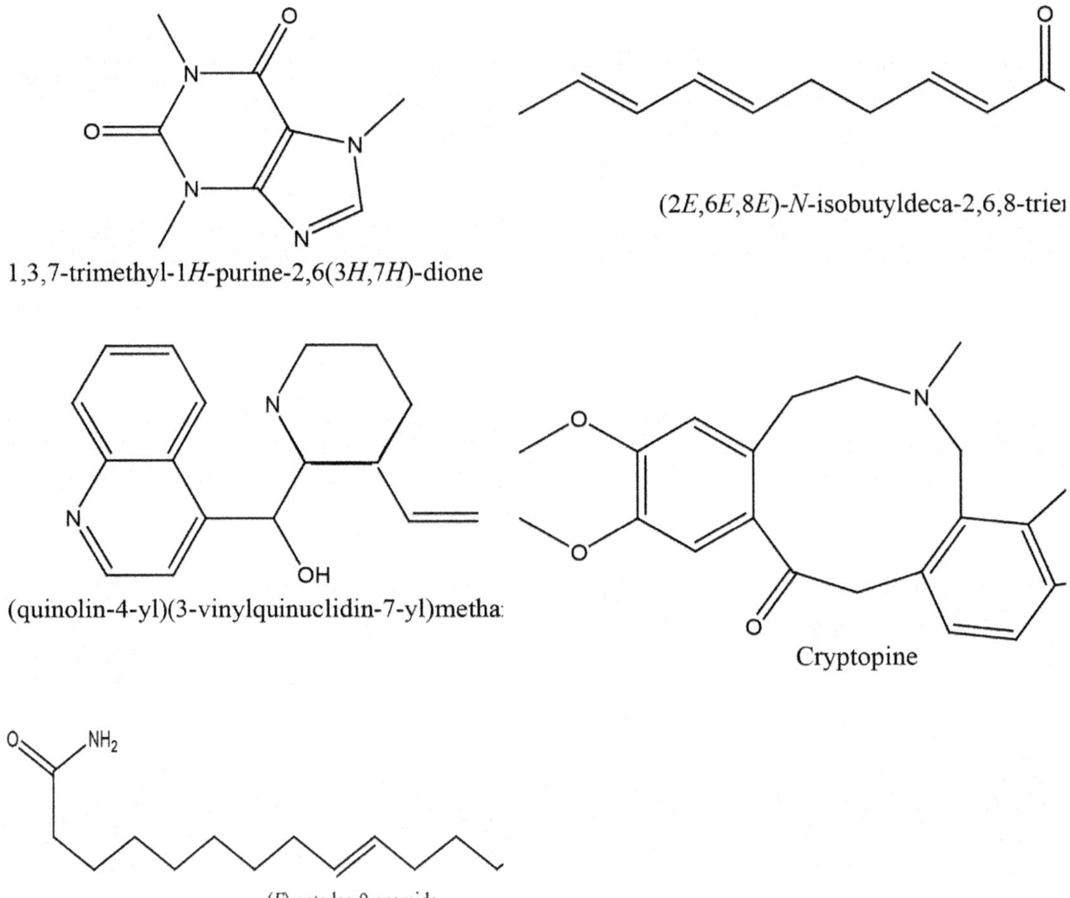

1,3,7-trimethyl-1*H*-purine-2,6(3*H*,7*H*)-dione

(2*E*,6*E*,8*E*)-*N*-isobutyldeca-2,6,8-trier

(quinolin-4-yl)(3-vinylquinuclidin-7-yl)metha:

Cryptopine

(*E*)-octadec-9-enamide

FIGURE 17.1 Alkaloids identified in different extracts of *Cola nitida* plant.

The presence of alkaloids in *C. nitida* may also contribute to its medicinal benefits, because humans have utilized alkaloid-containing plants for therapeutic and recreational purposes since ancient times (Aniszewski, 2007).

Caffeine is the major alkaloid reported in *C. nitida* (Erukainure et al., 2019a; Erukainure et al., 2019b) and one of the most often consumed dietary substances worldwide. It also occurs naturally in coffee beans, cacao beans, kola nuts, guarana berries, and yerba mate tea leaves. Caffeine's performance advantages include increased physical endurance, decreased tiredness, and increased mental alertness and focus (Heckman et al., 2010). Erukainure et al. (2017) reported that caffeine has therapeutic potential against T2D, neurodegeneration, oxidative stress, and toxicity using *in vitro, ex vivo, in vivo*, and in *silico* assays (Erukainure et al., 2019a; Erukainure et al., 2019b). HPLC analysis of *C. nitida* infusion revealed 80.08% of caffeine content, thus suggesting it is the main phytoconstituent of the plant (Erukainure et al., 2017).

17.4.2 PHENOLS

The phenolic compounds are a diverse group of plant compounds that include an aromatic ring with one or more hydroxyl substituents. Phenolic compounds (see Figure 17.2) are often water soluble due to their frequent association with sugar as glycosides and their location in the cell vacuole (Harborne, 1973). There has been a remarkable increase in research to describe the health-promoting qualities of numerous phenolic compounds with antioxidant capabilities in recent years. They may be used to treat and manage cancer, cardiovascular and neurological disorders, and are used in anti-aging and cosmetic products. However, several *in vitro* experiments have assessed the possible antioxidant activity of *Cola nitida* by quantifying and identifying its phenolic compounds. Hence, the high polyphenol content of this plant and its potential impacts on human health have

2-(3,4-dihydroxyphenyl)chroman-3,5,7-tr

2-(3,4-dihydroxyphenyl)chroman

5,7-dihydroxy-2-(4-hydroxyphenyl)-4*H*

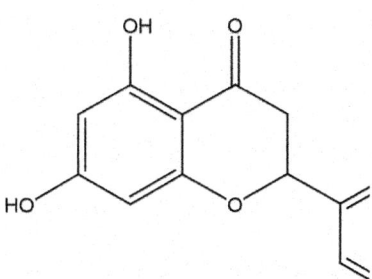

5,7-dihydroxy-2-(4-hydroxyphenyl)c

FIGURE 17.2 Phenolic compounds identified in different extracts of *Cola nitida* plant.

been well documented (Umoren et al., 2009). Finally, examination of soluble phenolic compounds reveals a high concentration catechin in *C. nitida* seeds.

17.4.3 FLAVONOIDS

Flavonoids (see Figure 17.3) are a kind of plant secondary metabolite with a polyphenolic structure. They are members of a family of low-molecular-weight phenolic compounds extensively dispersed across the plant kingdom. Furthermore, flavonoids are now well recognized as essential in a wide range of nutraceutical and pharmacological applications (Metodiewa et al., 1997). This is because of their antioxidative, anti-inflammatory, antimutagenic, and anticarcinogenic capabilities, as well as their ability to modulate important cellular enzyme performance. Phytochemical screening of *Cola nitida* revealed the existence of flavonoids that may inhibit the growth of *Streptococcus anginosus* bacteria, as reported by Muhammad et al. (2014).

17.4.4 SAPONINS

Saponins (see Figure 17.4) belong to the family of polyphenols composed of glycosides connected to a hydrophobic aglycone, which could be existed like triterpenoid or steroid in nature (Julkunen et al., 2009). Saponins' amphipathic nature has been connected to several pharmacological effects, including enhanced intestinal mucosal permeability, which facilitates the entry of chemicals into cells. Several studies have revealed that plant products have the capacity to improve glucose absorption, which is connected to the presence of saponins (Krogdahl et al., 2010).

17.4.5 TANNINS

Tannins (see Figure 17.5) are polyphenols found in practically all plant products and are water soluble. They have a relatively large molecular weight and the capacity to form complexes with carbohydrates and proteins. Consequently, fewer digestible complexes are formed, resulting in a

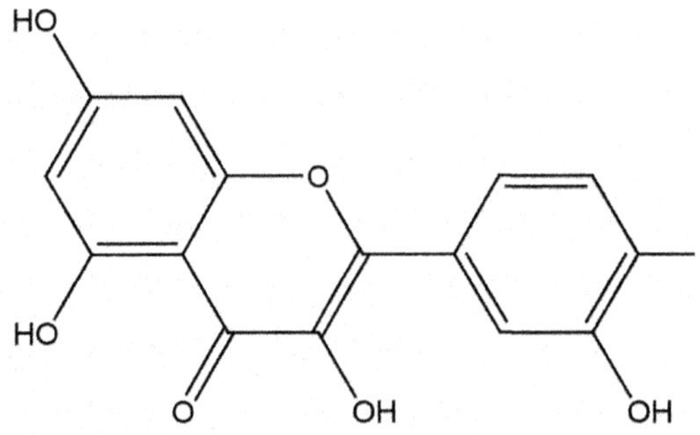

3,5,7-trihydroxy-2-(3,4-dihydroxyphenyl)-4*H*-chror

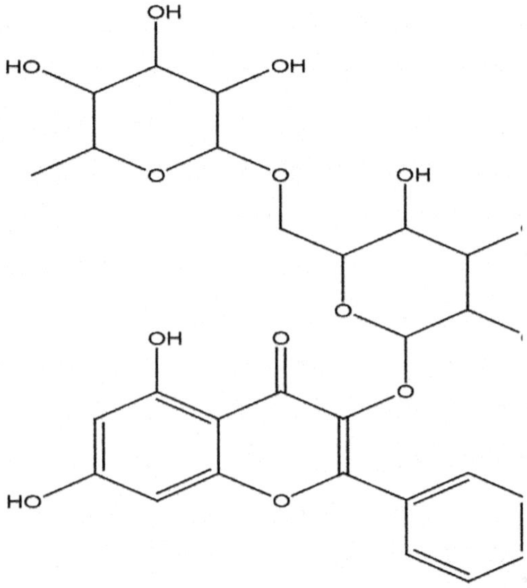

Rutin

FIGURE 17.3   Flavonoids identified in *Cola nitida* plant.

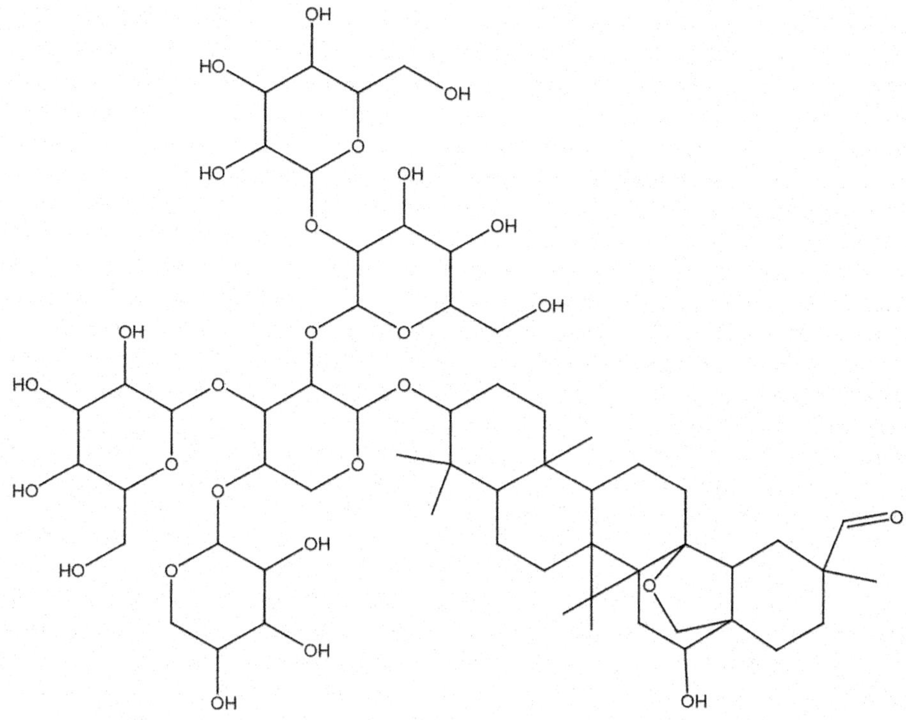

FIGURE 17.4 Saponin identified in *Cola nitida* plant.

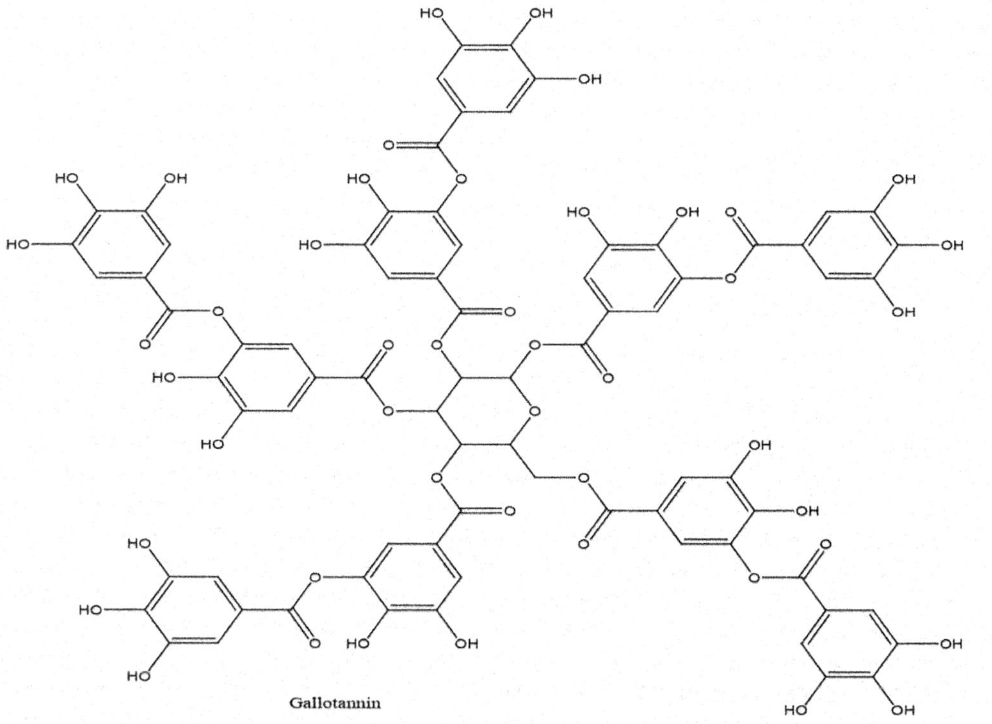

FIGURE 17.5 Tannins identified in *Cola nitida* plant.

decrease in postprandial blood glucose levels (Julkunen et al., 2009). Tannins have also been found to have various physiological effects, such as accelerating blood coagulation, lowering blood pressure, lowering serum cholesterol levels, causing liver necrosis, and modulating immune responses (Chung et al., 1998).

17.5 OXIDATIVE STRESS AND ANTIOXIDANT MECHANISM OF ACTIONS IN DIABETES

Oxidative stress is characterized as an increase in the formation of reactive oxygenated species (ROS) that cannot be counteracted by antioxidants, as well as a disruption in cell redox equilibrium (Pisoschi et al., 2015). ROS are oxygenated molecules that are represented by both free radicals and non-free radicals, such as hydrogen peroxide (H_2O_2), superoxide (O_2^-), and hydroxyl radical (OH^*). Other oxidants include reactive nitrogen, iron, copper, and sulfur (Islam, 2016). Moreover, free radicals are produced during aerobic interaction like cellular respiration, exposure to microbial infections that activate phagocytes, intense physical activity, or environmental pollution such as ionizing and UV radiation (Pisoschi et al., 2015). A wide range of biomolecules are affected by ROS, which can interact with practically every substrate in the cell. ROS are capable of oxidizing proteins on both their backbone and side chain, which further interacts with amino acid side chains to create carbonyl functionalities. These processes may result in DNA-protein crosslinking, strand breakage, and modification in the structure of purine and pyridine bases, with the resultant DNA mutations as a consequence (Gandhi et al., 2012). However, oxidative stress occurs when intrinsic antioxidant systems are unable to neutralize oxidants generated either internally or externally, resulting in an imbalance of oxidants and antioxidants. Furthermore, excess generation of oxidants, inadequate antioxidant levels, or insufficient antioxidant enzyme activity may result in oxidative stress, which may cause various diseases (Finaud et al., 2006).

Antioxidants are chemicals that either delay or prevent the oxidation of a substance's state. To exert their antioxidative effects, antioxidant chemicals may use a variety of chemical processes. These include (1) hydrogen atom transfer, (2) single-electron transfer, and (3) the capacity to chelate transition metals. In general, antioxidant compounds may respond either via various pathways or through a single dominating action method (Santos et al., 2019).

17.6 ROLES OF OXIDATIVE STRESS IN DIABETES PATHOLOGY

The majority of the food we consume is broken down into a simple molecule called glucose. Glucose is the primary source of energy for the body. After digestion, glucose enters our bloodstream, which is accessible for body cells to use for energy (Alberts et al., 2002). However, glucose cannot enter cells without the help of insulin and glucose transporters. Insulin is a hormone released by the pancreas that transports glucose from the blood into various cells throughout the body. If the pancreas does not create enough insulin or if the insulin produced does not function effectively, glucose cannot reach into the cells. As a result, glucose remains in blood cells, raising blood glucose levels (hyperglycemia). When hyperglycemia is left undiagnosed or untreated, it may result in various significant and sometimes life-threatening problems resulting from the diabetic complications (Soumya et al., 2011).

According to numerous scientific research, oxidative stress has a significant role in the etiology of both type 1 diabetes (T1D) and type 2 diabetes (T2D) (Bandeira et al., 2013). In diabetes, free radicals are produced in excess due to glucose oxidation, nonenzymatic protein glycation, and subsequent oxidative breakdown of glycated proteins. The free radical's overproduction may lead to severe cellular and enzyme damage, increased lipid peroxidation and enhanced insulin resistance. These ramifications of oxidative stress may contribute to diabetes-related problems, including microvascular and macrovascular diseases (Maritim et al., 2003).

17.7　EFFECTIVENESS OF *COLA NITIDA* AGAINST OXIDATIVE STRESS

For many years, scientists have been investigating the antioxidant properties of *C. nitida* and evaluating their therapeutic action against various diseases. Several studies have attempted to investigate the impact of *C. nitida* on preventing or treating metabolic illnesses such as diabetes and its complications.

The involvement of oxidative stress in the etiology and progression of T2D and its consequences has been extensively described in the scientific literature. According to the research, this has been related to an increase in hyperglycemia, which is accompanied by a reduction of the body's antioxidant system, resulting in a dysregulation of cellular metabolism (Pitocco et al., 2013). In previous studies, it has been proven that increased oxidative stress is caused by weakened antioxidant systems (reduced glutathione [GSH], superoxide dismutase [SOD], glutathione S-transferase [GST], and catalase [CAT]), as well as a simultaneous rise in malondialdehyde (MDA) (Feng et al., 2013). As a result, the increased production of ROS results in the development of oxidative toxicity or damage, both of which have negative consequences (Feng et al., 2013).

Accordingly, Erukainure et al. (2019a) reported that *C. nitida* caffeine-rich infusion treatment increased SOD and GSH levels. It decreased MDA levels in Fe^{2+}-induced oxidative hepatic tissues. Joshua et al. (2017) also reported that the ethanolic extract increased the activity of SOD. These findings show that *C. nitida* has intense antioxidant activities. These actions may be linked to the high caffeine level of the infusion that has been documented to have antioxidant properties.

Furthermore, Saliu et al. (2016) assessed the impact of *C. nitida* water extract on pro-oxidant–induced lipid peroxidation in rats' testes and its influence on arginase, a significant enzyme related to erectile dysfunction. The results confirmed that *C. nitida* water extract was shown to inhibit $FeSO_4$-induced lipid peroxidation and demonstrate its erectile function preventative measure in rat's testes. This is shown in its free radical scavenging actions, which are also effective. These actions may be linked to the high phytochemical contents, which have been reported as antioxidative molecules.

These results are also supported with *in vitro* experiment antioxidant activity of *C. nitida*, which may work in several pathways, including (1) by electron donation and (2) metal ion chelation. Hence, these results indicate that *C. nitida* has an intense antioxidative activity. This is corroborated by the ferric-reducing power (FRAP) of *C. nitida* previously reported (Erukainure et al., 2019b). Joshua et al. (2017) revealed that the caffeine-rich infusion extract and aqueous extracts of *C. nitida* had reduced the Fe^{+3} to Fe^{+2}, respectively. Onyeyilim et al. (2021) and Erukainure et al. (2019b) exhibited that the *C. nitida* caffeine-rich infusion showed strong scavenging activity of 2,2'-diphenyl-1-picrylhydrazyl (DPPH). Also, Fabunmi et al. (2015) informed that fermented samples of *C. nitida* exhibited high activity in scavenging DPPH radicals.

Based on the impact of *C. nitida* on fighting the ROS, we suggest that the antioxidants of *C. nitida* can work via two pathways: (1) direct scavenging of ROS, which reduces the amount of endogenous ROS produced; and (2) increasing the level of ROS scavenging enzymes.

17.8　ANTIDIABETIC PROPERTIES OF *COLA NITIDA*

The research for pharmaceutical drugs with a few side effects resulted in a radical shift toward traditional plants many years ago. Among many plants, the antidiabetic of *C. nitida* has been well investigated (Dorathy et al., 2014). Various scientific research reveals that *C. nitida* has intriguing antidiabetic capabilities, which seem to be significantly impacted by its capacity to alleviate diabetes-induced oxidative stress, enhance insulin secretion and activity, and inhibit metabolic disorders (Imam et al., 2018). Table 17.2 describes the impact of *C. nitida* on diabetes: molecular, cellular, and metabolic actions.

TABLE 17.2

The Impact of *Cola nitida* on Diabetes: Molecular, Cellular, and Metabolic Actions

Metabolites	Metabolic Activity	References
Proteins	• Unmodified amino acids	(Oboh et al., 2019)
	• Alternating overall changes	(Dah et al., 2015)
	• Stability of enzymes	
Lipids	• Suppress chain breakage	(Erukainure et al., 2021b)
	• Suppress peroxidation	(Oboh et al., 2019)
	• Protect the cell membrane	(Farombi, 2011)
	• Decrease membrane fluidity	(Ogunmefun et al., 2015)
Carbohydrates	• Improve the structure	(Erukainure et al., 2021a)
	• Suppress autooxidation	(Osukoya et al., 2016)
	• Promote nonenzymatic fragmentation	(Abou et al., 2016)
	• Enhance the function of cell surface receptor	
	• Suppress intercellular communication	

17.8.1 Effectiveness of *Cola nitida* against Hyperglycemia

Most human cells employ glucose as their principal substrate, which requires insulin for absorption. Insulin signaling is indeed crucial for the survival of these tissues. However, insulin resistance occurs when insulin sensitivity is decreased due to the disruption of numerous biochemical processes (Saltiel et al., 2001). Inadequate insulin production and action as a result of pancreatic β-cell depletion and malfunction, as well as insulin resistance in peripheral tissues, are the primary causes of chronic hyperglycemia in diabetes (Donath et al., 2004). For these reasons, there is a considerable need to develop acceptable, inexpensive, and safe blood glucose-lowering medicines that successfully treat diabetes mellitus while avoiding the significant side effects of presently used oral hypoglycemic medications. *C. nitida* has been suspected of having hypoglycemic effects, although this has not been well investigated (Mailloux, 2007). Accordingly, Erukainure et al. (2019b) reported that the treatment with *C. nitida* in hot water resulted in improved pancreatic β-cell activity and morphology, as well as restored pancreatic capillary networks. Likely, Dorathy et al. (2014) informed that *C. nitida* water extract decreased the blood glucose levels in diabetic rats from 599 ± 0.667 mg/dL (diabetic control) to 170 ± 0.577 mg/dL (extract-treated group). Thus, the extracts showed efficacy in lowering blood glucose levels in diabetic rats, which may be critical for avoiding long-term problems associated with hyperglycemia in diabetes mellitus. Furthermore, Dorathy et al. (2014) added that after 24 hours of therapy, *C. nitida* demonstrated a 26.04% decrease in blood glucose levels. The primary objective of diabetes mellitus treatment is to regulate increased blood glucose levels without generating abnormally low blood glucose levels (Dorathy et al., 2014).

As per the above-mentioned reports, *C. nitida* shows therapeutic benefits in diabetes by enhancing insulin production and decreasing apoptosis, improving pancreatic β cell proliferation, regulating glucose metabolism, and reducing muscle inflammation.

17.8.2 Effectiveness of *Cola nitida* against Carbohydrate-Digesting Enzyme Activity

Traditionally used medicinal plants have therapeutic properties attributed to an extensive collection of secondary metabolites, classified according to their structural and molecular compositions. The secondary metabolites may target cellular and molecular pathways involved in glucose metabolism and inhibit carbohydrate digestion and absorption. Studies have documented the enhancement of inhibition of *C. nitida* on α-glucosidase and α-amylase enzymes (Osukoya et al., 2016; Oboh et al., 2014).

α-Glucosidase and α-amylase are vital enzymes for regulating postprandial blood glucose levels in the treatment of T2D. These enzymes are involved in the hydrolysis of dietary starch into simple sugars such as glucose, increasing systemic glucose levels (Ahmad et al., 2021). Numerous phytoconstituents have been shown to reduce the activities of α-amylase and α-glucosidase and decrease intestinal glucose absorption, preventing postprandial hyperglycemia and maintaining a steady blood glucose level after a meal (Bharti et al., 2018). According to Erukainure et al. (2017), *C. nitida* caffeine-rich infusion extract has shown significant inhibitory activity against α-glucosidase, as well as α-amylase higher than the standard (acarbose). The plant inhibition demonstrates its capability to delay carbohydrate digestion. This is especially advantageous for people with diabetes who have poorly controlled glucose levels owing to abnormal glucose mechanistic metabolic machinery activity. Such drugs have been found to prevent or postpone the onset and progression of T2D and its accompanying problems. Furthermore, the presence of catechin, epicatechin, apigenin, and naringenin in the *C. nitida* might contribute to its enzyme inhibitory effects (Oboh et al., 2014). The phenolic rich extract's inhibition of carbohydrate enzyme activity agreed with previous reports on the inhibitory potential of widely used traditional plants against key enzymes related to treat diabetes.

17.8.3 Effectiveness of *Cola nitida* against Hepatic Enzyme Modification

Incessant hyperglycemia coupled with oxidative stress instigates diabetes-associated complications related to diabetes that possibly harm various vital organ systems. The liver is one of the body organs that could be affected by hyperglycemia-induced oxidative stress resulting in hepatic injury (Ayepola et al., 2013). The impact of *C. nitida* on hepatic enzyme function has been well documented (Zailani et al., 2020).

Na$^+$,K$^+$-ATPase, also known as the sodium pump, is a membrane-bound enzyme responsible for maintaining the Na$^+$ and K$^+$ gradients across the plasma membrane in an animal cell. Among the metabolic alterations associated with diabetes, abnormalities in Na$^+$,K$^+$-ATPase activity have been frequently described. Imam-Fulani et al. (2018) observed that Na$^+$,K$^+$-ATPase activity decreased significantly in the diabetic following *C. nitida* acetone extract treatment. This demonstrates the extract's ability to restore the reduced activity in diabetes enzymes.

The hepatic tissues produce aspartate aminotransferase transaminase (AST) and alanine aminotransferase transaminase (ALT), and an increase in these enzymes' blood levels indicates hepatic and cardiac injury, respectively. The reduction in ALT and AST levels in diabetic rats treated with various *C. nitida* extracts showed that the extract had no adverse impact on hepatic tissues and protected or ameliorated the cell membrane in alloxan-induced diabetic animals. However, in untreated diabetic rats, both enzymes increased significantly, suggesting that hepatic complications may have occurred, as reported by Dorathy et al. (2014). These findings point to *C. nitida*'s potential therapeutic role in hepatic enzymes function and antioxidant status in T2D patients.

17.8.4 Effectiveness of *Cola nitida* against Dyslipidemia

Quantitative and qualitative alterations in lipoproteins contribute to the increased risk of development in T2D individuals. In diabetic individuals, abnormal blood lipids include increased very-low-density lipoprotein (VLDL) and triglycerides and decreased high-density lipoprotein (HDL) (Vergès, 2015). These are linked to obesity and occur before the development of diabetes. Insulin resistance and hyperglycemia affect each lipid and lipoprotein component. The considerable decrease in serum lipid profile is consistent with prior research indicating that *C. nitida* treatment decreased triglyceride levels (Ogunmefun et al., 2015).

In T2D, impaired insulin production and action have been linked to lipid metabolism changes, resulting in diabetic dyslipidemia. It is often characterized by high total cholesterol, LDL cholesterol, triglycerides, and a decreased HDL cholesterol level (Boden et al., 2004). However, Salahdeen et al. (2015) and Erukainure et al. (2019b) reported that the *C. nitida* infusion extract significantly decreased blood glucose, serum triglycerides, LDL cholesterol, and HDL cholesterol levels. This is consistent with prior research in alloxan-induced diabetic rats as reported by Dorathy et al. (2014). Furthermore, the treatment of *C. nitida* hot water resulted in considerable depletion of diabetes-generated lipid metabolites, the production of fatty esters and steroids, and the deactivation of diabetes-activated pathways, as documented by Erukainure et al. (2021b).

17.8.5 MOLECULAR DOCKING STUDIES ON PHYTOCHEMICAL COMPOUNDS IN *COLA NITIDA*

Recently, molecular docking has been effectively used to investigate the mechanism of action of natural compounds. The molecular docking results are noteworthy and can be used as a tool for developing pharmacophore models, given that the chemicals are likely to be docked inside the enzymes' active pocket (Yan et al., 2014). As reported by Erukainure et al. (2019b), the molecular docking revealed that the ligands extracted from *C. nitida* showed strong interaction with caspase-3 and Nrf2.

17.9 TOXICITY ASSESSMENT OF *COLA NITIDA*

Burdock et al. (2009) investigated the effects of a fresh *C. nitida* extract on the postnatal development and behavior of mice. Pregnant Swiss-Webster albino mice (eight per dose group) were given the extract in their drinking water at reported doses of 0, 8, 16, or 32 mg/L. The study's findings show that the high-dose (32 mg/L) solution caused a substantial drop in pup body weights starting on day 4; the mid- and low-dose effects were less strong, not visible until the last week before weaning, and did not achieve statistical significance. When compared to controls, all three exposed groups had earlier eye opening and hair appearance. Furthermore, a research examined the acute toxicity of *C. nitida* methanol extract on liver enzymes and antioxidants in rats. For lethal dose (LD_{50}), administration of dosages up to 5000 mg/kg BW *C. nitida* resulted in no fatalities or apparent toxicity even after 48 hours. This provides evidence that the methanol extract of *C. nitida* is generally considered to be safe as reported by Emmanuel et al. (2016). While Erukainure et al. (2017) reported that caffeine's projected toxicity class and target might need prudence when using the infusion.

17.10 OTHER FOODS, HERBS, SPICES, AND BOTANICALS USED IN DIABETES

According to ethnobotanical data, about 800 plants may have antidiabetic properties. Numerous plants have been shown to have antidiabetic efficacy when evaluated using currently known experimental methodologies. various medicinal plants with antidiabetic properties and research on their methods of action were used, including *Brassica juncea, Origanum grosii, Combretum micranthum, Elephantopus scaber, Gymnema sylvestre, Liriope spicata, Parinari excelsa, Ricinus communis, Sarcopoterium spinosum, Smallanthus sonchifolius, Swertia punicea, Vernonia anthelmintica, Allium cepa* L., *Artemisia herba, Citrullus colocynthis, Ceratonia siliqua L*, and animal experimentation methods, as well as the medicinal efficacy of plant extracts (Arumugam et al., 2013; Skalli et al., 2019). The popularity of these plants has grown over time. Plants have the potential to be employed as a supplementary and alternative medicine, especially in metabolic illnesses like diabetes. These plants may potentially be useful in the creation of novel diabetic medications. The ways through which these plants affect glycemia vary. Some of them, such as sulfonylureas, inhibitors of hepatic neoglucogenesis, and glucosidase inhibitors, work similarly to traditional diabetes medications. It was also observed that combining plant extracts or their components may have synergistic benefits in treating diabetes. Likewise, several pharmaceuticals presently used to treat T2D are derived from plants, such as metformin, which was synthesized and developed from a biguanide compound discovered in French lilac (*Galega officinalis* L.). Indeed, traditional knowledge has been essential in the development of novel plant-based medications (Seetaloo et al., 2019).

Folkloric medicinal plants are usually employed in rural regions due to the abundance of medicinal plants in such places. As a result, treating diabetes mellitus using plant-derived chemicals that are readily available and do not need tedious pharmaceutical manufacturing seems particularly appealing.

17.11 CONCLUSIONS

The research on *Cola nitida* demonstrates promising antioxidant and antidiabetic properties. These properties are ascribed to the phytochemical elements of the plant, most notably alkaloids, which constitute the major phytochemicals of the plant. Thus, *C. nitida* can be used as a very effective functional food and nutraceutical in treating and managing diabetes and its complications. However, further research is needed to determine the molecular basis of the reported medicinal properties.

17.12 SUMMARY POINTS

- The effects of *Cola nitida* have shown promise as an antioxidant and antidiabetic agent.
- These characteristics are attributed to the phytochemical constituents of the plant, most notably alkaloids, which are the plant's primary phytochemicals and are responsible for these properties.
- *C. nitida* reduced the proportion of endogenous reactive oxygen species (ROS) generated while simultaneously increasing ROS scavenging enzymes.
- Treatment of *C. nitida* extracts resulted in a significant depletion of diabetes-derived lipid metabolites, the generation of fatty esters and steroids, and the deactivation of diabetes-related pathways.
- The plant may have therapeutic effects in diabetes by increasing insulin production and lowering apoptosis, increasing pancreatic beta-cell proliferation, modulating glucose metabolism, and decreasing muscle inflammation.
- Furthermore, *C. nitida* has the potential to be employed as a functional food and nutraceutical in the treatment and management of diabetes and its related complications.

17.13 CONFLICTS OF INTEREST

The authors declare no conflict of interests.

17.14 ACKNOWLEDGMENTS

The authors would like to acknowledge the Research Office, University of KwaZulu-Natal, Durban; and National Research Foundation (NRF), Pretoria, South Africa, for their financial supports.

REFERENCES

Abou, B., Houphouet, F., and Goueh, G. 2016. Effects of aqueous and ethanolic extracts of entandrophragma angolense, cola nitida and gomphrena celosioides against doxorubicin-induced cardiotoxicity in rats. *Journal of Advances in Medical and Pharmaceutical Sciences*, *10*(4): 1–13.

Adamu, A., Ingbian, I. N., Okhale, S. E., and Egharevba, H. O. 2020. Quantification of some phenolics acids and flavonoids in cola nitida, garcinia kola and buchholzia coriacea using high performance liquid chromatography-diode array detection (HPLC-DAD). *Journal of Medicinal Plants Research*, *14*(2): 81–87.

Adesanwo, J. K., Ogundele, S. B., Akinpelu, D. A., and McDonald, A. G. 2017. Chemical analyses, antimicrobial and antioxidant activities of extracts from cola nitida seed. *Journal of Exploratory Research in Pharmacology*, *2*(3): 67–77.

Agbor, A., Marie, Ebob, A., and Charles, N. 2019. Evaluation of the antimicrobial potentials and adverse effect of kolanut (Kola Nitida Malvaceae) on the oral cavity and the impact on cariogenic bacteria: A socio-demographic study. *Journal of Advances in Medical and Pharmaceutical Sciences* 20(1): 1–11.

Ahmad, J. B., Ajani, E. O., and Sabiu, S. 2021. Chemical group profiling, in vitro and in silico evaluation of Aristolochia ringens on α-amylase and α-glucosidase activity. *Evidence-Based Complementary and Alternative Medicine*, 2021.

Alberts, B., Johnson, A., Lewis, J., Raff, M., Roberts, K., and Walter, P. 2002. How cells obtain energy from food. In *Molecular Biology of the Cell*. 4th edition. Garland Science, New York.

Aniszewski, T. 2007. *Alkaloids-Secrets of Life: Aklaloid Chemistry, Biological Significance, Applications and Ecological Role*. Elsevier, Amsterdam, The Netherlands.

Arumugam, G., Manjula, P., and Paari, N. 2013. A review: Anti diabetic medicinal plants used for diabetes mellitus. *Journal of Acute Disease*, 2(3): 196–200.

Ayepola, O. R., Chegou, N. N., Brooks, N. L., and Oguntibeju, O. O. 2013. Kolaviron, a Garcinia biflavonoid complex ameliorates hyperglycemia-mediated hepatic injury in rats via suppression of inflammatory responses. *BMC Complementary and Alternative Medicine*, 13(1): 1–9.

Bandeira, D. M., Da Fonseca, L.J.S., Guedes, D. S., Rabelo, L. A., Goulart, M. O., and Vasconcelos, S.M.L. 2013. Oxidative stress as an underlying contributor in the development of chronic complications in diabetes mellitus. *International Journal of Molecular Sciences*, 14(2): 3265–3284.

Bharti, S. K., Krishnan, S., Kumar, A., and Kumar, A. 2018. Antidiabetic phytoconstituents and their mode of action on metabolic pathways. *Therapeutic Advances in Endocrinology and Metabolism*, 9(3): 81–100.

Boden, G., and Laakso, M. 2004. Lipids and glucose in type 2 diabetes: What is the cause and effect? *Diabetes Care*, 27(9): 2253–2259.

Boege, K. 2005. Herbivore attack in Casearia nitida influenced by plant ontogenetic variation in foliage quality and plant architecture. *Oecologia*, 143(1): 117–125.

Burdock, G. A., Carabin, I. G., and Crincoli, C. M. 2009. Safety assessment of kola nut extract as a food ingredient. *Food and Chemical Toxicology*, 47(8): 1725–1732.

Chung, K. T., Wong, T. Y., Wei, C. I., Huang, Y. W., and Lin, Y. 1998. Tannins and human health: A review. *Critical Reviews in Food Science and Nutrition*, 38(6): 421–464.

Dah-Nouvlessounon, D., Adjanohoun, A., Sina, H., Noumavo, P. A., Diarrasouba, N., Parkouda, C., and Baba-Moussa, L. 2015. Nutritional and anti-nutrient composition of three kola nuts (Cola nitida, Cola acuminata and Garcinia kola) produced in Benin. *Food and Nutrition Sciences*, 6(15): 1395.

Donath, M. Y., and Halban, P. A. 2004. Decreased beta-cell mass in diabetes: Significance, mechanisms and therapeutic implications. *Diabetologia*, 47(3): 581–589.

Dorathy, I. U., Okere, S. O., Daniel, E. E., and Liman, L. M. 2014. Phytochemical constitutents and anti-diabetic property of Cola nitida seeds on alloxan-induced diabetes mellitus in rats. *British Journal of Pharmaceutical Research*, 4(23): 2631.

Durand, D. N., Hubert, A. S., Nafan, D., Adolphe, A., Farid, B. M., Alphonse, S., and Lamine, B. M. 2015. Indigenous knowledge and socioeconomic values of three kola species (Cola nitida, Cola acuminata and Garcinia kola) used in southern Benin. *European Scientific Journal*, 11(36).

Emmanuel, E. U., Ebhohon, S. O., Adanma, O. C., Edith, O. C., Florence, O. N., Chioma, I., and Ndukaku, O. Y. 2016. Acute toxicity of methanol extract of cola nitida treatment on antioxidant capacity, Hepatic and renal functions in wistar rats. *International Journal of Biochemistry Research & Review*, 13(4): 1–6.

Erukainure, O. L., Ijomone, O. M., Oyebode, O. A., Chukwuma, C. I., Aschner, M., and Islam, M. S. 2019a. Hyperglycemia-induced oxidative brain injury: Therapeutic effects of Cola nitida infusion against redox imbalance, cerebellar neuronal insults, and upregulated Nrf2 expression in type 2 diabetic rats. *Food and Chemical Toxicology*, 127: 206–217.

Erukainure, O. L., Msomi, N. Z., Beseni, B. K., Salau, V. F., Ijomone, O. M., Koorbanally, N. A., and Islam, M. S. 2021a. Cola nitida infusion modulates cardiometabolic activities linked to cardiomyopathy in diabetic rats. *Food and Chemical Toxicology*, 154: 112335.

Erukainure, O. L., Oyebode, O. A., Sokhela, M. K., Koorbanally, N. A., and Islam, M. S. 2017. Caffeine-rich infusion from Cola nitida (kola nut) inhibits major carbohydrate catabolic enzymes; abates redox imbalance; and modulates oxidative dysregulated metabolic pathways and metabolites in Fe2+-induced hepatic toxicity. *Biomedicine and Pharmacotherapy*, 96: 1065–1074.

Erukainure, O. L., Sanni, O., Ijomone, O. M., Ibeji, C. U., Chukwuma, C. I., and Islam, M. S. 2019b. The antidiabetic properties of the hot water extract of kola nut (Cola nitida (Vent.) Schott and Endl.) in type 2 diabetic rats. *Journal of Ethnopharmacology*, 242: 112033.

Erukainure, O. L., Sanni, O., Salau, V. F., Koorbanally, N. A., and Islam, M. S. 2021b. Cola Nitida (Kola Nuts) Attenuates hepatic injury in type 2 diabetes by improving antioxidant and cholinergic dysfunctions and dysregulated lipid metabolism. *Endocrine, Metabolic and Immune Disorders-Drug Targets (Formerly Current Drug Targets-Immune, Endocrine and Metabolic Disorders)*, 21(4): 688–699.

Fabunmi, T. B., and Arotupin, D. J. 2015. Antioxidant properties of fermented kolanut husk and testa of three species of kolanut: Cola acuminata, Cola nitida and Cola verticillata. *British Biotechnology Journal*, 8(2): 1–13.

Farombi, E. O. 2011. Bitter kola (Garcinia kola) seeds and hepatoprotection. In *Nuts and Seeds in Health and Disease Prevention*: 221–228.

Feng, M., Qu, R., Wang, C., Wang, L., and Wang, Z. 2013. Comparative antioxidant status in freshwater fish Carassius auratus exposed to six current-use brominated flame retardants: A combined experimental and theoretical study. *Aquatic Toxicology*, 140: 314–323.

Finaud, J., Lac, G., and Filaire, E. 2006. Oxidative stress. *Sports medicine*, 36(4): 327–358.

Gandhi, S., and Abramov, A. Y. 2012. Mechanism of oxidative stress in neurodegeneration. *Oxidative Medicine and Cellular Longevity, 2012*.

Harborne, J. B. 1973. Phenolic compounds. In *Phytochemical Methods*: 33–88. Springer, Dordrecht, South Africa.

Heckman, M. A., Weil, J., and De Mejia, E. G. 2010. Caffeine (1, 3, 7-trimethylxanthine) in foods: A comprehensive review on consumption, functionality, safety, and regulatory matters. *Journal of Food Science*, 75(3): R77–R87.

IDF. 2021. *Diabetes Atlas. International Diabetes Federation*.10th edition. Brussels, Belgium.

Imam-Fulani, A. O., Sanusi, K. O., and Owoyele, B. V. 2018. Effects of acetone extract of Cola nitida on brain sodium-potassium adenosine triphosphatase activity and spatial memory in healthy and streptozotocin-induced diabetic female Wistar rats. *Journal of Basic and Clinical Physiology and Pharmacology*, 29(4): 411–416.

Islam, M. T. 2016. Concentration-dependent-activities of diterpenes: Achieving anti-/pro-oxidant links. *Asian Journal of Ethnopharmacology and Medicinal Foods*, 2, 12–15.

Joshua, P. E., Ukegbu, C. Y., Eze, C. S., Umeh, B. O., Oparandu, L. U., Okafor, J. O., and Ogara, A. 2017. Comparative studies on the possible antioxidant properties of ethanolic seed extracts of Cola nitida (kola nut) and Garcinia kola (bitter kola) on hydrogen peroxide induced oxidative stress in rats. *Journal of Medicinal Plants Research*, 12(22): 367–372.

Julkunen-Tiitto, R., and Haggman, H. 2009. Tannins and tannin agents. *Handbook of Natural Colorants*, 8: 201.

Kenny, H. C., and Abel, E. D. 2019. Heart failure in type 2 diabetes mellitus: Impact of glucose-lowering agents, heart failure therapies, and novel therapeutic strategies. *Circulation Research*, 124(1): 121–141.

Komlaga, G. A., Oduro, I., and Essel, E. M. 2019. Utilization of selected tropical crops (Cocoa, kola nuts, sorghum, millet, and shea butter). *Byproducts from Agriculture and Fisheries: Adding Value for Food, Feed, Pharma, and Fuels*: 563–580.

Krogdahl, Å., Penn, M., Thorsen, J., Refstie, S., and Bakke, A. M. 2010. Important antinutrients in plant feedstuffs for aquaculture: An update on recent findings regarding responses in salmonids. *Aquaculture Research*, 41(3): 333–344.

Mailloux, L. 2007. UpToDate dialysis in diabetic nephropathy. *UpToDate*. Retrieved, 12–07.

Maritim, A. C., Sanders, A., and Watkins Iii, J. B. 2003. Diabetes, oxidative stress, and antioxidants: A review. *Journal of Biochemical and Molecular Toxicology*, 17(1): 24–38.

Metodiewa, D., Kochman, A., and Karolczak, S. 1997. Evidence for antiradical and antioxidant properties of four biologically active N, N-Diethylaminoethyl ethers of flavaone oximes: A comparison with natural polyphenolic flavonoid rutin action. *IUBMB Life*, 41(5): 1067–1075.

Muhammad, S., and Fatima, A. 2014. Studies on phytochemical evaluation and antibacterial properties of two varieties of kolanut (Cola nitida) in Nigeria. *Journal of Biosciences and Medicines*, 2(3): 37–42.

Nwobodo, D. C., Ugwu, M. C., and Okoye, F.B.C. 2017. Screening of endophytic fungal secondary metabolites from Garcinia kola and Cola nitida for antioxidant properties. *Journal of Pharmaceutical Research*, 1: 000136.

Oboh, G., Ademosun, A. O., Ogunsuyi, O. B., Oyedola, E. T., Olasehinde, T. A., and Oyeleye, S. I. 2019. In vitro anticholinesterase, antimonoamine oxidase and antioxidant properties of alkaloid extracts from kola nuts (Cola acuminata and Cola nitida). *Journal of Complementary and Integrative Medicine*,16(1). https://doi.org/10.1515/jcim-2016-0155

Oboh, G., Nwokocha, K. E., Akinyemi, A. J., and Ademiluyi, A. O. 2014. Inhibitory effect of polyphenolic-rich extract from Cola nitida (Kolanut) seed on key enzyme linked to type 2 diabetes and Fe2+ induced lipid peroxidation in rat pancreas in vitro. *Asian Pacific Journal of Tropical Biomedicine*, 4: S405–S412.

Ogunmefun, O. T., Fasola, T. R., Saba, A. B., and Akinyemi, A. J. 2015. Inhibitory effect of Phragmanthera incana (Schum.) harvested from Cocoa (Theobroma Cacao) and Kolanut (Cola Nitida) trees on Fe2+ induced lipid oxidative stress in some rat tissues-in vitro. *International Journal of Biomedical Science: IJBS*, 11(1): 16.

Onyeyilim, E. L., Ugwu, E. E., Onugwu, A. L., Uzoewulu, C. P., and Otunomo, I. I. 2021. *Evaluation of Antioxidant Activity of Caffeine Extracted From Kolanut (Cola Nitida)*. Preprint at https://doi.org/10.21203/rs.3.rs-837364/v1

Osukoya, O., Agedah, A., Ozoemena, C. N., Onikanni, A., and Adewale, O. B. 2016. Physicochemical characterization of an hemagglutinating protein from the fruit of cola nitida, kolanut. *Innovare Journal of Science*, 4(4): 13–15.

Pereira, R. F., and Bartolo, P. J. 2016. Traditional therapies for skin wound healing. *Advances in Wound Care*, 5(5); 208–229.

Pisoschi, A. M., and Pop, A. 2015. The role of antioxidants in the chemistry of oxidative stress: A review. *European Journal of Medicinal Chemistry*, 97: 55–74.

Pitocco, D., Tesauro, M., Alessandro, R., Ghirlanda, G., and Cardillo, C. 2013. Oxidative stress in diabetes: Implications for vascular and other complications. *International Journal of Molecular Sciences*, 14(11): 21525–21550.

Quiroz-Garcia, D. L., Martinez-Hernandez, E., Palacios-Chavez, R., and Galindo-Miranda, N. E. 2001. Nest provisions and pollen foraging in three species of solitary bees (Hymenoptera: Apidae) from Jalisco, Mexico. *Journal of the Kansas Entomological Society*: 61–69.

Salahdeen, H. M., Omoaghe, A. O., Isehunwa, G. O., Murtala, B. A., and Alada, A. R. A. 2015. Gas chromatography mass spectrometry (GC-MS) analysis of ethanolic extracts of kolanut (*Cola nitida*)(vent) and its toxicity studies in rats. *Journal of Medicinal Plants Research*, 9(3): 56–70.

Saliu, J. A., Olabiyi, A. A., Adefegha, S. A., Oyeleye, S., and Olorunisola, O. O. 2016. Comparative evaluation of antioxidative properties and effects of aqueous extracts of Cola nitida and Vitex doniana on Fe2+-Generated oxidative stress in rat testes in vitro. *The International Journal of Biotechnology*, 5(2): 15–25.

Saltiel, A. R., and Kahn, C. R. 2001. Insulin signalling and the regulation of glucose and lipid metabolism. *Nature*, 414(6865): 799–806.

Santos-Sánchez, N. F., Salas-Coronado, R., Villanueva-Cañongo, C., and Hernández-Carlos, B. 2019. Antioxidant compounds and their antioxidant mechanism. *Antioxidants*: 10, 1–29.

Savi, M. K., Noumonvi, R., Chadaré, F. J., Daïnou, K., Salako, V. K., Idohou, R., and Glèlè Kakaï, R. 2019. Synergy between traditional knowledge of use and tree population structure for sustainability of Cola nitida (Vent.) Schott. and Endl in Benin (West Africa). *Environment, Development and Sustainability*, 21(3): 1357–1368.

Seetaloo, A. D., Aumeeruddy, M. Z., Kannan, R. R., and Mahomoodally, M. F. 2019. Potential of traditionally consumed medicinal herbs, spices, and food plants to inhibit key digestive enzymes geared towards diabetes mellitus management – A systematic review. *South African Journal of Botany*, 120: 3–24.

Skalli, S., Hassikou, R., and Arahou, M. 2019. An ethnobotanical survey of medicinal plants used for diabetes treatment in Rabat, Morocco. *Heliyon*, 5(3): e01421.

Soumya, D., and Srilatha, B. 2011. Late stage complications of diabetes and insulin resistance. *Journal of Diabetes & Metabolic*, 2(9): 1000167.

Umoren, E. B., Osim, E. E., and Udoh, P. B. 2009. The comparative effects of chronic consumption of kola nut (Cola nitida) and caffeine diets on locomotor behaviour and body weights in mice. *Nigerian Journal of Physiological Sciences*, 24(1).

Vergès, B. 2015. Pathophysiology of diabetic dyslipidaemia: Where are we? *Diabetologia*, 58(5): 886–899.

Yan, J., Zhang, G., Pan, J., and Wang, Y. 2014. α-Glucosidase inhibition by luteolin: Kinetics, interaction and molecular docking. *International Journal of Biological Macromolecules*, 64: 213–223.

Zailani, A. H., Iliyas, M. B., Benjamin, L., Ibrahim, B. A., Ubah, B., and Lamiya, A. 2020. Cola nitida leaf phytochemicals improve liver function indices of mice infected with Plasmodium berghei (NK-65). *Journal of Medicinal Plants*, 8(2): 143.

18 Mango (*Mangifera indica* L.) Phytochemical Profile, Nutritional Aspects and Potential Anti-Diabetic Therapeutics Studies

Heba A.S. El-Nashar, Shaza H. Aly, Lucian Hritcu and Omayma A. Eldahshan

CONTENTS

ABBREVIATIONS

AMPK   activated protein kinase
DM   diabetes mellitus
DPP-IV   dipeptidyl peptidase-IV
HbA_{1c} glycated hemoglobin
HFD   high-fat diet
GAE   gallic acid equivalent
STZ   streptozotocin
SIRT1   sirtuin 1

18.1 INTRODUCTION

Diabetes mellitus (DM) is a metabolic endocrine disorder characterized by glucose intolerance arising from insulin response impairment or lack of insulin secretion leading to abnormal metabolism of lipids and proteins (Sasi et al. 2020). Nowadays, the prevalence of DM is intensely enlarged as the response of the high-caloric food diets and sedentary lifestyles that are now common (Carpino and Goodwin 2010). Patients with diabetes are usually identified with having one of two forms: type 1 DM (insulin-dependent, most common) and type 2 DM (insulin-independent) (Niewczas et al. 2012). Long-term hyperglycemia leads to serious macrovascular and microangiopathy complications such as peripheral neuropathy, kidney damage, cataract, and coronary artery disorders (Agarwal et al. 2008). Current treatment regimens for DM embrace oral anti-diabetic medications like sulfonylureas, biguanides, α-glucosidase inhibitors, thiazolidinediones, and dipeptidyl peptidase-IV (DPP-IV) inhibitors that can be taken alone or in combination (Sola et al. 2015). These medicines are well-known for their disagreeable side effects, and some of them cannot accomplish glycemic control for patients with diabetes (Sola et al. 2015). The pathogenesis of DM comprises many factors and signaling pathways that requires the combination of various therapeutic applications involving multicomponent-based natural products (Wei et al. 2017). Therefore, researchers have focused their attention on developing anti-diabetic drugs that are safer and more effective. Interestingly, natural medicine has had an important role in treating diabetes for centuries worldwide. With the amazing growth of scientific research on different plant species, a large number of active constituents have been found to exhibit anti-diabetic properties that could be developed as new anti-diabetic drugs or supplements with the current synthetic medications.

Among these plants, *Mangifera indica* L. (Mango) is one of the most important edible fruits that belongs to the family Anacardiaceae distributed in many countries, particularly tropical regions (Ali et al. 2020). Mango fruits exhibited an imperative role in agricultural, food, pharmaceutical, and nutraceutical fields (Quintana et al. 2021). Moreover, mango fruit ranks second among industrial crops, after banana, in terms of production and coverage (Muchiri et al. 2012). Different parts of *M. indica* provide a rich source of different phytoconstituents, including flavonoids, xanthonoids, phenolic acids, and triterpenoids with potential value as functional molecules (Quintana et al. 2021). In addition, fruits supply the human body with vital components such as carbohydrates, proteins, fats, minerals, vitamins, essential amino acids, carotenoids, dietary fiber, and phenolic compounds (Jahurul et al. 2015). Traditionally, different organs of the mango plant have been used for several ailments as diarrhea, bloody dysentery, anemia, asthma, bronchitis, hypertension, insomnia, rheumatism, indigestion, hepatitis, tetanus, miscarriage, and hemorrhage (Ali et al. 2020).

This chapter accumulates biological studies (*in vitro* and *in vivo*) that describe the potential role of *M. indica* extracts and isolated bioactive compounds in the management of diabetes mellitus, focusing on the efficiency and mechanism of action. Additionally, we discuss the isolated bioactive compounds and their contribution to fight the disease. Hopefully, this chapter will encourage the scientists for further research to develop a new effective anti-diabetic drug.

18.2 BACKGROUND

Mangifera indica, or mango, is one of the most economically important and globally consumed fruits due to its diversity of macro- and micronutrients, the main consumable part; the mango pulp is rich with nutritional and functional compounds such as carbohydrates (16%–18%), proteins, amino acids, lipids, organic acids, and dietary fiber as macronutrients. The plant's micronutrients include the minerals calcium, phosphorus, iron, and the vitamins C and A. Besides, mango acts as a good source of energy and water (Lebaka et al. 2021). Studies investigate its beneficial role in health and its contribution in the management of diabetes mellitus, obesity, and related issues (Gondi et al. 2015). The composition of mango peel is mostly determined by the maturity stage, locale, variety, and climatic variables in the place of production. Vitamin C content varies greatly amongst cultivars, ranging from 188–2570 µg/g. Also, mango peel is a good source of vitamin E (205–509 µg/g), reflected in its use in the formulation of skin care products. Polyphenol levels in mango peel range from 55 to 110 mg/gm dry weight, with ripe peel having greater amounts than unripe peel (Ajila et al. 2007). One of the most important polyphenol compounds in the mango peel is mangiferin (1.69 g/kg dry weight) (Lebaka et al. 2021). The seed is high in nutrients, with 58%–80% carbohydrates, 6%–13% proteins, lipids, minerals, and vitamins. As mango peel, the seed is a rich source of polyphenols, about 112 mg gallic acid equivalent (GAE)/100 g peel of total polyphenols, and the total flavonoid content was about 3325 ± 120 mg catechin equivalent (CE)/100 g seed (Abdel-Aty et al. 2018). The mango kernel has higher antioxidant and polypheno-lic contents than the pulp and peel and is used for oil extraction; its possible usage along with corn and wheat flour in preparing nutraceuticals is being increasingly emphasized (Ajila et al. 2007). Mangoes are high in antioxidant micronutrients, including ascorbic acid, carotenoids, and pheno-lics. Additionally, the fruits are widely valued for their dietary fiber and their pleasing color, taste, and flavor. Carotenoids, primarily β-carotene, play an important role in mango nutritional quality as an antioxidant agent and prevention of leukemia and inhibiting progress of prostate, breast, and colon cancers (Lemmens et al. 2013). Different parts of mango have a long history of use in ancient traditional medicine to control different conditions, and many studies have explored its evidence-based biological effects as anti-inflammatory, antioxidant, anti-diabetic, antimicrobial, anticancer, antihyperlipemic, and immunomodulatory activities with fewer side effects and more benefits (Imran et al. 2017).

18.3 BIOACTIVE COMPOUNDS ISOLATED FROM *MANGIFERA INDICA*

18.3.1 FLAVONOIDS

Several compounds of flavonoid nature were isolated from *M. indica*, as illustrated in Figure 18.1. In-depth phytochemical study was conducted on the ethyl acetate fraction of 70% ethano-lic leaf extract (Pan et al. 2018). It revealed the purification of 12 flavonoids; quercetin (**1**),

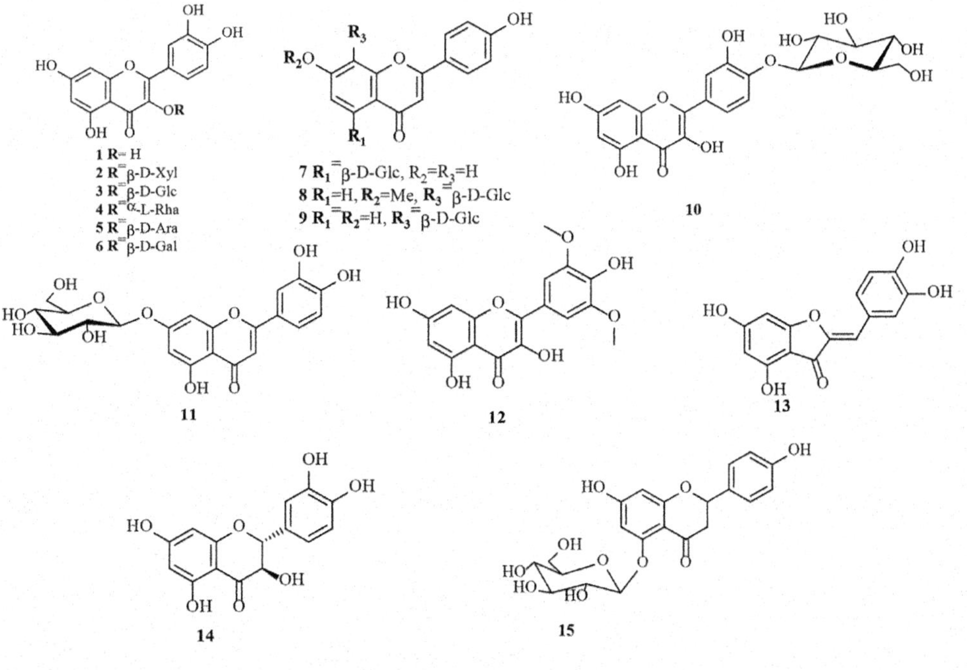

FIGURE 18.1   The structures of flavonoids (**1–27**) isolated from *Mangifera indica*.

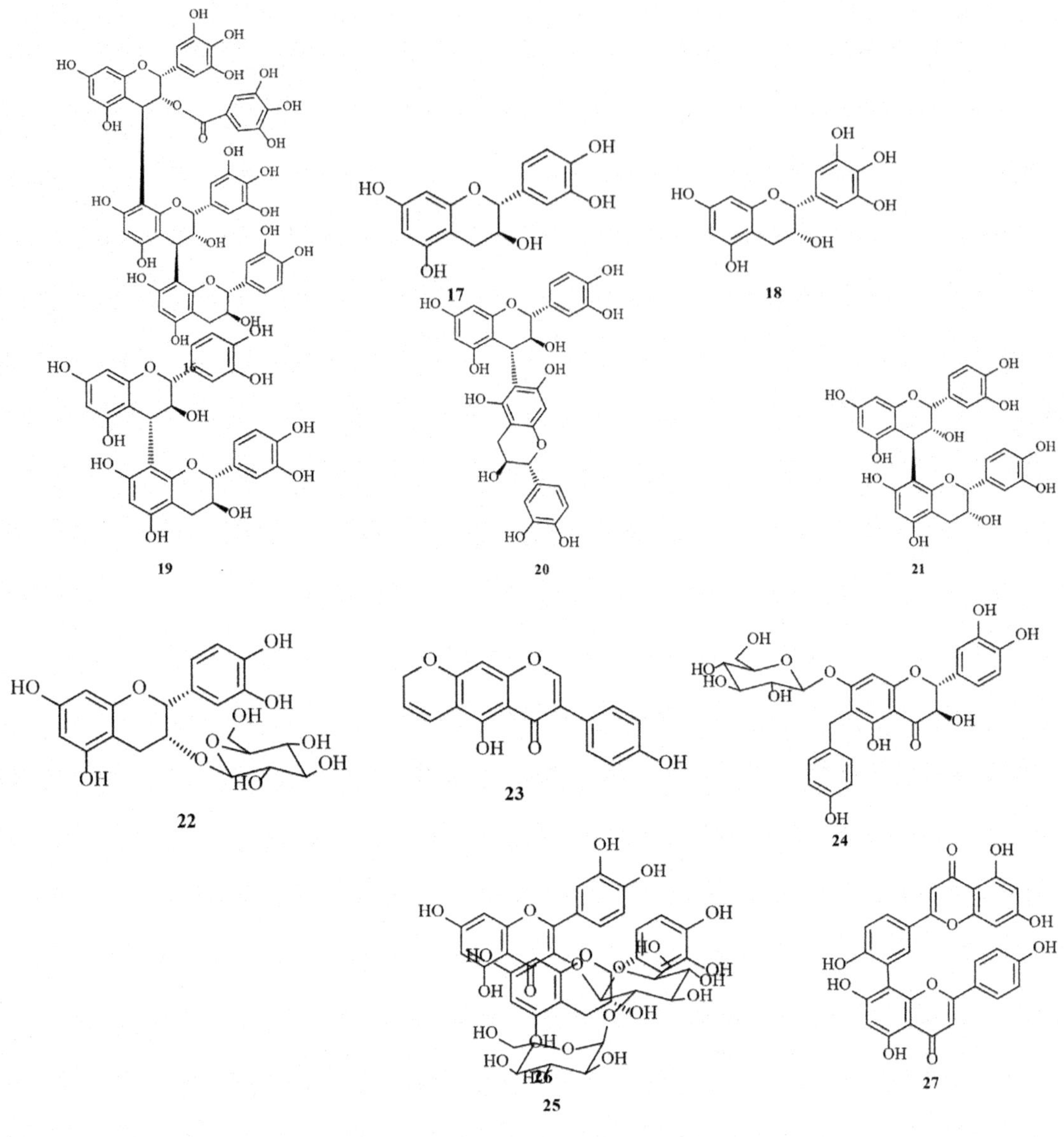

FIGURE 18.1 (Continued)

quercetin-3-O-β-D-xylopyranoside (**2**), quercetin-3-O-β-D-glucopyranoside (**3**), quercetin-3-O-α-L-rhamnpyranooside (**4**), quercetin-3-O-β-D-arabinoside (**5**), quercetine-3-O-β-D-galactpyranoside (**6**), isovitexin (**7**), isoswertisin (**8**), vitexin (**9**), quercetin-4′-O-β-D-glucopyranoside (**10**), luteolin-7-O-β-D-glucopyranoside (**11**), 3′,5′-dimethoxy-4′,5,7-trihydroxyflavone (**12**), sulfuretin (**13**), and taxifolin (**14**). In another study, naringenin 5-O-β-D-glucopyranoside (**15**) was obtained from fruit peels. Tawaha et al. (2010) has reported a new trimeric proanthocyanidin, namely, epigallocatechin-3-O-gallat-(4β→8)-epigallocatechin-(4β→8)-catechin (**16**) from the aqueous acetone extract of the leaves. Additionally, three known flavan-3-ols were identified as catechin (**17**) and epigallocatechin (**18**) with three dimeric proanthocyanidins such as catechin-(4α→8)-catechin (**19**), catechin-(4α→6)-catechin (**20**), and epicatechin-(4β→8)-catechin (**21**). In 2010, a group of researchers isolated five antifungal flavonoids from the methanol extract of leaves (Kanwal et al. 2010). These compounds were elucidated as (–)-epicatechin-3-O-β-glucopyranoside (**22**), 5-hydroxy-3-(4-hydroxylphenyl) pyrano [3,2-g]chromene-4(8H)-one (**23**), 6-(*p*-hydroxybenzyl)-taxifolin-7-*O*-β-D-glucoside (tricuspid, **24**), quercetin-3-*O*-β-glucopyranosyl-(1→2)-β-D-glucopyranoside (**25**), and (−)-epicatechin (**26**). On the other side, amentoflavone (**27**) was a biflavonoid identified from the ethyl acetate fraction of 70% ethanolic leaf extract (Pan et al. 2018).

18.3.2 XANTHONOIDS

Xanthonoids were predominant compounds reported in different parts of *Mangifera indica*, as illustrated in Figure 18.2. Mangiferin (**28**) was characterized as a major xanthone C-glycoside present in the different organs of *M. indica* (Pan et al. 2018). Another xanthone derivative, namely 4'-*O*-*p*-hydroxybenzoylmangiferin (**29**) was obtained from the ethyl acetate fraction of 70% ethanolic leaf extract (Pan et al. 2018). In anti-diabetic study published by (Amran et al. 2013), mangiferin structure with galloyl moiety was isolated and identified as 6-*O*-galloyl-5'-hydroxy mangiferin (**30**) from 90% aqueous methanol extract of seed kernels. Four new benzophenone glycosides were isolated from the ethyl acetate fraction of 70% ethanolic leaf extract (Pan et al. 2018). They were elucidated as 4',6-dihydroxy-4-methoxybenzophenone-2-*O*-(2''),3-C-(1'')-1''-desoxy-β-fructopyranoside (**31**), 4,4',6-trihydroxybenzophenone-2-*O*-(2''),3-C-(1'')-1''-desoxy-β-fructopyranoside (**32**), 4,4',6-trihydroxybenzophenone-2-*O*-(2''),3-C-(1'')-1''-desoxy-β-fructofuranoside (**33**), and 2,4',6-trihydroxy-4-methoxybenzophenone-3-C-(2-*O*-*p*-hydroxybenzoyl-*p*-hydroxybenzoyl)-α-D-galactopyranos

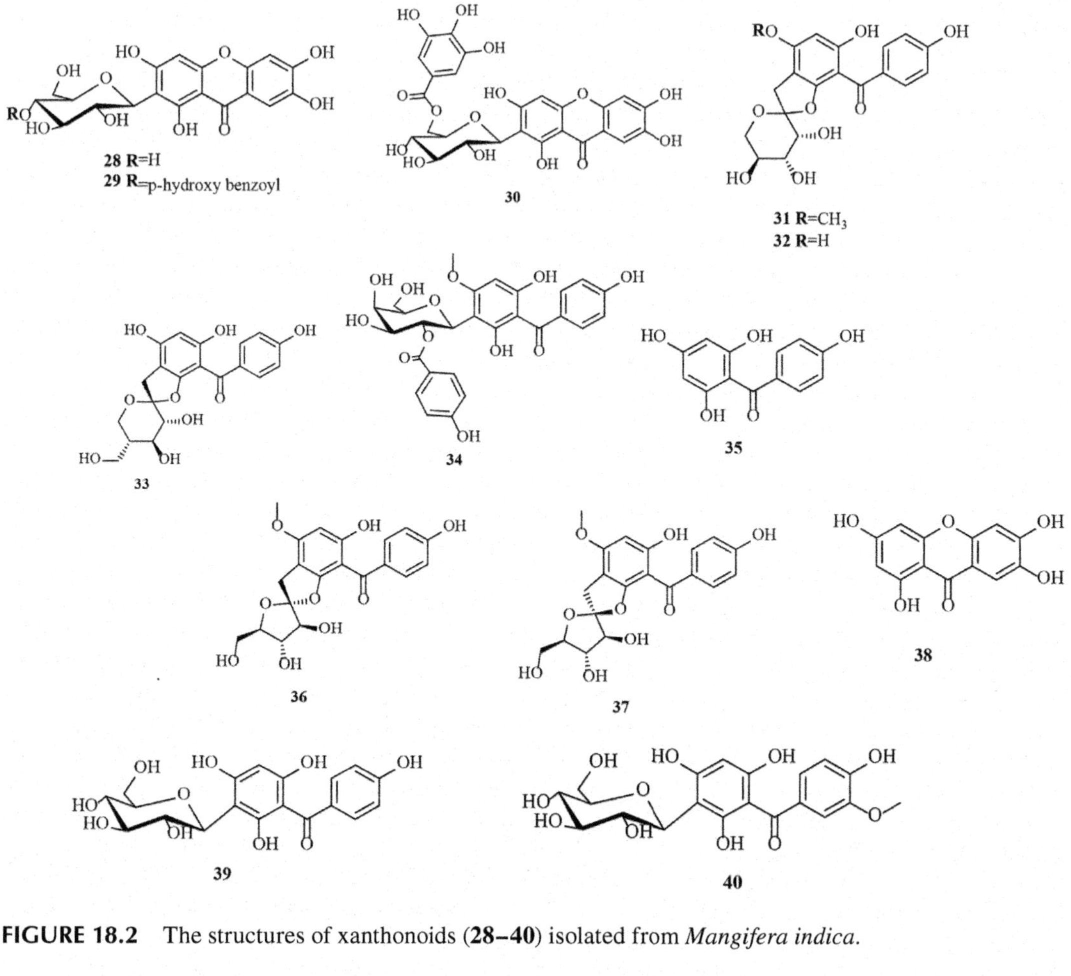

FIGURE 18.2 The structures of xanthonoids (**28–40**) isolated from *Mangifera indica*.

ide (**34**). In addition, iriflophene (**35**) was also isolated. Another study revealed isolation of four benzophenone derivatives from the leaf extract (Gu et al. 2019). Two of them were new compounds identified as manindicin A (**36**) and manindicin B (**37**). The other identified compounds were mangiferin (**28**) and norathyriol (**38**). In an attempt to investigate the cholesterol esterase inhibitory property of leaf extract, iriflophenone-3-β-C-glucopyranoside (**39**) was isolated from the ethyl acetate fraction of leaf extract (Gururaja et al. 2015). Another anti-diabetic study showed isolation of a novel benzophenone glycoside, namely 2,4,4′,6-tetrahydroxy-3′-methoxybenzophenone 3-C-β-D-glucopyranoside (**40**) from 70% ethanol extract of leaves of *M. indica* L. (Pan et al. 2016).

18.3.3 Phenolic Acids and Phenolic Acid Derivatives

Phenolic acids and their derivatives, isolated different parts of *Mangifera indica* are shown in Figure 18.3. Using two-step high-speed counter-current chromatography method, four phenolic acid derivatives – gallic acid (**41**), ethyl gallate (**42**), ethyl digallate (**43**), and ellagic acid (**44**) – were obtained from the ethanol extract of flowers (Shaheen et al. 2017). The phytochemical investigation of stem bark extract afforded the identification of gallic acid (**41**), methyl gallate (**45**), propyl gallate (**46**), mangiferin (**28**), 3,4-dihydroxy benzoic acid (**47**), benzoic acid (**48**), and propyl benzoate (**49**) (Núñez Sellés et al. 2002). Another four phenolic compounds, namely 1,4-benzenedicarboxylic acid-1,4-diethyl ester (**50**), 3,4-dihydroxy-5-methoxybenzoic acid ethyl ester (**51**) and 3-hydroxy-4,5-dimethoxybenzoic acid ethyl ester (**52**), were isolated from fruit peels (Jiang et al. 2019).

18.3.4 Triterpenes

Triterpenoids represent the main class of compounds isolated from *Mangifera indica* (Figure 18.4). Six triterpenoids of tetracyclic skeleton were isolated from the hexane extract of stem bark (Anjaneyulu et al. 1985). The isolated compounds were characterized as cycloart-24-ene-3β,26 diol (**53**), cycloart-25ene-3β,24,27-triol (**54**), cycloartane-3β,24,25-triol (**55**), cycloart-25-ene-3β,24-diol (**56**), 3β-hydroxycycloart-25-en-27-al (**57**), cycloartenol (**58**), α-amyrin (**59**), β-amyrin

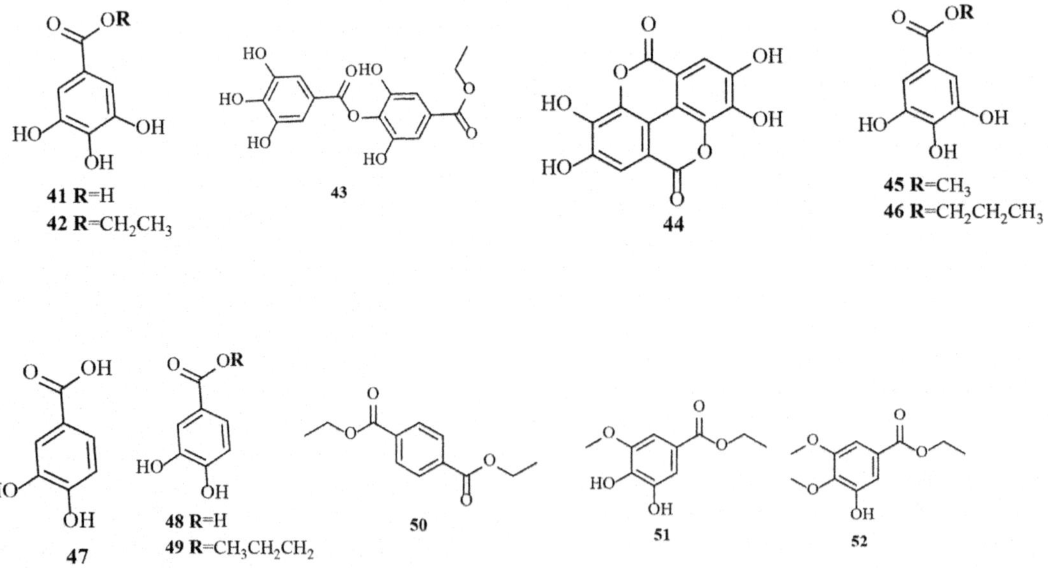

FIGURE 18.3 The structures of phenolic acids and phenolic acid derivatives (**41–52**) isolated from *Mangifera indica*.

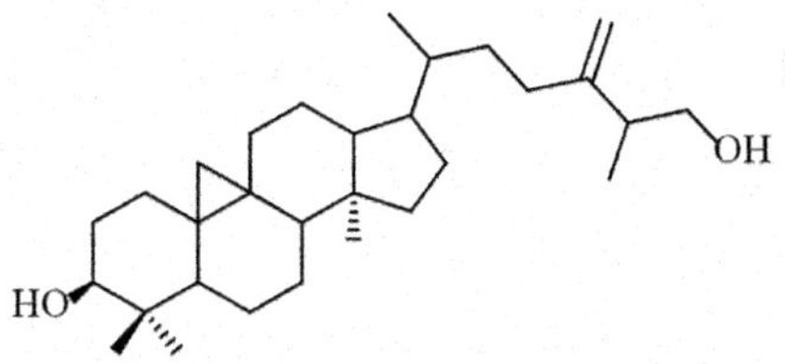

FIGURE 18.4 The structures of triterpenoids (**53–79**) isolated from *Mangifera indica*.

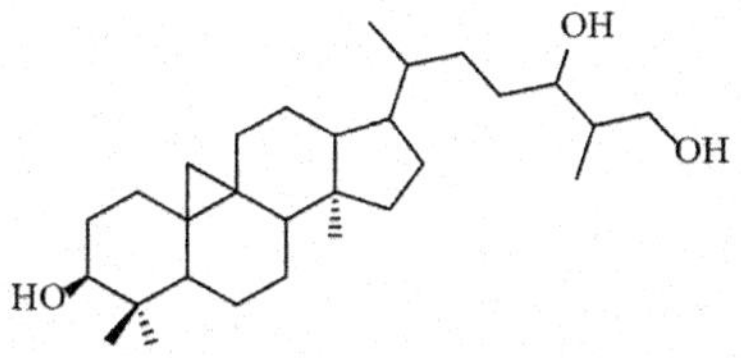

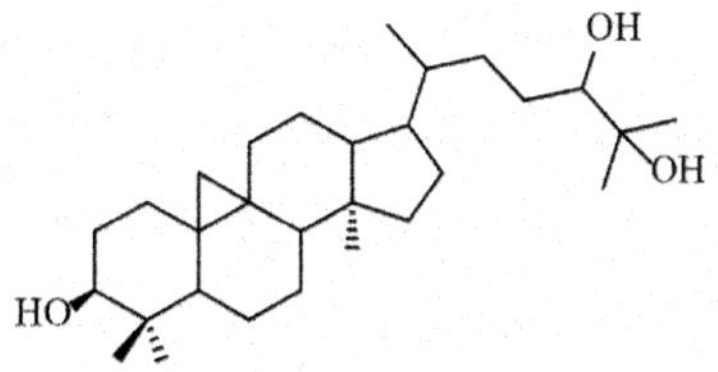

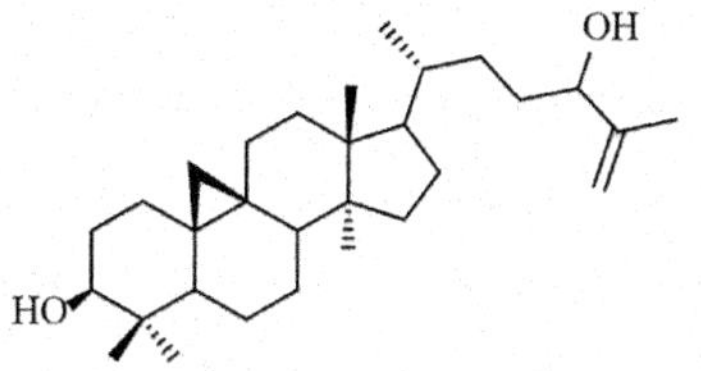

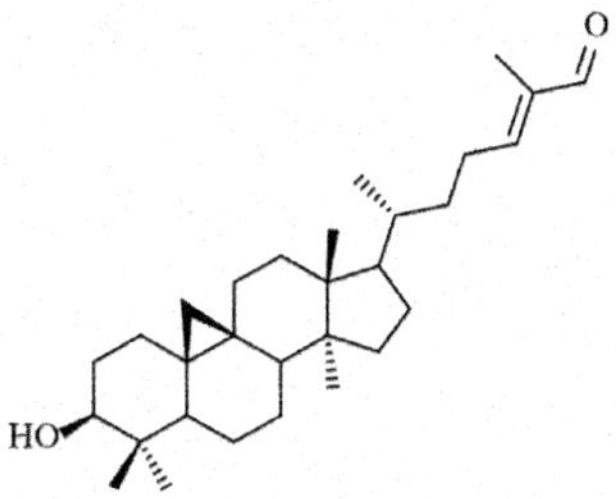

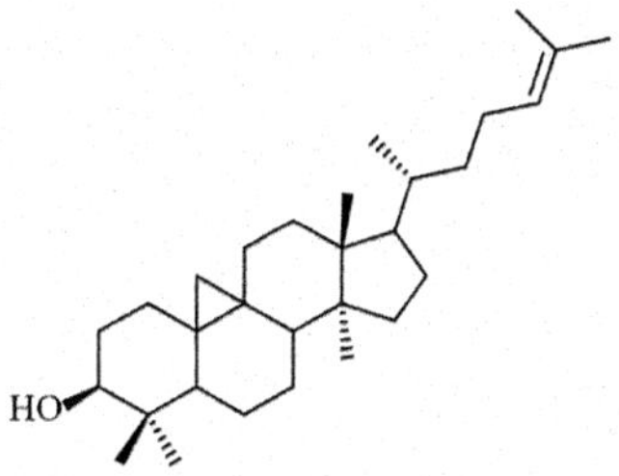

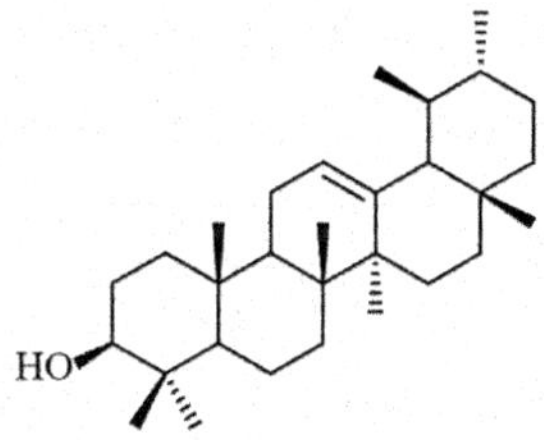

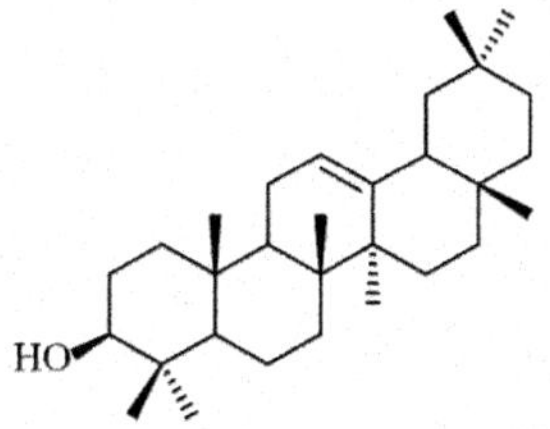

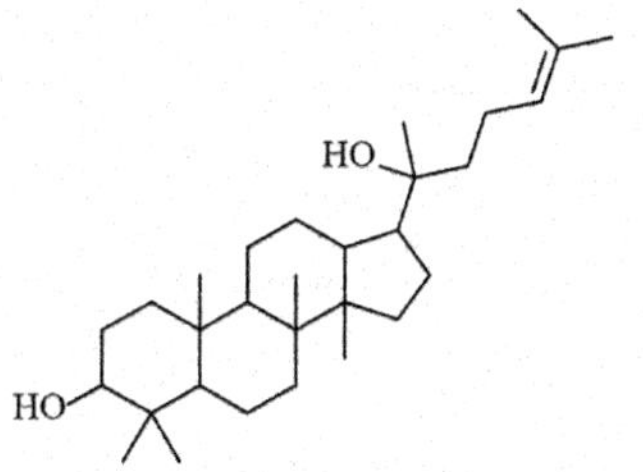

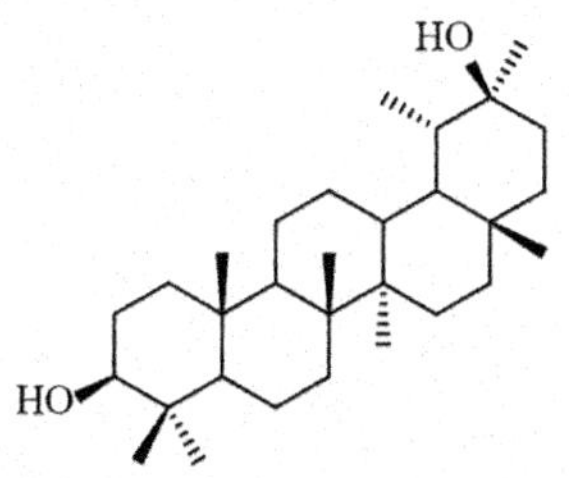

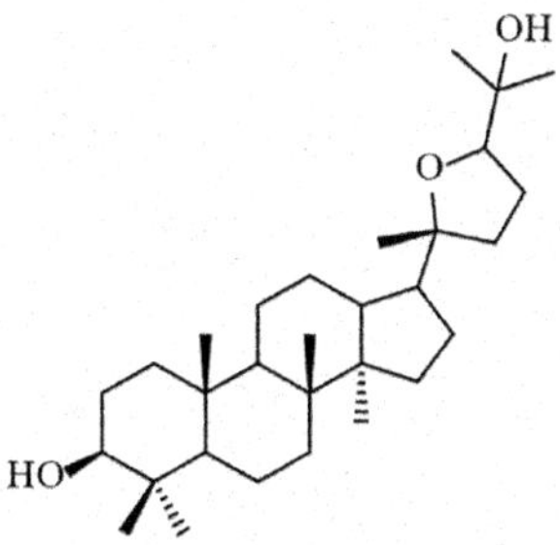

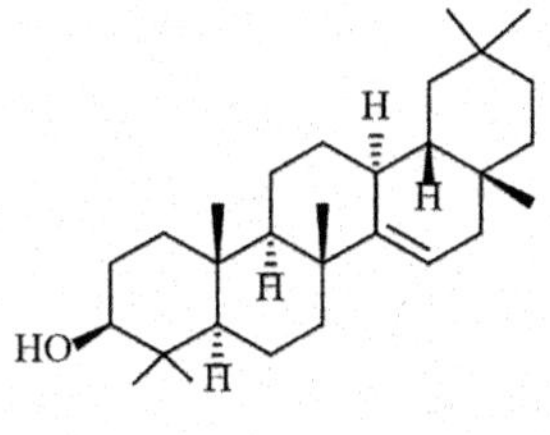

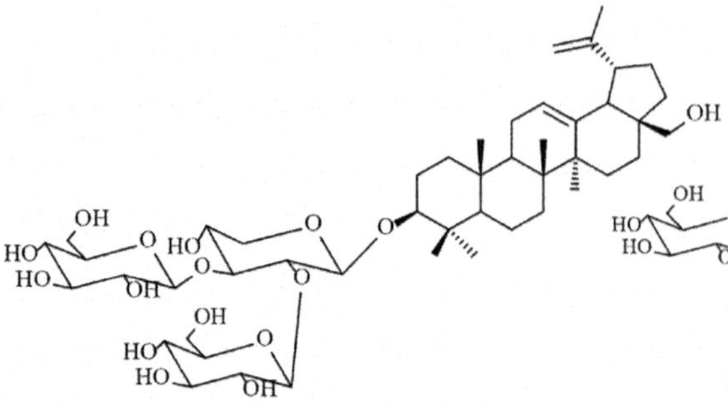

FIGURE 18.4 (Continued)

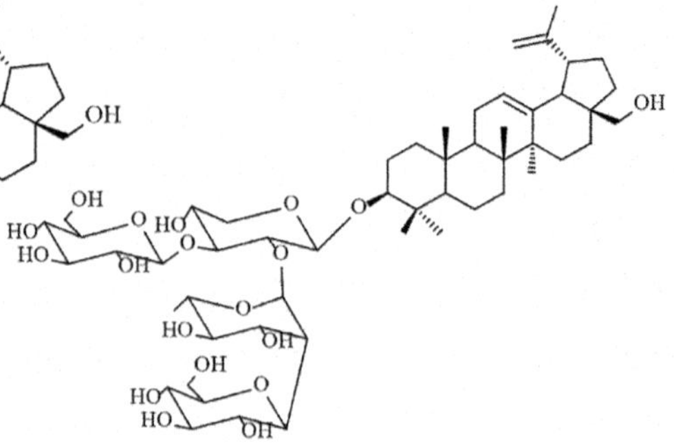

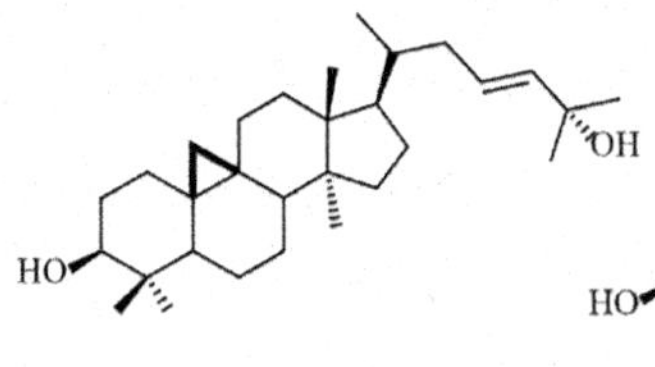

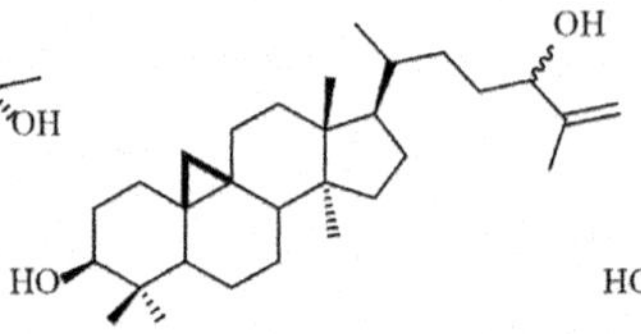

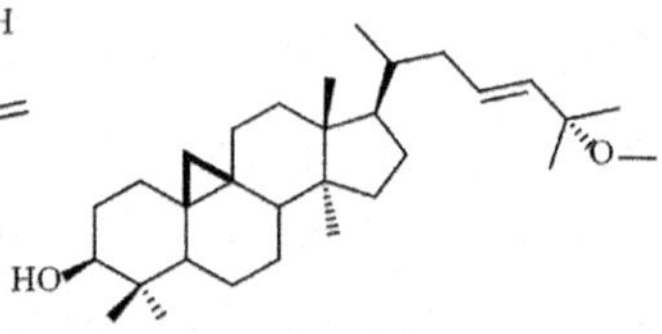

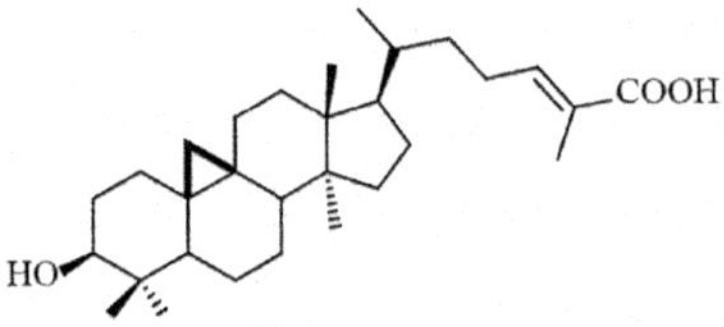

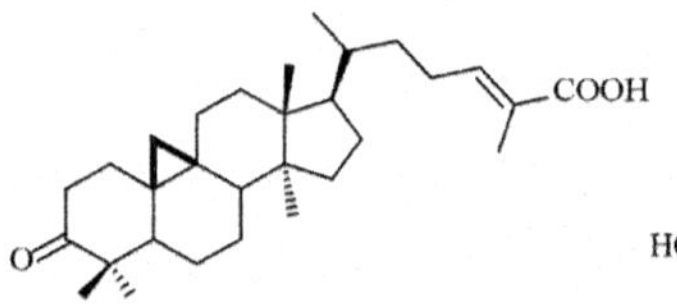

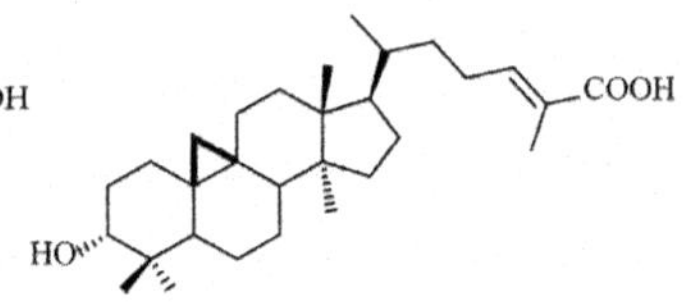

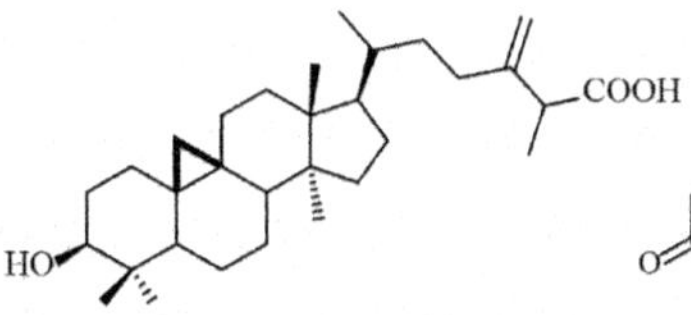

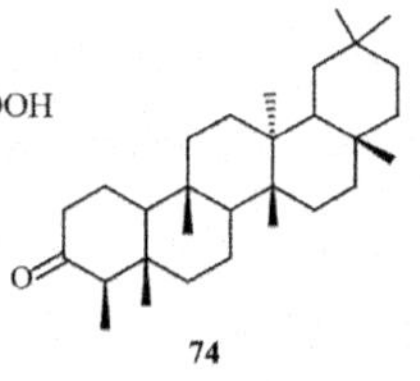

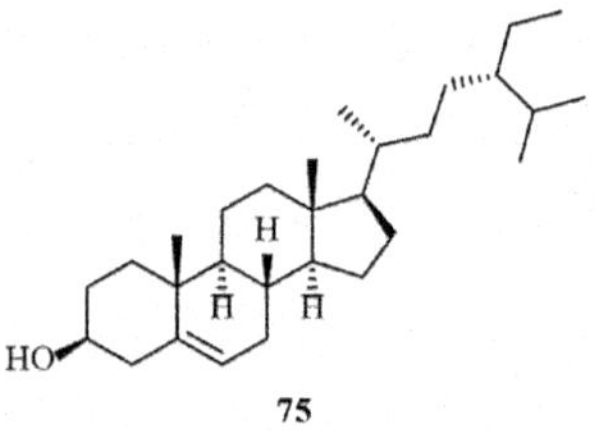

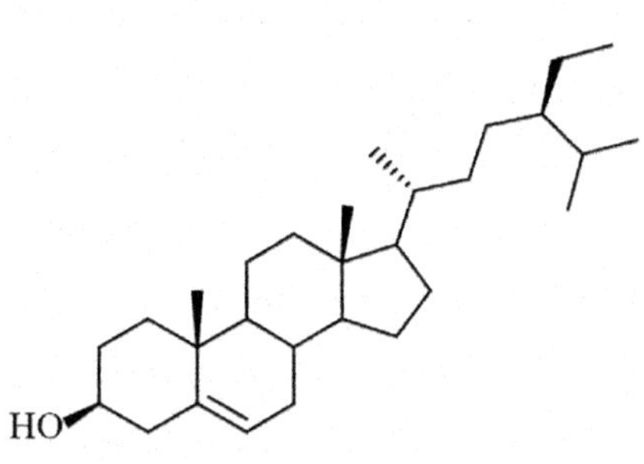

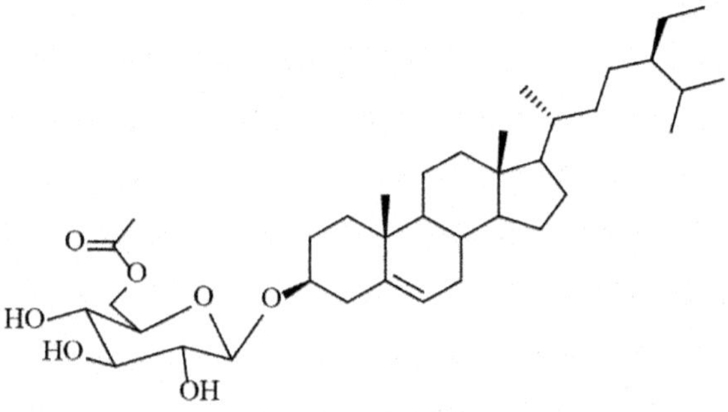

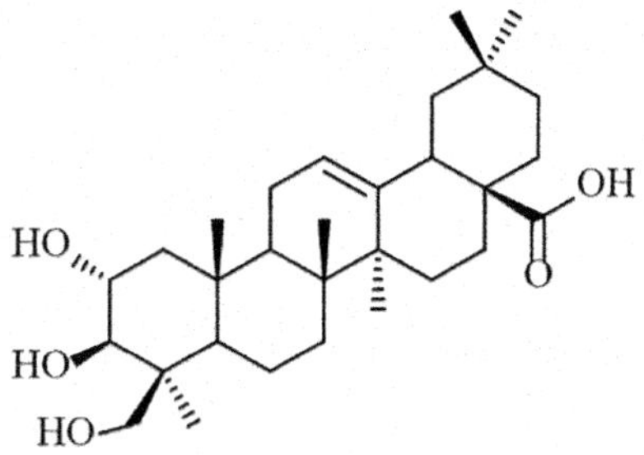

FIGURE 18.4 (Continued)

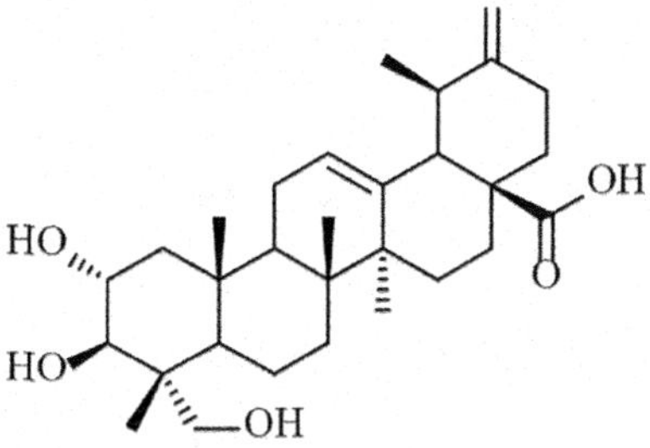

(**60**), dammarenediol II (**61**), Ψ-taraxastane-3β,20-diol (**62**), and ocotillol II (**63**). Another study published by Sangeetha et al. (2010) reported isolation of anti-diabetic compound of pentacyclic structure, namely 3β-taraxerol (**64**) from the ethyl acetate extract of plant leaves. Two triterpe-noidal saponins of lupene nulcus, namely indicoside A (**65**) and indicoside B (**66**), were isolated from the stem bark extract (Khan et al. 1993). They were characterized as 28-hydrorylupa-12,20(29)-diene-3-*O*-[β-glucopyranosyl-(1→2)][β-glucopyranosyl-(1→3)]-α-L-arabinopyranoside and 28-hydroxylupa-12,20(29)-diene-3-*O*-[β-glucopyranosyl-(1→3)-α-L-rhamnopyranosyl-(1→2)] [β-glucopyranosyl(1→3)]-α-L-arabinopyranoside. Escobedo-Martínez et al. (2012) examined the active constituents of the petroleum ether extract of *M. indica* stem bark. Seven triterpenoids of cycloartane-type were isolated by different column chromatographical technique. Among the isolated components, four compounds, namely cycloart-23-ene-3β,25-diol (**67**), 3β-hydroxy-25-methylenecycloartan-24-ol (**68**), 3β-hydroxy-cycloart-23-ene-25-methyl ether (**69**), and 3β-hydroxy-cycloart-24-ene-25-carboxylic acid (**70**) have been determined to be new triterpenoids. Additionally, mangiferonic acid (**71**), isomangiferolic acid (**72**), and ambolic acid (**73**) were reported to be known compounds along with pentacyclic triterpene, namely friedelin (**74**). Further, β-sitosterol (**75**), β-daucosterine (**76**), and 6′-*O*-acetyl-β-daucosterol (**77**) were isolated from fruit peels (Jiang et al. 2019). Another study showed isolation of two anti-diabetic triterpenoid acids, namely arjunolic acid (**78**) and actinidic acid (**79**) from 70% ethanol extract of leaves of *M. indica* L. (Pan et al. 2016).

18.3.5 Miscellaneous Compounds

Miscellaneous bioactive compounds were isolated from *Mangifera indica* and are clarified in Figure 18.5. Using bioassay guided-extraction, two anti-inflammatory phenolic compounds, namely 5-(11′Z-heptadecenyl)-resorcinol (**80**) and 5-(8′Z,11′Z-heptadecadienyl)-resorcinol (**81**), were purified from the 70% hydroethanolic peel extract of *M. indica* L. growing in Thailand (Knödler et al. 2008). Bioactivity-guided fractionation led to the isolation of anti-diabetic compounds, 1,2,3,4,6-penta-*O*-galloyl-β-D-glucose (**82**), and 1,2,3,4,6 penta-O-galloyl-α-D-glucose (**83**), from the methano-lic extract of leaves and seed kernels (Yang et al. 2020). Another phytochemical study showed the isolation of three phenolic compounds, 1,2,3-benzenetriol (**84**), 5-(hydroxymethyl) furfural (**85**), 3′,4-dihydroxy-5,5′-dimethoxybibenzyl (**86**), and crepidatin (**87**) from fruit peels (Jiang et al. 2019).

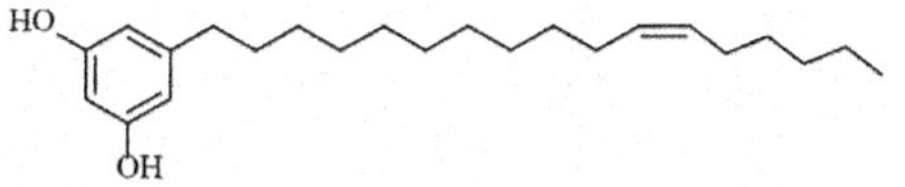

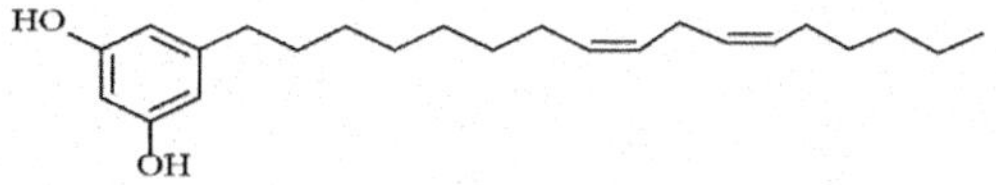

FIGURE 18.5 The structures of miscellaneous compounds (**80–87**) isolated from *Mangifera indica*.

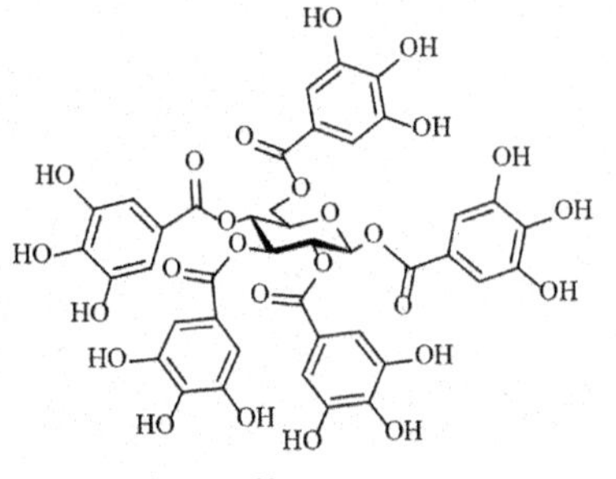

FIGURE 18.5 (Continued)

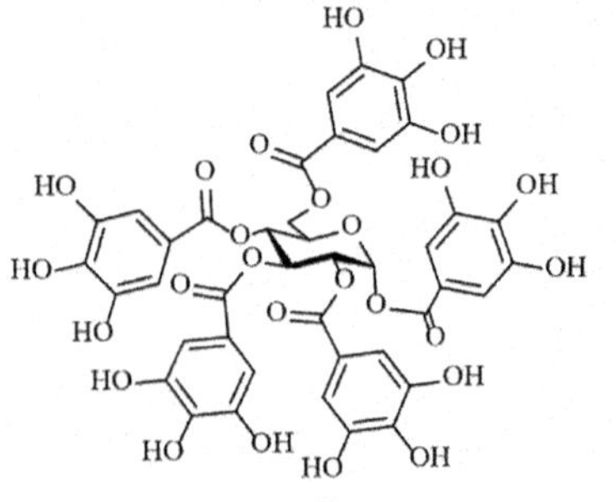

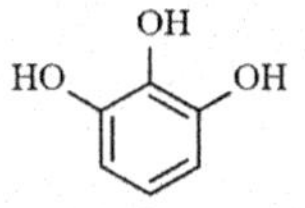

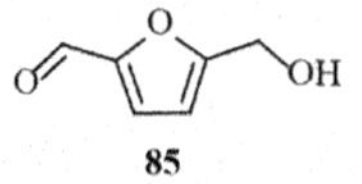

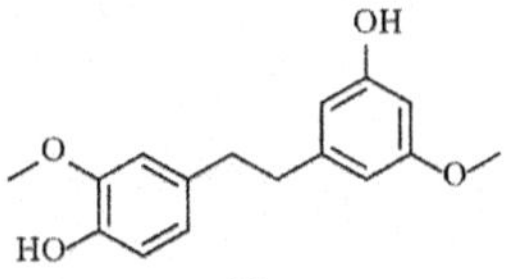

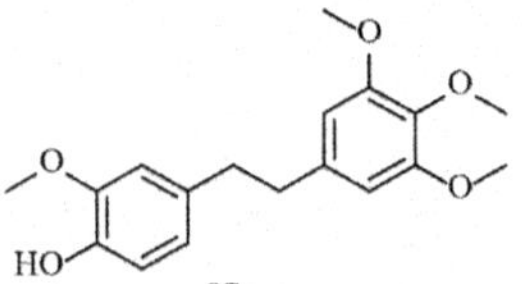

18.4 ANTI-DIABETIC STUDIES OF *MANGIFERA INDICA* EXTRACTS

18.4.1 *IN VITRO STUDIES*

Gondi and Rao investigated the inhibitory efficacy of 80% ethanolic extract of mango peel toward α-amylase and α-glucosidase enzymes. The peel extract showed IC_{50} values of 4 μg/mL and 3.5 μg/mL, respectively, in a concentration-dependent manner. That could be attributed to the presence of phenolic acids (gallic, protocatechuic, chlorogenic, and ferulic) identified in the peel ethanol extract by RP-HPLC (Gondi and Rao 2015). The fluorometric assay was used to investigate the dipeptidyl peptidase-IV (DPP-IV) inhibitory activity of seeds of *Mangifera indica* at a dose of 5000 μg/mL. It showed maximum inhibitory activity of the DPP-IV enzyme by 38 ± 4% compared with sitagliptin, vildagliptin, and diprotin A as inhibitors that decreased DPP-IV enzyme activity by up to 99 ± 2.0%, 99 ± 3%, and 95 ± 3%, respectively (Ansari et al. 2021). The ethanol extract of the bark of *M. indica* exhibited potent α-glucosidase inhibitory activity with an IC_{50} value of 314 μg/mL, as compared to reference acarbose with an IC_{50} value of 0.51 μg/mL (Prashanth et al. 2001). The ethanol extract of seeds of *M. indica* exerted α-glucosidase and α-amylase inhibition with IC_{50} values of 0.34 mg/mL and 0.71 mg/mL, respectively (Irondi et al. 2014). A bioactive phytochemical investigation of the 70% ethanol extract of leaves of *M. indica* L. resulted in isolation of 17 compounds belonging to benzophenones and triterpenoids. All isolated compounds were tested for their α-glucosidase inhibitory activity assay, with IC_{50} values ranging between 239.6 and 834.66 μM, compared with acarbose as the positive control with IC_{50} values of 185.25 ± 6.00 μM. Among the isolated compounds 2,4,4′,6-tetrahydroxy-3′-methoxybenzophenone 3-C-β-D-glucopyranoside (**40**), arjunolic acid (**78**), and actinidic acid (**79**) demonstrated the most potent α-glucosidase inhibitory activity with IC_{50} values of 284.93 ± 20.29 μM, 239.60 ± 25.00 μM, and 297.37 ± 8.12 μM, respectively (Pan et al. 2016). The authors attributed the effectiveness of compound (**40**) to the number of phenolic hydroxyl groups on the basic diphenyl ketone and absence of methoxy groups at C-4 (Beelders et al. 2014). Another study reported the *in vitro* enzyme inhibitory activity of solvent-partitioned fractions of *M. indica* leaves. The ethyl acetate fraction showed significant α-glucosidase and α-amylase inhibitory effects with IC_{50} values of 25.11 ± 0.01 μg/mL and 24.04 ± 0.12 μg/mL, respectively, compared with acarbose as reference drug (Ojo et al. 2018). A bioactivity guided isolation of methanol leaf extract of *M. indica* revealed the isolation of bioactive gallotannin identified as 1,2,3,4,6 penta-O-galloyl-β-D-glucose (PGG) (**82**) (Mohan et al. 2013). It showed the alleviation of all biochemical changes, including hyperglycemia, hypertriglyceridemia, elevated plasma insulin levels, and increased liver and white adipose mass with an increase in body weight was observed compared to normal control. Also, oral glucose tolerance was significantly improved compared to normal. Another phytochemical study on the different fractions of the seeds of *M. indica* L. revealed that petroleum ether and dichloromethane fractions showed moderate α-glucosidase inhibitory activity with IC_{50} values of 80.10 µg/mL and 83.58 µg/mL, respectively. The ethyl acetate fraction showed the best α-glucosidase inhibitory action with an IC_{50} value of 53.33 µg/mL. From the different fractions, 17 compounds were isolated. Among the isolated compounds, 1,2,3,4,6-penta-*O*-galloyl-β-D-glucoside (**82**) and 1,2,3,4,6-penta-*O*-galloyl-α-D-glucoside (**83**) exerted a significant α-glucosidase inhibitory activity with IC_{50} values of 0.60 ± 0.36 µM and 0.07 ± 0.10 µM, respectively, compared with acarbose with an IC_{50} value of 0.11 ± 0.01 µM. In the docking simulation study, results revealed that compound (**82**) inhibited α-glucosidase noncompetitively, whereas compound (**83**) acted competitively (Yang et al. 2020).

A phytochemical study of the ethyl acetate extract of *M. indica* leaves resulted in isolation and structure elucidation of bioactive compound, 3β-taraxerol (**64**). The isolated compound (100 ng/mL) exhibited translocation and activation of the glucose transporter (GLUT4) in an insulin receptor tyrosine kinase (IRTK) and phosphotidyl inositol 3-kinase (PI3K) dependent manner that resulted in insulin-stimulated glucose uptake followed by the activation of protein kinase B (PKB) and suppression of glycogen synthase kinase 3 (GSK3β) (Sangeetha et al. 2010).

The ethanol leaf extract of *M. indica* cv. Okrong and its bioactive compound mangiferin (**28**) showed anti-diabetic activities against yeast α-glucosidase α-glucosidase with IC_{50} values of 0.0503 mg/mL and 0.5813 mg/mL, respectively, and against rat intestinal α-glucosidase with the IC_{50} values of 1.4528 mg/mL and 0.4333 mg/mL, respectively, as compared to acarbose with the IC_{50} values of 11.9285 mg/mL and 0.4493 mg/mL, respectively (Ganogpichayagrai 2017).

18.4.2 *In Vivo* Studies

The aqueous extract of leaves of *Mangifera indica* at a dose of 1 g/kg revealed an absence of significant alterations in blood glucose level on normoglycemic rats between both control and treatment groups. In glucose-induced hyperglycemia, the aqueous extract significantly lowered the progressively increased glucose level compared to chlorpropamide (200 mg/kg) as a reference drug. However, the aqueous extract in STZ-induced hyperglycemia did not show a reduction in the blood glucose level and chlorpropamide (Aderibigbe et al. 1999).

Another study, the ethanolic extract of leaves of *M. indica* along with ethanolic extracts of stem bark of *Glycosmis pentaphylla* (Rutaceae) and whole plant of *Tridax procumbens* (Asteraceae) in the ratio of 1:2:2 was prepared as polyherbal formulation as capsules. The polyherbal capsule at a dose of (250 and 500 mg/kg) significantly reduced the fasting blood glucose level in the diabetic rats on days 7, 14, and 21, as compared to the diabetic control group using reference drug glibenclamide (0.25 mg/kg). Also, it showed elevation of insulin level and hemoglobin and HbA_{1c} levels returned to normal. It revealed normal glycogen and total protein levels in liver that would be attributed to stimulate insulin release from the β-cells that stimulates the glycogen synthase system. The polyherbal formulation exhibited mild congestion and a decrease in the number of islets of Langerhans with a normal β-cell population, indicating a considerable amount of recovery. Also, nearly normal hepatocytes appearance and less necrosis were observed (Petchi et al. 2014). Gondi and Rao investigated the hypoglycemic efficacy of 80% ethanolic extract of mango peel on oral glucose tolerance at doses of 100, 150, and 200 mg/kg b.w. (Gondi and Rao 2015). It showed a significant reduction in glucose levels by 15%, 23%, and 26%, respectively, compared with metformin (100 mg/kg) and gallic acid (100 mg/kg) as control drugs that showed a reduction in glucose levels by 13% and 29%, respectively, compared with the control group. Also, the authors investigated the ethanol mango peel extract using a STZ-induced diabetes model by using different doses of the peel extract; this showed a significant reduction in urine sugar and urine volume levels as compared to diabetic control rats.

Also, among the tested doses of the mango peel extract, a dose of 200 mg/kg b.w. showed significant reduction in the levels of glycated hemoglobin (HbA$_{1c}$) and fructosamine. Alongside, a dose of 200 mg/kg b.w. revealed the best improvement of blood glucose and insulin levels.

The aqueous extract of leaves of *M. indica* L. showed hypoglycemic effects in STZ-induced diabetic rats (Villas Boas et al. 2020). It showed a significant reduction in blood glucose levels at doses of 125, 250, 500, and 1000 mg/kg, exceeding glibenclamide 3 or 10 mg after 2 and 4 weeks of treatment, maintaining a long-term hypoglycemic effect. Also, the aqueous extract showed significant elevation in insulin plasma levels and insulin sensitivity of diabetic animals.

Another report based on using mango peel powder as a supplement in the basal diet, where an STZ-induced diabetic rat was fed with a diet supplemented with mango peel at 5% and 10% levels (Gondi et al. 2015). It improved all parameters associated with diabetes as an increase in urine sugar, urine volume, fasting blood glucose, total cholesterol, triglycerides, and low-density lipoprotein and a reduction in high-density lipoprotein. It improved the lipid profile and decreased lipid peroxidation in plasma. Sabater et al. (2017) investigated the efficacy of mango fruit powder obtained from *M. indica* on mice fed a moderate (45%) high-fat diet. The results of the administration of 54 mg/kg b.w./day of mango fruit powder revealed the protection from the early stages of insulin resistance and hepatic lipid deposition caused by a high-fat diet. Furthermore, AMP-activated protein kinase (AMPK) and sirtuin 1 (SIRT1) appear to be important regulators of improved fatty acid oxidation capacity, insulin sensitivity, and higher blood glucose uptake and metabolism through the glycolytic pathway capacity in the liver and skeletal muscle. Ansari et al. (2021) reported that hot water extract of *M. indica* 250 mg/5 ml/kg in high-fat–fed rats showed improvement in blood glucose tolerance test and insulin levels and decreased DPP-IV enzyme activity *in vivo*. Moreover, it showed an elevation in circulating active GLP-1 and improved glucose homeostasis. Another study investigated the anti-diabetic effects of 10% and 20% *M. indica* kernel flour (MIKF)-supplemented diets in a high-fat diet (HFD) and STZ-induced diabetes model using metformin (25 mg/kg b.w.) as a reference drug (Irondi et al. 2016). The results revealed the use of 10% and 20% MIKF in diabetic rats showed reduction in the fasting blood glucose levels by 60.02% and 64.95%, respectively. Also, hepatic glycogen, HbA$_{1c}$, lipid profile, plasma electrolytes, hepatic and pancreatic malonaldehyde, and liver function markers of the diabetic rats were improved compared to diabetic control rats. It was noticeable that the alleviation effect of 20% MIKF supplementation was comparable to metformin administration in the diabetic rats.

Mangiferin (**28**), a xanthone glucoside isolated from the leaves of *M. indica*, was evaluated for its effects on hyperglycemia and atherogenicity in STZ-diabetic rats at doses of 10 and 20 mg/kg (Muruganandan et al. 2005). Mangiferin showed anti-diabetic activity by a significant reduction in fasting plasma glucose levels, plasma total cholesterol, triglycerides, and low-density lipoprotein cholesterol (LDL-C) associated with an elevation of high-density lipoprotein cholesterol (HDL-C). Furthermore, it showed improvement in oral glucose tolerance in glucose-loaded normal rats the previous results suggesting mangiferin potent antihyperglycemic activity, antihyperlipidemic and anti-atherogenic activities. Another study reported the hypoglycemic effects of mangiferin (**28**) on diabetic insulin-resistant rat model using a high-fat/high-fructose diet and STZ induction (Saleh et al. 2014). Treatment with mangiferin (**28**) at a dose of (20 mg/kg, i.p.) relieved all changes occurred as obesity, hyperglycemia, and insulin resistance associated with a reduction in liver glycogen and dyslipidemia. Besides, it exerted improvement in TNF-α and adiponectin comparable to the reference drug rosiglitazone. Li et al. (2010) reported the protective effects of mangiferin (**28**) (15 and 45 mg/kg) on diabetic nephropathy in STZ-induced diabetic rats. It showed reduction in albuminuria excretion and malonaldehyde level. Also, it showed an elevation in activity of serum superoxide dismutase and glutathione peroxidase and creatinine clearance rate (Aswal et al. 2019). The hydro-alcoholic extract of leaves of *M. indica* L. cv. Anwar Ratol, the most famous cultivar of mango in South Asia, especially Pakistan, were also studied. An *in vivo* study on alloxan-induced diabetic mice showed that the leaf extract exerted a reduction in the postprandial blood glucose levels and interfered with the rise in blood glucose level using glucose tolerance test in diabetic mice (Saleem et al. 2019). Moreover, treatment of diabetic mice with the extract reduced the alloxan-induced loss in body weight and β cell mass and enhanced the lipid profile. The authors attributed the potency of the extract to the due to the presence of mangiferin (**28**) and other phenolic and flavonoid compounds. Another report showed that the aqueous extract of *M. indica* L. leaves showed improvement in the insulin and C-peptide levels and a reduction in central inflammation by lowering microglia burden, both in the cortex and hippocampus (Infante-Garcia et al. 2017); there was also a reduction in central spontaneous bleeding and cortical and hippocampal atrophy. These results suggest the use of *M. indica* in prevention of obesity-related central complications associated with Alzheimer disease (AD) and vascular dementia (VaD).

18.5   CONCLUSION

In this chapter, we explored the anti-diabetic potential of different extracts and isolated compounds of *Mangifera indica*. About ten *in vitro* and 14 *in vivo* studies were performed and revealed a remarkable anti-diabetic efficacy acting on different enzymes as α-amylase, α-glucosidase, and antioxidant defense mechanisms. Additionally, *in vivo* STZ and alloxan-induced diabetic models were used. Moreover, we explored the major bioactive compounds identified and isolated from different parts of *M. indica*, where 27 flavonoids and 27 triterpenoids represent the major identified classes, plus phenolic acids and xanthonoids. We conclude that isolated compounds would act as a good candidate for developing new promising anti-diabetic drugs. Thus, further studies are required for deep investigation of the isolated compounds and different extracts for their effectiveness, bioavailability, safety profile, and clinical trials as plant-derived anti-diabetic agents.

18.6   OTHER FOODS, HERBS, SPICES, AND BOTANICALS USED IN MANAGEMENT OF DIABETES MELLITUS

A diet rich in spices, herbs, vegetables and edible fruits is recognized as a precious cornerstone for management of diabetes mellitus based on *in vitro* and *in vivo* animal studies. These spices include *Nigella sativa* (black seed) and *Cuminum cyminum* (cumin seed), that showed marked regeneration of pancreatic β cells, an increase in insulin level, and a reduction in elevated blood glucose in an STZ-induced diabetic model (Mathur et al. 2011). Also, *Cinnamomum zeylanicum* (cinnamon) effectively decreased blood glucose coupled with increase in antioxidant effects in alloxan-induced diabetic rats (Beji et al. 2018). Further, the combined aqueous extracts of *Allium sativum* (garlic), *Zingiber officinale* (ginger), and *Capsicum frutescens* (cayenne pepper) demonstrated equipotent anti-diabetic effects similar to glibenclamide (Otunola and Afolayan 2015). Mohammed and Islam (2018) studied the anti-diabetic potential of several spices and their major bioactive components, such as capsaicin from *Capsicum* species, curcumin from *Curcuma longa* L., diosgenin from *Trigonella foenum-graecum* L. (fenugreek), eugenol from *Ocimum basilicum* L. (basil), gingerol from ginger, and piperine from *Piper nigrum* L. (black pepper). *Allium cepa* (onion), *Cuminum cyminum* (cumin), *Zingiber officinale* (ginger), *Brassica nigra* (black mustard), *Murraya koenigii* (curry leaves), and *Coriandrum sativum* (coriander) were documented to exert hypoglycemic effects in different diabetic animal models (Srinivasan 2005). Additionally, fruits such citrus, guava, pomegranate, blueberry, pamposia, kaki, mulberry, strawberry, bergamot, apple, prunes, grapefruit, apricots, raisins, peach and blackcurrant, figs, and banana are considered enriched resources of anti-diabetic nutrients and natural antioxidants that are highly recommended for patients with diabetes and prediabetes (El-Nashar et al. 2021).

18.7   TOXICITY AND CAUTIONARY NOTES

Regarding the toxicity studies of *Mangifera indica*, it was reported the lack of oral toxic effects of mango stem bark extract up to 2000 mg/kg containing mangiferin and there were no signs of maternal or developmental toxicity or dose-related effects in implantations, fetal viability, and development. Moreover, as evaluated by bone marrow cytogenetics in rodents, it does not appear to be embryotoxic or genotoxic (González et al. 2007). Additionally, the leaf extract of *M. indica* containing 60% mangiferin did not show any genotoxic activity or mortality in rats with a dose up to 2000 mg/kg (Reddeman et al. 2019). Another report by Villas-Boas et al. (2021) revealed that the aqueous leaves extract of *M. indica* did not show any deaths or clinical changes in the acute toxicity test, revealing that the LD_{50} is more than 2000 mg/kg. Regarding the previous reports, mango is considered safe during therapeutic use with no symptoms of drug-related toxicity found.

18.8 SUMMARY POINTS

- This chapter focuses on anti-diabetic potential of *Mangifera indica*.
- *M. indica* is characterized by rich nutritional value and medicinal aspects for human health.
- *M. indica* is a rich source of xanthonoids, flavonoids, triterpenoids, and phenolic acids.
- *M. indica* acts on different enzymes as α-amylase and α-glucosidase.
- Therefore, we can develop a new plant-derived anti-diabetic agent from *M. indica*.

REFERENCES

Abdel-Aty, A. M., W. H. Salama, M. B. Hamed, A. S. Fahmy and S. A. Mohamed. 2018. Phenolic-antioxidant capacity of mango seed kernels: Therapeutic effect against viper venoms. *Revista Brasileira de Farmacognosia* 28:594–601.

Aderibigbe, A. O., T. S. Emudianughe and B.A.S. Lawal. 1999. Antihyperglycaemic effect of mangifera indica in rat. *Phytotherapy Research* 13:504–507.

Agarwal, S., P. Venkatesh and N. Tandon. 2008. The kidney and the eye in people with diabetes mellitus. *The National Medical Journal of India* 21:82.

Ajila, C. M., S. G. Bhat and U.J.S. Prasada Rao. 2007. Valuable components of raw and ripe peels from two Indian mango varieties. *Food Chemistry* 102:1006–1011.

Ali, B. A., A. A. Alfa, K. B. Tijani, E. T. Idris, U. S. Unoyiza and Y. Junaidu. 2020. Nutritional health benefits and bioactive compounds of mangifera indica L (Mango) leaves methanolic extracts. *Asian Plant Research Journal*:41–51.

Amran, M. S., M. Z. Sultan, A. Rahman and M. A. Rashid. 2013. Antidiabetic activity of compounds isolated from the kernel of Mangifera indica in alloxan induced diabetic rats. *Dhaka University Journal of Pharmaceutical Sciences* 12:77–81.

Anjaneyulu, V., K. H. Prasad, K. Ravi and J. Connolly. 1985. Triterpenoids from mangifera indica. *Phytochemistry* 24:2359–2367.

Ansari, P., M. P. Hannon-fletcher, P. R. Flatt and Y.H.A. Abdel-Wahab. 2021. Effects of 22 traditional anti-diabetic medicinal plants on DPP-IV enzyme activity and glucose homeostasis in high-fat fed obese diabetic rats. *Bioscience Reports* 41:1–15.

Aswal, S., A. Kumar, A. Chauhan, R. B. Semwal, A. Kumar and D. K. Semwal. 2019. A Molecular approach on the protective effects of mangiferin against diabetes and diabetes-related complications. *Current Diabetes Reviews* 16:690–698.

Beelders, T., D. J. Brand, D. De Beer, C. J. Malherbe, S. E. Mazibuko, C.J.F. Muller and E. Joubert. 2014. Benzophenone C- and O-glucosides from Cyclopia genistoides (Honeybush) inhibit mammalian α-glucosidase. *Journal of Natural Products* 77:2694–2699.

Beji, R. S., S. Khemir, W. A. Wannes, K. Ayari and R. Ksouri. 2018. Antidiabetic, antihyperlipidemic and antioxidant influences of the spice cinnamon (Cinnamomum zeylanicumon) in experimental rats. *Brazilian Journal of Pharmaceutical Sciences* 54.

Carpino, P. A. and B. Goodwin. 2010. Diabetes area participation analysis: a review of companies and targets described in the 2008–2010 patent literature. *Expert Opinion on Therapeutic Patents* 20:1627–1651.

El-Nashar, H. A., W. M. Eldehna, S. T. Al-Rashood, A. Alharbi, R. O. Eskandrani and S. H. Aly. 2021. GC/MS analysis of essential oil and enzyme inhibitory activities of Syzygium cumini (Pamposia) grown in Egypt: Chemical characterization and molecular docking studies. *Molecules* 26:6984.

Escobedo-Martínez, C., M. Concepción Lozada, S. Hernández-Ortega, M. L. Villarreal, D. Gnecco, R. G. Enríquez and W. Reynolds. 2012. 1H and 13C NMR characterization of new cycloartane triterpenes from Mangifera indica. *Magnetic Resonance in Chemistry* 50:52–57.

Ganogpichayagrai, A. 2017. Antidiabetic and anticancer activities of Mangifera indica cv. Okrong leaves. *Journal of Advanced Pharmaceutical Technology & Research* 8:19–24.

Gondi, M., S. A. Basha, J. J. Bhaskar, P. V. Salimath and A.U.J.S.P. Rao. 2015. Anti-diabetic effect of dietary mango (Mangifera indica L.) peel in streptozotocin-induced diabetic rats. *Journal of the Science of Food and Agriculture* 95:991–999.

Gondi, M. and U.J.S.P. Rao. 2015. Ethanol extract of mango (Mangifera indica L.) peel inhibits α-amylase and α-glucosidase activities, and ameliorates diabetes related biochemical parameters in streptozotocin (STZ)-induced diabetic rats. *Journal of Food Science and Technology* 52:7883–7893.

González, J., M. Rodríguez, I. Rodeiro, J. Morffi, E. Guerra, F. Leal, H. García, E. Goicochea, S. Guerrero and G. Garrido. 2007. Lack of in vivo embryotoxic and genotoxic activities of orally administered stem bark aqueous extract of Mangifera indica L.(Vimang®). *Food and Chemical Toxicology* 45:2526–2532.

Gu, C., M. Yang, Z. Zhou, A. Khan, J. Cao and G. Cheng. 2019. Purification and characterization of four benzophenone derivatives from Mangifera indica L. leaves and their antioxidant, immunosuppressive and α-glucosidase inhibitory activities. *Journal of Functional Foods* 52:709–714.

Gururaja, G., D. Mundkinajeddu, S. M. Dethe, G. K. Sangli, K. Abhilash and A. Agarwal. 2015. Cholesterol esterase inhibitory activity of bioactives from leaves of Mangifera indica L. *Pharmacognosy Research* 7:355.

Imran, M., M. S. Arshad, M. S. Butt, J. H. Kwon, M. U. Arshad and M. T. Sultan. 2017. Mangiferin: A natural miracle bioactive compound against lifestyle related disorders. *Lipids in Health and Disease* 16:1–17.

Infante-Garcia, C., J. J. Ramos-Rodriguez, Y. Marin-Zambrana, M. T. Fernandez-Ponce, L. Casas, C. Mantell and M. Garcia-Alloza. 2017. Mango leaf extract improves central pathology and cognitive impairment in a type 2 diabetes mouse model. *Brain Pathology* 27:449–507.

Irondi, E. A., G. Oboh and A. A. Akindahunsi. 2016. Antidiabetic effects of Mangifera indica kernel flour-supplemented diet in streptozotocin-induced type 2 diabetes in rats. *Food Science and Nutrition* 4:828–839.

Irondi, E. A., G. Oboh, A. A. Akindahunsi, A. A. Boligon and M. L. Athayde. 2014. Phenolic composition and inhibitory activity of Mangifera indica and Mucuna urens seeds extracts against key enzymes linked to the pathology and complications of type 2 diabetes. *Asian Pacific Journal of Tropical Biomedicine* 4:903–910.

Jahurul, M., I. Zaidul, K. Ghafoor, F. Y. Al-Juhaimi, K.-L. Nyam, N. Norulaini, F. Sahena and A. M. Omar. 2015. Mango (Mangifera indica L.) by-products and their valuable components: A review. *Food Chemistry* 183:173–180.

Jiang, H.-Z., J.-J. Yuan, Q.-Y. Ma, X.-F. Ma and Y.-X. Zhao. 2019. Phenolic compounds from Mangifera indica. *Chemistry of Natural Compounds* 55:147–150.

Kanwal, Q., I. Hussain, H. Latif Siddiqui and A. Javaid. 2010. Antifungal activity of flavonoids isolated from mango (Mangifera indica L.) leaves. *Natural Product Research* 24:1907–1914.

Khan, M.N.I., S. S. Nizami, M. A. Khan and Z. Ahmed. 1993. New saponins from Mangifera indica. *Journal of Natural Products* 56:767–770.

Knödler, M., J. Conrad, E. M. Wenzig, R. Bauer, M. Lacorn, U. Beifuss, R. Carle and A. Schieber. 2008. Anti-inflammatory 5-(11′Z-heptadecenyl)- and 5-(8′Z,11′Z-heptadecadienyl)-resorcinols from mango (Mangifera indica L.) peels. *Phytochemistry* 69:988–993.

Lebaka, V. R., Y. J. Wee, W. Ye and M. Korivi. 2021. Nutritional composition and bioactive compounds in three different parts of mango fruit. *International Journal of Environmental Research and Public Health* 18:1–20.

Lemmens, L., E. S. Tchuenche, A. M. van Loey and M. E. Hendrickx. 2013. Beta-carotene isomerisation in mango puree as influenced by thermal processing and high-pressure homogenisation. *European Food Research and Technology* 236:155–163.

Li, X., X. Cui, X. Sun, X. Li, Q. Zhu and W. Li. 2010. Mangiferin prevents diabetic nephropathy progression in streptozotocin-induced diabetic rats. *Phytotherapy Research* 24:893–899.

Mathur, M. L., J. Gaur, R. Sharma and K. R. Haldiya. 2011. Antidiabetic properties of a spice plant Nigella sativa. *Journal of Endocrinology and Metabolism* 1:1–8.

Mohammed, A. and M. Islam. 2018. Spice-derived bioactive ingredients: Potential agents or food adjuvant in the management of diabetes mellitus. *Frontiers in Pharmacology* 9:893.

Mohan, C. G., G. L. Viswanatha, G. Savinay, C. E. Rajendra and P. D. Halemani. 2013. 1,2,3,4,6 Penta-O-galloyl-β-d-glucose, a bioactivity guided isolated compound from Mangifera indica inhibits 11β-HSD-1 and ameliorates high fat diet-induced diabetes in C57BL/6 mice. *Phytomedicine* 20:417–426.

Muchiri, D. R., S. M. Mahungu and S. N. Gituanja. 2012. Studies on mango (Mangifera indica, L.) kernel fat of some Kenyan varieties in Meru. *Journal of the American Oil Chemists' Society* 89:1567–1575.

Muruganandan, S., K. Srinivasan, S. Gupta, P. K. Gupta and J. Lal. 2005. Effect of mangiferin on hyperglycemia and atherogenicity in streptozotocin diabetic rats. *Journal of Ethnopharmacology* 97:497–501.

Niewczas, M. A., T. Gohda, J. Skupien, A. M. Smiles, W. H. Walker, F. Rosetti, X. Cullere, J. H. Eckfeldt, A. Doria and T. N. Mayadas. 2012. Circulating TNF receptors 1 and 2 predict ESRD in type 2 diabetes. *Journal of the American Society of Nephrology* 23:507–515.

Núñez Sellés, A. J., H. T. Vélez Castro, J. Agüero-Agüero, J. González-González, F. Naddeo, F. De Simone and L. Rastrelli. 2002. Isolation and quantitative analysis of phenolic antioxidants, free sugars, and polyols from mango (Mangifera indica L.) stem bark aqueous decoction used in Cuba as a nutritional supplement. *Journal of Agricultural and Food Chemistry* 50:762–766.

Ojo, O. A., A. A. Afon, A. Busola and O. Id. 2018. Inhibitory effects of solvent-partitioned fractions of two Nigerian herbs (Spondias mombin Linn. and Mangifera indica L.) on α-Amylase and α-Glucosidase. *Antioxidants* 7:73.

Otunola, G. A. and A. J. Afolayan. 2015. Antidiabetic effect of combined spices of Allium sativum, Zingiber officinale and Capsicum frutescens in alloxan-induced diabetic rats. *Frontiers in Life Science* 8:314–323.

Pan, J., X. Yi, Y. Wang, G. Chen and X. He. 2016. Benzophenones from mango leaves exhibit α-Glucosidase and NO inhibitory activities. *Journal of Agricultural and Food Chemistry* 64:7475–7480.

Pan, J., X. Yi, S. Zhang, J. Cheng, Y. Wang, C. Liu and X. He. 2018. Bioactive phenolics from mango leaves (Mangifera indica L.). *Industrial Crops and Products* 111:400–406.

Petchi, R. R., C. Vijaya and S. Parasuraman. 2014. Antidiabetic activity of polyherbal formulation in streptozotocin – Nicotinamide induced diabetic wistar rats. *Journal of Traditional and Complementary Medicine* 4:108–117.

Prashanth, D. U., A. Amit, D. S. Samiulla, M. K. Asha and R. Padmaja. 2001. α-Glucosidase inhibitory activity of Mangifera indica bark. *Fitoterapia* 72:686–688.

Quintana, S. E., S. Salas and L. A. García-Zapateiro. 2021. Bioactive compounds of mango (Mangifera indica): A review of extraction technologies and chemical constituents. *Journal of the Science of Food and Agriculture* 101:6186–6192.

Reddeman, R. A., R. Glávits, J. R. Endres, A. E. Clewell, G. Hirka, A. Vértesi, E. Béres and I. P. Szakonyiné. 2019. A toxicological evaluation of mango leaf extract (Mangifera indica) containing 60% mangiferin. *Journal of Toxicology*, 2019.

Sabater, A. G., J. Ribot, T. Priego, I. Vazquez, S. Frank, A. Palou and S. Buchwald-Werner. 2017. Consumption of a mango fruit powder protects mice from high-fat induced insulin resistance and hepatic fat accumulation. *Cellular Physiology and Biochemistry* 42:564–578.

Saleem, M., M. Tanvir, M. F. Akhtar and M. Iqbal. 2019. Antidiabetic potential of mangifera indica L. cv. anwar ratol leaves: Medicinal application of food wastes. *Medicina* 55:353.

Saleh, S., N. El-Maraghy, E. Reda and W. Barakat. 2014. Modulation of diabetes and dyslipidemia in diabetic insulin-resistant rats by mangiferin: Role of adiponectin and TNF-α. *Anais da Academia Brasileira de Ciencias* 86:1935–1947.

Sangeetha, K. N., S. Sujatha, V. S. Muthusamy, S. Anand, N. Nithya, D. Velmurugan, A. Balakrishnan and B. S. Lakshmi. 2010. 3beta-taraxerol of Mangifera indica, a PI3K dependent dual activator of glucose transport and glycogen synthesis in 3T3-L1 adipocytes. *Biochim Biophys Acta* 1800:359–366.

Sasi, U.S.S., S. Ganapathy, S. R. Palayyan and R. K. Gopal. 2020. Mitochondria associated membranes (MAMs): Emerging drug targets for diabetes. *Current Medicinal Chemistry* 27:3362–3385.

Shaheen, N., Y. Lu, P. Geng, Q. Shao and Y. Wei. 2017. Isolation of four phenolic compounds from Mangifera indica L. flowers by using normal phase combined with elution extrusion two-step high speed counter-current chromatography. *Journal of Chromatography B: Analytical Technologies in the Biomedical and Life Sciences* 1046:211–217.

Sola, D., L. Rossi, G.P.C. Schianca, P. Maffioli, M. Bigliocca, R. Mella, F. Corlianò, G. P. Fra, E. Bartoli and G. Derosa. 2015. Sulfonylureas and their use in clinical practice. *Archives of Medical Science: AMS* 11:840.

Srinivasan, K. 2005. Plant foods in the management of diabetes mellitus: spices as beneficial antidiabetic food adjuncts. *International Journal of Food Sciences and Nutrition* 56:399–414.

Tawaha, K., R. Sadi, F. Qa'dan, K. Z. Matalka and A. Nahrstedt. 2010. A bioactive prodelphinidin from Mangifera indica leaf extract. *Zeitschrift für Naturforschung C* 65:322–326.

Villas-Boas, G. R., J.O.M.R. Lemos, M. W. De Oliveira, R. C. Dos Santos, A.P.S. Da Silveira, F. B. Bacha, C.N.A. Ito, E. B. Cornelius, F. B. Lima, A.M.S. Rodrigues, N. B. Costa, F. F. Bittencourt, F. F. Fe Lima, M. M. Paes, P. Gubert and S. A. Oesterreich. 2020. Aqueous extract from Mangifera indica Linn. (Anacardiaceae) leaves exerts long-term hypoglycemic effect, increases insulin sensitivity and plasma insulin levels on diabetic Wistar rats. *PLoS ONE* 15:1–19.

Villas-Boas, G. R., M. M. Paes, P. Gubert and S. A. Oesterreich. 2021. Evaluation of the toxic potential of the aqueous extract from Mangifera indica Linn.(Anacardiaceae) in rats submitted to experimental models of acute and subacute oral toxicity. *Journal of Ethnopharmacology* 275:114100.

Wei, C. K., Y. H. Tsai, M. Korinek, P. H. Hung, M. El-Shazly, Y. B. Cheng, Y. C. Wu, T. J. Hsieh and F. R. Chang. 2017. 6-Paradol and 6-shogaol, the pungent compounds of ginger, promote glucose utilization in adipocytes and myotubes, and 6-paradol reduces blood glucose in high-fat diet-fed mice. *International Journal of Molecular Sciences* 18.

Yang, D., X. Chen, X. Liu, N. Han, Z. Liu, S. Li, J. Zhai and J. Yin. 2020. Antioxidant and α-glucosidase inhibitory activities guided isolation and identification of components from mango seed kernel. *Oxidative Medicine and Cellular Longevity* 2020.

19 Hemp Vine, *Mikania cordata* (Asteraceae) Use in Diabetes

Pavithra L. Jayatilake and Helani Munasinghe

CONTENTS

ABBREVIATIONS

BMI	body mass index
CVD	cardiovascular disease
DKA	diabetic ketoacidosis
DM	diabetes mellitus
HbA_{1c}	hemoglobin A_{1c}
HDI	herb-drug interaction
OGTT	oral glucose tolerance test
T1DM	type 1 diabetes mellitus
T2DM	type 2 diabetes mellitus
VLDL	very low-density lipoproteins
WHO	World Health Organization

19.1 INTRODUCTION

Diabetes, as described by the World Health Organization (WHO), is considered one of the most prevalent chronic metabolic diseases among the world's population and its case numbers are increasing all over the world. The causative factors for diabetes mellitus have been identified as either malfunction or deficiency in insulin production, insulin's mode of action, or a combination of both. The insulin deficiency is a consequence of the destruction of β cells in the pancreas and hindered action of insulin due to its abnormalities in mode of action. Hence, this results in abnormal or inadequate metabolism of carbohydrates, fats, and proteins within target tissues (Kharroubi 2015).

DOI: 10.1201/9781003220930-21

When uncontrolled diabetes can lead to several long-term complications, including nephropathy, neuropathy, retinopathy, compromised immunity, increased risk of microvascular and macrovascular disease including stroke, ischemic heart disease, foot ulcers, amputation, and dementia. Diabetes or its medications could even affect patients in a life-threatening manner in terms of hypoglycemia, ketoacidosis, or nonketotic hyperosmolar syndrome (American Diabetes Association 2009).

Diabetes mellitus (DM) is considered an autoimmune disease where the β cells located in the pancreatic islets are destroyed, which in turn causes the deficiency of insulin, an essential anabolic hormone. Patients with type 1 diabetes (T1DM) require insulin replacement early in the course of illness due to prominent pancreatic failure and also to avoid diabetic ketoacidosis (DKA), an increased concentration of body ketones due to uncontrolled hyperglycemia. Even though it has been identified that T1DM has genetic origins, some other environmental factors too have been identified that supports and triggers the autoimmune destruction of β cells which include maternal age, psychological stress, and intestinal microbiota (Rewers and Ludvigsson 2016).

Type 2 diabetes mellitus (T2DM), which is outlined by insulin resistance, accounts for approximately 90% of all diabetic cases. Older age, obesity, inadequate physical activity, and intensive high-calorie diets are among the long list of causative agents of T2DM (Zheng et al. 2017).

Both T1DM and T2DM can be diagnosed from hemoglobin A_{1c} criteria (HbA_{1c}) or by the concentration of glucose in the plasma (performed under fasted conditions or via OGTT test which is an oral glucose tolerance test). HbA_{1c} could annotate results as a mean value of blood glucose levels over the past couple of months where a result greater than 6.5% would categorize a diagnosis of DM. The OGTT captures the level of glucose in the plasma prior to taking the glucose solution and 2 hours after the ingestion of 75 g of glucose. A plasma glucose level of more than 200 mg/dL would conclude the diagnosis of DM at the completion of OGTT. The diagnosis and management of DM demands lifestyle changes where the patients are encouraged to have a balanced diet, keep up a regular exercise routine, and maintain weight within the healthy range calculated according to body mass index (BMI), as the complications from DM could hinder quality of life (Lim et al. 2018).

19.2 BACKGROUND

Herbal medicine has traditionally been used over a long period of time for a myriad of ailments, chronic, and acute diseases. Plants and herbs serve as natural reservoirs of a vast array of medicinal properties where further exploration of this traditional trade is essential to battle DM. Meanwhile, the discovery of novel therapeutic substances has expanded through the boundaries of continents and the interests have been aroused to explore them from around the globe. Few of the main reasons for the greater tendency of using traditional herbal medicine over allopathic medicine (medicine prepared by isolating the active ingredient, which is the widely used method in most of the existing health systems) by the patients who are diagnosed particularly with DM is the relatively immense amount of side effects of allopathic medicine when used over a long period of time and patient preference (Rehani et al. 2019). A few of the side effects include dehydration and kidney failure, renal or hepatic impairment, and acute congestive heart failure owing to a long-term regimen of diabetes medication (Cefalu et al. 2011). Another reason could be outlined as the affordability and availability of herbal medicine when compared with the prices of allopathic medicine. A considerably large population of the world relies on plant-based natural medication for diabetes, cancer, microbial infections, and so forth. Naturally occurring phytochemicals could be either primary or secondary metabolites of the plant (Tran et al. 2020). Primary metabolites are directly involved in plant growth and reproduction while the secondary metabolites aren't essential for the growth but, could be macromolecules or smaller molecules which are biosynthesized within the plants. Secondary metabolites are generally formed as a response to stress. These could be alkaloids, steroids, glycosides, and so on. Most of the secondary metabolites show pharmaceutical properties. *Mikania cordata* is one such resource that is awaiting exclusive exploration for its medicinal properties but is known to be used massively in traditional practice (Kiang et al. 1968).

19.3 HERBS AND CROPS UTILIZED IN TRADITIONAL MEDICINE AS TREATMENT FOR DIABETES

Bitter melon (*Momordica charantia*), which is cultivated in abundance in Asian and Southeast Asian countries (a member of the Cucurbitaceae family), is renowned for its antioxidant activities and antihyperglycemic activities in the field of Asian folk medicine. Hence, it has been advised to include bitter melon as a vegetable in the daily diet. Akhtat et al. (2011) reported that charantin, polypeptide-p, and vicine, which were extracted into ethanol from the whole fruit of *M. charantia*, showed a reduction of blood glucose levels, inhibited absorption of glucose in the intestine, and reduced hepatic gluconeogenesis in alloxan-induced diabetic rabbits by 200 mg/kg. Singh et al. (2008) showed that the β cells present in the islets of Langerhans of the pancreas were recovered by doses of 25 mg, 50 mg, and 75 mg of the alcoholic extract of *M. charantia* when tested on alloxan-induced diabetic albino rats. The saponins 3-hydroxycucurbita-5,24-dien-19-al-7,23-di-O-β-glucopyranoside (4) and momordicine II isolated from *M. charantia* have demonstrated remarkable insulin releasing activity in β cells of the pancreatic islets at concentrations of 10 and 25 μg/mL (Keller et al. 2011).

Some other most commonly used herbs and crops in traditional medicine (Table 19.1) to battle diabetes are ginger (*Zingiber officinale*), fenugreek (*Trigonella foenum-graecum*), and *Euphorbia hirta*.

The ethanolic extract of *E. hirta* was orally tested *in vivo* for 21 days on adult alloxan-induced diabetic mice to demonstrate a significant inhibition of triglycerides and alkaline phosphatase levels. It has further shown a free-radical scavenging effect which has been subjected to an in-depth analysis in order to confirm the antioxidant potential of the herb (Kumar et al. 2010).

Artemisia absinthium is used as traditional herbal medicine for diabetes in some regions of South Africa; particularly, the leaves and bark are prepared into an aqueous extract. Even though *Mangifera indica* is not used entirely as an antidiabetic therapeutic agent, the fruit shows properties of lowering blood glucose levels along with triglycerides and very-low-density lipoproteins (VLDL) (Salehi et al. 2019).

It has been shown that the aqueous extract of *Aloe vera* significantly increased the amount of insulin that was secreted and the overall activity of β cells when treated on diabetic mice that were induced by streptozotocin (Noor et al. 2017).

TABLE 19.1
Botanicals Used as Antidiabetic Therapeutics

Species	Country/Geographic Zone	Therapeutic Property	Reference
Acacia arabica	India	Hypoglycemic and antihyperglycemic	Yasir et al. 2010
Aloe vera	Many Southeast Asian countries like Sri Lanka, India	α-amylase inhibitor, hypoglycemic	Noor et al. 2017
Aralia elata	Japan, Korea, traditional Chinese medicine	α-glucosidase inhibitor	Shikov et al. 2016
Artemisia dracunculus	Asia	Antidiabetic	Ota and Ulrih 2017
Curcuma longa	India, Sri Lanka, Bangladesh	Antidiabetic	Marton et al. 2021
Terminalia corticosa	Vietnam	Antidiabetic	Nguyen et al. 2016

Note: This table lists a few other most commonly used herbs in treating high blood glucose levels.

Cinnamomum zeylanicum bark includes tannins and flavonoids which have reverse inhibitory action on human α-glucosidase as shown in *in vitro* studies conducted by Mohamed et al. (2011).

19.4 PHYTOTHERAPEUTIC ACTIVITY OF *MIKANIA*

The genus *Mikania* houses a large variety of species (approximately 430 identified) which are concentrated largely in the tropical regions of the world. It is estimated that about 12% of *Mikania* species have been studied and analyzed for their chemical composition. Coumarins, sesquiterpenes, diterpenes, flavonoids, and alkaloids are among the major groups of chemical compounds categorized according to their therapeutic uses. A detailed analysis showed the presence of acids and organic esters that are of pharmacological importance within the genus *Mikania*. A wide range of antimicrobials, anti-inflammatory, anticoagulant, and antioxidant isolated from the *Mikania* genus have been identified as coumarins and their derivatives. One such example is 1,2-benzopyran, dihydrocoumarin, and O-coumaric acid isolated and identified from extracts of *M. glomerata* (Rufatto et al. 2012).

Similarly, the derivatives of the dilactones mikanolide and miscandenin depict properties of analgesic activities, anticancer and antimicrobial properties in most of the species within the genus of *Mikania* (Ahmed et al. 2001). Cinnamoylgrandifloric acid obtained from the aerial parts of *M. oblongifolia* and the flavonoids such as kaempferol 3-O-β-D-glucopyranoside isolated from its leaves show antibacterial properties (Yatsuda et al. 2005). It has also been found that the chlorogenic acid and caffeic acid have the ability to battle cardiovascular diseases and chronic inflammation (3,5-di-O-caffeoylquinic acid n-butyl ester, which is a derivative of caffeic and quinic acids from *M. micrantha*) (Rufatto et al. 2012).

M. glomerata is very commonly used to treat respiratory diseases and disorders such as asthma, cough, and even bronchitis. It is owing to the presence of the coumarins that causes the dilating of the bronchi via the smooth muscle relaxation (Agra et al. 2008).

The antimicrobial effects of *M. micrantha* leaf pulp have been well-known empirically for decades. Its potassium mikanin 3-sulfate has depicted inhibition against parainfluenza virus type 3. Diterpene *ent*-kaur-16-en-19-oic acid extracted into ethanol from *M. obtusata* has been identified for its trypanocidal activity against *Trypanosoma cruzi* (Muelas-Serrano et al. 2000).

Fernandes and Vargas (2003) reported the antimutagenic activity of *M. laevigata* plant extract which caused the inhibition of the mutagenic effect that was imparted by sodium azide.

The hydromethanol leaf extract of *M. scandens* and *M. cordata* showed strong analgesic activity when assessed by tail immersion method in mice (Hasan et al. 2009).

19.5 *MIKANIA CORDATA* (BURM.F.) B. L. ROBINSON

M. cordata (Asteraceae) is one such perennial vine which harbors a vast number of bioactive compounds that possess properties of actioning as antimicrobial, antidiabetic, antioxidant compounds. *M. cordata*, commonly known as the heartleaf hemp vine, is the only species of the genus *Mikania* that is Asiatic. It was first mistakenly characterized to be conspecific with *M. scandens*. The credit of reidentification of *M. cordata* as a separate Asiatic species is given to B. L. Robinson. *M. cordata* is native and widespread in Sri Lanka, Bangladesh, China, Thailand, Malaysia, and many other Asian and Southeast Asian countries (Kiang et al. 1968). *M. cordata* is a rapidly growing vine with cordate-shaped foliage arranged in an opposite pattern (Rufatto et al. 2012).

The leaf blade (Figure 19.1) is 3–12 cm long bearing entire or slightly dentate margins and three to seven palmate veins from the base. The leaf surface is glabrous. Flowers are white and are borne in corymbose panicles. The panicles contain a four-flowered group. Seed dispersal by wind and rooting by nodes are the main modes of propagation. This is a heavy seed producing perennial vine and the long distant dispersal of the seeds is owing to the pappus. Flowering is seasonal and is observed from December to March (Kiang et al. 1968). This vine acts as a sunlight barrier to other

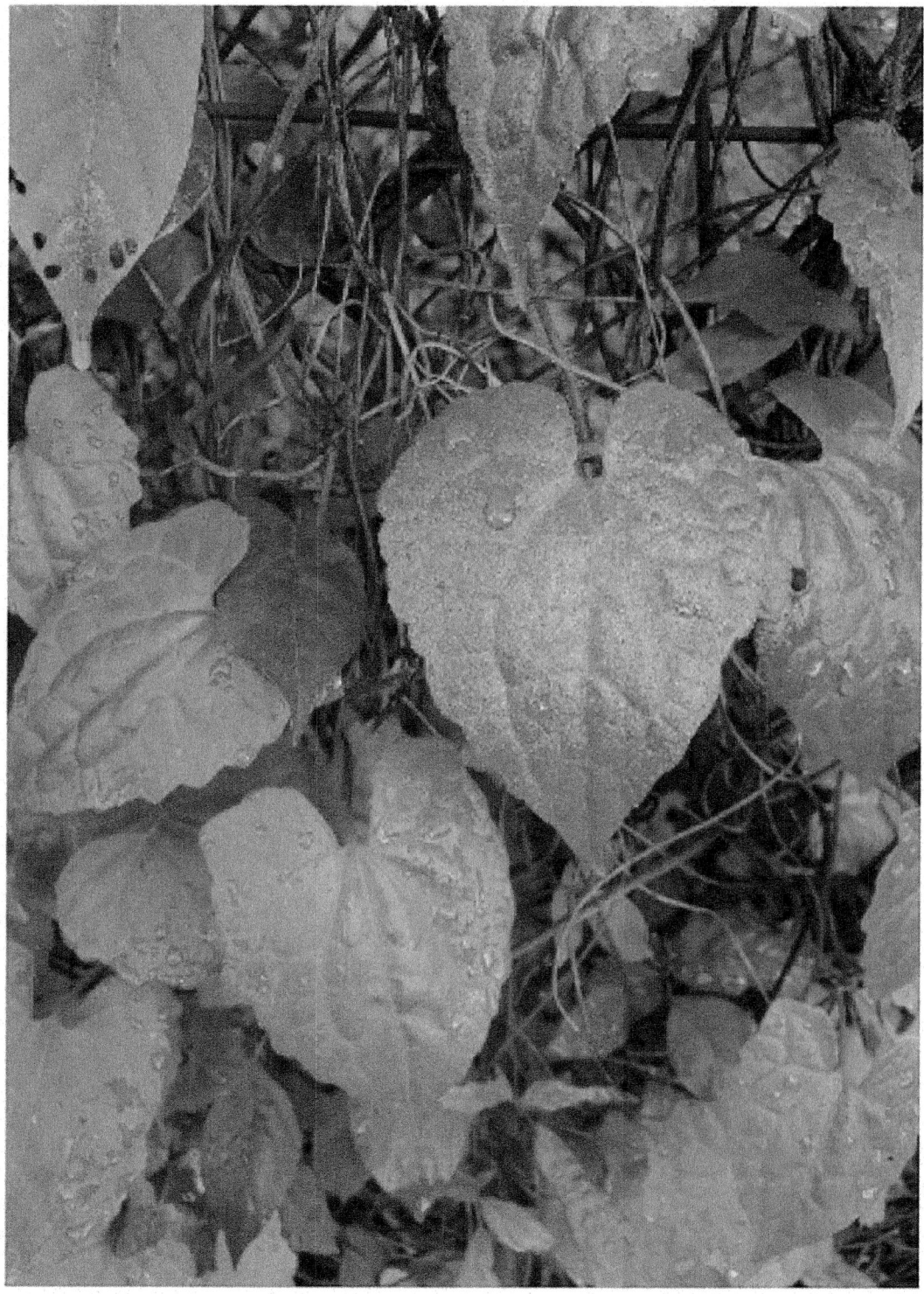

FIGURE 19.1   Leaves of *Mikania cordata*.

Source: Photographed by P.H.A.P.L. Jayatilake on February 08, 2019.

vegetation due to its dense growth. Owing to this reason, *M. cordata* is commonly known as "mile-a-minute." The vine would be destroyed at the beginning of its flowering season to avoid overgrowth and becoming an extremely devastating weed (de Almeida et al. 2017).

19.6 COMMON USES OF *MIKANIA CORDATA* IN TRADITIONAL HERBAL MEDICINE

M. cordata is commonly used in the field of traditional medicine. The raw leaf extract of *M. cordata* is widely used to treat coughs, various gastrointestinal infections, ophthalmic conditions such as eye sores, insect and scorpion stings, and snake bites. The leaf pulp is commonly used on open wounds in the form of a poultice which will speed up the process of healing. The decoction of *M. cordata* leaves is highly effective in curing ulcers and dysentery. The pulp of leaves is used as a remedy for itching. The ointment containing essential oils of the consortium of *M. cordata* leaves and twigs is commonly used to relieve the discomfort caused due to bee stings and ant bites (Paul et al. 2000). Bhattacharya et al. (1992) demonstrated that the root extract of *M. cordata* possess anti-inflammatory effects.

19.7 ANTIDIABETIC PROPERTIES OF *MIKANIA CORDATA*

Herbal remedies for diabetes are in the search as most of the therapeutic agents that are currently been used are associated with numerous side effects. Some herbal remedies depict insufficient activity, while many others like *Cinnamomum zeylanicum* and *Trigonella foenum-graecum* (fenugreek) have shown promising hypoglycemic effects. The *in vitro* glucose uptake by yeast (*Saccharomyces cerevisiae*) is an effective preliminary means of identifying potential hypoglycemic ability when screening for novel bioactive compounds. The glucose transport occurs via facilitated diffusion in yeast cells. There are stereospecific carriers (Hxt1, 2, 3, 4, 6 and 7) that transport glucose across a concentration gradient. Therefore, an effective uptake of glucose will occur only if there is an efficient removal of intracellular glucose. That is, metabolism will cause the removal of intracellular glucose which favors further uptake of extracellular glucose. This assay is a cost-effective and a convenient analysis method to screen bioactive compounds for antidiabetic property before allocating time and implementing intensive research (Woldemariam and Van Winkle 2015).

M. cordata leaf compounds extracted into a medium of methyl acetate have exhibited a similar trend in taking up glucose in the solution as the most commonly used pharmaceutical drug, metformin, when assayed using the yeast cell glucose uptake method. The maximum hypoglycemic effect was observed at 25 mM concentration of glucose, which was 1.6 times greater than which was observed at 10 mM and nine times higher than what was observed at a glucose concentration of 5 mM. It conforms to the initial hypothesis that the leaves of *M. cordata* are a promising source of antidiabetic compounds (Jayatilake and Munasinghe 2020).

19.8 *MIKANIA SCANDENS* AND ITS ANTIDIABETIC PROPERTIES

M. scandens leaf pulp is commonly used as a therapeutic agent for treating stomach ulcers and skin wounds in many Asian countries like India and Bangladesh. The ethanolic extract of *M. scandens* leaves has revealed its antidiabetic properties in alloxan-induced diabetic rats. The chemical analysis of the ethanolic extract has also confirmed the phytochemicals responsible for the antidiabetic activities were alkaloids, saponins, flavonoids, and tannins, which are also found in the ethanolic extract of *M. cordata*, which could also suggest that these classes of compounds could be responsible for the antidiabetic properties depicted by *M. cordata*. The histopathological observations made during the same study showed the rapid accelerated regeneration of the hepatic cells upon the treatment of ethanolic extract of *M. scandens* leaves. Lipid peroxidation is one of the most interesting features and effects of chronic diabetes. It was also observed during this study that the treatment of *M. scandens* decoction decreased the degree of lipid peroxidation, indicating the highly effective antioxidant property of this naturally derived drug. The rapid increase of the oxidative stress in the form of reduced glutathione (used by glutathione peroxidase) has also been observed in alloxan-induced diabetic rats. Hence, it was hypothesized that the antioxidant potential of *M. scandens* inactivated glutathione peroxidase by reducing the level of glucose in blood. The enhanced expression of the antioxidant enzymes in chemically induced diabetic rats that were treated with the leaf extracts of *M. scandens* depicts the reactivated oxidant defense via the increased oxy radical scavenging mechanisms (Baishya et al. 2018).

19.9 TOXICITY AND CAUTIONARY NOTES, HERB-DRUG INTERACTION (HDI)

A change or alteration in the mode of interaction when two or more drugs are administered together could lead to an inhibition or increase in effectiveness or even cause severe devastating adverse effects. The outcome may mostly depend on the physiochemical nature of the drugs and their effect on each other in terms of pharmacodynamic (qualitative alteration) and pharmacokinetic (quantitative alteration) properties. Therefore, similar interactions could be observed when herbal drugs are involved and they tend to be even more complex. The natural drug molecules found in the components of the herbal concoctions could affect clinical safety and its efficacy in either synergistically or antagonistically.

Altered renal clearance, drug distribution, and mechanism of adsorption could be associated with pharmacokinetic HDIs while the pharmacodynamic HDIs could alter the drug-herb actions in receptor sites of enzymes. It has been found that most of the antidiabetic drugs are acting as substrates for the cytochrome P_{450} (CYP_{450}) isoenzyme family, hence it is identified as a common pathway for pharmacokinetic HDIs. An example for this would be the inhibition of $CYP2C_{19}$ by gingko's antidiabetic compounds (Gupta et al. 2017).

Fenugreek's (*Trigonella foenum-graecum* at 150 mg/kg) interaction with metformin (100 mg/kg) has shown a significant decrease in the plasma glucose level by 20.7% in T2DM-induced animal models (Neha et al. 2015).

It is worth pointing out, however, that drug efficacy, safety, and mode of interaction with commercially available pharmaceuticals should be studied in detail for *M. cordata*. Particularly, the herb-herb interactions and herb-drug interactions should be analyzed, and that would be critical information to formulate the clinical use of antidiabetic components isolated from *M. cordata* acting individually or in combination with other herbal therapeutics in order to achieve a more organic and natural therapy for T2DM.

It is necessary to continuously identify and research the potential risks involved with herbal preparations and gather data based on clinical trials, especially from cohorts of elderly patient populations, to analyze the risk-benefit ratio associated with herb-drug interactions as it is acting as double-edged sword when concerning patients and healthcare professionals. Clinical data would therefore be critical to formulate guidelines so that there will be better outcomes in people's health.

19.10 SUMMARY POINTS

- This chapter focuses on *Mikania cordata* herb and its applications in traditional medicine with attention to its potential antidiabetic properties.
- The methyl acetate extract of *M. cordata* leaves analyzed in an *in vitro* study depicted a similar trend in action to the commercially available metformin which is used to treat T2DM.
- *M. cordata* leaves are chewed often when sensing or having symptoms of high glucose levels in blood by many people in the Asian countries and has become a practice in folk medicine.

- *M. cordata* is often found as a fast-growing vine in Southeast Asian countries and is found to be extremely fast spreading during its flowering season.
- The antimicrobial, antidiabetic, wound-healing compounds of *M. cordata* have only yet been analyzed at a rather preliminary level hence, a huge research opportunity would be to further analyze these constituents to gain understanding and knowledge of their mechanism of action, herb-drug interactions, and efficacy.

REFERENCES

Agra, M. D., K. N. Silva, I.J.L.D. Basílio, P. F. Freitas, and J. M. Barbosa-Filho. 2008. "Survey of Medicinal Plants Used in the Region Northeast of Brazil." *Revista Brasileira De Farmacognosia* 18 (3): 472–508.

Ahmed, M., M. T. Rahman, M. Alimuzzaman, and J. A. Shilpi. 2001. "Analgesic Sesquiterpene Dilactone From Mikania Cordata." *Fitoterapia* 72 (8): 919–921.

Akhtar, N., B. A. Khan, A. Majid, H.M.S. Khan, T. Mahmood, and G. T. Saeed. 2011. "Pharmaceutical and Biopharmaceutical Evaluation of Extracts from Different Plant Parts of Indigenous Origin for Their Hypoglycaemic Responses in Rabbits." *Acta Poloniae Pharmaceutica* 68: 919–925.

American Diabetes Association. 2009. "Diagnosis and Classification of Diabetes Mellitus." *Diabetes Care* 32 (Supplement 1): S62–S67.

Baishya, R., A. Adhikari, S. Biswas, and S. Banerjee. 2018. "Antidiabetic Effect of Mikania Scandens on Alloxan-Induced Rat Model." *Asian Journal of Pharmaceutical and Clinical Research* 11 (3): 109.

Bhattacharya, S., S. Pal, and A. K. Nag Chaudhuri. 1992. "Pharmacological Studies of the Antiinflammatory Profile Ofmikania Cordata (Burm) B. L. Robinson Root Extract in Rodents." *Phytotherapy Research* 6 (5): 255–260.

Cefalu, W. T., J. M. Stephens, and D. M. Ribnicky. 2011. "Diabetes and Herbal (Botanical) Medicine." In *Herbal Medicine: Biomolecular and Clinical Aspects*, 2nd ed. Boca Raton: CRC Press/Taylor & Francis.

de Almeida, V. P., A. A. Hirt, P. A. Raeski, B. E. Mika, B. Justus, V.L.P. dos Santos, C.R.C. Franco, J. P. de Paula, P. V. Farago, and J. M. Budel. 2017. "Comparative Morphoanatomical Analysis of Mikania Species." *Revista Brasileira De Farmacognosia* 27 (1): 9–19.

Fernandes, J.B.F., and V.M.F. Vargas. 2003. "Mutagenic and Antimutagenic Potential of the Medicinal Plants M. Laevigata and C. Xanthocarpa." *Phytotherapy Research* 17 (3): 269–273.

Gupta, R. C., D. Chang, S. Nammi, A. Bensoussan, K. Bilinski, and B.L.D. Roufogalis. 2017. "Interactions Between Antidiabetic Drugs and Herbs: An Overview of Mechanisms of Action and Clinical Implications." *Diabetology & Metabolic Syndrome* 9 (1).

Hasan, S.M.R., M. Jamila, M. M. Majumder, R. Akter, M. M. Hossain, M.E.H. Mazumder, and M. A. Alam. 2009. "Analgesic and Antioxidant Activity of the Hydromethanolic Extract of Mikania Scandens (L.) Willd. Leaves." *American Journal of Pharmacology and Toxicology* 4 (1): 1–7.

Jayatilake, Pavithra L., and H. Munasinghe. 2020. "In vitro Determination of Antimicrobial And Hypoglycemic Activities of *Mikania Cordata* (Asteraceae) Leaf Extracts." *Biochemistry Research International* 2020: 1–7.

Keller, A. C., J. Ma, A. Kavalier, K. He, A.M.B. Brillantes, and E. J. Kennelly. 2011. "Saponins From The Traditional Medicinal Plant Momordica Charantia Stimulate Insulin Secretion In vitro." *Phytomedicine* 19 (1): 32–37.

Kharroubi, A. T. 2015. "Diabetes Mellitus: The Epidemic of the Century." *World Journal of Diabetes* 6 (6): 850.

Kiang, A. K., K. Y. Sim, and S. W. Yoong. 1968. "Constituents of *Mikania Cordata* (Burm. F.) B. L. Robinson (Compositae)-II." *Phytochemistry* 7 (6): 1035–1037.

Kumar, S., R. Malhotra, and D. Kumar. 2010. "Antidiabetic and Free Radicals Scavenging Potential of Euphorbia Hirta Flower Extract." *Indian Journal of Pharmaceutical Sciences* 72 (4): 533.

Lim, W. Y., S. Ma, D. Heng, E. S. Tai, C. M. Khoo, and T. P. Loh. 2018. "Screening for Diabetes with Hba1c: Test Performance of Hba1c Compared to Fasting Plasma Glucose Among Chinese, Malay and Indian Community Residents in Singapore." *Scientific Reports* 8 (1).

Marton, L. T., L. M. Pescinini-e-Salzedas, M.E.C. Camargo, S. M. Barbalho, J. F. dos Santos Haber, R. V. Sinatora, C.R.P. Detregiachi, R.J.S. Girio, D. V. Buchaim, and P. C. dos Santos Bueno. 2021. "The Effects of Curcumin on Diabetes Mellitus: A Systematic Review." *Frontiers in Endocrinology* 12.

Mohamed S. S., H. D. Hansi, and K. Thirumurugan. 2011. "Cinnamon Extract Inhibits A-Glucosidase Activity and Dampens Postprandial Glucose Excursion in Diabetic Rats." *Nutrition & Metabolism* 8 (1).

Muelas-Serrano, S., J. J. Nogal, R. A. Martínez-Díaz, J. A. Escario, A. R. Martínez-Fernández, and A. Gómez-Barrio. 2000. "In Vitro Screening of American Plant Extracts on Trypanosoma Cruzi and Trichomonas Vaginalis." *Journal of Ethnopharmacology* 71 (1–2): 101–107.

Neha, S., K. Anand, and P. Sunanda. 2015. "Administration of Fenugreek Seed Extract Produces Better Effects in Glibenclamide-Induced Inhibition in Hepatic Lipid Peroxidation: An In vitro Study." *Chinese Journal of Integrative Medicine* 25 (4): 278–284.

Nguyen, Q., V. B. Nguyen, J. Eun, S. Wang, D. H. Nguyen, T. N. Tran, and A. D. Nguyen. 2016. "Anti-Oxidant and Antidiabetic Effect of Some Medicinal Plants Belong to Terminalia Species Collected in Dak Lak Province, Vietnam." *Research on Chemical Intermediates* 42 (6): 5859–5871.

Noor, A., S. Gunasekaran, and M. A. Vijayalakshmi. 2017. "Improvement of Insulin Secretion and Pancreatic B-Cell Function in Streptozotocin-Induced Diabetic Rats Treated with Aloe Vera Extract." *Pharmacognosy Research* 9 (5): 99.

Ota, A., and N. P. Ulrih. 2017. "An Overview of Herbal Products and Secondary Metabolites Used for Management of Type Two Diabetes." *Frontiers in Pharmacology* 8: 436.

Paul, R. K., A. Jabbar, and M. A. Rashid. 2000. "Antiulcer Activity of *Mikania Cordata*." *Fitoterapia* 71 (6): 701–703.

Rehani, P. R., H. Iftikhar, M. Nakajima, T. Tanaka, Z. Jabbar, and R. N. Rehani. 2019. "Safety and Mode of Action of Diabetes Medications in Comparison with 5-Aminolevulinic Acid (5-ALA)." *Journal of Diabetes Research* 2019: 1–10.

Rewers, M., and J. Ludvigsson. 2016. "Environmental Risk Factors for Type 1 Diabetes." *The Lancet* 387 (10035): 2340–2348.

Rufatto, L. C., A. Gower, J. Schwambach, and S. Moura. 2012. "Genus Mikania: Chemical Composition and Phytotherapeutical Activity." *Revista Brasileira De Farmacognosia* 22 (6): 1384–1403.

Salehi, A, V. A. Kumar, Sharopov, R. Alarcón, R. Ortega, and A. Ayatollahi. 2019. "Antidiabetic Potential of Medicinal Plants and Their Active Components." *Biomolecules* 9 (10): 551.

Shikov, A. N., O. N. Pozharitskaya, and V. G. Makarov. 2016. "Aralia Elata Var. Mandshurica (Rupr. &Amp; Maxim.) J.Wen: An Overview of Pharmacological Studies." *Phytomedicine* 23 (12): 1409–1421.

Singh, N., M. Gupta, P. Sirohi, and Varsha. 2008. "Effects of Alcoholic Extract of *Momordica charantia* (Linn.) Whole Fruit Powder on the Pancreatic Islets of Alloxan Diabetic Albino Rats." *Journal of Environmental Biology* 29: 101–106.

Tran, N., B. Pham, and L. Le. 2020. "Bioactive Compounds in Anti-Diabetic Plants: From Herbal Medicine to Modern Drug Discovery." *Biology* 9 (9): 252.

Woldemariam, T., and J. Van Winkle. 2015. "*In Vitro* Hypoglycemic Effect of *Salvia Hispanica* Using a Yeast Glucose Uptake Model." *Journal of Pharmaceutical Sciences and Pharmacology* 2 (2): 119–122.

Yasir, M., P. Jain, D. jyoti, and M. D. Kharya. 2010. "Hypoglycemic and Antihyperglycemic Effect of Different Extracts of *Acacia Arabica Lamk* Bark in Normal and Alloxan Induced Diabetic Rats." *International Journal of Phytomedicine* 2 (2): 133–138.

Yatsuda, R., P. L. Rosalen, J. A. Cury, R. M. Murata, V.L.G. Rehder, L. V. Melo, and H. Koo. 2005. "Effects of Mikania Genus Plants on Growth and Cell Adherence of Mutans Streptococci." *Journal of Ethnopharmacology* 97 (2): 183–189.

Zheng, Y., S. H. Ley, and F. B. Hu. 2017. "Global Aetiology and Epidemiology of Type 2 Diabetes Mellitus and its Complications." *Nature Reviews Endocrinology* 14 (2): 88–98.

20 Mint Family Herbs (Lamiaceae) and Antidiabetic Potential

Snezana Agatonovic-Kustrin, Davoud Babazadeh Ortakand and David W. Morton

CONTENTS

ABBREVIATIONS

nAChR   nicotinic acetylcholine receptor
ROS   reactive oxygen species

20.1 INTRODUCTION

Diabetes is a serious chronic metabolic disease characterized by elevated blood glucose levels or hyperglycemia. The prevalence of hyperglycemia and non–insulin-dependent type 2 diabetes have increased dramatically over the last two decades due to increased obesity, lack of physical activity, unhealthy diet, and an aging population (van Dam et al. 2002). If not controlled, hyperglycemia can cause serious long-term complications that can be attributed to oxidative stress and inflammation (Giacco and Brownlee 2010). Under diabetic conditions, chronic hyperglycemia generates excessive reactive oxygen species (ROS) in the vascular environment. The main concern with diabetes is to avoid the development of long-term cardiovascular chronic complications. ROS cause membrane lipid peroxidation and degradation and lead to many diabetes complications, including vascular atherosclerosis which is the major cause of mortality and significant morbidity in diabetes and hypertension. Left untreated, excess blood sugar can decrease blood vessel elasticity resulting in a narrowing of blood vessels and a reduction in blood flow. Furthermore, this reduction of blood flow can cause damage to vital organs such as the kidneys (renal neuropathy). Cardiovascular complications, such as hypertension, are a result of rigidity and loss of elasticity in both small and large blood vessels. Thus, the major objective for diabetic patients is to improve the metabolic elements leading to the development and progression of complications, by maintaining the recommended levels for blood pressure, glycemia, and lipids. Healthy lifestyle and diet are considered as important factors for the prevention and the slowing of the progression of diabetes. In addition to a healthy diet, phytotherapy with herbal medicines may help to maintain glucose levels at normal levels (Moradi et al. 2018).

DOI: 10.1201/9781003220930-22

Blood sugar comes mostly from intestinal absorption of digested carbohydrates, since only mono-saccharides, such as glucose, galactose, and fructose, can be absorbed by enterocytes lining the villi of the small intestine (Levin 1994). Therefore, dietary polysaccharides must be digested into monosaccharides before they can be absorbed. This is performed by hydrolytic enzymes, α-amylase (starch digestive enzyme) and α-glucosidases (glycoside hydrolases). Inhibition of these enzymes plays an important role in the management of type 2 diabetes by delaying glucose absorption and lowering after meal glucose levels (Liu et al. 2011). Although synthetic inhibitors of carbohydrate digestive enzymes, like acarbose, offer good control of postprandial hyperglycemia, plant-based α-amylase and α-glucosidase inhibitors potentially have fewer adverse side effects. However, they cannot replace either oral or insulin therapeutic agents that are used to treat diabetes. Most herbal medicines that are used for their hypoglycemic effect in the treatment of diabetes also contain large amounts of natural antioxidants, such as flavonoids and polyphenolic acids, which also have beneficial health effects. Because of reported health benefits in the use of herbal medicines in diabetes treatment, there is much interest among many diabetic patients to incorporate them into their treatment regime.

20.2 MINT FAMILY

The mint family (Lamiaceae, formerly called Labiatae) includes flowering plants that are distributed throughout the world. It is one of the largest families with more than 7000 species assigned to 236 genera (Harley et al. 2004).

Mint typically grows in warm and temperate Mediterranean-type climates. The health benefits of the Mediterranean diet are credited to a high intake of antioxidants from fresh fruits and vegetables, nuts, monounsaturated fatty acids from olive oil, omega-3 fatty acids from fish, and moderate intake of wine during meals. However, the beneficial effects of this diet could also be attributed to the use of culinary herbs of the Mediterranean region. Many Lamiaceae species are grown for edible leaves and several are widely used as culinary herbs, such as basil (*Ocimum* spp.); lavender (*Lavandula angustifolia* Mill.); marjoram (*Origanum majorana* L.); mint (e.g., peppermint (*Mentha* × *piperita* L.), spearmint (*M. spicata* L.)); oregano (*Origanum vulgare* L.); rosemary (*Rosmarinus officinalis* L.); common sage (*Salvia officinalis* L.); and thyme (*Thymus vulgaris* L.). These herbs are abundant in phenolic compounds with potent antioxidant activities (Frankel et al. 1996). In addition to common plant antioxidants, these herbs also contain specific antioxidants, like carnosic acid, carvacrol, and rosmarinic acid (Suhaj 2006). Lamiaceae plants have been used in various cultures for centuries. Peppermint is among the oldest medicinal herbs in the world, with documented use in ancient Egypt, Greece, Rome, and Persia. Studies on the antidiabetic effects of mint are rare, despite their significant phenolic content. Water extracts of peppermint have been shown to improve glycemia and lipidemia in streptozotocin-induced diabetic rats (Barbalho et al. 2011). Both extracts and isolated antioxidants have been found to have potential antidiabetic properties. Moreover, extracts of basil, marjoram, oregano, sage, and thyme have been found to significantly inhibit α-amylase and α-glucosidase, two key enzymes of carbohydrate digestion, both *in vitro* (Cazzola, Camerotto, and Cestaro 2011; Agatonovic-Kustrin, Kustrin, et al. 2020) and *in vivo* (Koga et al. 2006).

20.3 ANTIOXIDANTS

Medicinal plants and herbs in the family Lamiaceae that are used as spices and aromatic herbs are well-known as good sources of natural antioxidants, especially phenolic antioxidants. Phenolic phytochemicals in general have potential to provide protection against chronic oxidation linked complications, such as cardiovascular diseases and type 2 diabetes. Most of the Lamiaceae plants that are a good source of antioxidants belong to the subfamily Nepetoideae. This includes basil, lemon balm, marjoram, mint, oregano, rosemary, and sage, and their antioxidant activities have been widely reported (Gonçalves et al. 2009; Trakoontivakorn, Tangkanakul, and Nakahara 2012; Lagouri and Alexandri

2013; Skotti et al. 2014; Trivellini et al. 2016). In particular, sage, marjoram, thyme, and rosemary are known to have strong antioxidant activity. In a study by Kaefer and Milner, marjoram, rosemary, sage, and thyme had the greatest antioxidant capacity of the herbs investigated (Malmir et al. 2015).

Common sage is a member of the *Salvia* genus, the largest genus of the Lamiaceae family with about 900 species. Many *Salvia* species have been used in traditional medicine, but common sage is the most widely used since antiquity, as suggested by its genus name *Salvia*, derived from the Latin word *salvare*, meaning "to heal" or "to cure," and its species name *officinalis*, meaning "medicinal" (Mathew and Thoppil 2011). Common sage has a wide range of biological activities, including many antioxidative properties (Škrovánková, Mišurcová, and Machů 2012) and hypoglycemic (Alarcon-Aguilar et al. 2002) and anti-inflammatory effects (Chohan et al. 2012).

Extracts of rosemary were the first natural antioxidants used in commercial food products. The plants in the Lamiaceae family contain specific terpenoids, such as the phenolic diterpenes, labiatic acid, and carnosic acid (Loussouarn et al. 2017); the monoterpene carvacrol; various methyl and ethyl esters of these substances; and derivatives of phenolic acids, such as rosmarinic acid (Figure 20.1).

Caffeic acid, rosmarinic acid (caffeic acid ester), and their derivatives are the most reported phenolic acids in rosemary (Frezza et al. 2019). Natural antioxidants like rosmarinic acid provide protection against oxidation linked disorders in general (Petersen and Simmonds 2003). Rosmarinic acid, first isolated from *Rosmarinus officinalis* L. (Cela 2015), is a caffeic acid ester. Both aqueous and lipid rosemary extracts show significant antioxidant activity due to the presence of a catechol group in the aromatic ring of phenolic terpenes, and catechols conjugated with a carboxylic acid group in rosmarinic acid. It is also found other plants from the Lamiaceae family including common sage, Spanish sage (*Salvia lavandulifolia*), basil (*Ocimum basilicum*), oregano (*Origanum vulgare*), marjoram (*Origanum majorana*), and lemon balm (*Melissa officinalis*). Thus, the high antioxidant activity generally seen for sage and marjoram may be due to the presence of rosmarinic acid. Carnosic acid and carnosol are phenolic diterpenes, which contribute to both the antioxidant and anti-inflammatory activity observed in rosemary extracts (Chang et al. 2008).

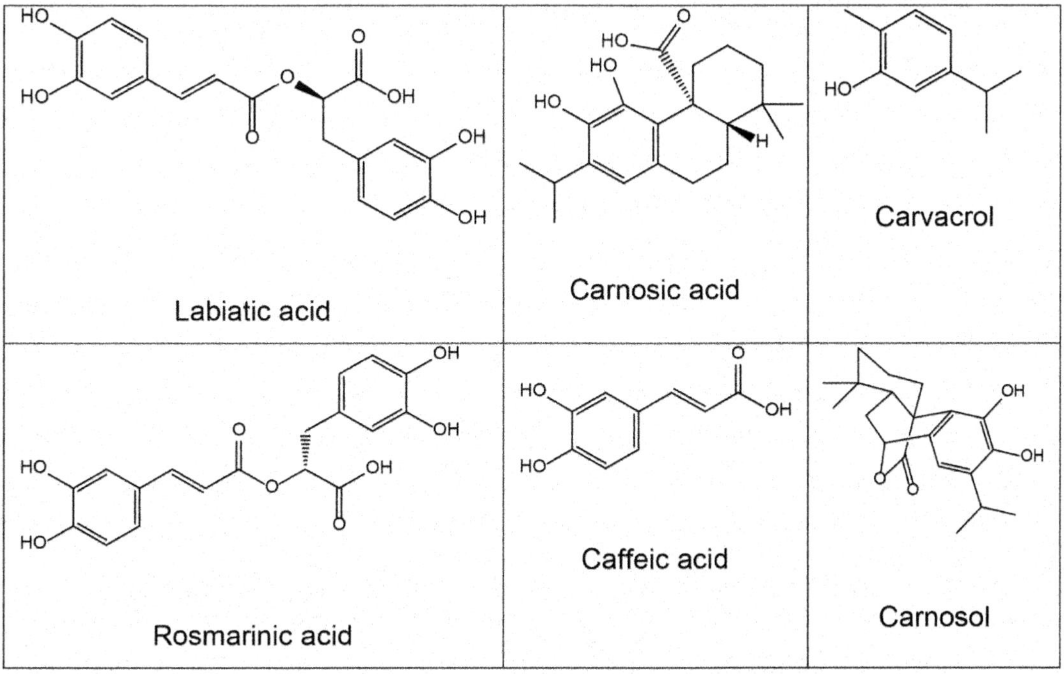

FIGURE 20.1 Main antioxidants found in extracts from herbs in the Lamiaceae plant family.

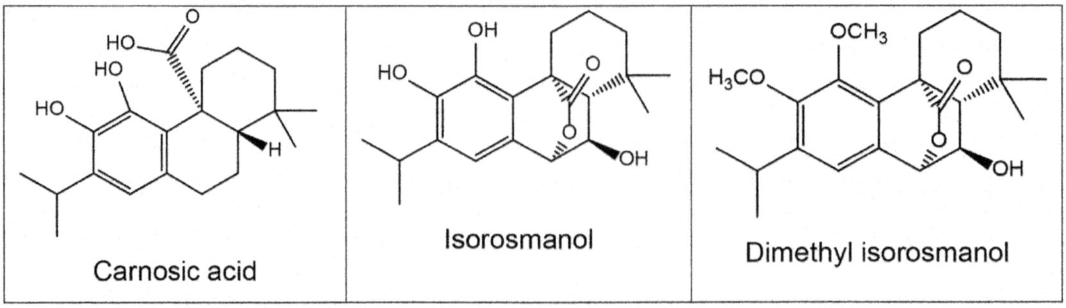

FIGURE 20.2 Carnosic acid and its abietane diterpene oxidation products, isorosmanol and dimethyl isorosmanol.

Both plant extracts and isolated antioxidants are reported to have potential antidiabetic properties (Agatonovic-Kustrin, Kustrin, et al. 2020; Agatonovic-Kustrin, Kustrin, and Morton 2019). Carnosic acid is a benzenediol abietane diterpene found only in the Lamiaceae family, with significant amounts in both rosemary (*Rosmarinus officinalis*) and common sage (Schwarz and Ternes 1992). It is a strong antioxidant, likely due to the presence of an o-diphenol structure (catechol), and is able to efficiently protect lipids from oxidation, both *in vitro* (lipid solutions) and *in vivo* (biomembranes). Carnosic acid acts as a scavenger of reactive oxygen species (ROS) or lipid radicals and can reduce toxic ROS through its oxidation. Thus, it is readily oxidized by ROS, resulting in the formation of a range of metabolites (Loussouarn et al. 2017). Carnosol is the major oxidation product of carnosic acid, produced by a spontaneous oxidation rather than by an enzymatic reaction. It is as efficient as carnosic acid as an antioxidant and lipid protector (Aruoma et al. 1992), and together with carnosic acid accounts for more than 90% of the antioxidant activity of a rosemary leaf extract.

Rosemary also contains other related diphenolic abietane diterpenes, rosmanol, epirosmanol, isorosmanol, rosmaridiphenol, and rosmariquinone, in low quantities (Nakatani and Inatani 1984; Kähkönen et al. 1999). Carnosic acid is very unstable, due to the presence of a catechol (two phenol groups in the *ortho* position) and can be easily oxidized by enzymatic dehydrogenation and scavenging of activated oxygen, to abietane diterpenes such as isorosmanol, dimethyl isorosmanol (Figure 20.2), and other related compounds (Escuder et al. 2002; Tada 2000; Sergi, Karin, and Leonor 1999).

These highly oxidized carnosic acid metabolites also possess some antioxidant activity (Y. Zhang et al. 2012; Escuder et al. 2002). Thus, when scavenging ROS, carnosic acid can generate a range of secondary antioxidants. This chain-type process increases the antioxidative power of carnosic acid and makes an effective defence mechanism against damage by ROS.

20.4 PHENOLIC ANTIOXIDANTS

Lowering the blood glucose level to normal levels is the most important part of treating persistent hyperglycemia seen in diabetes patients. This can be achieved by reducing carbohydrate digestion rate and slowing the glucose absorption by inhibiting α-glucosidase enzymes in the gastrointestinal tract. Herbs in the family Lamiaceae are known to be a rich source of phenolic antioxidants, with a number of them containing a high inhibition of carbohydrate hydrolyzing enzymes (Kwon, Vattem, and Shetty 2006). This suggests that the use of Lamiaceae herbs as food flavorings and food preservation also has potential health benefits, in terms of prevention of hyperglycemia seen in type 2 diabetes. Of the three major classes of plant secondary metabolites (alkaloids, polyphenolics, and terpenoids), phenolics are the most studied (Harborne 1999). One of the problems is that most of the extractions are performed using aqueous and alcoholic solvents leading to extracts rich in phenolics and flavonoids (Zengin et al. 2018). Furthermore, whole extracts are evaluated for biological activity without previous fractionalization or separation and further identification of the biologically active constituents. As a result, many studies have associated phenolic compounds as potential α-amylase inhibitors in the treatment of diabetes (Moein et al. 2017). For example, McCue et al. compared the *in vitro* inhibitory effect of oregano extracts containing rosmarinic acid on porcine pancreatic α-amylase activity to purified rosmarinic acid. Oregano extracts yielded higher than expected α-amylase inhibition than similar amounts of purified rosmarinic acid, suggesting that other phenolic compounds present contribute to this higher α-amylase inhibitory activity (McCue, Vattem, and Shetty 2004). Plants from the Lamiaceae family contain characteristic phenolic monoterpene alcohols such as carvacrol, diterpene antioxidants such as carnosic acid, and derivatives of phenolic acids such as rosmarinic acid. Several studies have shown that the monoterpene components enhance the antioxidative potential of extracts. The potent antioxidant activity of oregano essential oil is mostly attributed to the presence of polyphenolic acids and γ-terpinene. High amounts of δ- and γ-terpinene and oxygenated monoterpenes such as terpinen-4-ol and thymol in oregano essential oil are the main contributors to its antioxidant activity (Asensio, Grosso, and Juliani 2015).

The beneficial effects of polyphenolic compounds, besides their antioxidant activity, are associated to their inhibitory activity against digestive enzymes (Martinez-Gonzalez et al. 2017). Flavonoids are recognized as being able to regulate food digestion through interaction with digestive enzymes. Digestive enzymes such as α-amylase have been inhibited in the presence of polyphenolic compounds and plant phenolic extracts (Hemalatha et al. 2016; Yang and Kong 2016). Although a mixed-type inhibition has been reported for most polyphenolic compounds, the interaction mechanism is unclear. Flavonoids exhibit higher inhibitory effect, compared to other polyphenolic compounds (Narita and Inouye 2011; Tadera et al. 2006). Docking analysis showed that flavonoids bind near to enzyme active site, while acarbose, an antidiabetic drug, binds at another site behind the catalytic triad (Martinez-Gonzalez et al. 2019). Extrinsic fluorescence analysis, together with docking analysis, suggests that hydrophobic interactions regulate the flavonoid-α-amylase interactions. Therefore, Lamiaceae herbs contain certain phenolic compounds such as rosmarinic acid, caffeic acid, and rutin that show promise in assisting in hyperglycemia management, due to their high α-glucosidase inhibitory activities. Inclusion of these herbs in our diet may reduce blood glucose concentration and lengthen the duration of carbohydrate absorption (Yeh et al. 2003).

Several studies have reported that the high antioxidant activity of sage is associated with the presence of phenolic compounds (Škrovánková, Mišurcová, and Machů 2012; Bozin et al. 2007), especially rosmarinic acid (Generalić et al. 2012). Lima et al. (Lima et al. 2006) reported on dose-dependent antidiabetic activity of sage tea, and showed that it was similar to the antidiabetic activity of the antidiabetic drug metformin (glibenclamide). Greek oregano (*Origanum vulgare*) and marjoram (*Oregano majorana*) have been grown in the Mediterranean, North Africa, and Middle East for thousands of years and were traditionally used in diabetes control and treatment (Cazzola and Cestaro 2014; Bouyahya et al. 2020; Skalli, Hassikou, and Arahou 2019; Rouzbehan et al. 2017). *In vitro* studies have shown there is a correlation of the potential antidiabetic effect of oregano to its antioxidant content (Kwon, Vattem, and Shetty 2006; Škrovánková, Mišurcová, and Machů 2012) and inhibition of carbohydrate-digesting enzymes (Soliman, Abdo Nassan, and Ismail 2016; McCue, Vattem, and Shetty 2004). Lemhadri et al. reported that an aqueous extract from oregano leaves significantly decreased blood glucose levels in rats with streptozotocin-induced diabetes. Its antihyperglycemic activity was comparable to the reference drug (sodium vanadate) used in the study (Lemhadri et al. 2004).

Studies on the antidiabetic effects of Lamiaceae plant extracts have shown that basil, marjoram, oregano, sage, and thyme significantly decrease activity of α-amylase and α-glucosidase (Kwon, Vattem, and Shetty 2006). Since these are key enzymes responsible for the breakdown of dietary carbohydrates, their inhibition can significantly suppress the postprandial glycemic response after a carbohydrate rich food intake. Flavonoids, a large family of naturally occurring polyphenolic antioxidants widely distributed in plants, have been described as glucosidase inhibitors. They target disaccharidases enzymes (glycoside hydrolases) that are involved in the regulation of glucose absorption and therefore glucose homeostasis (Pereira et al. 2011). A variety of individual flavonoids, like quercetin, have shown favorable mechanisms in blood sugar control. The inhibitory activity of eight selected Korean edible plants from the Lamiaceae family against α-glucosidases, maltase, and sucrase (Kim et al. 2009) was correlated to their quercetin content. Quercetin is a potent antioxidant flavonoid. The gastrointestinal absorption of dietary carbohydrates such as maltose and sucrose is carried out by a group of α-glucosidases that include intestinal sucrase and maltase. All the extracts showed a similar inhibition of the sucrase but did not have significant inhibitory activity against maltase. Extracts with a high quercetin content had the most potent sucrase inhibitory activity. The sucrase inhibitory activity of the sample extracts correlated with quercetin content which individually demonstrated high inhibition of α-glucosidase.

Antioxidant activity and α-amylase inhibitory activity of extracts from herbs commonly used in Mediterranean diet, fresh basil, lavender, oregano, rosemary, sage, and thyme were analyzed and compared *in vitro* by Agatonovic-Kustrin et al. They found that the highest antioxidant activity in this group of herbs was observed in ethyl acetate extracts of oregano leaf. All extracts except lavender leaf and lavender flower extracts showed significant α-amylase inhibition. The compound responsible for α-amylase inhibition in the extracts, was characterized via an integrated HPTLC-ATR/FTIR approach (Agatonovic-Kustrin, Ramenskaya, et al. 2020), and was found to be oleanolic acid or its derivative (Agatonovic-Kustrin, Kustrin, et al. 2020). Oleanolic acid is a natural pentacyclic triterpenoid that has been isolated from several medicinal plants. The antidiabetic activity of oleanolic acid and related pentacyclic triterpenes has been previously reported (Castellano et al. 2013). Triterpenoids, a large class of natural products with more than 20,000 found in nature, are a rich source of potential drug candidates (Dzubak et al. 2006). They are composed of six isoprene $(C_5H_8)_6$ units, and based on their structure they can be classified into two chemical types, either tetracyclic or pentacyclic.

Numerous studies have suggested that some triterpenoids (tetracyclic and pentacyclic triterpenoids) from plants exhibit antidiabetic activity in normal and/or diabetic animal models. Triterpenoids have been shown to lower the plasma glucose level and improve glucose tolerance of experimental animals (Tan et al. 2008; Kako et al. 1997; Matsuda et al. 1998; De Tommasi et al. 1991). Kinetic studies have shown that corosolic acid and oleanolic acid exhibit non-competitive α-amylase inhibition, synergistic to acarbose (B.W. Zhang et al. 2017). Oleanolic acid has also been investigated for use in cancer treatment. Liby et al. synthesized a number of oleanane triterpenoid derivatives based on oleanolic acid, in an attempt to increase its potency and investigated them as treatments for cancer (Liby, Yore, and Sporn 2007).

20.5 ESSENTIAL OILS

Most of the species from the Lamiaceae family are highly aromatic plants that are particularly abundant in odorous, volatile, lipophilic, and highly concentrated volatile or essential oils (or ethereal oils), produced in the external glandular structures (Giuliani and Bini 2008). Essential oils are responsible for their scent or fragrance. Their main function is to attract pollinator insects and/or deter herbivores. Their small molecular size combined with their high lipophilicity make monoterpenes the most abundant components of essential oils. Thus, many of the plants from this family plants are distilled to produce essential oils with a high level of pharmacologically active terpenoids with biological and medical applications (Uritu et al. 2018). The essential oils of Lamiaceae family plants are especially rich in volatile monoterpenes, diterpenes, sesquiterpenes, and fatty acids (Panizzi et al. 1993).

Direct antioxidant activity and radical scavenging (ROS) are mainly a function of polyphenolic compounds, that are poorly represented in monoterpenes. Thus, antioxidant activity is not the major mechanism that accounts for the antidiabetic activity of monoterpenes, except for thymol and carvacrol (Figure 20.3).

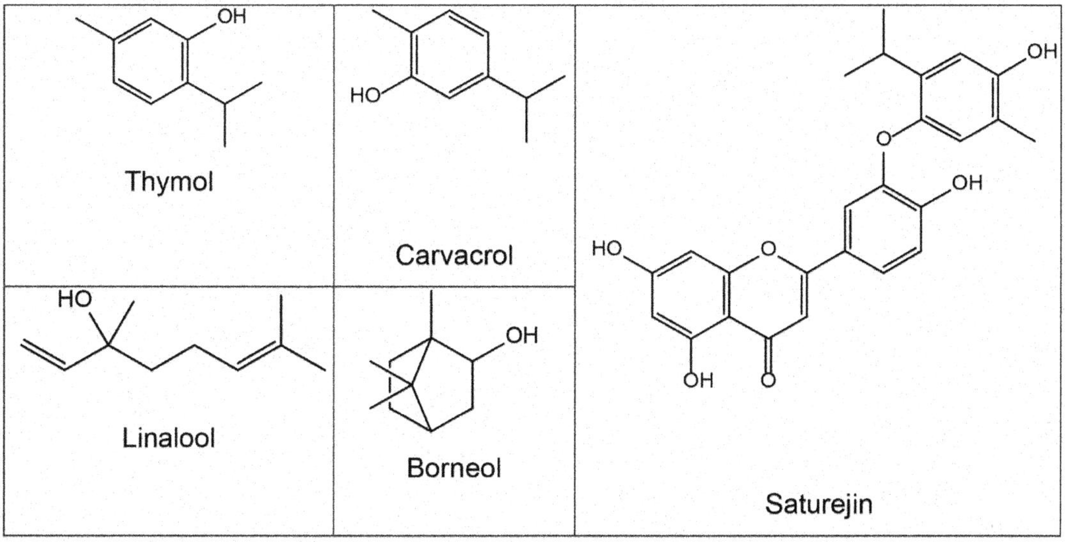

FIGURE 20.3 Bioactive monoterpenes and saturejin (flavonoid) found in Lamiaceae essential oils.

Carvacrol and thymol, the main bioactive monoterpenes found in the essential oils of plants from the Lamiaceae family are phenolic in nature (have phenolic skeleton) (Rúa et al. 2019). They have exhibited similar antioxidant activities when compared to commercial phenolic antioxidants, butylated hydroxyanisole (BHA) and butylated hydroxytoluene (BHT), and higher antioxidant power than α-tocopherol in linoleic acid emulsion test at different concentrations (Yildiz et al. 2021).

The general mechanism of action of monoterpenes has been related to their volatile nature that enables them to freely move across biological membranes and interact with various biological macromolecules (Agatonovic-Kustrin, Chan, et al. 2020). For example, the anticonvulsant mode of action of linalool (Figure 20.3) includes a direct interaction with the N-methyl-d-aspartate receptors (NMDA receptor complex) (Agatonovic-Kustrin, Chan, et al. 2020). Borneol (Figure 20.3), one of the main components of the essential oil prepared from aerial parts of sage (Länger, Mechtler, and Jurenitsch 1996) specifically inhibits nicotinic acetylcholine receptor (nAChR) mediated effects in a non-competitive way (Park et al. 2003). This inhibitory effect by borneol is stronger than the effect by lidocaine, a local anesthetic agent commonly used for local and topical anesthesia. In recent years antidiabetic effects of monoterpenes have also been reported. When monoterpenes get incorporated into other structural groups like flavonoids, much better direct antioxidant and enzyme inhibitory effects have been achieved, as shown by the flavonoid saturejin (Figure 20.3) (Malmir et al. 2015). The numerous *in vitro* and *in vivo* studies suggest that monoterpenes, despite their structural simplicity, have the potential to be considered as antidiabetic lead agents, either on their own or as a structural part in complex structures.

The effects of many monoterpenes as modulators of metabolic pathways responsible for the glucose homeostasis have been reported. Recent studies by Rocamora et al. support the idea that the common constituents of essential oils, especially monoterpene hydrocarbons, significantly inhibit α-amylase activity. Essential oils from the Lamiaceae family, basil, lavender, oregano, rosemary, sage, and thyme essential oils have shown ability to counteract oxidative stress and to inhibit α-amylase activity. Given the lipophilic nature of essential oils, significant α-amylase inhibition could not be related to polyphenolic content. Oregano essential oil exhibited the highest antioxidant activity followed by peppermint and sage. The strongest antioxidant activity of oregano leaf extract was associated with the high levels of polyphenolic acids, while the highest α-amylase inhibition of lemon myrtle and rosemary extracts was attributed to the presence of monoterpenes. Antioxidant activity in terms of free radical

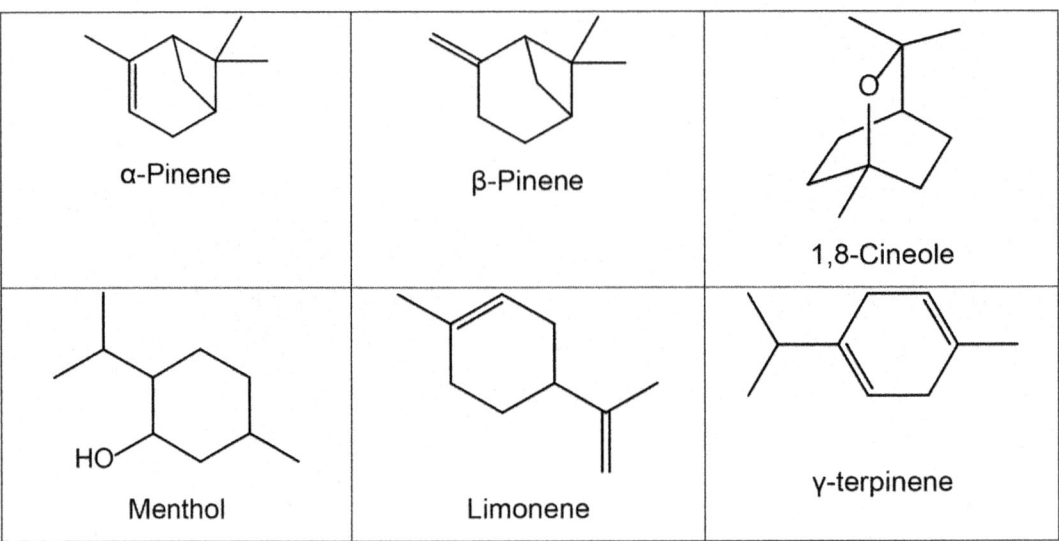

FIGURE 20.4 The main monoterpenes found in Lamiaceae plants.

scavenging capacity was positively related to phenolic content ($R = 0.49$), while α-amylase inhibitory activity was related to terpenoid/sterol content ($R = 0.31$) (Rocamora et al. 2020).

Most plants from the *Organum vulgare* species are characterized by the presence of aromatic monoterpenes carvacrol, p-cymene, thymol, and γ-terpinene as the main terpene compounds (Lawrence 1984). They are easily oxidized by the common atmospheric oxidants such as ozone (O_3), hydroxyl and nitrate radicals (OH and NO_3), and thus exhibit short lifetimes from minutes to hours (Atkinson and Arey 2003). γ-Terpinene and polyphenolic acids, like caffeic acid and rosmarinic acid, are components responsible for oregano antioxidant activity (Panizzi et al. 1993). Monoterpene hydrocarbons exhibit significant antioxidant activities, with γ-terpinene showing the highest activity (Foti and Ingold 2003). The most reported phenolic acids found in the Lamiaceae family are caffeic acid and its ester, and rosmarinic acids and their derivatives (Frezza et al. 2019).

The main monoterpenes found in Lamiaceae plants family are α-pinene, β-pinene, 1,8-cineole, menthol, limonene, and γ-terpinene (Figure 20.4).

Terpenes with endo-double bonds (internal unsaturated carbons), like γ-terpinene, are more easily oxidized, mostly to a C10 aldehyde, because oxidation does not necessarily result in carbon loss. The antioxidant effectiveness of γ-terpinene (non-conjugated diene), is higher than the conjugated diene, α-terpinene (Li and Liu 2009). Both γ-terpinene and α-terpinene can scavenge radicals directly (Li and Liu 2009). A terpinene with an exocyclic double bond will form a Criegee intermediate and a formaldehyde or ketone, while a structure with endocyclic unsaturation, will form two Criegee intermediates with aldehydic ends. The formed aldehyde can easily be autoxidized to a mixture of oxidation products.

Combination of these monoterpenes with structurally different flavonoids is an interesting concept in developing potential antidiabetic therapeutic effects (Malmir et al. 2015). Flavonoids are potent antioxidants that can prevent diabetes-induced glycation, hyperglycemic complications, and oxidative injuries. In silico studies for lead discovery and prediction and lead optimization could be used to optimize bioavailability and general pharmacokinetic profiles of terpenoids due to their extremely non-polar nature. An exemplary model for identifying antidiabetic natural products by filtering and mapping discriminative physicochemical properties has been reported (Zeidan et al. 2017). Thus, monoterpenes could be used as antidiabetic lead compounds through multiple mechanisms as demonstrated from *in vitro* and *in vivo* studies.

20.6 CONCLUSION

Plants from the Lamiaceae family are a potential source of therapeutic agents for the management of metabolic disorders, such as diabetes. However, there are currently no comprehensive human/clinical studies reported to support their use as therapeutic agents. Therefore, further preclinical and clinical studies are required in order to see whether the use of the Lamiaceae species in the management of diabetes can be effective. Further work should focus on investigating and determining their potential therapeutic use both in the prevention of diabetes and related complications.

20.7 OTHER FOODS, HERBS, AND SPICES USED IN DIABETES

The use of plants in the treatment of diabetes dates from around 1550 BC, and descriptions have been found in ancient Egyptian, Chinese, Indian, Greek and Arab literature (Karamanou et al. 2016). The positive effects of over 1200 herbal drugs in reducing blood glucose levels or complications due to hyperglycemia have been reported.

Some herbal remedies act by reducing the absorption of sugars, while some promote gastric motility and emptying and lower postprandial blood glucose levels. Prickly pear cactus, or nopal, a traditional Mexican herbal medicine, is thought to lower blood glucose by preventing the absorption of sugars in the gastrointestinal tract (GIT) due to its high soluble polysaccharide fiber and pectin content (Bacardi-Gascon, Dueñas-Mena, and Jimenez-Cruz 2007). Gurmar (*Gymnema sylvestre*), a slow growing herb found in central and southern India and tropical Africa, is commonly used to treat diabetes and is a natural anti-obesity medication. It is thought to lower blood glucose levels by reducing uptake from the GIT and promoting the regeneration of insulin-producing islet cells (Pothuraju et al. 2014).

Fenugreek (*Trigonella foenum-graecum*), a plant cultivated in India and North Africa, has a long history of medicinal and culinary use (Basch et al. 2003). Its seeds are widely used as a flavoring ingredient in many cuisines. They contain high amounts of protein and fiber that promote gastric emptying, resulting in lowering postprandial glucose levels (Kong and Horowitz 1999). It is also suggested that 4-hydroxyisoleucine present in fenugreek seeds also lowers glucose levels in the body (Broca et al. 2000). Bitter melon (*Momordica charantia*) has been used to treat diabetes and other diseases in Asia, India, South Africa, and East Africa; with the glucose-lowering effects of some actives present due to their structural similarities to insulin. The main hypoglycemic compounds in bitter melon are charantin, polypeptide-p, and vicine (Joseph and Jini 2013).

Although many studies have recommended ginseng as a natural remedy to control diabetes claiming that it lowers blood glucose, results of human studies remain inconclusive due to contradictory results (Yuan et al. 2012). Controlled trials (Vogler, Pittler, and Ernst 1999) of extracts from Asian (*Panax ginseng*) and American ginseng (*P. quinquefolius*) do not support the efficacy for lipid or glycemic indications. Some studies have suggested a positive effect of cinnamon on glycemia or lipids. However, the outcome of studies have been mixed. This may be due to the relatively small numbers of patients in trials and trial design. More work needs to be done to confirm if cinnamon can be beneficial in assisting in controlling diabetes (Pham, Kourlas, and Pham 2007).

Unlike French tarragon, which is mainly used for culinary purposes, Russian or wild tarragon has been traditionally used to treat a variety of diseases. It has been found to contain a number of antidiabetic compounds; extracts of wild tarragon have shown to be active in several different pathways associated with diabetes (Eisenman et al. 2011). Although enhanced insulin receptor signaling with a tarragon extract has been reported in mice (Zang et al. 2010), a human trial reported a non-statistically significant lowering of blood glucose in response to a dextrose load (Bloomer, Canale, and Pischel 2011).

Aloe vera has also been used as a traditional treatment for diabetes. It improves carbohydrate metabolism and metabolic condition in obese prediabetes and early nontreated diabetic patients by reducing body weight, body fat mass, fasting blood glucose, and fasting serum insulin in obese individuals (Choi et al. 2013). The gel obtained from the inner portion of the leaves contains glu-comannan, a water-soluble fiber, with reportedly hypoglycemic and insulin-sensitizing actions (Vuksan et al. 2000). A review of reported trials by Suksomboon et al. found that *A. vera* provides some glycemic control in prediabetes and type 2 diabetes. However, further work is needed to quantify and determine its actual therapeutic benefits (Suksomboon, Poolsup, and Punthanitisarn 2016).

Although there has been extensive historical use of botanicals to treat diabetes and its related symptoms, there is currently not enough reliable data available to clearly understand their mode of action or to be confident in their efficacy and safety.

20.8 TOXICITY AND CAUTIONARY NOTES

Medicinal plants from the Lamiaceae family are among the safest to use for therapeutic purposes. Despite their use for many centuries, there are no reports on significant side effects on the use of these plants for therapeutic purposes. For example, sage is has been used as a natural treatment for diabetes. A group of healthy volunteers drinking common sage tea (300 mL, twice a day) showed an increase in the activity of antioxidant enzymes in the body and an improved lipid profile without causing any side effects (Sá et al. 2009). However, excessive use of common sage may result in adverse effects due to the high amounts of thujone present (Lachenmeier and Uebelacker 2010). Levels of thujone in sage leaves can vary between the locations where they are grown and also between different species (Hamidpour et al. 2014). Both common sage and Spanish sage have similar chemical compositions, but the advantage of Spanish sage is that it does not contain thujone. This may make it a better option for therapeutic use if taken over a long period of time and in significant amounts (Hamidpour et al. 2014).

Rosemary has also been reported to lower glucose levels in diabetic patients (Quirarte-Báez et al. 2019). It is found that the toxicity of phytochemicals present in rosemary is very low. The oral LD_{50} for rosemary leaves is >2 g/kg (Anadón et al. 2008), for rosemary leaf extract is >8.5 g/kg, and for rosemary oil is 5.5 g/kg (Fahim et al. 1999). No serious poisoning by rosemary leaves or its essential oil has been reported. However, ingestion of large amounts of rosemary oil can cause gastroenteritis and nephritis (Fiume et al. 2018). Acute toxicity by rosemary extract has not been observed in animals, although there were increases in absolute and relative liver-to-body weights in repeated-dose toxicity studies. These changes were shown to be reversible, and no other signs of toxicity were observed. Oral administration of rosemary leaf essential oil also affected liver weights (Younes et al. 2018).

20.9 SUMMARY POINTS

- This chapter focuses on the selected plants in the Lamiaceae family.
- They are a potential source of therapeutic agents for the management of diabetes.
- They contain α-amylase and α-glucosidase inhibitors.
- They contain large amounts of natural antioxidants (flavonoids and polyphenolic acids).
- Currently there are no comprehensive human/clinical studies reported to support their use as therapeutic agents.

REFERENCES

Agatonovic-Kustrin, S., C.K.Y. Chan, V. Gegechkori, and D.W. Morton. 2020. "Models for skin and brain penetration of major components from essential oils used in aromatherapy for dementia patients." *J. Biomol. Struct. Dyn.* 38 (8): 2402–2411.

Agatonovic-Kustrin, S., E. Kustrin, V. Gegechkori, and D.W. Morton. 2020. "Bioassay-guided identification of α-amylase inhibitors in herbal extracts." *J. Chromatogr. A* 1620: 460970.

Agatonovic-Kustrin, S., E. Kustrin, and D.W. Morton. 2019. "Essential oils and functional herbs for healthy aging." *Neural Regen. Res.* 14 (3): 441–445.

Agatonovic-Kustrin, S., G. Ramenskaya, E. Kustrin, D.B. Ortakand, and D.W. Morton. 2020. "A new integrated HPTLC–ATR/FTIR approach in marine algae bioprofiling." *J. Pharm. Biomed. Anal.* 189: 113488.

Alarcon-Aguilar, F.J., R. Roman-Ramos, J.L. Flores-Saenz, and F. Aguirre-Garcia. 2002. "Investigation on the hypoglycaemic effects of extracts of four Mexican medicinal plants in normal and Alloxan-diabetic mice." *J. Phytother. Res.* 16 (4): 383–386.

Anadón, A., M.R. Martínez-Larrañaga, M.A. Martínez, I. Ares, M.R. García-Risco, F.J. Señoráns, and G. Reglero. 2008. "Acute oral safety study of rosemary extracts in rats." *J. Food Prot.* 71 (4): 790–795.

Aruoma, O.I., B. Halliwell, R. Aeschbach, and J. Löligers. 1992. "Antioxidant and pro-oxidant properties of active rosemary constituents: Carnosol and carnosic acid." *Xenobiotica* 22 (2): 257–268. https://doi.org/10.3109/00498259209046624.

Asensio, C.M., N.R. Grosso, and H.R. Juliani. 2015. "Quality characters, chemical composition and biological activities of oregano (Origanum spp.) essential oils from Central and Southern Argentina." *Ind. Crops Prod.* 63: 203–213.

Atkinson, R., and J. Arey. 2003. "Gas-phase tropospheric chemistry of biogenic volatile organic compounds: A review." *Atoms. Environ.* 37: 197–219.

Bacardi-Gascon, M., D. Dueñas-Mena, and A. Jimenez-Cruz. 2007. "Lowering effect on postprandial glycemic response of nopales added to Mexican breakfasts." *Diabetes Care* 30 (5): 1264–1265.

Barbalho, S.M., D.C. Damasceno, A.P.M. Spada, V.S. da Silva, K.A. Martuchi, F. Machado, M.V. Farinazzi, and C.G. Mendes. 2011. "Metabolic profile of offspring from diabetic Wistar rats treated with Mentha piperita (peppermint)." *Evid. Based Complement. Alternat. Med.* 2011: 430237.

Basch, E., C. Ulbricht, G. Kuo, P. Szapary, and M. Smith. 2003. "Therapeutic applications of fenugreek." *Altern. Med. Rev.* 8 (1): 20–27.

Bloomer, R.J., R.E. Canale, and I. Pischel. 2011. "Effect of an aqueous russian tarragon extract on glucose tolerance in response to an oral dextrose load in non-diabetic men." *J. Diet. Suppl.* 3: 43–49.

Bouyahya, A., I. Chamkhi, T. Benali, F. Guaouguaou, A. Balahbib, N. El Omari, D. Taha, O. Belmehdi, Z. Ghokhan, and N. El Menyiy. 2020. "Traditional use, phytochemistry, toxicology, and pharmacology of *Origanum majorana* L." *J. Ethnopharmacol.* 265: 113318.

Bozin, B., N. Mimica-Dukic, I. Samojlik, and E. Jovin. 2007. "Antimicrobial and antioxidant properties of rosemary and sage (*Rosmarinus officinalis* L. and *Salvia officinalis* L., Lamiaceae) essential oils." *J. Agric. Food Chem.* 55 (19): 7879–7885. https://doi.org/10.1021/jf0715323.

Broca, C, M. Manteghetti, R. Gross, Y. Baissac, M. Jacob, P. Petit, Y. Sauvaire, and G. Ribes. 2000. "4-Hydroxyisoleucine: Effects of synthetic and natural analogues on insulin secretion." *Eur. J. Pharmacol.* 390 (3): 339–245.

Castellano, J.M., A. Guinda, T. Delgado, M. Rada, and J.A. Cayuela. 2013. "Biochemical basis of the antidiabetic activity of oleanolic acid and related pentacyclic triterpenes." *Diabetes* 62 (6): 1791. https://doi.org/10.2337/db12-1215.

Cazzola, R., C. Camerotto, and B. Cestaro. 2011. "Anti-oxidant, anti-glycant, and inhibitory activity against α-amylase and α-glucosidase of selected spices and culinary herbs." *Int. J. Food Sci. Nutr.* 62 (2): 175–184. https://doi.org/10.3109/09637486.2010.529068.

Cazzola, R., and B. Cestaro. 2014. "Antioxidant spices and herbs used in diabetes." In *Diabetes Oxidative Stress and Dietary Antioxidants*, edited by V.R. Preedy. Amsterdam: Elsevier.

Cela, F. 2015. "Effects of boron and mycorrhizic mushrooms on basil (Ocimum Basilicum L.), with particular reference to the accumulation of secondary metabolites (Rosmarinic Acid)." MSc, Department of Agricultural, Food and Agro-Environmental Sciences, University of Pisa.

Chang, C.-H., C.-C. Chyau, C.-L. Hsieh, Y.-Y. Wu, Y.-B. Ker, H.-Y. Tsen, and R.Y. Peng. 2008. "Relevance of phenolic diterpene constituents to antioxidant activity of supercritical CO_2 extract from the leaves of rosemary." *Nat. Prod. Res.* 22 (1): 76–90.

Chohan, M., D.P. Naughton, L. Jones, and E.I. Opara. 2012. "An investigation of the relationship between the anti-inflammatory activity, polyphenolic content, and antioxidant activities of cooked and in vitro digested culinary herbs." *Oxid. Med. Cell Longev.* 2012: Article ID 627843.

Choi, H.-C., S.-J. Kim, K.-Y. Son, B.-J. Oh, and B.-L. Cho. 2013. "Metabolic effects of aloe vera gel complex in obese prediabetes and early non-treated diabetic patients: Randomized controlled trial." *Nutrition* 29: 1110–1114.

De Tommasi, N., F. De Simone, G. Cirino, C. Cicala, and C. Pizza. 1991. "Hypoglycemic effects of sesquiterpene glycosides and polyhydroxylated triterpenoids of *Eriobotrya japonica*." *Planta Med.* 57 (5): 414–416.

Dzubak, P., M. Hajduch, D. Vydra, A. Hustova, M. Kvasnica, D. Biedermann, L. Markova, M. Urban, and J. Sarek. 2006. "Pharmacological activities of natural triterpenoids and their therapeutic implications." *J. Nat. Prod.* 23 (3): 394–411.

Eisenman, S.W., A. Poulev, L. Struwe, I. Raskin, and D.M. Ribnicky. 2011. "Qualitative variation of anti-diabetic compounds in different tarragon (*Artemisia dracunculus* L.) cytotypes." *Fitoterapia*. 82 (7): 1062–1074.

Escuder, B., R. Torres, E. Lissi, C. Labbé, and F. Faini. 2002. "Antioxidant capacity of abietanes from *Sphacele salviae*." *Nat. Prod. Lett.* 16 (4): 277–281.

Fahim, F., A. Esmat, H. Fadel, and K. Hassan. 1999. "Allied studies on the effect of *Rosmarinus officinalis* L. on experimental hepatotoxicity and mutagenesis." *Int. J. Food Sci. Nutr.* 50 (6): 413–427.

Fiume, M.M., W.F. Bergfeld, D.V. Belsito, R.A. Hill, C.D. Klaassen, D.C. Liebler, J.G. Marks Jr, R.C. Shank, T.J. Slaga, P.W. Snyder, L.J. Gill, and B. Heldreth. 2018. "Safety assessment of *Rosmarinus officinalis* (rosemary)-derived ingredients as used in cosmetics." *Int. J. Toxicol.* 37 (3): 12S–50S.

Foti, M.C., and K.U. Ingold. 2003. "Mechanism of inhibition of lipid peroxidation by γ-terpinene, an unusual and potentially useful hydrocarbon antioxidant." *J. Agric. Food Chem.* 51 (9): 2758–2765.

Frankel, E.N., S.-W. Huang, R. Aeschbach, and E. Prior. 1996. "Antioxidant activity of a rosemary extract and its constituents, carnosic acid, carnosol, and rosmarinic acid, in bulk oil and oil-in-water emulsion." *J. Agric. Food Chem.* 44 (1): 131–135.

Frezza, C., A. Venditti, M. Serafini, and A. Bianco. 2019. "Phytochemistry, chemotaxonomy, ethnopharmacology, and nutraceutics of *Lamiaceae*." In *Studies in Natural Products Chemistry*, edited by Atta-ur-Rahman, 125–178. Amsterdam: Elsevier.

Generalić, I., D. Skroza, J. Šurjak, S.S. Možina, I. Ljubenkov, A. Katalinić, V. Šimat, and V. Katalinić. 2012. "Seasonal variations of phenolic compounds and biological properties in sage (*Salvia officinalis* L.)." *Chem. Biodivers.* 9 (2): 441–457. https://doi.org/10.1002/cbdv.201100219.

Giacco, F., and M. Brownlee. 2010. "Oxidative stress and diabetic complications." *Circ. Res.* 107 (9): 1058–1070. https://doi.org/10.1161/CIRCRESAHA.110.223545.

Giuliani, C., and L.M. Bini. 2008. "Insight into the structure and chemistry of glandular trichomes of Labiatae, with emphasis on subfamily Lamioideae." *Plant Syst. Evol.* 276 (3): 199–208.

Gonçalves, R.S., A. Battistin, G. Pauletti, L. Rota, and L.A. Serafini. 2009. "Antioxidant properties of essential oils from Mentha species evidenced by electrochemical methods." *Rev. Bras. de Plantas Medicinais* 11: 372–382.

Hamidpour, M., R. Hamidpour, S. Hamidpour, and M. Shahlari. 2014. "Chemistry, pharmacology, and medicinal property of sage (*Salvia*) to prevent and cure illnesses such as obesity, diabetes, depression, dementia, lupus, autism, heart disease, and cancer." *J. Tradit. Complement. Med.* 4 (2): 82–88.

Harborne, J. 1999. "Classes and functions of secondary products from plants." In *Chemicals from Plants*, edited by N.J. Walton and D.E. Brown, 1–25. London: Imperial College Press.

Harley, R.M., S. Atkins, A. Budantsev, P.D. Cantino, B. Conn, R.J. Grayer, M.M. Harley, R. De Kok, T. Krestovskaja, and A. Morales. 2004. "Labiatae." In *The Families and Genera of Vascular Plants, VII Flowering Plants • Dicotyledons Lamiales (except Acanthaceae including Avicenniaceae)*, edited by J.W. Kadereit. Berlin: Springer-Verlag.

Hemalatha, P., D.P. Bomzan, B.V. Sathyendra Rao, and Y.N. Sreerama. 2016. "Distribution of phenolic antioxidants in whole and milled fractions of quinoa and their inhibitory effects on α-amylase and α-glucosidase activities." *Food Chem.* 199: 330–338. https://doi.org/10.1016/j.foodchem.2015.12.025.

Joseph, B., and D. Jini. 2013. "Antidiabetic effects of *Momordica charantia* (bitter melon) and its medicinal potency." *Asian Pac. J. Trop. Dis.* 3 (2): 93–102.

Kähkönen, M.P., A.I. Hopia, H.J. Vuorela, J.-P. Rauha, K. Pihlaja, T.S. Kujala, and M. Heinonen. 1999. "Antioxidant activity of plant extracts containing phenolic compounds." *J. Agric. Food Chem.* 47 (10): 3954–3962.

Kako, M., T. Miura, Y. Nishiyama, M. Ichimaru, M. Moriyasu, and A. Kato. 1997. "Hypoglycemic activity of some triterpenoid glycosides." *J. Nat. Prod.* 60 (6): 604–605.

Karamanou, M., A. Protogerou, G. Tsoucalas, G. Androutsos, and E. Poulakou-Rebelakou. 2016. "Milestones in the history of diabetes mellitus: The main contributors." *World J. Diabetes* 7 (1): 1–7.

Kim, D.-S., H. Kwon, H. Jang, and Y.-I. Kwon. 2009. "In vitro α-glucosidase inhibitory potential and antioxidant activity of selected Lamiaceae species inhabited in Korean Peninsula." *Food Sci. Biotechnol.* 18: 239–244.

Koga, K., H. Shibata, K. Yoshino, and K. Nomoto. 2006. "Effects of 50% ethanol extract from rosemary (*Rosmarinus officinalis*) on α-glucosidase inhibitory activity and the elevation of plasma glucose level in rats, and its active compound." *J. Food Sci.* 71 (7): S507–S512. https://doi.org/10.1111/j.1750-3841.2006.00125.x.

Kong, M.F., and M. Horowitz. 1999. "Gastric emptying in diabetes mellitus: Relationship to blood-glucose control." *Clin. Geriatr. Med.* 15 (2): 321–338.

Kwon, Y.I., D.A.Vattem, and K. Shetty. 2006. "Evaluation of clonal herbs of Lamiaceae species for management of diabetes and hypertension." *Asia Pac. J. Clin. Nutr.* 15 (1): 107–118.

Lachenmeier, D.W., and M. Uebelacker. 2010. "Risk assessment of thujone in foods and medicines containing sage and wormwood – Evidence for a need of regulatory changes?" *Regul. Toxicol. Pharmacol.* 58: 437–443.

Lagouri, V., and G. Alexandri. 2013. "Antioxidant properties of Greek *O. dictamnus* and *R. officinalis* methanol and aqueous extracts – HPLC determination of phenolic acids." *Int. J. Food Prop.* 16 (3): 549–562. https://doi.org/10.1080/10942912.2010.535185.

Länger, R., Ch. Mechtler, and J. Jurenitsch. 1996. "Composition of the essential oils of commercial samples of *Salvia officinalis* L. and *S. fruticosa* Miller: A comparison of oils obtained by extraction and steam distillation." *Phytochem. Anal.* 7 (6): 289–293.

Lawrence, B.M. 1984. "The botanical and chemical aspects of oregano." *Perfum. Flavor.* 9: 41–52.

Lemhadri, A., N. A. Zeggwagh, M. Maghrani, H. Jouad, and M. Eddouks. 2004. "Anti-hyperglycaemic activity of the aqueous extract of *Origanum vulgare* growing wild in Tafilalet region." *J. Ethnopharmacol.* 92 (2–3): 251–256. https://doi.org/10.1016/j.jep.2004.02.026.

Levin, R.J. 1994. "Digestion and absorption of carbohydrates-from molecules and membranes to humans." *Am. J. Clin. Nutr.* 59 (3): 690S–698S. https://doi.org/10.1093/ajcn/59.3.690S.

Li, G.X., and Z.Q. Liu. 2009. "Unusual antioxidant behavior of alpha- and gamma-terpinene in protecting methyl linoleate, DNA, and erythrocyte." *J. Agric. Food Chem.* 57 (9): 3943–3948. https://doi.org/10.1021/jf803358g.

Liby, K.T., M.M. Yore, and M.B. Sporn. 2007. "Triterpenoids and rexinoids as multifunctional agents for the prevention and treatment of cancer." *Nat. Rev. Cancer* 7 (5): 357–369.

Lima, C.F., M.F. Azevedo, R. Araujo, M. Fernandes-Ferreira, and C. Pereira-Wilson. 2006. "Metformin-like effect of *Salvia officinalis* (common sage): Is it useful in diabetes prevention?" *Br. J. Nutr.* 96 (2): 326–333. https://doi.org/10.1079/BJN20061832.

Liu, L., M.A. Deseo, C. Morris, K.M. Winter, and D.N. Leach. 2011. "Investigation of α-glucosidase inhibitory activity of wheat bran and germ." *J. Food Chem.* 126 (2): 553–561.

Loussouarn, M., A. Krieger-Liszkay, L. Svilar, A. Bily, S. Birtić, and M. Havaux. 2017. "Carnosic acid and carnosol, two major antioxidants of rosemary, act through different mechanisms." *Plant Physiol.* 175 (3): 1381–1394. https://doi.org/10.1104/pp.17.01183.

Malmir, M., A.R. Gohari, S. Saeidnia, and O. Silva. 2015. "A new bioactive monoterpene – flavonoid from *Satureja khuzistanica*." *Fitoterapia* 105: 107–112.

Martinez-Gonzalez, A.I., Á.G. Díaz-Sánchez, L.A. de la Rosa, I. Bustos-Jaimes, and E. Alvarez-Parrilla. 2019. "Inhibition of α-amylase by flavonoids: Structure activity relationship (SAR)." *Spectrochim. Acta A Mol. Biomol. Spectrosc.* 206: 437–447. https://doi.org/10.1016/j.saa.2018.08.057.

Martinez-Gonzalez, A.I., A.G. Díaz-Sánchez, L.A. De La Rosa, C.L. Vargas-Requena, I. Bustos-Jaimes, and E. Alvarez-Parrilla. 2017. "Polyphenolic compounds and digestive enzymes: In vitro non-covalent interactions." *Molecules* 22 (4): 669. https://doi.org/10.3390/molecules22040669.

Mathew, J., and J.E. Thoppil. 2011. "Chemical composition and mosquito larvicidal activities of *Salvia* essential oils." *Pharm. Biol.* 49 (5): 456–463.

Matsuda, H., Y. Li, T. Murakami, N. Matsumura, J. Yamahara, and M. Yoshikawa. 1998. "Antidiabetic principles of natural medicines. III. Structure-related inhibitory activity and action mode of oleanolic acid glycosides on hypoglycemic activity." *Chem. Pharm. Bull. (Tokyo).* 46 (9): 1399–1403.

McCue, P., D. Vattem, and K. Shetty. 2004. "Inhibitory effect of clonal oregano extracts against porcine pancreatic amylase in vitro." *Asia Pac. J. Clin. Nutr.* 13 (4): 401–408.

Moein, S., E. Pimoradloo, M. Moein, and M. Vessal. 2017. "Evaluation of antioxidant potentials and ◘-amylase inhibition of different fractions of labiatae plants extracts: As a model of antidiabetic compounds properties." *BioMed Res. Int.* 2017: Article ID 7319504. https://doi.org/10.1155/2017/7319504.

Moradi, B., S. Abbaszadeh, S. Shahsavari, M. Alizadeh, and F. Beyranvand. 2018. "The most useful medicinal herbs to treat diabetes." *Biomed. Res. Ther.* 5 (8): 2538–2551.

Nakatani, N., and R. Inatani. 1984. "Two Antioxidative Diterpenes from Rosemary (*Rosmarinus officinalis* L.) and a Revised Structure for Rosmanol†." *Agr. Biol. Chem.* 48 (8): 2081–2085. https://doi.org/10.1080/00021369.1984.10866436.

Narita, Y., and K. Inouye. 2011. "Inhibitory effects of chlorogenic acids from green coffee beans and cinnamate derivatives on the activity of porcine pancreas α-amylase isozyme I." *Food Chem.* 127 (4): 1532–1539. https://doi.org/10.1016/j.foodchem.2011.02.013.

Panizzi, L., G. Flamini, P. L. Cioni, and I. Morelli. 1993. "Composition and antimicrobial properties of essential oils of four Mediterranean Lamiaceae." *J. Ethnopharmacol.* 39 (3): 167–170. https://doi.org/10.1016/0378-8741(93)90032-Z.

Park, T.J., Y.S. Park, T.G. Lee, H. Ha, and K.T. Kim. 2003. "Inhibition of acetylcholine-mediated effects by borneol." *Biochem. Pharmacol.* 65 (1): 83–90. https://doi.org/10.1016/s0006-2952(02)01444-2.

Pereira, D.F., L.H. Cazarolli, C. Lavado, V. Mengatto, M.S. Figueiredo, A. Guedes, M.G. Pizzolatti, and F.R. Silva. 2011. "Effects of flavonoids on α-glucosidase activity: Potential targets for glucose homeostasis." *Nutrition.* 27 (11–12): 1161–1167. https://doi.org/10.1016/j.nut.2011.01.008.

Petersen, M., and M.S.J. Simmonds. 2003. "Rosmarinic acid." *Phytochemistry* 62 (2): 121–125.

Pham, A.Q., H. Kourlas, and D.Q. Pham. 2007. "Cinnamon supplementation in patients with type 2 diabetes mellitus." *Pharmacotherapy* 27 (4): 595–599.

Pothuraju, R., R.K. Sharma, J. Chagalamarri, S. Jangra, and P.K. Kavadi. 2014. "A systematic review of *Gymnema sylvestre* in obesity and diabetes management." *J. Sci. Food Agric.* 94 (5): 834–840.

Quirarte-Báez, S.M., A.L. Zamora-Perez, C.A. Reyes-Estrada, R. Gutiérrez-Hernández, M. Sosa-Macías, C. Galaviz-Hernández, G.G.G. Manríquez, and B.P. Lazalde-Ramos. 2019. "A shortened treatment with rosemary tea (*rosmarinus officinalis*) instead of glucose in patients with diabetes mellitus type 2 (TSD)." *J. Popul. Ther. Clin. Pharmacol.* 26 (4): e18–e28.

Rocamora, C.R., K. Ramasamy, S.M. Lim, A.B.A. Majeed, and S. Agatonovic-Kustrin. 2020. "HPTLC based approach for bioassay-guided evaluation of antidiabetic and neuroprotective effects of eight essential oils of the Lamiaceae family plants." *J. Pharm. Biomed. Anal.* 178: 112909.

Rouzbehan, S., S. Moein, A. Homaei, and M.R. Moein. 2017. "Kinetics of α-glucosidase inhibition by different fractions of three species of Labiatae extracts: A new diabetes treatment model." *Pharm. Biol.* 55 (1): 1483–1488. https://doi.org/10.1080/13880209.2017.1306569.

Rúa, J., P. Del Valle, D. de Arriaga, L. Fernández-Álvarez, and M.R. García-Armesto. 2019. "Combination of carvacrol and thymol: Antimicrobial activity against *Staphylococcus aureus* and antioxidant activity." *Foodborne Pathog. Dis.* 16 (9): 622–629.

Sá, C.M., A.A. Ramos, M.F. Azevedo, C.F. Lima, M. Fernandes-Ferreira, and C. Pereira-Wilson. 2009. "Sage tea drinking improves lipid profile and Antioxidant defences in humans." *Int. J. Mol. Sci.* 10: 3937–3950.

Schwarz, K., and W. Ternes. 1992. "Antioxidative constituents of *Rosmarinus officinalis* and *Salvia officinalis*. II. Isolation of carnosic acid and formation of other phenolic diterpenes." *Z. Lebensm. Unters. Forsch.* 195 (2): 99–103. https://doi.org/10.1007/BF01201766.

Sergi, M.-B., S. Karin, and A. Leonor. 1999. "Enhanced formation of α-tocopherol and highly oxidized abietane diterpenes in water-stressed rosemary plants." *Plant Physiol.* 121 (3): 1047–1052. https://doi.org/10.1104/pp.121.3.1047.

Skalli, S., R. Hassikou, and M. Arahou. 2019. "An ethnobotanical survey of medicinal plants used for diabetes treatment in Rabat, Morocco." *Heliyon* 5 (3): e01421.

Skotti, E., E. Anastasaki, G. Kanellou, M. Polissiou, and P.A. Tarantilis. 2014. "Total phenolic content, antioxidant activity and toxicity of aqueous extracts from selected Greek medicinal and aromatic plants." *Ind. Crops Prod.* 53: 46–54. https://doi.org/10.1016/j.indcrop.2013.12.013.

Škrovánková, S., L. Mišurcová, and L. Machů. 2012. "Chapter three – Antioxidant activity and protecting health effects of common medicinal plants." In *Advances in Food and Nutrition Research*, edited by J. Henry, 75–139. Waltham: Elsevier.

Soliman, M.M., M. Abdo Nassan, and T.A. Ismail. 2016. "Origanum majoranum extract modulates gene expression, hepatic and renal changes in a rat model of type 2 diabetes." *Iran. J. Pharm. Sci.* 15 (Suppl): 45–54.

Suhaj, M. 2006. "Spice antioxidants isolation and their antiradical activity: A review." *J. Food Compos. Anal.* 19 (6): 531–537. https://doi.org/10.1016/j.jfca.2004.11.005.

Suksomboon, N., N. Poolsup, and S. Punthanitisarn. 2016. "Effect of *Aloe vera* on glycaemic control in prediabetes and type 2 diabetes: A systematic review and meta-analysis." *J. Clin. Pharm. Ther.* 41: 180–188.

Tada, M. 2000. "Biological activities of antioxidants from herbs in Labiatae." *Foods Food Ingredients J. Jpn.* 184: 33–39.

Tadera, K., Y. Minami, K. Takamatsu, and T. Matsuoka. 2006. "Inhibition of α-glucosidase and α-amylase by flavonoids." *J. Nutr. Sci. Vitaminol.* 52 (2): 149–153. https://doi.org/10.3177/jnsv.52.149.

Tan, M.-J., J.-M. Ye, N. Turner, C. Hohnen-Behrens, C.-Q. Ke, C.-P. Tang, T. Chen, H.-C. Weiss, E.-R. Gesing, and A. Rowland. 2008. "Antidiabetic activities of triterpenoids isolated from bitter melon associated with activation of the AMPK pathway." *Chem. Biol.* 15 (3): 263–273.

Trakoontivakorn, G., P. Tangkanakul, and K. Nakahara. 2012. "Changes of antioxidant capacity and phenolics in Ocimum herbs after various cooking methods." *Jpn. Agric. Res. Q.* 46 (4): 347–353.

Trivellini, A., M. Lucchesini, R. Maggini, H. Mosadegh, T.S.S. Villamarin, P. Vernieri, A. Mensuali-Sodi, and A. Pardossi. 2016. "Lamiaceae phenols as multifaceted compounds: Bioactivity, industrial prospects and role of 'positive-stress.'" *Ind. Crops Prod.* 83: 241–254. https://doi.org/10.1016/j.indcrop.2015.12.039.

Uritu, C.M., C.T. Mihai, G.D. Stanciu, G. Dodi, T. Alexa-Stratulat, A. Luca, M.M. Leon-Constantin, R. Stefanescu, V. Bild, S. Melnic, and B.I. Tamba. 2018. "Medicinal plants of the family lamiaceae in pain therapy: A review." *Pain Res. Manag.* 2018: 7801543. https://doi.org/10.1155/2018/7801543.

van Dam, R.M., E.B. Rimm, W.C. Willett, M.J. Stampfer, and F.B. Hu. 2002. "Dietary patterns and risk for type 2 diabetes mellitus in U.S. men." *Ann. Intern. Med.* 136 (3): 201–209.

Vogler, B.K., M.H. Pittler, and E. Ernst. 1999. "The efficacy of ginseng. A systematic review of randomised clinical trials." *Eur. J. Clin. Pharmacol.* 55 (8): 567–575.

Vuksan, V., J.L. Sievenpiper, R. Owen, J.A. Swilley, P. Spadafora, D.J. Jenkins, E. Vidgen, F. Brighenti, R.G. Josse, L.A. Leiter, Z. Xu, and R. Novokmet. 2000. "Beneficial effects of viscous dietary fiber from Konjac-mannan in subjects with the insulin resistance syndrome: Results of a controlled metabolic trial." *Diabetes Care* 23 (1): 9–14.

Yang, X., and F. Kong. 2016. "Effects of tea polyphenols and different teas on pancreatic α-amylase activity in vitro." *LWT – Food Sci. Technol.* 66: 232–238. https://doi.org/10.1016/j.lwt.2015.10.035.

Yeh, G.Y., D.M. Eisenberg, T.J. Kaptchuk, and R.S. Phillips. 2003. "Systematic review of herbs and dietary supplements for glycemic control in diabetes." *Diabetes Care* 26 (4): 1277–1294.

Yildiz, S., S. Turan, M. Kiralan, and M.F. Ramadan. 2021. "Antioxidant properties of thymol, carvacrol, and thymoquinone and its efficiencies on the stabilization of refined and stripped corn oils." *J. Food Meas. Charact.* 15 (1): 621–632. https://doi.org/10.1007/s11694-020-00665-0.

Younes, M., P. Aggett, F. Aguilar, R. Crebelli, B. Dusemund, M. Filipic, M.J. Frutos, P. Galtier, D. Gott, U. Gundert-Remy, G.G. Kuhnle, C. Lambre, I.T. Lillegaard, P. Moldeus, A. Mortensen, A. Oskarsson, I. Stankovic, I. Waalkens-Berendsen, R.A. Woutersen, M. Wright, P. Boon, O. Lindtner, C. Tlustos, A. Tard, and J.-C. Leblanc. 2018. "Refined exposure assessment of extracts of rosemary(E 392) from its use as food additive." *EFSA J.* 16 (8): 5373.

Yuan, H.-D., J.T. Kim, S.H. Kim, and S.H. Chung. 2012. "Ginseng and diabetes: The evidences from in vitro, animal and human studies." *J. Ginseng Res.* 36 (1): 27–29.

Zang, Z.Q., D. Ribnicky, X.H. Zhang, A. Zuberi, I. Raskin, Y. Yu, and W.T. Cefalu. 2010. "An extract of *Artemisia dracunculus* L. enhances insulin receptor signaling and modulates gene expression in skel-muscle in KK-A(y) mice." *J. Nutr. Biochem.* 22 (1): 71–78.

Zeidan, M., M. Rayan, N. Zeidan, M. Falah, and A. Rayan. 2017. "Indexing natural products for their potential anti-diabetic activity: Filtering and mapping discriminative physicochemical properties." *Molecules* 22 (9): 1563.

Zengin, G., I. Senkardes, A. Mollica, C.M.N. Picot-Allain, G. Bulut, A. Dogan, and M.F. Mahomoodally. 2018. "New insights into the in vitro biological effects, in silico docking and chemical profile of clary sage – *Salvia sclarea* L." *Comput. Biol. Chem.* 75: 111–119. https://doi.org/10.1016/j.compbiolchem.2018.05.005.

Zhang, B.W., Y. Xing, C. Wen, X.X. Yu, W.L. Sun, Z.L. Xiu, and Y.S. Dong. 2017. "Pentacyclic triterpenes as alpha-glucosidase and alpha-amylase inhibitors: Structure-activity relationships and the synergism with acarbose." *Bioorg. Med. Chem. Lett.* 27 (22): 5065–5070. https://doi.org/10.1016/j.bmcl.2017.09.027.

Zhang, Y., J.P. Smuts, E. Dodbiba, R. Rangarajan, J.C. Lang, and D.W. Armstrong. 2012. "Degradation study of carnosic acid, carnosol, rosmarinic acid, and rosemary extract (*Rosmarinus officinalis* L.) assessed using HPLC." *J. Agric. Food Chem.* 60 (36): 9305–9314. https://doi.org/10.1021/jf302179c.

21 Northern Groundcone (*Boschniakia rossica*) and Use in Diabetes via Glucagon-Like Peptide-1

Keng-Chang Tsai and Hui-Kang Liu

CONTENTS

ABBREVIATIONS

A_{1c}	hemoglobin A_{1c}
AGEs	advanced glycation end products
ALT	alanine aminotransferase
ALP	alkaline phosphatase
ADA	American Diabetes Association
AST	aspartic transaminase
BUN	blood urea nitrogen
CaR	calcium-sensing receptor
CREA	creatinine
cAMP	cyclic adenosine monophosphate
DPP4	dipeptidyl peptidase 4
ECD	extracellular domain
FDA	US Food and Drug Administration
FPG	fasting plasma glucose
GLP-1	glucagon like peptide-1
GLP-1R	glucagon like peptide-1 receptor

DOI: 10.1201/9781003220930-23

GLP-1RAs	GLP-1R agonists
GPR119	cannabinoid receptor
GPCR	G-protein coupled receptor
GPRs	fatty acid receptors
HOMA-IR	Homeostatic Model Assessment for Insulin Resistance
HOMA-B%	Homeostatic Model Assessment for β cell function
HBA	hydrogen bond acceptor
HBD	hydrogen bond donor
HYD	hydrophobic domain
NMR	nuclear magnetic resonance
OGTT	oral glucose tolerance test
PG	plasma glucose
Pos	positive ion
PDB	Protein Data Bank
STD	saturation transfer difference
T1/2Rs	sweet and bitter taste receptor
T2D	type 2 diabetes
TBIL	total bilirubin
TGR5	bile acid receptor

21.1 INTRODUCTION

Boschniakia rossica, also known as northern groundcone, belongs to the Orobanchaceae family and is a holoparasitic plant grown on the roots from the genus *Alnus* with up to three stems per plant to a height of 6–12 inches. The morphology looks like a pine cone vertically growing on the ground with color ranging from reddish brown to dark maroon. *B. rossica* appears to be found only in the northern latitudes of the Northern Hemisphere. This plant is widespread in China, Russia, Korea, Japan, US, and Canada. It has various common names including cao-cong-rong (China), bu lao cao (Chia), herb of Russian boschniakia, oniku (Japan), orinamudcobusali (Korea), du'iinahshèe (Gwichya Gwich'in), doo'iinahshìh/Ts'eedichi (Teetå'it Gwich'in), tuluk-kam nauligaafa (Inuit), uktschutsch (Kamtschadalis), and poque. The whole plant of *B. rossica* is usually harvested for medicinal use (Royal Botanic Gardens 2020; Wang 2021; Elven et al. 2006). In China, *B. rossica* is distributed among the Changbai Mountains and the northern area of Daxinganling. Due to its great medical and economical value, previously intensive harvest for this parasitic herb in the wild caused *B. rossica* to become endangered. Now, *B. rossica* is the second class of national protected plants in the list of rare and endangered plants in China (Fan and Ren 2019).

21.2 BACKGROUND

The earliest use of *Boschniakia rossica* dates back to AD 659 in the Tang dynasty in China. In traditional Chinese medicine, *B. rossica* is prescribed to invigorate the kidney and strengthen yang, to moisturize the intestines and serve as a laxative, to stop hemostatic activity, to improve kidney deficiency, impotence, cold pain in the waist and knees, to treat habitual constipation in the elderly and cystitis, and to enhance longevity (Fan and Ren 2019). From the book *Shí yī xīn jìng*, written by Blame Yin in the Tang dynasty, ground *B. rossica* immersed in alcohol was used to treat impotence. In the book, *Kāi bǎo běncǎo*, similar preparation was identified to tonify the kidney. Northern Native Americans would use the mixed plant powder to treat skin rashes. The groundcone roots were mixed with tobacco and smoked in a pipe (Andre and Fehr 2002).

Currently, characterization of chemical constituents in *B. rossica* using chromatography reveals over 70 compounds including phenylpropanoid glycosides, iridoids, polysaccharides, organic acids and alkaloids. Among those chemicals, phenylpropanoid glycosides, iridoids, polysaccharides, and the resinous exudates receive more attention for research and development. Because *B. rossica* contains phenylpropanoid glycoside rossicaside B, it has been also regarded as a substitute for Cistanche (*Cistanche deserticola* Ma) (Lin and Chen 2004; Lin et al. 2006).

Although *B. rossica* is clinically used to treat kidney problems and organ hemorrhage and relieve pain and constipation, various biological effects have been discovered from modern pharmacological investigation including immune enhancement (Fan and Ren 2019), anti-aging, antitumor (Yao et al. 2017; Wang et al. 2014), antioxidant (Tsuda et al. 1994), anti-inflammation (Quan et al. 2014), anti-atherosclerosis, hepatoprotective (Quan et al. 2009; Quan et al. 2013), neuroprotective, memory enhancement, and anti-diabetes activities (Lin et al. 2019; Liu, Tsai, and Lin 2018). Water extract, ethanol extract, iridoid glycosides, phenylpropanoid glycosides, and polysaccharide are the major preparations used in those studies.

In terms of the iridoid compounds from *B. rossica*, several iridoid compounds were identified (Yim et al. 2004; Yin et al. 1999; Lin and Chen 2004; Lin et al. 2006; Murai and Tagawa 1982). To the best of our knowledge, boschnaloside is the major constituent from *B. rossica* studied for anti-diabetes activity *in vivo*. Acteoside, a phenylethanoid glycoside also found in *B. rossica*, provided an inhibitory effect on the formation of advanced glycation end products (AGEs) *in vitro* (Liu et al. 2013). In the following sections, pharmacological effects of boschnaloside on the type 2 diabetes mice model are further elaborated.

21.3 TYPE 2 DIABETES

Type 2 diabetes mellitus (T2D) is a multifactorial chronic disease caused by hyperglycemia. Currently, the prevalence of diabetes mellitus is over 415 million people worldwide and could further increase to 624 million people by 2040 (Ogurtsova et al. 2017). T2D accounts for 95% of the diabetic population. According to the standard published by American Diabetes Association (ADA), the classification of T2D is related to a progressive loss of proper β cell insulin secretion against the background of insulin resistance. In terms of the criteria for diagnosing diabetes, 8-hour fasting plasma glucose (FPG) values over 126 mg/dL (7.0 mmol/L), 2-hour plasma glucose (PG) values after the execution of oral glucose tolerance test (OGTT) over 200 mg/dL (11.1 mmol/L), hemoglobin A_{1c} (A_{1c}) values over 6.5% (48 mmol/mol), or patients with classic symptoms of diabetes with random plasma glucose at least 200 mg/dL (11.1 mmol/L) are the main criteria for diabetes diagnosis (American Diabetes 2021). It was noted that nearly half of the T2D population remain to achieve the targeted HbA_{1c} level under 7% (Ali et al. 2013). Therefore, an effective therapeutic regime for the general T2D population is still in demand.

During T2D pathogenesis, insulin resistance usually occurs at early stage before the onset of T2D. Compensation for such resistance would lead to hyperinsulinemia and islet hypertrophy. After onset, islet/β cell dysfunction and failure would exacerbate the T2D progression (Do et al. 2016). Therefore, in addition to attenuating insulin resistance, preservation and/or restoration of β cell function and mass are regarded as the ultimate goals for T2D therapy. Among current anti-diabetes drugs, incretin-based therapeutics belong to a class of drugs which can promote β cell function and mass for T2D subjects via elevating endogenous glucagon like peptide-1 (GLP-1) levels or activating GLP-1 receptor (GLP-1R) signaling via GLP-1R activation.

21.4 GLUCAGON-LIKE PEPTIDE-1 AND ITS BIOLOGICAL ACTIVITIES

GLP-1 is a gut hormone mainly secreted from L cells in the intestine, although a small amount of GLP-1 is secreted from neurons in the hypothalamus. Different from pancreatic a cells, the proglucagon gene product is converted into glicentin, oxyntomodulin, GLP-1, intervening peptide, and GLP-2 through differential posttranslational process. Once entering into circulation, GLP-1(7–36) amide is the active form secreted from L cells. It can be rapidly degraded by enzyme dipeptidyl peptidase

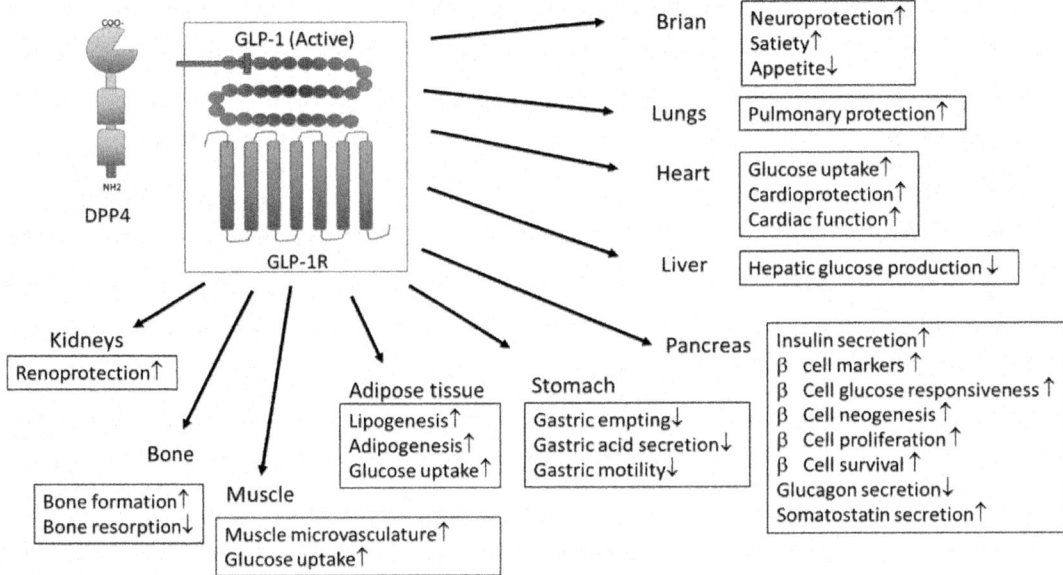

FIGURE 21.1 A summary for the multiple biological effects of GLP-1.

4 (DPP4; T1/2=1.5–2.1min) to become GLP-1(19–36) amide, which acts like a GLP-1R antagonist. GLP-1(19–36) amide can be further degraded into GLP-1(28–36) amide, which transforms into GLP-1(7–36) amide mimetics (Almasri, Taha, and Mohammad 2013; Kim and Jang 2015).

The expression of GLP-1R can be found in pancreatic islets, heart, gastrointestinal tract, brain, and various organs. Activation of GLP-1R, a class B G-protein coupled receptor (GPCR), and multiple biological activities have been observed (Edwards 2005). Figure 21.1 summarizes various biological effects by organ.

Through binding to glucagon like peptide-1 receptor (GLP-1R), GLP-1 could provide multiple biological effects on GLP-1R–expressing organs. The activity of GLP-1 can be largely attenuated by dipeptidyl-peptidase 4 (DPP4).

GLP-1 provides protective effects on brain, lung, heart, pancreatic islets, bone structure, and kidney function. It also regulates energy expenditure and glucose homeostasis through brain, stomach, liver, pancreas, and muscle. To pancreatic islet b cells, activation of GLP-1R would lead to a glucose-dependent insulinotropic effect and promote b function for insulin secretion and glucose responsiveness. In addition, GLP-1 also promotes b cell neogenesis and survival. As a result, modulating GLP-1 activity could result in various beneficial health outcomes.

21.5 GLP-1–BASED THERAPEUTICS FOR TREATING DIABETES

In terms of current available incretin based therapeutics for treating type 2 diabetes, both GLP-1 receptor agonists and DPP4 inhibitors have been applied on type 2 diabetic subjects (Kang and Jung 2016; Patel et al. 2020). To classify DPP4-resistant GLP-1R agonists (GLP-1RAs), dulaglutide (QW; weekly) and albiglutide (QW), liraglutide (QD; daily) and semaglutide (QW) are using human GLP-1 backbone. In contrast, exenatide BID (twice a day), exenatide QW, and lixisenatide (QD) are using exendin-4 as a backbone molecule. On the other hand, sitagliptin, vildagliptin, saxagliptin, linagliptin, trelagliptin, gemigliptin, omarigliptin, alogliptin, and teneligliptin are FDA-approved DPP4 inhibitors on the market (Turdu et al. 2018; Nauck 2011).

An oral version of semaglutide (Ozempic) is the first oral GLP-1RA on the drug market (Nordisk 2018). Apart from that, orthosteric or allosteric GLP-1RA small molecules have been also developed

(Chen et al. 2007; Willard, Bueno, and Sloop 2012; He et al. 2012; Su et al. 2008). However, none of them passed the phase III clinical trials. Similarly, GLP-1 secretogagus small molecules also belong to investigational therapeutics or supplements for treating type 2 diabetes (Lee et al. 2021; Gonzalez-Abuin et al. 2014; Bianchini et al. 2021; Drzazga et al. 2021; Guo et al. 2021; Suzuki and Aoe 2021; Yang et al. 2021).

21.6   BOSCHNALOSIDE FROM *B. ROSSICA* IS A GLP-1 RECEPTOR AGONIST

The claim that boschnaloside is a GLP-1R agonist is supported by the following experiments (Lin et al. 2019). As shown in Figure 21.2, the interaction between boschnaloside and the extracellular domain of GLP-1R recombinant protein was shown by performing saturation transfer difference (STD) nuclear magnetic resonance (NMR) analysis. By comparing 1D^{3}H reference spectrum with 1D STD spectrum, positive signals at δ_H 5.55 (H-1), 3.36, 3.28, and 3.13 (sugar protons, H-2¢ to H-5¢) representing both glycosyl and aglycone regions of boschnaloside were identified. In response to a ligand stimulus binds to GLP-1R, activated GLP-1R would result in a conformational change to transduce signal to intracellular heterotrimeric G protein complex. The activated G$_s$ alpha subunit would attract and activate adenylyl cyclase to convert ATP into cyclic adenosine monophosphate (cAMP). In pancreatic b-cells, the increment of cAMP further activates protein kinase A and promotes insulin exocytosis (McClenaghan 2007). In comparing to GLP-1R transfected cAMP/protein kinase A equipped with a reporter system, the advantage of using GLP-1R expressed insulin secreting cells is a direct connection from GLP-R signaling transduction to insulin secretory function (Liu et al. 2007). Based on the results from our investigation, the interaction between boschnaloside and the extracellular domain of GLP-1R was observed by performing ligand-observed NMR experiment (Lin et al. 2019). In addition, treating BRIN-BD11 cells with boschnaloside further increased cAMP production and stimulated insulin secretion in a dose-dependent manner. Finally, boschnaloside stimulated insulin secretion was inhibited by the GLP-1R antagonist exendin$_{9-39}$.

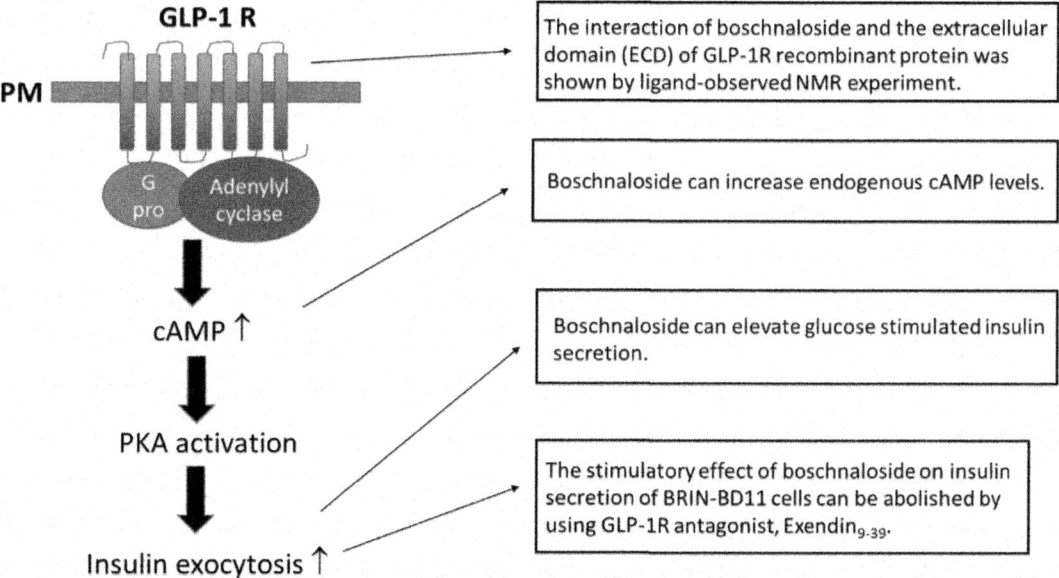

FIGURE 21.2   Current evidence to support that boschnaloside is a GLP-1R agonist. By employing NMR and GLP-1R expressed BRIN-BD11 cells, effects of boschnaloside on binding to ECD of GLP-1R, inducing cAMP production, and stimulating insulin secretion in GLP-1R dependent manner were shown. PM, plasma membrane; G pro, G protein.

21.7 PROPOSED PHARMACOPHORE FOR THE INTERACTION BETWEEN BOSCHNALOSIDE AND GLP-1 RECEPTOR

Although the crystal structure evidence for the complex of GLP-1R and boschnaloside or other iridoid glycosides is unavailable, the proposed interaction between boschnaloside and GLP-1R has been presented in a conference (Liu, Tsai, and Lin 2018). In Figure 21.3A and 21.3B, by employing the crystal structure data (id=3IOL) of GLP-1 in complex with the extracellular domain of the GLP-1 receptor downloaded from the RCSB Protein Data Bank (PDB), the GLP-1 Receptor-GLP-1 pharmacophore was generated by using the "receptor-ligand pharmacophore generation module" in BIOVIA Discovery Studio software (Dassault Systèmes BIOVIA, USA). Based on the receptor-ligand interactions, the following ligand features were considered, including hydrogen bond acceptor (HB_ACCEPTOR), hydrogen bond donor (HB_DONOR), hydrophobic feature (HYDROPHOBIC), negative ionizable feature (NEG_IONIZABLE), positive ionizable feature (POS_IONIZABLE), and Aromatic ring (RING_AROMATIC) (Figure 21.3C) (Tseng et al. 2016). By applying the 3D structure of boschnaloside or its derivative, the "screen library module" in BIOVIA Discovery Studio software was executed to map the imported compound structure in the established pharmacophore on the basis of one compound with at least 300 types of conformations. Hit value and hit features from the conformation which fits into the features of pharmacophore were

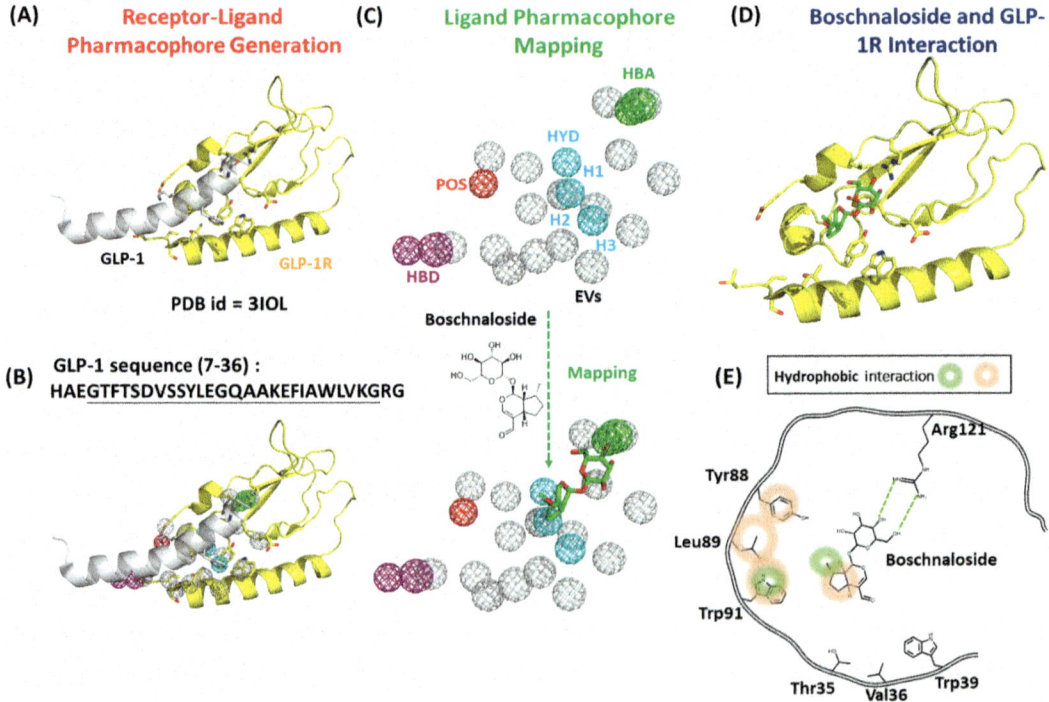

FIGURE 21.3 Computer modeling for the potential interaction between boschnaloside and the extracellular domain of GLP-1R. (A) The illustration of the ligand (GLP-1)-receptor pharmacophore established from x-ray crystallographic data (PDB id: 3IOL). (B) The illustration of the established ligand (GLP-1) pharmacophore with various binding features. (C) The illustration of the ligand (boschnaloside) pharmacophore mapping result. Major features including exclusion volume (EV), hydrophobic domain (HYD), hydrogen bond acceptor (HBA), hydrogen bond donor (HBD), and positive ion (Pos) were color-coded. (F) The illustration of predicted amino acid residues of GLP-1R which interact with Bosl. Hydrophobic interaction is labeled with blue circles and hydrogen bond formation is labeled with green dotted lines.

Source: Liu, Tsai, and Lin (2018).

displayed. By docking boschnaloside into extracted pharmacophore features, fitting result indicated that boschnaloside interacts with three features of pharmacophore, including one HBA (hydrogen bond acceptor) and two HYD (hydrophobic domain H1 and H2). The putative interaction amino acid residues of GLP-1R were arginine 121 (HBA) and tyrosine 88, leucine 89, and tryptophan 91 (HYD), in Figure 21.3D and 21.3E.

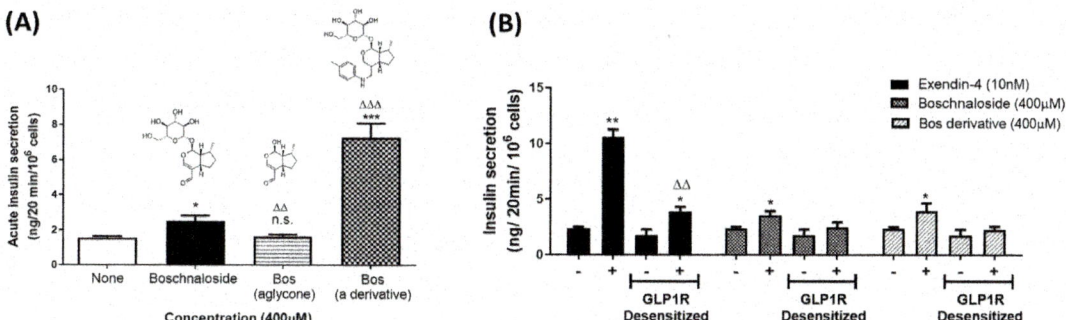

FIGURE 21.4   A structure and activity relationship established by using boschnaloside and derivatives stimulated insulin secretory activities. (A) Acute insulin secretion of BRIN-BD11 cells in response to boschnaloside, boschnaloside aglycone, and benzyl residue added boschnaloside derivative (400 μM) in the presence of 16.7 mM glucose was measured. (B) Insulin secretion of BRIN-BD11 cells in response to exendin-4 (10 nM), boschnaloside (400 μM), and benzyl residue added boschnaloside derivative (400 μM) in the presence or absence of GLP-1R desensitization. Data represents mean ± S.E.M ($n = 8$). *$p < 0.05$; **$p < 0.01$; ***$p < 0.001$, when compared with none group. ${}^{\Delta\Delta}p < 0.01$ and ${}^{\Delta\Delta\Delta}p$ 33< 0.001, when compared with boschnaloside (400 μM) group.

Source: Liu, Tsai, and Lin (2018).

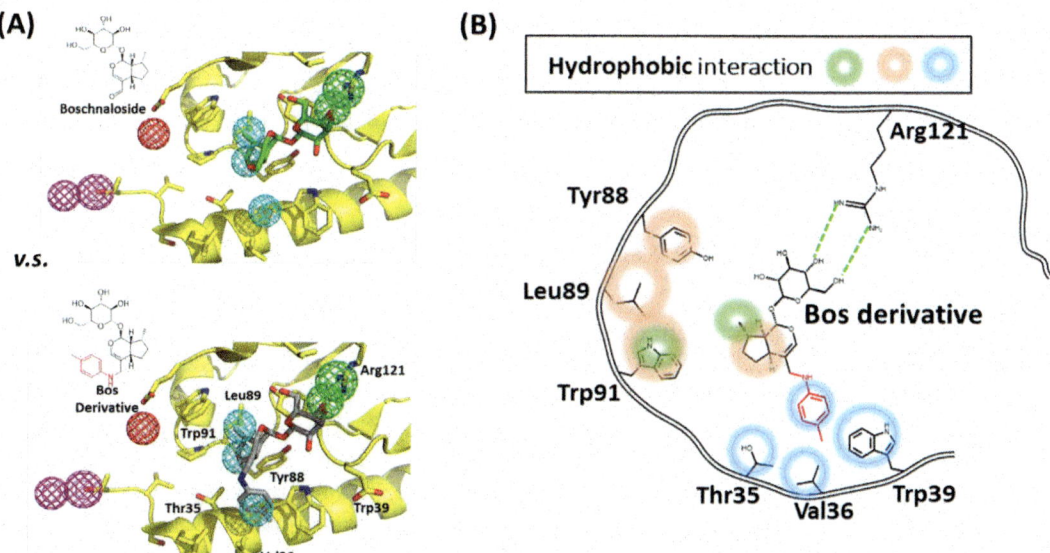

FIGURE 21.5   Illustrations of the predicted amino acid residues of GLP-1R which interacts with boschnaloside and its derivative. (A) Comparison of ligand pharmacophore mapping results between boschnaloside and its derivative. Hydrophobic interaction was labeled with blue circles and hydrogen bond formation was labeled with green dotted lines. (B) Hydrophobic interaction between benzyl residue added boschaloside derivative and amino acid residues of GLP-1 receptor.

Source: Liu, Tsai, and Lin (2018).

The structure and activity relationships were further illustrated by comparing insulin secretory activities among boschnaloside, boschnaloside aglycone, and benzyl residue added boschnaloside derivative (Figure 21.4A). In the presence of 16.7 mM glucose condition (none), insulin secretion was significantly increased in cells treated with boschnaloside and boschnaloside derivative at 400 μM. In addition, there was nearly 2.5- or 3.5-fold increase of insulin secretion from cells treated with boschnaloside derivative when comparing with the parent boschnaloside. In contrast, boschnaloside aglycone clearly lost the insulinotropic activity. By employing GLP-1R desensitization method in which cells were cultured with exendine-4 (400 nM) for 24 hours prior to performing acute insulin secretion, the insulinotropic effect of exendin-4 was significantly reduced ($p < 0.01$) under GLP-1R desensitized condition. Under the same condition, both boschnaloside and boschnaloside derivatives were unable to stimulate insulin secretion (Figure 21.4B).

Based on the pharmacophore mapping of boschnaloside and its benzyl residue added derivative, the benzyl residue addition resulted in an additional feature (HYD H3) fitting at the positions Thr35, Val36, and Trp39 of GLP-1R. In contrast, HBA feature was lost in boschnaloside aglycone due to the lack of hydrogen bond formation (Figure 21.5A and 21.5B).

21.8 ADDITIONAL EFFECTS OF BOSCHNALOSIDE RELATED TO ENDOGENOUS GLP-1 LEVEL MODULATION

Reduced plasma GLP-1 levels indicated potential risk for diseases like type 2 diabetes, non-alcoholic fatty liver disease, and polycystic ovary syndrome. In addition, the GLP-1 effects on targeted organs are also associated with endogenous GLP-1 levels (Wang et al. 2015). In addition to being rapidly degraded by DPP4, stimulation of GLP-1 secretion from L-cells can be achieved by various nutrients, drugs, bariatric surgery, and other factors. In general, combination of the inhibition of DPP4 activity and stimulation of GLP-1 secretion results in a synergistic effect on modulation of plasma GLP-1 levels. Such combination was also observed from boschnaloside-treated *db/db* mice. Inhibition of DPP4 enzyme activity and increased GLP-1 secretion in STC-1 cells after 24-hour treatment of boschnaloside suggested a potential synergistic effect occurred after boschnaloside treatment for *db/db* mice (Lin et al. 2019).

21.9 ANTI-DIABETIC EFFECTS OF ORAL BOSCHNALOSIDE TREATMENT ON TYPE 2 DIABETIC MICE

A summary of the anti-diabetic effects after oral boschnaloside treatment for *db/db* mice for 4 weeks is shown in Table 21.1. When diabetic *db/db* mice suffered from severe hyperglycemia (FPG > 400 mg/dL and HbA$_{1c}$ > 10%), once-daily oral administration of boschnaloside at a dose of 300 mg/kg for 4 weeks resulted in following improvement. Comparing to untreated diabetic mice, HbA$_{1c}$ level reduced 80%, FPG, hyperinsulinemia, Homeostatic Model Assessment for Insulin Resistance (HOMA-IR), and urination reduced 70%, quantitative oral glucose tolerance test (OGTT) data by using area under curve, as well as food and water intake reduced 50%. On the other hand, serum adiponectin and serum GLP-1 level increased 1.5- and 3.5-fold, respectively, while Homeostatic Model Assessment for β cell function (HOMA-B%) increased twofold (Lin et al. 2019). It should be emphasized that once-daily oral administration regime is more friendly to patients in comparison with the daily peptide injection regime. Since oral version of Victoza (liraglutide) is FDA approved, comparative pharmacology between oral version of Victoza and boschnaloside could be performed in order to find out the similarities and differences between these two drugs.

TABLE 21.1

ANTI-DIABETIC EFFECTS OF BOSCHNALOSIDE ON TYPE 2 DIABETIC MICE

Therapeutic index part 1.	Improvement
HbA1c	80%
FPG	70%
OGTT/PG	50%
Hyperinsulinemia	70%
HOMA-IR	70%
Food intake	50%
Water intake	50%
Urination	70%
Therapeutic index part 2.	**Increment**
HOMA-B%	200%
Serum GLP-1$_{active}$ level	350%
Serum adiponectin level	150%

A summary of anti-diabetic effects of oral boschnaloside (300 mg/kg/day) administration on type 2 diabetic *db/db* mice after 4 weeks of treatment. The improvement and increment levels represent the difference between untreated diabetic *db/db* mice and boschnaloside-treated diabetic *db/db* mice.

Source: (Lin et al. 2019)

21.10 OTHER FOODS, HERBS, AND SPICES AND BOTANICALS USED IN DIABETES

In addition to *Boschniakia rossica*, *B. himalaica* is the other plant belonging to the genus *Boschniakia* in China. Both herbs appear to have similar chemical constituents (Zhang, Zhao, et al. 2016).

A wide range of nature materials can be used for diabetes treatment. In the current review, we emphasized the mechanisms of anti-diabetes activities of boschnaloside related to GLP-1R activation, the increment of GLP-1 secretion, and the inhibition of DPP4 activity. Similarly, many iridoid glycosides in nature were also reported as GLP-1R agonists and can be used for treating diabetes, neuron disorder, and pain. For examples, geniposide (an iridoid glycoside from *Gardenia jasminoides* fruits), morroniside (a secoiridoid glycoside from *Cornus officinalis*), and iridoid glycosides from *Lamiophlomis* rotate (an orally available Tibetan herbal painkiller) have all been reported as GLP-1R agonists (Xu et al. 2017; Zhang, Ding, et al. 2016; Zhu et al. 2014).

There are various nutrient sensors expressed in the enteroendocrine L cells, such as sweet and bitter taste receptors (T1R2–T1R3 and T2Rs), cannabinoid receptor (GPR119), bile acid receptor (TGR5), fatty acid receptors (GPR40/GPR120, GPR41/GPR43), the calcium-sensing receptor (CaR), and so on. Many plant derived GLP-1 secretagogues activating those nutrient sensors include in ginsenosides and compound K from *Panax ginseng*, gordonoside F from *Hoodia* extract, quinine from *Plasmodium falciparum*, rutin from tartary buckwheat, loganic acid from *Gentiana scabra*, cucurbitane-type triterpenoids from the vines of *Momordica charantia*, and so on (Kim and Jang 2015; Lee et al. 2021; Liaw et al. 2021).

Phytochemicals which inhibit DPP4 activity are expected to stabilize or even increase plasma GLP-1 levels. When combining with GLP-1 secretagogues, dual activities due to such combinations would lead to significantly increased plasma GLP-1 levels and therefore promote stronger

GLP-1 activities. Currently, many plant-derived DPP4 inhibitors have also been identified. There are bioactive peptides from *Vigna unguiculata*; alkaloid, sterol, and flavonoid from *Urena lobata*; smilachinin, bismilachinone, vitexin, and rutin from *Smilax china* L.; quinovic acid and derivatives from *Fagonia cretica* L.; 16,17-dihydro-17b-hydroxy from *Mitragyna parvifolia*; berberine from *Coptis chinensis*; castanospermine, australine, and 7-deoxy-6-epi-castanospermine from *Castanospermum austral* Cunn.; and *Mangifera indica* L. extracts (Turdu et al. 2018).

21.11   TOXICITY AND CAUTIONARY NOTES

Based on the China standard "Procedures and Methods for Toxicological Assessment: On Food Safety" (GB15193–2003), the toxicology of *Boschniakia rossica* related to acute and inherent toxicity was investigated. Serial tests including maximum tolerated dose, micronucleus of bone marrow in mice, and sperm abnormality in mice were executed. As a result, the LD_{50} of *B. rossica* was over 24 g/kg. The maximum tolerance dose was 30 g/kg. Finally, no significant difference in the micronucleus and the sperm abnormality rate of mice treated with *B. rossica* was found. The conclusion is that *B. rossica* is classified as an herb with first-class non-toxicity and without mutagenic action. It is considered safe to be used in clinic (Shen-yang 2008). However, it should be noted that information about herb-drug interactions from *B. rossica* is not available. A rigorous investigation for this scope is in demand.

There is no enough information about the toxicity of non-polysaccharide phytochemicals from *B. rossica*. One study focused on the cytotoxicity of phenolic glycosides from the whole plant of *B. himalaica*. Cell lines including A549 (human lung carcinoma) and P388 (murine leukemia) were used and shown a modest cytotoxicity with IC_{50} ranging from 32.5 to 72.5 mM (Zhang, Zhao, et al. 2016).

Considering geniposide can be regarded as a surrogate boschnaloside, liver toxicity appears to be the major issue of boschnaloside for its safety. The acute toxicity study indicated that geniposide could induce oxidative stress related hepatotoxicity in rats within 48 hours after oral administration of geniposide at dose of 574 mg/kg (Shan et al. 2017). However, hepatotoxicity was not shown in rats orally administered geniposide less than 24.3 mg/kg for consecutive 90 days (Ding et al. 2013). Intranasal treatment provided the least toxicity when compared to intravenous, intragastrical, or intramuscular administration. Interestingly, induced toxicity appears to be species sensitive because only SD or Wistar rats, not ICR mice, treated with geniposide would lead to an obvious hepatotoxicity. In addition to liver damage, the increment of alanine aminotransferase (ALT), aspartic transaminase (AST), alkaline phosphatase (ALP), total bilirubin (TBIL), blood urea nitrogen (BUN), and creatinine (CREA) activities in serum of rats treated with geniposide (1.2 g/kg; i.g.) indicated serious pathological damage in the kidney (Cheng et al. 2015). As a result, a rigorous investigation for the toxicity of boschnaloside is also in demand.

21.12   SUMMARY POINTS

- *Boschniakia rossica* is a parasitic plant that grows on the tree roots of the genus *Alnus*.
- The earliest use of *B. rossica* dates back to AD 659 in the Tang dynasty in China.
- The ancient text from the Tang *Materia Medica* suggested that *B. rossica* is a substitute of Cistanche (*Cistanche deserticola* Ma).
- Purposes of *B. rossica* prescription are to tonify kidney, improve impotence, attenuate constipation, and enhance longevity.
- Iridoid glycosides, such as boschnaloside, from *B. rossica* are potent anti-diabetes phytochemicals.
- The important mechanisms of action for boschnaloside include the activation of glucagon like peptide-1 receptor, the promotion of GLP-1 secretion, and the inhibition of DPP4 enzyme activity.

- Consumption of boschnaloside improved several diabetes-related biomarkers and features including fasting blood sugar, glucose tolerance, HbA_{1c}, insulin sensitivity, and b cell functions in type 2 diabetic *db/db* mice.
- Computer modeling results suggest that boschnaloside interacts with the extracellular domain of GLP-1R, and both hydrophobic domain and hydrogen bond acceptor domains from GLP-1R potentially interact with boschnaloside.
- Based on the China standard "Procedures and Methods for Toxicological Assessment: On Food Safety" (GB15193–2003), *B. rossica* is classified as an herb with first-class non-toxicity and without mutagenic action.
- Boschnaloside-related iridoid glycoside, geniposide, provided hepatotoxicity and kidney damages in rats at dose of 574 mg/kg and above, so a rigorous investigation for the toxicity of boschnaloside is in demand.

REFERENCES

Ali, M. K., K. M. Bullard, J. B. Saaddine, C. C. Cowie, G. Imperatore, and E. W. Gregg. 2013. "Achievement of goals in U.S. diabetes care, 1999–2010." *N Engl J Med* 368 (17):1613–1624. https://doi.org/10.1056/NEJMsa1213829.

Almasri, I. M., M. O. Taha, and M. K. Mohammad. 2013. "New leads for DPP IV inhibition: Structure-based pharmacophore mapping and virtual screening study." *Arch Pharm Res* 36 (11):1326–1337. https://doi.org/10.1007/s12272-013-0224-1.

American Diabetes, Association. 2021. "2. Classification and diagnosis of diabetes: Standards of medical care in diabetes-2021." *Diabetes Care* 44 (Suppl 1):S15–S33. https://doi.org/10.2337/dc21-S002.

Andre, A., and A. Fehr. 2002. *Gwich'in Ethnobotany*. 2nd ed. Gwich&in Social and Cultural Institute and Aurora Research Institute, Tsiigehtchic and Inuvik, Canada.

Bianchini, G., C. Nigro, A. Sirico, R. Novelli, I. Prevenzano, C. Miele, F. Beguinot, and A. Aramini. 2021. "A new synthetic dual agonist of GPR120/GPR40 induces GLP-1 secretion and improves glucose homeostasis in mice." *Biomed Pharmacother* 139:111613. https://doi.org/10.1016/j.biopha.2021.111613.

Chen, D., J. Liao, N. Li, C. Zhou, Q. Liu, G. Wang, R. Zhang, S. Zhang, L. Lin, K. Chen, X. Xie, F. Nan, A. A. Young, and M. W. Wang. 2007. "A nonpeptidic agonist of glucagon-like peptide 1 receptors with efficacy in diabetic db/db mice." *Proc Natl Acad Sci U S A* 104 (3):943–948. https://doi.org/10.1073/pnas.0610173104.

Cheng, S. H., Y. Y. Zhang, H. F. Li, and J. P. Wei. 2015. "Acute hepatotoxicity and nephrotoxicity study of geniposide on jaundice rats." *Chin J Exp Tradit Med Formuae* 21:174–178.

Ding, Y., T. Zhang, J. S. Tao, L. Y. Zhang, J. R. Shi, and G. Ji. 2013. "Potential hepatotoxicity of geniposide, the major iridoid glycoside in dried ripe fruits of Gardenia jasminoides (Zhi-zi)." *Nat Prod Res* 27 (10):929–933. https://doi.org/10.1080/14786419.2012.673604.

Do, O. H., J. E. Gunton, H. Y. Gaisano, and P. Thorn. 2016. "Changes in beta cell function occur in prediabetes and early disease in the Lepr (db) mouse model of diabetes." *Diabetologia* 59 (6):1222–1230. https://doi.org/10.1007/s00125-016-3942-3.

Drzazga, A., D. Kaminska, A. Gliszczynska, and E. Gendaszewska-Darmach. 2021. "Isoprenoid derivatives of lysophosphatidylcholines enhance insulin and GLP-1 secretion through lipid-binding GPCRs." *Int J Mol Sci* 22 (11). https://doi.org/10.3390/ijms22115748.

Edwards, C. M. 2005. "The GLP-1 system as a therapeutic target." *Ann Med* 37 (5):314–322. https://doi.org/10.1080/07853890510037400.

Elven, R., D. F. Murray, V. Y. Razzhivin, and B. A. Yurtsev. 2006. Checklist of the panarctic flora (PAF). In *Vascular plants*: University of Oslo, Oslo.

Fan, L., and J. Ren. 2019. "Traditional uses, chemical constituents and pharmacological effects of Boschniakia rossica: A systematic review." *Trop J of Pharm Res* 18 (12):2643–2651.

Gonzalez-Abuin, N., N. Martinez-Micaelo, M. Blay, B. D. Green, M. Pinent, and A. Ardevol. 2014. "Grape-seed procyanidins modulate cellular membrane potential and nutrient-induced GLP-1 secretion in STC-1 cells." *Am J Physiol Cell Physiol* 306 (5):C485–C492. https://doi.org/10.1152/ajpcell.00355.2013.

Guo, S., T. Yan, L. Shi, A. Liu, T. Zhang, Y. Xu, W. Jiang, Q. Yang, L. Yang, L. Liu, R. Zhao, and S. Zhang. 2021. "Matrine, as a CaSR agonist promotes intestinal GLP-1 secretion and improves insulin resistance in diabetes mellitus." *Phytomedicine* 84:153507. https://doi.org/10.1016/j.phymed.2021.153507.

He, M., N. Guan, W. W. Gao, Q. Liu, X. Y. Wu, D. W. Ma, D. F. Zhong, G. B. Ge, C. Li, X. Y. Chen, L. Yang, J. Y. Liao, and M. W. Wang. 2012. "A continued saga of Boc5, the first non-peptidic glucagon-like peptide-1 receptor agonist with in vivo activities." *Acta Pharmacol Sin* 33 (2):148–154. https://doi.org/10.1038/aps.2011.169.

Kang, Y. M., and C. H. Jung. 2016. "Cardiovascular effects of glucagon-like peptide-1 receptor agonists." *Endocrinol Metab (Seoul)* 31 (2):258–274. https://doi.org/10.3803/EnM.2016.31.2.258.

Kim, K. S., and H. J. Jang. 2015. "Medicinal plants qua glucagon-like peptide-1 secretagogue via intestinal nutrient sensors." *Evid Based Complement Alternat Med* 2015:171742. https://doi.org/10.1155/2015/171742.

Lee, L. C., Y. C. Hou, Y. Y. Hsieh, Y. H. Chen, Y. C. Shen, I. J. Lee, M.C.M. Shih, W. C. Hou, and H. K. Liu. 2021. "Dietary supplementation of rutin and rutin-rich buckwheat elevates endogenous glucagon-like peptide 1 levels to facilitate glycemic control in type 2 diabetic mice." *J of Funct Foods* 85:104653.

Liaw, C. C., H. T. Huang, H. K. Liu, Y. C. Lin, L. J. Zhang, W. C. Wei, C. C. Shen, C. L. Wu, C. Y. Huang, and Y. H. Kuo. 2021. "Cucurbitane-type triterpenoids from the vines of Momordica charantia and their anti-inflammatory, cytotoxic, and antidiabetic activity." *Phytochemistry* 195:113026. https://doi.org/10.1016/j.phytochem.2021.113026.

Lin, L. C., and K. T. Chen. 2004. "New Phenylpropanoid Glycoside from Boschniakia rossica." *Chinese Pharm J* 56 (2):77–85. https://doi.org/10.7019/CPJ.200404.0077.

Lin, L. C., L. C. Lee, C. Huang, C. T. Chen, J. S. Song, Y. J. Shiao, and H. K. Liu. 2019. "Effects of boschnaloside from Boschniakia rossica on dysglycemia and islet dysfunction in severely diabetic mice through modulating the action of glucagon-like peptide-1." *Phytomedicine* 62:152946. https://doi.org/10.1016/j.phymed.2019.152946.

Lin, L. C., Y. H. Wang, Y. C. Hou, S. Chang, K. T. Liou, Y. C. Chou, W. Y. Wang, and Y. C. Shen. 2006. "The inhibitory effect of phenylpropanoid glycosides and iridoid glucosides on free radical production and beta2 integrin expression in human leucocytes." *J Pharm Pharmacol* 58 (1):129–135. https://doi.org/10.1211/jpp.58.1.0016.

Liu, H. K., K. C. Tsai, and L. C. Lin. 2018. "Oral administration of boschnaloside, a GLP-1 receptor activator from herbal medicine Boschniakia rossica (the northern groundcone), improved diabetic conditions and modulated incretin hormone levels in db/db mice." *18th World Congress of Basic and Clinical Pharmacology*, Kyoto, Japan.

Liu, J., F. Yin, X. Zheng, J. Jing, and Y. Hu. 2007. "Geniposide, a novel agonist for GLP-1 receptor, prevents PC12 cells from oxidative damage via MAP kinase pathway." *Neurochem Int* 51 (6–7):361–369. https://doi.org/10.1016/j.neuint.2007.04.021.

Liu, Y. H., Y. L. Lu, C. H. Han, and W. C. Hou. 2013. "Inhibitory activities of acteoside, isoacteoside, and its structural constituents against protein glycation in vitro." *Bot Stud* 54 (1):6. https://doi.org/10.1186/1999-3110-54-6.

McClenaghan, N. H. 2007. "Physiological regulation of the pancreatic (beta)-cell: Functional insights for understanding and therapy of diabetes." *Exp Physiol* 92 (3):481–496. https://doi.org/10.1113/expphysiol.2006.034835.

Murai, F., and M. Tagawa. 1982. "8-Epi-iridodial glucoside from Boschniakia rossica." *Planta Med* 46 (1):45–47. https://doi.org/10.1055/s-2007-970017.

Nauck, M. A. 2011. "Incretin-based therapies for type 2 diabetes mellitus: Properties, functions, and clinical implications." *Am J Med* 124 (1 Suppl):S3–18. https://doi.org/10.1016/j.amjmed.2010.11.002.

Nordisk, Novo. 2018. "Novo Nordisk successfully completes the first phase 3a trial, PIONEER 1, with oral semaglutide." *Novo Nordisk*. www.novonordisk.com/media/news-details.2170941.html.

Ogurtsova, K., J. D. da Rocha Fernandes, Y. Huang, U. Linnenkamp, L. Guariguata, N. H. Cho, D. Cavan, J. E. Shaw, and L. E. Makaroff. 2017. "IDF diabetes atlas: Global estimates for the prevalence of diabetes for 2015 and 2040." *Diabetes Res Clin Pract* 128:40–50. https://doi.org/10.1016/j.diabres.2017.03.024.

Patel, K. V., A. Sarraju, I. J. Neeland, and D. K. McGuire. 2020. "Cardiovascular effects of dipeptidyl peptidase-4 inhibitors and glucagon-like peptide-1 receptor agonists: A review for the general cardiologist." *Curr Cardiol Rep* 22 (10):105. https://doi.org/10.1007/s11886-020-01355-5.

Quan, J., M. Jin, H. Xu, D. Qiu, and X. Yin. 2014. "BRP, a polysaccharide fraction isolated from Boschniakia rossica, protects against galactosamine and lipopolysaccharide induced hepatic failure in mice." *J Clin Biochem Nutr* 54 (3):181–189. https://doi.org/10.3164/jcbn.13-105.

Quan, J., T. Li, W. Zhao, H. Xu, D. Qiu, and X. Yin. 2013. "Hepatoprotective effect of polysaccharides from Boschniakia rossica on carbon tetrachloride-induced toxicity in mice." *J Clin Biochem Nutr* 52 (3):244–252. https://doi.org/10.3164/jcbn.12-96.

Quan, J., L. Piao, H. Xu, T. Li, and X. Yin. 2009. "Protective effect of iridoid glucosides from Boschniakia rossica on acute liver injury induced by carbon tetrachloride in rats." *Biosci Biotechnol Biochem* 73 (4):849–854. https://doi.org/10.1271/bbb.80757.

Royal Botanic Gardens, Kew. 2020. *Boschniakia rossica* (Cham. & Schltdl.) B. Fedtsch. In *Plants of the World Online*. Royal Botanic Gardens, Kew.

Shan, M., S. Yu, H. Yan, S. Guo, W. Xiao, Z. Wang, L. Zhang, A. Ding, Q. Wu, and S.F.Y. Li. 2017. "A review on the phytochemistry, pharmacology, pharmacokinetics and toxicology of geniposide, a natural product." *Molecules* 22 (10). https://doi.org/10.3390/molecules22101689.

Shen-yang, Xing. 2008. "Toxicity of polysaccharides of Boschniakia rossica." *J Northeast Normal Univ.* 40(2):98–100.

Su, H., M. He, H. Li, Q. Liu, J. Wang, Y. Wang, W. Gao, L. Zhou, J. Liao, A. A. Young, and M. W. Wang. 2008. "Boc5, a non-peptidic glucagon-like Peptide-1 receptor agonist, invokes sustained glycemic control and weight loss in diabetic mice." *PLoS ONE* 3 (8):e2892. https://doi.org/10.1371/journal.pone.0002892.

Suzuki, S., and S. Aoe. 2021. "High beta-glucan barley supplementation improves glucose tolerance by increasing GLP-1 secretion in diet-induced obesity mice." *Nutrients* 13 (2). https://doi.org/10.3390/nu13020527.

Tseng, T. S., S. M. Chuang, N. W. Hsiao, Y. W. Chen, Y. C. Lee, C. C. Lin, C. Huang, and K. C. Tsai. 2016. "Discovery of a potent cyclooxygenase-2 inhibitor, S4, through docking-based pharmacophore screening, in vivo and in vitro estimations." *Mol Biosyst* 12 (8):2541–2551. https://doi.org/10.1039/c6mb00229c.

Tsuda, T. S., A. Sugaya, Y. Z. Liu, K. Katoh, H. Tanaka, H. Kawazura, E. Sugaya, M. Kusai, and M. Kohno. 1994. "Radical scavenger effect of Boschniakia rossica." *J Ethnopharmacol* 41 (1–2):85–90. https://doi.org/10.1016/0378-8741(94)90062-0.

Turdu, G., H. Gao, Y. Jiang, and M. Kabas. 2018. "Plant dipeptidyl peptidase-IV inhibitors as antidiabetic agents: A brief review." *Future Med Chem* 10 (10):1229–1239. https://doi.org/10.4155/fmc-2017-0235.

Wang, X., H. Liu, J. Chen, Y. Li, and S. Qu. 2015. "Multiple factors related to the secretion of glucagon-like peptide-1." *Int J Endocrinol* 2015:651757. https://doi.org/10.1155/2015/651757.

Wang, Y. H. 2021. "Traditional uses, chemical constituents, pharmacological activities, and toxicological effects of Dendrobium leaves: A review." *J Ethnopharmacol* 270:113851. https://doi.org/10.1016/j.jep.2021.113851.

Wang, Z., C. Lu, C. Wu, M. Xu, X. Kou, D. Kong, and G. Jing. 2014. "Polysaccharide of Boschniakia rossica induces apoptosis on laryngeal carcinoma Hep2 cells." *Gene* 536 (1):203–206. https://doi.org/10.1016/j.gene.2013.11.090.

Willard, F. S., A. B. Bueno, and K. W. Sloop. 2012. "Small molecule drug discovery at the glucagon-like peptide-1 receptor." *Exp Diabetes Res* 2012:709893. https://doi.org/10.1155/2012/709893.

Xu, M., H. Y. Wu, H. Liu, N. Gong, Y. R. Wang, and Y. X. Wang. 2017. "Morroniside, a secoiridoid glycoside from Cornus officinalis, attenuates neuropathic pain by activation of spinal glucagon-like peptide-1 receptors." *Br J Pharmacol* 174 (7):580–590. https://doi.org/10.1111/bph.13720.

Yang, Y., A. Tian, Z. Wu, Y. Wei, X. Hu, and J. Guo. 2021. "Finger citron extract ameliorates glycolipid metabolism and inflammation by regulating GLP-1 secretion via TGR5 receptors in obese rats." *Evid Based Complement Alternat Med* 2021:6623379. https://doi.org/10.1155/2021/6623379.

Yao, C., X. Cao, Z. Fu, J. Tian, W. Dong, J. Xu, K. An, L. Zhai, and J. Yu. 2017. "Boschniakia rossica polysaccharide triggers laryngeal carcinoma cell apoptosis by regulating expression of Bcl-2, Caspase-3, and P53." *Med Sci Monit* 23:2059–2064. https://doi.org/10.12659/msm.901381.

Yim, S. H., H. J. Kim, Y. Z. Liu, and I. S. Lee. 2004. "A novel iridoid from Boschniakia rossica." *Chem Pharm Bull (Tokyo)* 52 (2):289–290. https://doi.org/10.1248/cpb.52.289.

Yin, Z. Z., H. S. Kim, Y. H. Kim, and J. J. Lee. 1999. "Iridoid compounds from Boschniakia rossica." *Arch Pharm Res* 22 (1):78–80. https://doi.org/10.1007/BF02976441.

Zhang, L., Y. Zhao, Z. A. Wang, K. Wei, B. Qiu, C. Zhang, Q. Wang-Muller, and M. Li. 2016. "The genus Boschniakia in China: An ethnopharmacological and phytochemical review." *J Ethnopharmacol* 194:987–1004. https://doi.org/10.1016/j.jep.2016.10.051.

Zhang, Y., Y. Ding, X. Zhong, Q. Guo, H. Wang, J. Gao, T. Bai, L. Ren, Y. Guo, X. Jiao, and Y. Liu. 2016. "Geniposide acutely stimulates insulin secretion in pancreatic beta-cells by regulating GLP-1 receptor/cAMP signaling and ion channels." *Mol Cell Endocrinol* 430:89–96. https://doi.org/10.1016/j.mce.2016.04.020.

Zhu, B., N. Gong, H. Fan, C. S. Peng, X. J. Ding, Y. Jiang, and Y. X. Wang. 2014. "Lamiophlomis rotata, an orally available Tibetan herbal painkiller, specifically reduces pain hypersensitivity states through the activation of spinal glucagon-like peptide-1 receptors." *Anesthesiology* 121 (4):835–851. https://doi.org/10.1097/ALN.0000000000000320.

22 Okra (*Abelmoschus esculentus* L.) Derived Abscisic Acid and Use in Diabetes

Patricia Daliu and Antonello Santini

CONTENTS

Abbreviations

ABA	abscisic acid
cAMP	cyclic adenosine monophosphate
GLP-1	glucagon peptide 1
PKA	protein kinase A
STZ	streptozotocin
TAA	total antioxidant activity
TPC	total phenolic content
TD2	type 2 diabetes

22.1 INTRODUCTION

Food and nutrition are closely associated with human health. In the past few decades, science has made great efforts to unravel how nutrients and functional ingredients modulate human physiology and responses. Traditional medicines from plants have been used with an holistic approach for a long time and play still today in some places of the world an important role as alternative medicines. Plants are continously studied worldwide for novel possible use and as sources for pharmaceuticals, nutraceuticals, cosmetics, and food supplements, and also as a source of new traditional medicines, which may play a vital role for the prescription drugs in allopathic medicine (Vats et al. 2022; Hermanson et al. 2021; Chauhan et al. 2010). Now there is more demand for the use of plant and natural products rather than synthetic medicines. Alternative treatments for diabetes, for example, become increasingly popular in recent years, including the use of medicinal herbs, nutritional supplements, and even acupuncture

DOI: 10.1201/9781003220930-24

(Guariguata et al. 2014). Diabetes is a health conditions often associated to other health conditions clustered in the metabolic syndrome. It is characterized by hyperglycemia, together with polyuria, polydipsia, and polyphagia. Type 2 diabetes mellitus, in particular, is characterized by peripheral insulin resistance and the pharmacologic approach is currently used. Natural products and nutraceuticals nonetheless can be an alternative tool to complement the conventional therapeutic approach, especially in subjects who do not qualify for a pharmacological treatment (Viera et al. 2019; Santini et al. 2014). Many conventional drugs are based on molecules present in medicinal plants. Metformin, an effective drug for lowering glucose level, has been developed based on the compunds contained in *Galega officinalis* used to treat diabetes (Rasekh et al. 2008). *Galega officinalis* is rich in guanidine, the hypoglycemic component, and experience with guanidine and biguanides stimulated the development of metformin. On this field, plenty of plants from different regions of the world have been investigated for antidiabetic effects, including also other less common, like the Hawthorn (Nazhand et al. 2020). Among them, there is the Okra, *Abelmoschus esculentus* (L.) Moench, also known as lady's fingers, *gombo*, or *bamje*, an annual plant belonging to the *Malvaceae* family (Kumar et al. 2013) which has interesting properties and beneficial effect on health other than its nutritional interest (Elkhalifa, et al. 2021). Its synonym is the *Hibiscus esculentus* L. About one hundred plant name records match this name according to the Plant List available online ("The Plant List. A Working List of All Plant Species",available online at: http://www.theplantlist.org); among these we selected *Abelmoschus esculentus* L., widely diffused and popular in West Africa, India, Brazil, East Europe, and in the Balkans (Roy et al. 2014). The first use of the word *Okra* (alternatively *okro* or *ochro*) appeared in 1679 in the British Colony of Virginia (USA). The Okra fruit/pod is a greenish capsule with length of 10–30 cm long and a diameter of 1–4 cm, it is slightly curved and tapers to a blunt point, a six-chambered pod of fibrous texture as shown in Figure 22.1A. A new variety named red bhindi, *Kashi Lalima*, or red velvet Okra (shown in Figure 22.1B) was recently developed by agricultural experts at the Indian Institute of Vegetable Research (IIVR) in Varanasi (India). This red lady's finger is much more nutritious and healthy compared to the green vegetal, and it has been proposed as a novel botanical source of bioactive compounds (Reddy et al. 2016). Specifically, red Okra pods contain xenobiotics antioxidants (anthocyanins), which are responsible for the pods' red color. Extracts from purple Okra contain anthocyanins with an higher antioxidant and quercetin content with respect to green Okra; hence, plants containing anthocyanins are more effective than the plant devoided of this compound (Irshad et al. 2017).

Since ancient times, Okra is used as a food, for the nutritional value and beneficial properties for health (Petropolous et al. 2023; Liu et al. 2021). The infusions and decoctions of *A. esculentus*

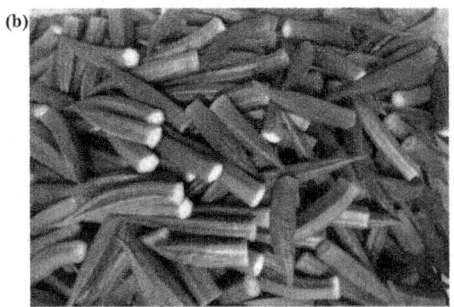 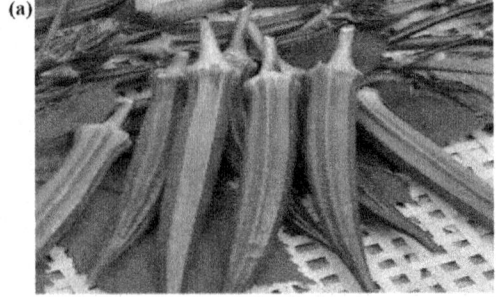

FIGURE 22.1 (A) Okra green pods obtained by a local market in Albania; (B) a new variety named red bhindi or *Kashi Lalima*.

fruits (pods) have been used in folk medicine as a diuretic and for treating diarrhea, acute inflammation, stomach and bowel irritation, catarrhal infections, gonorrhea and dysuria, dental ailments, bronchitis, and pneumonia (Arapitsas 2008). A survey of the ethnobotanical literature revealed that Okra has been used for more than 1000 years in traditional medicine, and the ethnopharmacological and scientific evidence of this seems to be highly effective in treatment of diabetes mellitus (Durazzo et al. 2018) and in improving insulinemia, postprandial glycemia, and satiety (Yang at al. 2023). Okra is known for its good palatability among different regions, and its culinary uses are wide. Its immature green seed pods are eaten fresh as a vegetable, while the extract obtained from the fruit is used to thicken stews, soups, and sauces to improve their consistency (Islam, 2019).

22.1.1 HEALTH BENEFITS AND NOVEL STUDIES

The control of glucose homeostasis is the main goal for both the prevention and management of Type 2 diabetes (TD2M) and prediabetes. Evidences indicates that eating Okra or Okra extracts is an optimal tools for the glycemic control and also that the daily diet plays an important role in the prevention of T2DM (Kabelo.et al. 2023; Nikpayam et al. 2021; Tian et al. 2015). Among the main effects attributed to Okra, its antidiabetic property is the focus. Traditional holistic medicine for centuries has directly associated this plant and its parts to a beneficial health hypoglycemic effect. Different research suggests that Okra may provide antifatigue and antioxidant effects related with antidiabetics properties (Hu et al. 2014). Okra beneficial health properties have been associated to its high polysaccharide content (Khan et al. 2023), which exhibits significant antihyperglycemic activity on STZ-induced diabetic mice by inhibiting the lipid peroxidation chain reaction (Zhang et al. 2018). Summaries of the benefits are shown in Figure 22.2. Further studies are required to explore the details of the mechanisms of action and to clarify the dose and dosage form.

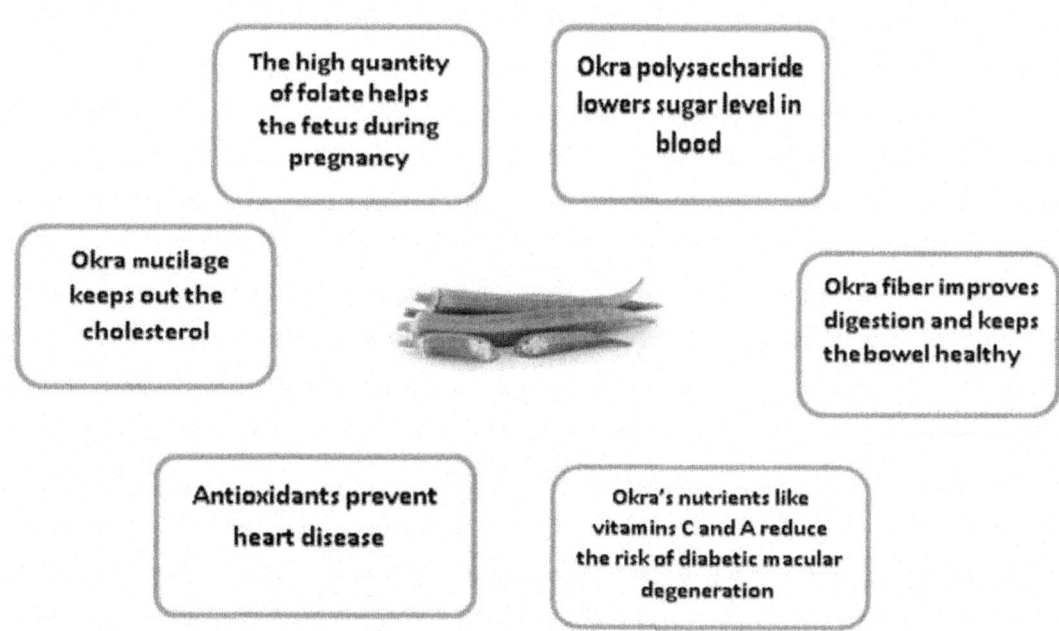

FIGURE 22.2 Okra health benefits.

22.1.2 Biologically Active Components in Okra

Okra is a high-value crop since it represents a source of nutrients that are important to human health, such as vitamins, potassium, calcium, carbohydrates, dietary fiber, and unsaturated fatty acids such as linolenic and oleic acids, and also bioactive compounds. Recent studies on this vegetable lead to identify and quantify for the first time in Okra, the abscisic acid (ABA) (Daliu et al. 2019). Abscisic acid stimulates the glucose uptake by increasing glucose transporter 4 (GLUT4) translocation in myoblasts and adipocytes (Bruzzone et al. 2012). At the same time, ABA also induces glucagon peptide 1 (GLP-1) release in the human L cell line through a cAMP/PKA-dependent mechanism. The possible addition of Okra extracts in food or food additives could suggest to exploit the topic in developing a sustainable and novel nutraceutical taking advantage of ABA health beneficial effect as an alternatives or complement tool for diabetes management. Recent evidence (Zocchi et al. 2017) has been provided on the effects of a low dose of ABA intake from fruit or vegetable extracts. Nonetheless, there is still a lack of data regarding ABA bioaccessibility. From this point of view, once assessed that Okra contains abscisic acid, and with the aim of taking advantage of its hypoglycemic effect, the possibility to use it as nutraceutical to prevent or treat the postprandial glucose level, the bioaccessibility of ABA by *in vitro* studies at gastric and duodenal stages has been performed. The total antioxidant activity (TAA) on three different varieties of Okra cultivated in Albania, Africa, and China were carried out using the 1,1-diphenyl 1–2-picrylhydrazl (DPPH) method. The total phenolic content (TPC) was carried out using the Folin-Ciocalteu method. Okra, besides its medicinal value in antidiabetic, anticarcinogenic, hypocholesterolemic, antioxidant, and immunological activities, it is also used as a component of various food product developments, as a food stabilizer, adhesive, and emulsifying agent. These peculiarities are mainly attributed to the intrinsic dietary fiber and polysaccharides, in particular of mucilage content of the Okra (Liu et al. 2018). The relationship and possible interaction between ABA plant hormone are associated with the other antioxidant compounds present in Okra, which prevent histological damage of the β cells caused by oxidative stress (Majd et al. 2018). The above-mentioned studies on this vegetable seem to suggest that the functional, nutritional, and therapeutic characteristics of Okra can be exploited further in the development of healthy food products, functional foods (Dantas et al. 2021), and nutraceuticals (Daliu et al. 2019).

22.1.3 Other Foods, Herbs, and Botanicals from Albania and Other Countries Used in Diabetes

In Albania and in other Mediterranean Countries, there are many other traditional herbs and plant that are rich in active principles that can improve the diabetes health condition. Aromatic and medicinal plants in Albania are distinguished not only by a relatively wide variety of forms and types but also by the high content of aromatic and pharmacological substances. Being authentic and rare medicinal plants, the evidence is the only source of traditional medicine. Clinical studies for nutraceutical uses of these traditional herbs have enhanced the potential and enhanced the development of the pharmaceutical industry and advanced scientific studies. Among the medicinal plants with health properties can be considered the *Cornus mas* L., the *Cornelian* cherry (Thana) from the *Cornaceae* family (Figure 22.3A). Cornelian cherry fruits have potential cardiovascular, lipid-lowering, and hypoglycemic bioactivities (Kazimierski et al. 2019). *Arbutus unedo* is an evergreen shrub of the *Ericaceae* family (Figure 22.3B). Its edible fruits are used in the production of traditional products such as jam, jelly, and alcoholic beverages (Allali et al. 2013).

Another traditional plant is the Mushmolla (*Mespilus germanica*). It is a large shrub or small tree which belongs to the *Rosaceae* family. It is known also as Medlar, and the fruit of this tree has been cultivated for centuries. The ripened fruit is appreciated for its specific taste and flavor, and it possesses antioxidant and antimicrobial biological properties (Rop et al. 2011, Güçlü et al. 2022, Katanić Stanković,et al. 2022). The fruits are similar to those of the wild rose but are larger in size

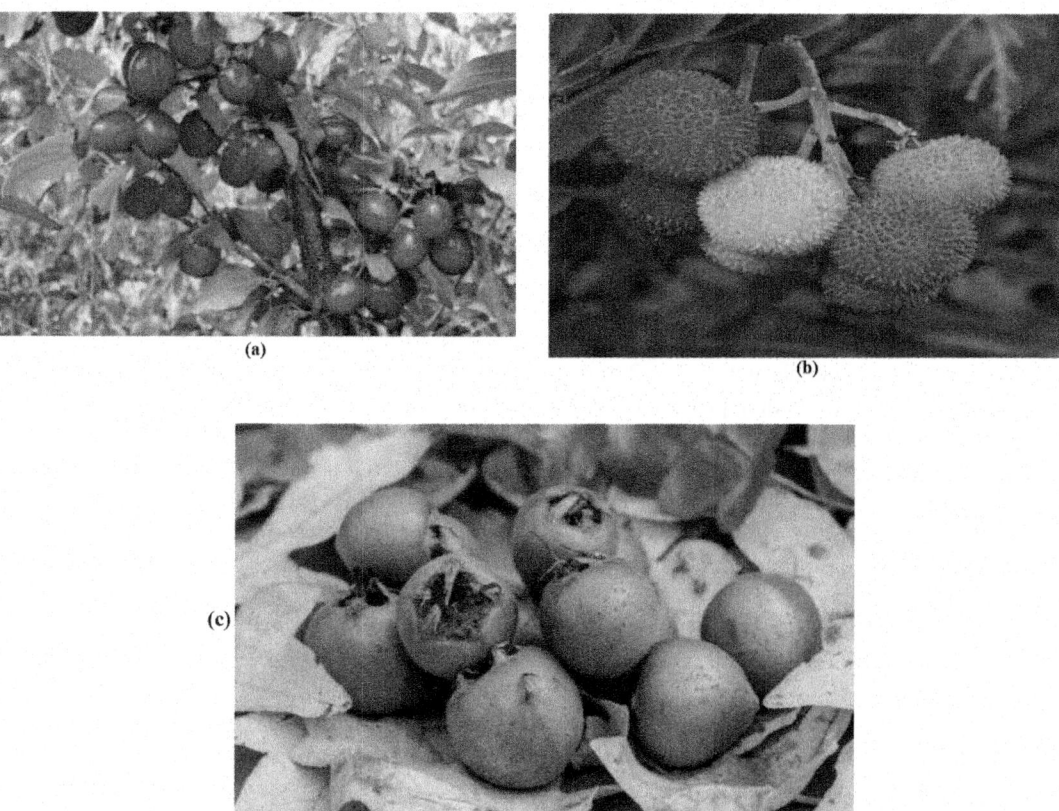

FIGURE 22.3   (A) Fruits of *Cornus mas*; (B) fruits of *Arbutus unedo*; (C) fruits of medlar (*Mespilus germanica*).

(Figure 22.3C). Herbs and supplements may provide relief from diabetes symptoms and reduce the risk of complication alone or in combination with conventional treatment.

Some other herbal supplements well known and diffused wordwide and which show promising results in treating Type 2 diabetes include the ones here briefly reported in the following:

Curcumin: The compound curcumin, which is found in the spice turmeric, has been shown to both boost blood sugar control and help prevent the disease (Zeng et al. 2023). In a 9-month study of 240 adults with prediabetes, those who took curcumin capsules (which are available over the counter) completely avoided developing diabetes, whereas only one-sixth of patients in the placebo group did (Yousef et al. 2008).

Ginseng: Ginseng has been used as a traditional medicine for more than 2000 years. Studies suggest that both Asian and American ginseng may help lower blood sugar in people with diabetes (Li et al. 2023). One study realized by Cheon et al. (2015) found that extract from the ginseng berry was able to normalize blood sugar and improve insulin sensitivity in mice who were bred to develop diabetes.

Fenugreek. This herb has been used as a medicine and as a spice for thousands of years in the Middle East. Benefits of fenugreek for diabetes have been demonstrated in both animal and human trials (Shabil et al. 2023). In one study of 25 people with type 2 diabetes, fenugreek was found to have a significant effect on controlling blood sugar (Gupta et al. 2001).

Psyllium. This plant fiber is found in common bulk laxatives and fiber supplements. Psyllium has also been used historically to treat diabetes (Giri et al. 2023). Studies show that people with type 2 diabetes who take 10 g of psyllium every day can improve their blood sugar and lower blood cholesterol (Wolfram and Ismail-Beigi 2010).

Cinnamon. Cinnamon is a fragrant spice that comes from the bark of a tree. It is a popular ingredient in sweets and baked goods, as well as some savory dishes. This spice may add sweetness to a dish, limiting the need for sugar. It is popular among people with type 2 diabetes for this reason alone, but it may also have other benefits (Błaszczyk et al. 2021). Qin et al. (2010) found evidence from studies in humans that cinnamon may improve levels of glucose, insulin and insulin sensitivity, lipids in the blood, antioxidants, blood pressure, and digestion.

Aloe vera: This plant has been used for thousands of years for its healing properties (Gao et al. 2019). A recent study suggests that the juice from the *Aloe vera* plant can help lower blood sugar in people with types 2 diabetes (Sánchez et al. 2020). The findings suggested that Aloe vera might help protect and repair the β cells in the pancreas that produce insulin. The researchers believed that this might be due to aloe's antioxidant effects.

Bitter melon: Momordica charantia is a medicinal fruit and a popular ingredient of Asian cooking and traditional Chinese medicine. It is believed to relieve thirst and fatigue, which are possible symptoms of type 2 diabetes and Alzheimer's disease (Richter et al.). More recently, researchers have been looking into its properties Massounga Bora et al. 2023). There is some evidence that bitter melon may help manage diabetes (Joseph and Jini 2013). In the reported study, ninety participants received either bitter melon extract or a placebo, those who took the extract had lower fasting blood glucose levels after 12 weeks.

Milk thistle: This flowering herb is found around the Mediterranean Sea. It has been used for its medicinal properties for thousands of years (Samee et al. 2023; Abenavoli et al. 2018). Silymarin, the extract from milk thistle that has received the most attention from scientists, is a compound with antioxidant and anti-inflammatory properties. These are what may make milk thistle a useful herb for people with diabetes. Many results of investigations into the effects of silymarin have been promising, to recommend the herb or its extract alone for diabetes care. Milk thistle may reduce insulin resistance in people with type 2 diabetes who also have liver disease (Soto et al. 2014).

Holy basil: This herb is commonly used in India as a traditional medicine for diabetes Anandhi, 2023; Sahu, 2023). Studies in animals suggest that holy basil may increase the secretion of insulin. (Singh and Chaudhuri 2018). A controlled trial of holy basil in people with type 2 diabetes showed a positive effect on fasting blood sugar and on blood sugar following a meal (Cohen and Tulsi 2014).

A plethora of scientific evidence on the antidiabetic potency of these herbs exists to date, through which it is apparent that they could be promoted as alternative therapies for diabetes.

22.1.4 TOXICITY AND CAUTIONARY NOTES

Data on the safety and toxicity of Okra fruits are limited notwhitstanding its use in many areas is growing (Das et al. 2023). Nonetheless, it seems reasonable to consider that the fruit and seeds of Okra are nontoxic at normal levels of consumption. However, Okra contains a toxic alkaloid, namely the solanine (Sinisterra.Hunter et al. 2018), which may exacerbate symptoms such as *pain* and inflammation in people with joint disorders such as *arthritis* but further clinical studies and research are required on this edible medicinal plant in the context of nutraceutical and functional food development, food excipients, and drug discovery (Jarret et al. 2011). Additionally, being nontoxic in nature, this fruit could be easily tested in human trials rather than in animal models. An Okra-based antidiabetic food with a rich antioxidant formulation can be thus easily be realized and tested with safety and clinical trials for proper formulation, dose and efficacy assessment. These aspects may lead to better value addition for Okra and its wider use and commercialization in the near future and avoiding a limited use as a food only.

22.2 SUMMARY POINTS

- Okra, *Abelmoschus esculentus* L. (Moench), also known as lady's fingers, *gombo*, or *bamje*, is an annual plant belonging to the *Malvaceae* family which is widely diffused in West Africa, India, Brazil, East Europe, and in the Balkans.
- This chapter focuses on the functional and health beneficial properties of Okra, traditional claims, scientific evidence, as well as on other medicinal plants.
- Okra can be recommended and should be taken as a part of a daily diet as its liberal use can be considered safe and various health benefits can be drawn from this natural plant.
- Okra extracts can be used in nutraceutical formulations.

REFERENCES

Abenavoli, L., Izzo, A.A., Milić, N., Cicala, C., Santini, A, Capasso, R. 2018. Milk thistle (Silybum marianum): A concise overview on its chemistry, pharmacological, and nutraceutical uses in liver diseases. *Phytother Res.* 32(11): 2202-2213. doi: 10.1002/ptr.6171.

Anandhi, D., Rajeswari, J., Edwin, J.L. Effects of holy basil leaves extract on blood sugar. 2023. IJCSPUB 13(1), 223-229. Arapitsas, P. 2008. Identification and quantification of polyphenolic compounds from Okra seeds and skins. *Food Chem* 110: 1041–1045.

Bruzzone, S., Battaglia, F., Mannino, E., Parodi, A., Fruscione, F., Basile, G., Salis, A., Sturla, L., Negrini, S., Kalli, F., Stringara, S. 2012. Abscisic acid ameliorates the systemic sclerosis fibroblast phenotype in vitro. *Biochem Biophys Res Commun* 422: 70–74.

Chauhan, A., Sharma, P. K., Srivastava, P., Kumar, N. 2010. Plants having potential antidiabetic activity: A review. *Der Pharm Lett* 2: 369–387.

Cheon, J. M., Kim, D. I., Kim, K. S. 2015. Insulin sensitivity improvement of fermented Korean red ginseng (*Panax ginseng*) mediated by insulin resistance hallmarks in old-aged ob/ob mice. *J Ginseng Res* 39: 331–337.

Cohen, M., Tulsi, M. 2014. *Ocimum sanctum*: A herb for all reasons. *J Ayurveda Integr Med.* 5: 251–259. https://doi.org/10.4103/0975–9476.146554

Daliu, P., Annunziata, G., Tenore, G. C., Santini, A. 2019. Abscisic acid identification in Okra, *Abelmoschus esculentus* L. (Moench): Perspective nutraceutical use for the treatment of diabetes. *Nat Prod Res* 34: 3–9. https://doi.org/10.1080/14786419.2019.1637874.

Dantas, T.L, Alonso Buriti, F.C, Florentino, E.R. 2021. Okra (Abelmoschus esculentus L.) as a Potential Functional Food Source of Mucilage and Bioactive Compounds with Technological Applications and Health Benefits. Plants 10(8): 1683. doi: 10.3390/plants10081683.

Das, S., Sarkar, D., Sen, A.K., Sen, D.B., Das, R. Jha, S.K. 2023. Innovative Pharmaceutical Excipient and Their Evaluation: A Study on Okra Fruit. *Current Overview on Pharmaceutical Sci* 5: 55–74. https://doi.org/10.9734/bpi/cops/v5/3751C.

Dib, L.M.A., Allali, H., Bendiabdellah, A., Melianim, N., Tabti, B. 2013. Anti-microbial activity and phytochemical screening of Arbutus unedo. L. *J Saudi Chem Soc* 17: 381–385.

Durazzo, A., Lucarini,M., Novellino, E., Souto, E.B., Daliu, P., Santini, A. 2018. *Abelmoschus esculentus* (L.): Bioactive Components' Beneficial Properties—Focused on Antidiabetic Role—For Sustainable Health Applications. *Molecules.* 24(1), 38. https://doi.org/ 10.3390/molecules24010038.

Elkhalifa, A.E.O., Alshammari, E., Adnan, M., Alcantara, J.C., Awadelkareem, A.M., Eltoum, N.E., Mehmood, K., Panda, B.P., Ashraf, S.A. 2021. Okra (Abelmoschus Esculentus) as a Potential Dietary Medicine with Nutraceutical Importance for Sustainable Health Applications. Molecules 26, 696. https://doi.org/10.3390/molecules26030696.

Gao, Y., Kuok, K.I., Jin, Y., Wang, R. 2019. Biomedical applications of Aloe vera. 2019. Critical Reviews in Food Science and Nutrition 59: S244-S256. https://doi.org/10.1080/10408398.2018.1496320.

Giri S., Sahoo, J., Roy, A., Kamalanathan, S., Naik, D. 2023. Treatment on Nature's lap: Use of herbal products in the management of hyperglycemia. *World J Diabetes*. 14(4): 412–423. https://doi.org/10.4239/wjd. v14.i4.412.

Guariguata, L., Whiting, D., Hambleton, I., Beagley, J., Linnenkamp, U., Shaw, J. 2014. Global estimates of diabetes prevalence for 2013 and projections for 2035. *Diabetes Res. Clin. Pract*. 103: 137–149.

Güçlü, S. F., Koyuncu, F., Atay, E. 2022. Organic acid, phenolic acid and flavonoids of medlar during different maturation stages. *Akademik Ziraat Dergisi* 11(2), 207-212. https://doi.org/10.29278/azd.1061365.

Gupta, A., Gupta, R., Lal, B. 2001. Effect of Trigonella foenum-graecum (fenugreek) seeds on glycaemic control and insulin resistance in type 2 diabetes mellitus: A double blind placebo controlled study. *J Assoc Physicians India* 49: 1057–1061.

Hu, L., Yu, W., Li, Y., Prasad, N., Tang, Z. 2014. Antioxidant activity of extract and its major constituents from Okra seed on rat hepatocytes injured by carbon tetrachloride. *Biomed Res Int*, Article ID: 341291 120.

Irshad, M., Shuang, L., Bezhu, H., Debnath, S., Min, L., Rizwan, H. M., Dongliang, Q. 2017. In vitro regeneration of *Abelmoschus esculentus* L. cv. Wufu: Influence of anti-browning additives on phenolic secretion and callus formation frequency in explants. *Hortic Environ Biotechnol* 58: 503–513.

Islam, M. T. 2019. Phytochemical information and pharmacological activities of Okra (Abelmoschus esculentus): A literature-based review. *Phytother Res* 33: 72–80.

Jarret, R. L., Wang, M. L., Levy, I. J. 2011. Seed oil and fatty acid content in Okra (Abelmoschus esculentus) and related species. J Agric Food Chem 59: 4019–4024.

Joseph, B., Jini, D. 2013. Antidiabetic effects of Momordica charantia (bitter melon) and its medicinal potency. Asian Pac J Trop Dis 3: 93–102.

Hermanson, S., Pujari, A., Williams, B., Blackmore, C., & Kaplan, G. 2021. Successes and challenges of implementing an integrative medicine practice in an allopathic medical center. In: Healthcare Vol. 9, No. 2, p. 100457. Elsevier (Amsterdam, The Netherlands).

Kabelo, M., Lucky, L.S., Perpetua, M., Saba, G. 2023. Okra ameliorates hyperglycaemia in pre diabetic and type 2 diabetic patients: A systematic review and meta-analysis of the clinical evidence. Fron. Pharmacol 14: 1132650. https://doi.org/10.3389/fphar.2023.1132650.

Katanić Stanković, J.S., Mićanović, N., Grozdanić, N., Kostić, A.Ž., Gašić, U., Stanojković, T., Popović-Djordjević, J.B. 2022. Polyphenolic Profile, Antioxidant and Antidiabetic Potential of Medlar (Mespilus germanica L.), Blackthorn (Prunus spinosa L.) and Common Hawthorn (Crataegus monogyna Jacq.) Fruit Extracts from Serbia. *Horticulturae* 8: 1053. https://doi.org/10.3390/horticulturae8111053.

Kazimierski, M., Regula, J., Molska, M. 2019. Cornelian cherry (Cornus mas L.) – Characteristics, nutritional and pro-health properties. Acta Sci Pol Technol Aliment 18: 5–12.

Khan, S., Gul, H., Ahmed, A., & Shireen, F. 2023. Anti-diabetic potential of water-soluble polysaccharide from okra pods mucilage diabetes. International Journal of Health Sciences 6(S9), 4795–4802. https://doi.org/10.53730/ijhs.v6nS9.14064.

Kumar, D. S., Tony, D. E., Kumar, A. P., Kumar, K. A., Rao, D.B.S., Nadendla, R. 2013. A review on: Abelmoschus Esculentus (okra). Int Res J Pharm App Sci 3: 129–132.

Li, M., Jin, Mh., Hu, R., Tang, S., Li, K., Gong, X.J., Sun, Y., Wang, Y., Li, W. 2023. Exploring the mechanism of active components from ginseng to manage diabetes mellitus based on network pharmacology and molecular docking. *Sci Rep* 13, 793. https://doi.org/10.1038/s41598-023-27540-4

Liu, J., Zhao, Y., Wu, Q., John, A., Jiang, Y., Yang, J., Liu, H., Yang, B. 2018. Structure characterisation of polysaccharides in vegetable "Okra" and evaluation of hypoglycemic activity. *Food Chem* 242: 211–216.

Majd, N. E, Tabandeh, R. M, Shahriari, A., Soleimani, Z. 2018. Okra (Abelmoscus esculentus) improved islets structure, and down regulated ppars gene expression in pancreas of high-fat diet and streptozotocin-induced diabetic rats. *Cell J* 20: 31–40.

Massounga Bora, A.F., Eric-Parfait Kouame K.J., Li, X., Liu, L., Pan, Y. 2023. New insights into the bioactive polysaccharides, proteins, and triterpenoids isolated from bitter melon (Momordica charantia) and their relevance for nutraceutical and food application: A review. Biological Macromolecules 231, 123173. https://doi.org/10.1016/j.ijbiomac.2023.123173.

Nazhand, A., Lucarini, M., Durazzo, A., Zaccardelli, M., Cristarella, S., Souto, S.B., Silva, A.M., Severino, P., Souto, E.B., Santini, A. 2020. Hawthorn (Crataegus spp.): An Updated Overview on Its Beneficial Properties. Forests 11, 564. https://doi.org/10.3390/f11050564.

Nikpayam, O., Safaei,E., Bahreini, N., Saghafi-Asl, M. 2021. The effects of Okra (Abelmoschus esculentus L.) products on glycemic control and lipid profile: A comprehensive systematic review. J of Functional Foods 87: 104795. https://doi.org/10.1016/j.jff.2021.104795.

Qin, B., Panickar, K. S., Anderson R. A. 2010. Cinnamon: Potential role in the prevention of insulin resistance, metabolic syndrome, and type 2 diabetes. *J Diabetes Sci Technol* 4:685–693.

Rasekh, H. R., Nazari, P., Kamli-Nejad, M., Hosseinzadeh, L. 2008. Acute and subchronic oral toxicity of *Galega officinalis* in rats. *J Ethnopharmacol* 116:21–26.

Richter, E., Geetha, T., Burnett, D., Broderick, T.L., Babu, J.R. 2023. The Effects of Momordica charantia on Type 2 Diabetes Mellitus and Alzheimer's Disease. Int J Mol Sci 24: 4643. https://doi.org/10.3390/ijms24054643.

Petropoulos, S., Fernandes, A., Barros, L., C.F.R. Ferreira, I. 2018. Chemical composition, nutritional value and antioxidant properties of Mediterranean okra genotypes in relation to harvest stage. Food Chemistry 242, 466-474. https://doi.org/10.1016/j.foodchem.2017.09.082.

Reddy M.T., Pandravada S.R., Sivaraj N., Sunil, N. 2016. Characterization of Indian landrace germplast and morphological traits desiderable for designing a customer-driven variety in Okra. (Abelmoschus esculentus L. Moench). Journal of Global Agriculture and Ecology 6(1): 7-34. ISSN: 2454-4205.

Rop, O., Sochor, J., Jurikova, T., Zitka, O., Skutkova, H., Mlcek, J., Salas, P., Krska, B., Babula, P., Adam, V. 2011. Effect of five different stages of ripening on chemical compounds in medlar (*Mespilus germanica* L.). *Molecules* 16: 74–91.

Roy, A., Shrivastava, S. L., Mandal, S. M. 2014. Functional properties of Okra Abelmoschus esculentus L. (Moench): Traditional claims and scientific evidences. *Plant Sci Today* 1: 121–130.

Sahu, S.C. 2023. Holy Basil: A Medicinal Plant in India from Ancient Vedic Times. Ann Clin Case Stud 5(3): 1081. ISSN: 2688-1241.

Sánchez, M., González-Burgos, E., Iglesias I, and Gómez-Serranillos, M. P. 2020. Pharmacological update properties of *Aloe Vera* and its major active constituents. *Molecules* 25:1324. https://doi.org/10.3390/molecules250613241.

Samee, A., Muhammad Amir, R., Ahmad, A., Masoud Watto, F., Ali, M., Azam, M.T., Sheeraz, M., Fatima, F., Zahoor, Z., Zahid, M., Ashraf, H. 2023. Effectiveness of Milk Thistle on Human Body against Diseases: A Comprehensive Review. Sch Bull, 9(2): 8-18. https://doi.org/10.36348/sb.2023.v09i02.002.

Santini, A., Novellino, E. 2014. Nutraceuticals: Beyond the Diet Before the Drugs. Current Bioactive Compounds 10(1). https://dx.doi.org/10.2174/157340721001140724145924.

Singh, D., Chaudhuri, P. K. 2018. A review on phytochemical and pharmacological properties of Holy basil (Ocimum sanctum L.). *Ind Crops Prod* 118: 367–382.

Shabil, M., Bushi, G., Bodige, P.K., Maradi, P.S., Patra, B.P., Padhi, B.K., Khubchandani, J. 2023. Effect of Fenugreek on Hyperglycemia: A Systematic Review and Meta-Analysis. *Medicina* 59: 248. https://doi.org/10.3390/medicina59020248.

Sinisterra-Hunter, X., Hunter, W.B. 2018. Towards a holistic integrated pest management lessons learned from plant-insect mechanisms in the field. In: The Biology of Plant-Insect Interactions. Emani C. Ed., pp. 204–226. CRC Press, Boca Raton, FL,USA.

Soto, C., Raya, L., Perez, J., Gonzalez, I., Perez, S. 2014. Silymarin induces expression of pancreatic Nkx6.1 transcription factor and beta-cell neogenesis in a pancreatectomy model. Molecules 19: 4654–4668.

Tian, Z. H., Miao, F. T., Zhang, X., Wang, Q. H., Lei, N., Guo, L. Ch. 2015. Therapeutic effect of Okra extract on gestational diabetes mellitus rats induced by streptozotocin. *Asian Pacific J Trop Med* 8:1038–1042.

The Plant List. 2013. Version 1.1. Published on the Internet; http://www.theplantlist.org/. (accessed April 27, 2022).

Vats, V., Kaushik, N., Sharma, L., Arora, K., Verma, P.K. 2022. A Review on Traditional Systems of Medicine. Journal of Pharmaceutical Research & Reports 3(4), 1-6. ISSN: 2754-5008.

Vieira, R., Souto, S.B., Sánchez-López, E., López Machado, A., Severino, P., Jose, S., Santini, A., Silva, A.M., Fortuna, A., García, M.L., Souto, E.B. 2019. Sugar-Lowering Drugs for Type 2 Diabetes Mellitus and Metabolic Syndrome—Strategies for In Vivo Administration: Part-II. J Cli. Med 8, 1332. https://doi.org/10.3390/jcm8091332.

Wolfram, T., Ismail-Beigi, F. 2010. Efficacy of high-fiber diets in the management of type 2 diabetes mellitus. *Endocr Pract* 17:132–142.

Yousef, M. I., El-Demerdash, F. M., Radwan F.M.E. 2008. Sodium arsenite induced biochemical perturbations in rats: Ameliorating effect of curcumin. *Food and Chem Toxicol* 46:3506–3511.

Zhang,T., Xiang, J., Zheng, G.,Yan, R., Min, X. 2018. Preliminary characterization and anti-hyperglycemic activity of a pectic polysaccharide from Okra (*Abelmoschus esculentus* (L.) Moench). *Journal of
Functional Food* 41: 9-14.

Zeng, Y., Luo, Y.; Wang, L., Zhang, K., Peng, J., Fan, G. 2023. Therapeutic Effect of Curcumin on Metabolic
Diseases: Evidence from Clinical Studies. *Int. J. Mol. Sci.* 24, 3323. https://doi.org/10.3390/ijms24043323.

Zocchi, E., Hontecillas, R., Leberm A., Einerhand, A., Carbo, A., Bruzzone, S., Tubau-Juni, N., Philipson, N.,
Zoccoli-Rodriguez, V., Sturla, E., Bassaganya-Riera, J. 2017. Abscisic acid: A novel nutraceutical for
glycemic control. *Front Nutr* 13: 4–24.

23 Scarlet Gourd (*Coccinia grandis* L. Voigt)
Use in Diabetes, Molecular, Cellular Metabolic Effects

Keddagoda Gamage Piyumi Wasana and Anoja Priyadarshani Attanayake

CONTENTS

ABBREVIATIONS

ALP	alkaline phosphatase
ALT	alanine aminotransferase
AST	aspartate aminotransferase
FPG	fasting plasma glucose
HbA_{1c}	glycated hemoglobin
HOMA-IR	homeostasis model assessment for insulin resistance
MCH	mean corpuscular hemoglobin
MCHC	mean corpuscular hemoglobin concentration
MCV	mean corpuscular volume
OGTT	oral glucose tolerance test
PCV	packed cell volume
RBC	red blood cells

DOI: 10.1201/9781003220930-25

TC	total cholesterol
TG	triglycerides
VLDL-C	very low-density lipoprotein cholesterol
WBC	white blood cells
γ-GT	γ-glutamyl transferase

23.1 INTRODUCTION

23.1.1 MORPHOLOGY

Coccinia grandis (L.) Voigt (Cucurbitaceae) is an edible perennial herbaceous climber with a large tuberous root, cylindrical glabrous stems, and simple tendrils. *C. indica* and *C. cordifolia* are synonyms for *C. grandis*. The plant *C. grandis* is called scarlet gourd in English, *kowakka* or *kem-wel* in Sinhala, and *kovai* or *kwai* in Tamil. This plant can be widely found in Sri Lanka, India, Malaya, and tropical Africa. It is widely naturalized in these regions of the world, as the plant is able to thrive well in warm, humid, and tropical areas. Its simple, alternate, 5–10 cm long dull green leaves are glabrous on both sides with glaucous beneath. The regular, unisexual, star-shaped white flowers of *C. grandis* are dioecious, solitary, and axillary, and its fusiform, ovoid, and cylindrical fruits are marked with white streaks when immature and becomes bright scarlet when fully ripe. The plant *C. grandis* exerts a high growth rate by readily covering small trees and shrubs. Seeds typically germinate in 2–4 weeks at 20°C. The eye-catching nature of the flora leads to its use as a garden ornament. Figure 23.1 shows fresh leaves, flowers, raw, and ripe fruits of *C. grandis*.

23.2 BACKGROUND

23.2.1 PHYTOMEDICINES TO MANAGE DIABETES MELLITUS

Diabetes mellitus, a chronic disease, affected 463 million adults (20–79 years) around the world in 2019. The prevalence of diabetes mellitus is steadily increasing and is projected to reach 700 million by 2045 (IDF 2019). Several oral hypoglycemic agents with various mechanisms of action are available to treat diabetes mellitus. These mechanisms of action include (a) slowing carbohydrate

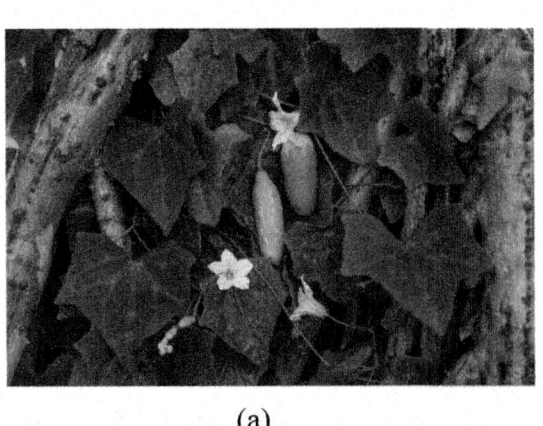

(a)

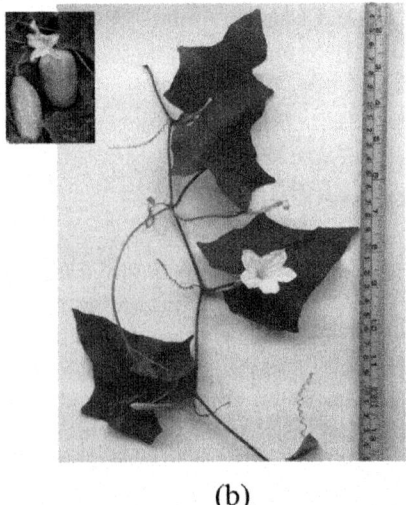

(b)

FIGURE 23.1   Fresh leaves, flowers, raw, and ripe fruits of *Coccinia grandis* (A) in natural habitat; (B) close view of aerial parts of the climber.

absorption from the intestine by α-glucosidase, (b) reduction of liver gluconeogenesis by biguanides, (c) stimulating insulin synthesis by sulfonylurea and nonsulfonylurea secretagogues, and (d) reduction of liver glucose production by thiazolidinediones (Bösenberg and Van Zyl 2008). However, these medications have several side effects such as hypoglycemia, weight gain, lactic acidosis, edema, acute pancreatitis, renal dysfunction, risk of bladder cancer, vitamin B_{12} and folate deficiencies, and gastrointestinal effects including nausea, vomiting, diarrhea, and flatulence (Chaudhury et al. 2017). Furthermore, these agents have not significantly reduced the mortality rate, and some are associated with diabetic complications. The growing impact of diabetes mellitus and its complications lead to one death every 8 seconds in the world (IDF 2019). Due to these facts, focus on therapeutic agents derived from natural sources has gained much interest all over the world.

Phytomedicines, as one of the largest natural sources, have never been obsolete and still play an important role in human health care. More than 1,200 plants have been recognized as potential remedies for the management of diabetes mellitus. Among them, over 400 plants and 700 recipes and compounds have been scientifically evaluated for their antidiabetic properties (Chang et al. 2013). To date, phytomedicines have focused on in-depth pathophysiology of diabetes mellitus through multiple mechanisms such as glucose-lowering, anti-inflammatory, antioxidant, and lipid-lowering activities (Kasole et al. 2019; Salehi et al. 2019).

23.3 *COCCINIA GRANDIS* AS A FOOD-CUM-MEDICINE

From time immemorial, each part of *C. grandis*, predominantly the leaves and fruits, have been used in indigenous medicine systems for the treatment of diabetes mellitus. In effect, this medicinal plant is considered a reservoir of antidiabetic effects. According to ethnobotanical surveys, *C. grandis* leaves are known to be of great importance in complementary medicine for the treatment of diabetes mellitus in Sri Lanka and India (Medagama et al. 2014; Das et al. 2019). It is recommended to use 22.5 g of fresh leaves of *C. grandis* per day as *mallum* or *sambol* for the treatment of mild hyperglycemia in Sri Lankan traditional and Ayurvedic medicine (Anonymous 1979). Young leaves, immature fruits, and long, slender stems of *C. grandis* are cooked as a curry or added to make porridge. Raw and ripe fruits are prominent ingredients in salads. In India, the fruit is frequently supplemented to prepare *sambhar*, which is the name for the South Indian lentil-based vegetable soup. Thai natives use the fruit to prepare several culinary dishes (Das et al. 2019).

The fresh leaf of *C. grandis* or its juice is applied for skin eruptions, such as in ringworm infections. Leaves are used internally as decoctions in the management of gonorrhea (Jayaweera 1980). *C. grandis* is also useful in acute and chronic pyelitis and strangury. It has antilithic properties and is employed for urinary gravel and calculi (Jayaweera 1980). Leaves and fruits are also utilized in healing of snakebites. The stem of *C. grandis* is recommended for asthma, bronchitis, gastrointestinal disturbances, and intermittent glycosuria (Jayaweera 1980). Stems are also dipped into the eye to treat cataract. Patients are advised to use root decoction for pain relief in joints, skin lesions, and aphthous ulcers. Raw or ripe fruit is endorsed as an ingredient in salads for patients with diabetes. Accordingly, the plant exerts immense medicinal significance by means of the management of several diseases in traditional medicine.

As mentioned earlier, *C. grandis* is one of the most often used plants in herbal medicine to manage diabetes mellitus. Despite its use in traditional health care systems around the world, it is important to scientifically assess the efficacy and safety of this plant with regard to its antidiabetic activities. Next, the eminence of *C. grandis* is described with an aim to introduce it as a promising antidiabetic agent.

23.4 ANTIDIABETIC ACTIVITY: PRECLINICAL STUDIES

Based on important records of *Coccinia grandis* as an antidiabetic agent in traditional health care systems, several preclinical studies have been performed to assess its efficacy and safety. Although people believe that *C. grandis* preparations/isolated bioactive compounds are safer than allopathic drugs, perhaps these agents can be toxic for several reasons, such as overdose, contamination with toxic metals, adulteration, misidentification, substitution of herbal ingredients, and improper processing methods. Therefore, it is important to assess the toxicity of *C. grandis* extracts in addition to their potential efficacy before recommending them for primary health care needs.

Meenatchi et al. (2017) have studied the cytoprotective effect of the methanolic extract of *C. grandis* fruit against alloxan-induced diabetic cell death using MTT assay. In general, alloxan, a free radical-producing agent, is reported to decrease the number of RINm5F cells. The results of the MTT assay revealed that *C. grandis* fruit extract was able to protect against alloxan-induced RINm5F cell damage (Meenatchi et al. 2017). Furthermore, the study revealed concentration-dependent *in vitro* insulin secretory potential of the methanolic extract of *C. grandis* fruit in RINm5F cells. A sudden increase in blood glucose concentration after a meal occurs mainly due to starch hydrolysis by pancreatic α-amylase and glucose uptake by intestinal α-glucosidase. The products of starch hydrolysis are not absorbed in the duodenum and upper jejunum and therefore are further hydrolyzed into glucose by α-glucosidase. Glucose is transported from the intestinal lumen into the bloodstream via the carrier of glucose, the Na+/glucose cotransporter. Therefore, inhibition of the enzymes α-amylase and α-glucosidase suppresses carbohydrate digestion, delays glucose uptake, and thus reduces the blood glucose level. The transport of glucose through the yeast cell membrane may involve facilitated diffusion. The concentration within the cell is decreased upon conversion of glucose to other metabolites. This phenomenon inspires high uptake of glucose within cells and further supports antidiabetic activity. Several *in vitro* studies have reported the antidiabetic activity of several parts of *C. grandis* via the assessment of α-amylase and α-glucosidase inhibitory activities, the potential of glucose uptake, and so forth (Raja et al. 2014; Patel and Ishnava 2015; Poongunran et al. 2015; Pulbutr et al. 2017). Furthermore, it has been given an account to exert remarkable *in vitro* antidiabetic activity of synthesizing silver nanoparticles of *C. grandis* hydroalcoholic stem extract, and therefore, Momin and Yeligar (2021) have proposed to utilize silver nanoparticles as the vehicle in the drug delivery system in the development of the novel drug leads. Inhibition of the formation of advanced glycated end products is one of the target therapies against the development and progression of diabetes mellitus and its associated complications. Indeed, advanced glycated end product formation instigates under hyperglycemic conditions and is characterized by the conversion of reversible Schiff-base adducts to covalently bound Amadori products, which undergo further rearrangements in the formation of irreversibly bound advanced glycated end products. An *in vitro* study reported the potency of the formation of glycated end products by the methanol extract of *C. grandis* fruit through the assessment of biochemical parameters (Meenatchi et al. 2017).

In summary, efficacy and toxicity evaluations were performed in alloxan-induced diabetic male Wistar rats, and the results revealed that aqueous leaf extract of *C. grandis* at a dose of 0.75 mg/kg exerts optimal glucose-lowering activity (Attanayake et al. 2013). An acute toxicity study of the aqueous leaf extract of *C. grandis* was shown to be safe in healthy Wistar rats up to a dose of 2 g/kg. A subchronic toxicity study revealed that oral administration of *C. grandis* aqueous leaf extract (0.75 g/kg per day) for 30 days was not associated with adverse effects reflected in general condition, growth, body, and relative weight of organs such as heart, lung, small intestine, liver, spleen, pancreas, and kidney. The toxicity studies have further revealed that there were no statistically significant differences in the liver and kidney function tests and hematological parameters. The histopathological findings revealed the absence of treatment-related cellular changes in hematoxylin and eosin–stained sections of the heart, lung, small intestine, liver, spleen, pancreas, and kidney (Attanayake et al. 2013). Consequently, several studies have testified to the remarkable antidiabetic activity and safety of different extracts of *C. grandis* in chemically induced diabetic rats (Attanayake et al. 2015a; Mohammed et al. 2016; Doss and Dhanabalan 2008; Suryawanshi et al. 2020; Packirisamy et al. 2018).

The antidiabetic activity of *C. grandis* is presumably by its antioxidant, anti-inflammatory, and lipid-lowering activities, among others. To date, several promising reports on potent antioxidant, anti-inflammatory, and lipid-lowering activities of *C. grandis* are available; therefore they could be used to control the development and progression of diabetes-associated complications (Doss and Dhanabalan 2008; Deshpande et al. 2011; Attanayake et al. 2015b; Mohammed et al. 2016).

23.5 SYNERGISTIC EFFECT OF *COCCINIA GRANDIS* ON THE MANAGEMENT OF DIABETES MELLITUS: PRECLINICAL STUDIES

The antidiabetic activity of a plant extract could be improved by combining it with other plant extracts or drugs that have comparable activity. By the same token, the extracts of *C. grandis* have shown an increased antidiabetic activity with safety in the form of combined plant mixtures. Administration of combined aqueous extracts of *C. grandis* leaves and *Abroma augusta* L. (Malvaceae) root (300 mg/kg body weight) for 8 weeks resulted in better antihyperglycemic and antihyperlipidemic activities in streptozotocin-induced diabetic rats than its administration as a single preparation (Eshrat 2003). Synergism was also stated by Rajesh et al. (2010), with the administration of an aqueous extract of *C. grandis* and *Morinda citrifolia* L. (Rubiaceae) fruits (300 mg/kg body weight) in alloxan-induced diabetic rats for 30 days. The results of the study denoted a reduction in serum glucose concentration and an increase in serum insulin concentration (Rajesh et al. 2010). Similarly, *C. grandis* extracts have shown enhanced antidiabetic activity with the combination of several plant extracts (Mallick et al. 2007; Mallick et al. 2009; Saklani et al. 2012). Drug combinations of *C. grandis* extract with allopathic oral hypoglycemic agents such as acarbose, glibenclamide, and pioglitazone have resulted in improved efficacy and safety in chemically induced diabetic rat models (Jose and Usha 2011; Kohli and Kumar 2014; Basavarajappa et al. 2020).

23.6 ANTIDIABETIC ACTIVITY: CLINICAL STUDIES

Even though herbal preparations are widely used in the management of several diseases, the assurance of the risk-benefit ratio of herbal preparations is infrequent. The actual benefits and risks of herbal preparations are evaluated via clinical trials according to the standards of modern clinical science. Clinical trials are studies that prospectively assign human participants to one or more health-associated interventions to determine the influences on health outcomes. Most of the clinical trials of herbal medicines have focused on the standardized extract of a single medicinal plant or a mixture of several plant extracts. Generally, the goal of a clinical trial is to evaluate efficacy, safety, or risk-benefit ratio.

Several scientific studies have been conducted on the evaluation of the efficacy and safety of *C. grandis* in exploiting its antidiabetic effects in human subjects. The hypoglycemic effect of *C. grandis* has been assessed in healthy subjects through a phase I double-blind, randomized, placebo-controlled clinical trial (Munasinghe et al. 2011). A total of 61 healthy volunteers received a test meal of 20 g of *C. grandis* leaves mixed with the measured amount of scraped coconut and table salt. Another 61 healthy volunteers received a placebo meal consisting of scraped coconut and salt. The test meal of fresh *C. grandis* was able to significantly reduce the postprandial blood glucose concentration measured by OGTT (75 g) compared to a placebo meal (Munasinghe et al. 2011) by implicating an improvement in glucose tolerance by *C. grandis* leaves in healthy individuals. Furthermore, Munasinghe et al. (2011) suggested that the hypoglycemic activity of *C. grandis* leaves could cause an increase in insulin synthesis and glucose uptake by muscle cells and adipocytes, a reduction in glucose release from the liver, and the rate of glucose absorption from the gut.

To date, dual action therapy with respect to antihyperglycemic activity and lipid-lowering potential of *C. grandis* leaves has been reported through a phase II double-blind, randomized, placebo-controlled clinical trial of newly diagnosed patients with type 2 diabetes mellitus (Wasana et al. 2021a). In this study, 79 patients received an herbal capsule of *C. grandis* and 79 patients received a placebo capsule of corn starch. The herbal capsule consisted of 100% genuine freeze-dried powder of hot water extract of *C. grandis* leaves. The study revealed that the administration of herbal capsule *C. grandis* (500 mg/day) for 3 months was able to significantly improve glycemic parameters; HbA_{1c}, FPG concentration, serum concentration of fructosamine, insulin, HOMA-IR, and lipid profile parameters; TG and VLDL-C with well-tolerated safety in patients with newly diagnosed type 2 diabetes mellitus. Apart from intensive glycemic and lipid profile control, achieving tight control of oxidative stress and inflammation in patients with type 2 diabetes mellitus has occurred upon the administration of the herbal capsule *C. grandis* (Wasana et al. 2021b). It was evident through the significant increment of the serum activity of glutathione reductase and the significant decrement of serum concentrations of malonaldehyde and interleukin-6 (Wasana et al. 2021b). Importantly, one of the end points in the clinical trial showed that administration of the herbal capsule *C. grandis* for 3 months in patients with diabetes mellitus patients was safe after evaluation of several parameters on renal toxicity; creatinine, liver toxicity; AST, ALT, ALP, γ-GT, and hematotoxicity; WBC, RBC, hemoglobin, platelet count, PCV, MCV, MCH, MCHC (Wasana et al. 2021a).

According to a study carried out by Khan et al. (1980), maturity-onset diabetic patients have received the tablet made out of the homogenized freeze-dried powder of *C. indica* leaves or placebo tablets made out of chlorophyll for 6 weeks. At the end of 6 weeks of a double-blind controlled trial, a significant reduction in FPG concentration and OGTT (50 g) with well-tolerated safety were observed in the test group, compared to the placebo tablet–treated group.

The potent hypoglycemic activity of *C. cordifolia* was assessed via a double-blind, randomized, placebo-controlled clinical trial (Kuriyan et al. 2008). In the study, 60 newly detected diabetic patients were randomized equally into groups to receive test capsules or placebo capsules at 1 g/day for 3 months. The test capsule consisted of alcoholic extract of the aerial parts of *C. cordifolia* (fruits and leaves), whereas the placebo capsules consisted of maltodextrin. The study results revealed a significant decrement in FPG concentration, postprandial blood glucose, and HbA_{1c} in the test capsule–treated group when compared to the placebo capsule–treated group. However, the study did not report changes in the lipid profile after administration of the test capsule (Kuriyan et al. 2008).

Administration of dried extract of *C. indica* for 6 weeks in patients with diabetes was able to restore the activity of the lipoprotein lipase enzyme and reduce glucose-6-phosphatase and lactate dehydrogenase (Kamble et al. 1998). Therefore, it could conclude that dry extract of *C. indica* mimics the insulin action.

It was reported as a remarkable decrement of blood glucose concentration upon the administration of beverage prepared by Indian variety of ivy gourd leaf in patients with diabetes (Lu et al. 2018). In the study, three embodiments of the leaf beverage were assessed: (1) a mixture of ivy gourd aqueous leaf extract, 1 g stevioside, and 0.1 g potassium sorbate; (2) a mixture of ivy gourd aqueous leaf extract, 1.5 g stevioside, and 0.15 g potassium sorbate; and (3) a mixture of ivy gourd aqueous leaf extract, 2 g stevioside, and 0.2 g potassium sorbate. All three embodiments resulted in a decrease in blood glucose concentration. Furthermore, it was confirmed that the potential of glucose-lowering activity of ivy gourd leaf beverage is preferable to that of fresh leaves of ivy gourd (Lu et al. 2018).

23.7 SYNERGISTIC EFFECT OF *COCCINIA GRANDIS* IN HERBAL MIXTURES TO MANAGE DIABETES MELLITUS: CLINICAL STUDIES

The synergetic effect of *C. grandis* has been clinically substantiated to a limited degree. The organic extract of *C. indica* (250–300 mg/day) together with the organic extract of *Salacia chinensis* L. (Celastraceae) (400–550 mg/day) resulted in a reduction of FPG concentration and postprandial glucose concentration in patients with diabetes (Dubey et al. 2009). The administration of organic extracts of *C. indica* (200–300 mg/day) along with *Hippophae rhamnoides* L. (Elaeagnaceae) (250–450 mg/day) was able to reduce TC and TG in diabetic patients (Dubey et al. 2009). Administration of the mixture of organic extracts of *C. indica* (200–300 mg/day), *H. rhamnoides* (250–450 mg/day), and *S. chinensis* (400–650 mg/day) was able to significantly improve FPG concentration, postprandial blood glucose concentration, and manage TC, TG, and LDL-C in diabetic patients (Dubey et al. 2009). Based on the mentioned facts, *C. grandis* could be lucratively blended with a sense of modern science to develop novel antidiabetic agents to treat diabetes mellitus and its complications.

After the successful completion of clinical trials and based on the records of the use of medicinal flora for thousands of years, advances in medicinal plant research have promoted novel herbal preparations as medicines for diabetes mellitus. To date, several herbal products of *C. grandis* are available on the market. The renowned formulated herbal drug diasulin consists of ten plant ingredients, including *C. indica* fruits. The aquoeus leaf extract of *C. grandis* extract from Sri Lanka has been standardized and a new herbal capsule has been developed using the freeze-dried powder of the standardized aqueous extract for the treatment of the development of type 2 diabetes mellitus (Attanayake et al. 2016a; Wasana et al. 2021a).

23.8   TOXICITY AND CAUTIONARY NOTES

Despite numerous advantages associated with *C. grandis* in the treatment of diabetes mellitus, there is obvious concern about its toxicity and cautionary notes. Herbal preparations of *C. grandis* have a high chance of microbes and heavy metal contamination that could unfavorably affect human health (Okaiyeto and Oguntibeju 2021). However, plant preparations are prominently contaminated with microbes. Therefore, recommended quality control guidelines are needed regarding the potential health risks associated with the use of preparations of *C. grandis*. In fact, the standardized form of *C. grandis* is highly recommended for human consumption (Attanayake et al. 2016a; Wasana et al. 2021a). There is a general notion that the toxicity of medicinal plants varies with their chemical composition. The potential toxicity of *C. grandis* could be raised from acute or chronic exposure even with extracts of low toxicity. Clinical trials and several studies on *in vitro* cytotoxicity, acute toxicity, repeated dose toxicity, subchronic toxicity, and chronic toxicity in experimental animals revealed the safety of *C. grandis* (Khan et al. 1980; Attanayake et al. 2013; Mohammed et al. 2016; Meenatchi et al. 2017; Packirisamy et al. 2018; Wasana et al. 2021a). To date, no toxicity and cautionary notes of *C. grandis* have been reported based on the scientific investigations.

23.9   ANTIDIABETIC DRUG LEADS: ACTIVE PHYTOCONSTITUENTS OF *COCCINIA GRANDIS*

There is renewed interest in the isolation and characterization of pharmacologically active compounds from medicinal plants and in the discovery of new drugs by applying new technologies. Thus far, several studies reported the presence of bioactive phytoconstituents such as polyphenols, alkaloids, flavonoids, and saponins in *C. grandis*, and these metabolites involve bioactivities including antidiabetic, antioxidant, and anti-inflammatory activities via several mechanisms (Attanayake et al. 2015b; Attanayake et al. 2016b; Sunny et al. 2020).

Cucurbitacins B (Figure 23.2(1)) and D (Figure 23.2(2)), cephalandrol, cephalandrin A and B, and related analogs were identified as drug leads responsible for the glucose-lowering potential in the standardized extract of *C. grandis* (Subbiah 2008). However, to date, the exact underlying mechanisms of these compounds in connection with reported bioactivities have not been explored.

The bioactive compound of C_{60}-polyprenol (Figure 23.3) has been isolated from the ethanol extract of *C. grandis* and has been tested in high-fat–fed hamsters (Singh et al. 2007). Administration

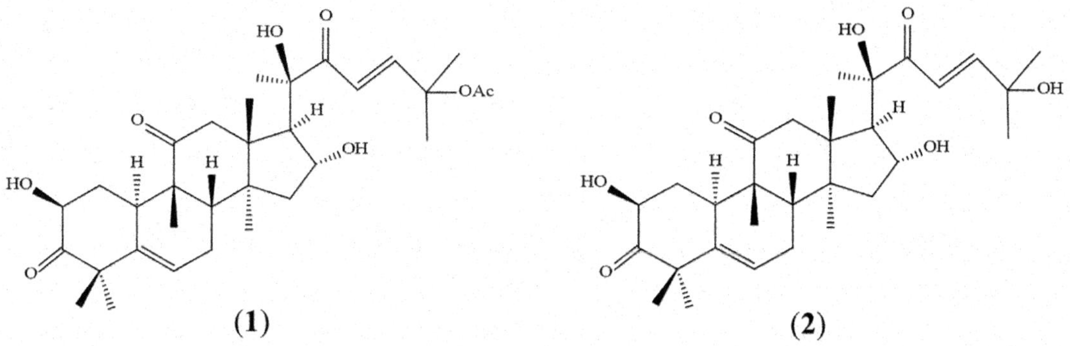

FIGURE 23.2   Molecular structures of (1) cucurbitacins B and (2) cucurbitacins D.

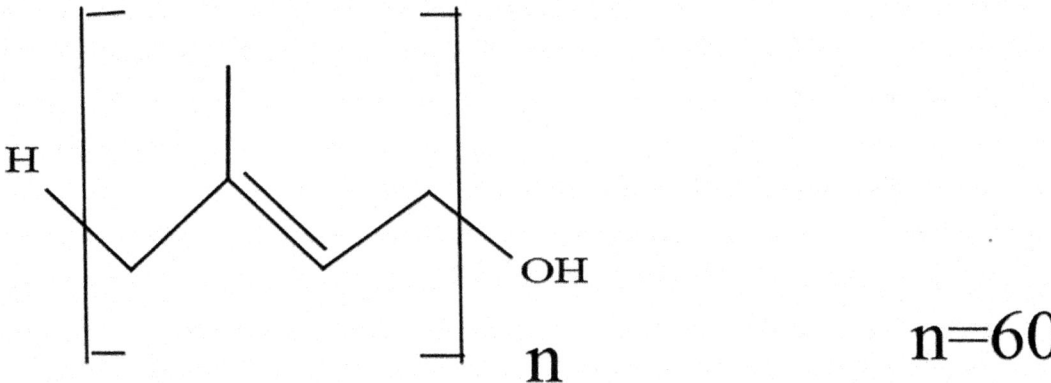

FIGURE 23.3 Molecular structure of C_{60}-polyprenol.

of suspended C_{60}-polyprenol (50 mg/kg per day) in the vehicle that had 1% methylcellulose for 1 week was able to significantly reduce serum triglyceride by 42%, TC by 25%, and glycerol by 12%, accompanied by ratio of HDL-C/TC by 26% in high-fat–fed dyslipidemic hamsters, implicating a marked reverse in dyslipidemia. Furthermore, the results of the study revealed that these favorable outcomes were comparable to the standard drug fenofibrate at a dose of 108 mg/kg.

Phytoconstituents such as lupeol, β-sitosterol, ferulic acid, and trans-p-coumaric acid were isolated from the plant, and these isolated compounds are well documented to exert medicinal properties including hypoglycemic, antioxidant, and anti-inflammatory activities (Ohnishi et al. 2004; Gupta et al. 2011; Niture et al. 2014; Amalan et al. 2016). The prominent bioactive compounds isolated from the different parts of *C. grandis* are shown in Table 23.1.

To date, the bioactivities of isolated compounds have been evaluated through *in vitro* studies and *in vivo* studies on experimental animal models. Therefore, it is urgently necessary to assess the clinical efficacy and safety of these compounds and thus develop novel antidiabetic drugs/drug leads for the management of diabetes mellitus and its complications.

TABLE 23.1

Isolated Bioactive Phytoconstituents of *Coccinia grandis*

Parts of the Plant	Extract	Isolated Compound	Reference
Fruit	n-Butanolic	Lupeol	Meenatch et al. 2018

Parts of the Plant	Extract	Isolated Compound	Reference
Fruit	n-Butanolic or methanolic	β-Sitosterol	Meenatch et al. 2018
Leaves	Methanol	Ferulic acid	Al-Madhagy et al. 2019a
Leaves	Methanol	Kaempferol-3-O-rutinoside	Al-Madhagy et al. 2019b
Leaves	Methanol	Kaempferol-3-O-β-D-glucoside	Al-Madhagy et al. 2019a
Leaves	Methanol	Trans-p-coumaric acid	Al-Madhagy et al. 2019a

(*Continued*)

TABLE 23.1
(Continued)

Parts of the Plant	Extract	Isolated Compound	Reference
Leaves	Methanol	Ligstroside	Al-Madhagy et al. 2019a
Leaves	Methanol	Methyl caffeate	Al-Madhagy et al. 2019a
Leaves	Methanol	Oleuropein	Al-Madhagy et al. 2019b
Leaves	Methanol	Quercetin-3-O-neohesperidoside	Al-Madhagy et al. 2019b

Parts of the Plant	Extract	Isolated Compound	Reference
Leaves	Methanol		Al-Madhagy et al. 2019b

Rutin

| Whole plant | Dichloromethane | | Gantait et al. 2010 |

Taraxerol

23.10 CELLULAR AND MOLECULAR MECHANISMS OF *COCCINIA GRANDIS* EXTRACTS

It is important to review cellular and molecular mechanisms of action and specific molecular targets of *C. grandis* extracts and their isolated compounds in the development of novel antidiabetic drugs with proper dosing. Administration of *C. grandis* aqueous leaf extract (0.75 g/kg) in alloxan-induced diabetic rats for 30 days has produced a significant β cell regeneration potential via increment of the number of islets and percentage of insulin-secreting β cells (Attanayake et al. 2019). Similar findings were also observed with the treatment of *C. grandis* aqueous leaf extract at the same dose in streptozotocin-induced diabetic rats (Attanayake et al. 2015a). Insulin-dependent glucose removal from the bloodstream into skeletal muscle is an important determinant of proper glycemic control in patients with diabetes mellitus. In that process, insulin recruits glucose transporter 4 (GLUT4) to the plasma membrane to promote the uptake of glucose. The water extract of the *C. indica* stem promoted glucose uptake by increasing the amount of GLUT4 on the cell membrane and increasing the production of GLUT1 in rat L8 myotubes (Purintrapiban et al. 2006). Oral administration of the ethanolic leaf extract of *C. indica* depressed the glucose-6-phosphatase and fructose-1,6-bisphosphatase enzyme activities and thereby slowing down the process of gluconeogenesis in streptozotocin-induced diabetic rats after 18 hours of fasting (Shibib et al. 1993). Furthermore, the study revealed the glucose oxidation potential of *C. indica* leaves (Shibib et al. 1993). A similar observation as depression of glucose-6-phosphatase and fructose-1,6-bisphosphatase enzyme activities was also observed upon the administration of ethanolic extract of *C. grandis* unripe fruit (125–750 mg/kg of body weight) in streptozotocin-induced diabetic rats (Packirisamy et al. 2018). Another study reported the enzymes; glucose-6-phosphatase and fructose-1,6-bisphosphatase, inhibition activities, and improvement of glucose uptake by stimulating hepatic hexokinase in the glycolytic pathway upon the administration of the ethanolic extract of *C. grandis* leaves (200 mg/kg body weight) in streptozotocin-induced diabetic rats (Venkateswaran and Pari 2002). In the investigation of underlined mechanisms of action related to the glucose-lowering potential of *C. grandis*, attention has also been paid to evaluating the mechanisms related to the potential for lipid-lowering. Pochhi (2019) reported a significant reduction of lipid metabolizing enzymes such as HMG CoA-reductase and lecithin cholesterol acyltransferase upon the administration of the aqueous extract of *C. indica* leaves (200 mg/kg) in alloxan-induced diabetic rats. A molecular coupling study carried out by Udayasankar and Santhi (2020) revealed that *C. indica* had potential inhibitors; pectin, ellagic acid, and cucurbitacin for the catalytic subunit of the human 5′-AMP-activated protein kinase catalytic subunit $α_2$, a diabetic target that implicates its antidiabetic approaches.

Furthermore, pectin isolated from the fruit of *C. indica* exerted hypoglycemic activity and occurred through an enhanced process of glycolysis by activating the activity of the hexokinase enzyme, increased glycogenesis, and decreased glycogenolysis (Kumar et al. 1993). Administration of pectin (200 mg/100 g body weight) in normal rats showed a significant reduction in blood glucose concentration (Kumar et al. 1993). Consequently, the experimental findings on the cellular mechanisms of action and target of *C. grandis* describe the way that biological parts collaborate to provide an effective and safe antidiabetic medicine.

23.11 OTHER FOODS, HERBS, SPICES, AND BOTANICALS USED IN DIABETES MELLITUS

In addition to the use of *C. grandis*, several other medicinal herbs, spices, and food supplements are used in the management of diabetes mellitus mostly where indigenous medicines are well established. Examples include seeds of *Syzygium cumini* L. Skeels (Myrtaceae); root bark of *Salacia reticulate* var. b-diandra Weight (Celestraceae); fruit of *Phyllanthus emblica* L. (Euphorbiaceae); stem bark of *Ficus religiosa* L. (Moraceae); whole plant of *Scoparia dulcis* L. (Scrophulariaceae); leaves of *Gymnema sylvestre* R. Br (Apocynaceae); fruit of *Terminalia chebula* Retz. (Combretaceae); rhizome of *Alpinia galangal* L. Willd (Zingiberaceae); leaves of *Adhathoda vasica* L. (Acanthaceae); fruit of *Terminalia bellirica* (Gaertn.) Roxb. (Combretaceae); and roots of *Oryza sativa* L. (Poaceae). Plant preparations are in different forms, such as decoctions, porridge, powders, pastes, and juices. The formation of decoctions may involve a single medicinal plant or mixture of plants. Most of the time, the decoctions of polyherbal mixtures consist of *Aloe vera* L. Burm.f. (Asphodelaceae) and *Cyperus rotundus* L. (Cyperaceae). *A. vera* is used to minimize hypoglycemic complications derived from allopathic drugs (Ediriweera and Ratnasooriya 2009). The fruit of *Momordica charantia* L. (Cucurbitaceae) in the form of salad or curry is recommended for patients with diabetes and complications. In particular, cinnamon is advised as a dietary supplement or spice for patients with diabetes mellitus who have coexisting hypertension (Howard and White 2013). The fruits of *Terminalia chebula*, *T. bellirica*, and *Phyllanthus emblica* are collectively combined to form Triphala, which is widely used in the treatment of diabetes mellitus. Triphala delivers fine advantages in patients with diabetes, such as bowel movement and blood detoxification potential. In addition, several herbal products such as diabecon, diasulin, 180 cp pancreatic tonic, diabeta, gurmar powder, and dia-care have been formulated for the management of diabetes mellitus using various medicinal botanicals (Modak et al. 2007; Choudhury et al. 2018). In most cases, the world population uses these products as dietary supplements or as alternative medicines as adjuvants to existing oral hypoglycemic agents.

To date, antidiabetic activity in terms of efficacy and safety of foods, herbs, spices, and botanicals has been scientifically assessed. *In vitro* studies including α-amylase, α-glucosidase, dipeptidyl peptidase-IV enzymes, inhibitory activities, and glucose uptake rate were carried out on the aqueous leaf extracts of *Murraya koenigii* L. Spreng., *Catharanthus roseus* L., *Gardenia latifolia* Ait., and the methanol extract of *Indianthus virgatus* (Roxb.) (Bhutkar et al. 2018; Tamilselvi et al. 2018; Sangeetha and Rajamani 2019). Antidiabetic activity and acute and long-term toxicity of several extracts of medicinal botanicals such as leaf latex extract of *Aloe megalacantha* Baker, aqueous bark extract of *Fraxinus floribunda* Wall., methanol extract of the entire plant of *Lindernia ciliata* (Colsm.) Pennell, and methanol extract of the aerial parts of *Atylosia albicans* (Wight & Arn.) Benth. have been estimated in chemically induced diabetic rat models (Hammeso et al. 2019; Subba et al. 2019; Reddy and Rani 2020; Umasankar 2020).

A few clinical studies have been conducted on the medicinal botanicals and food cum medicines, including *Zingiber officinale* Roscoe rhizome powder, 70% ethanol fruit extract of *Cornus mas* L., aqueous bark extract of *Cinnamomum cassia*, and 70% ethanol extract of *Balanites aegyptiaca* L. Delile pericarps with an aim to investigate clinical effectiveness and safety against diabetes mellitus (Attari et al. 2015; Soltani et al. 2015; Anderson et al. 2016; Rashad et al. 2017). Based on strong evidence of the antidiabetic activity of medicinal flora, foods, and spices, scientists have isolated several active compounds that could be introduced as lead drug molecules for the treatment of diabetes mellitus. The isolated active compounds include salacinol, kotanalol, gymnemic acid, gallic acid, eugenol, umbelliferone acid, ellagic acid, eucalyptol, ursolic acid, and oleanolic acid (Yoshikawa et al. 1997; Poongunran et al. 2017; Wasana et al. 2021c). Furthermore, the mechanisms of actions related to antidiabetic activity have been explored. Common mechanisms of action included intestinal α-glucosidase inhibitory activity, decreased glucose absorption from the gut, increase in insulin synthesis, reduction in glucose release from the liver, and increase in glucose uptake by adipocytes and muscle cells (Wasana et al. 2021c). Collectively, all these facts signify the importance of medicinal flora and food cum medicine (foods/spices) in the management of diabetes mellitus. Therefore, it is imperative to develop new therapeutic agents from natural resources and thereby deliver an explanation for the economic burden associated with the management of diabetes mellitus.

23.12 CONCLUSIONS AND WAY FORWARD

Coccinia grandis is a high-value medicinal plant that has been used in traditional health care systems to manage diabetes mellitus since ancient times. Preclinical and clinical studies affirmed that different extracts of *C. grandis* and their synergistic potentials were efficacious, effective, and safe against diabetes mellitus and associated diabetic complications, thus recommending their use. Several compounds have been isolated as new drug leads from *C. grandis*. The antidiabetic, antioxidant, and anti-inflammatory potential of these isolated drug lead molecules were investigated through preclinical studies. To date, the efficacy and safety of the isolated drug leads of *C. grandis* have not been pronounced. The reported molecular and cellular mechanisms of action could be utilized in the development of novel antidiabetic agents of *C. grandis*. It is important to conduct clinical trials on different extracts/isolated drug lead molecules of the plant to introduce innovative antidiabetic agents with improved efficacy and safety. In this way, the overall antidiabetic potential of *C. grandis* could be fully understood.

23.13 SUMMARY POINTS

- This chapter focuses on scarlet gourd (*Coccinia grandis* L. Voigt) and its use in diabetes, as well as its molecular and cellular metabolic effects.
- *C. grandis* is widely distributed in warm, humid, and tropical areas including Sri Lanka, India, Malaya, and tropical Africa.
- Every part of *C. grandis* exerts medicinal properties.
- From time immemorial, *C. grandis* has been used to manage diabetes mellitus in traditional health care systems.

- The efficacy and safety of the different extracts of *C. grandis* against diabetes mellitus and its complications have been assessed through preclinical and clinical studies.
- The synergistic effect of *C. grandis* in herbal mixtures delivers improved efficacy and safety against the development and progression of diabetes mellitus.
- Active compounds that exert antidiabetic, antilipidemic, antioxidant, and anti-inflammatory potential have been isolated from *C. grandis*.
- Cellular and molecular mechanisms of action behind the antidiabetic activity of *C. grandis* have been investigated.
- The plant *C. grandis* is a reservoir of antidiabetic activity and other medicinal properties that could be effective in the management of diabetes mellitus.

23.14 ACKNOWLEDGMENT

The research project that has been funded by the World Bank under the Accelerating Higher Education Expansion and Development-AHEAD project (AHEAD/DOR STEM-15), Sri Lanka, is acknowledged for providing financial support for the bioactivity and toxicological studies of *Coccinia grandis* in our research laboratory.

REFERENCES

Al-Madhagy, S., Mostafa, N.M., Youssef, F.S., Awad, G., Eldahshan, O.A. and Singab, A.N.B. 2019a. Isolation and structure elucidation of compounds from *Coccinia grandis* leaves extract. *Egyptian Journal of Chemistry* 62:1869–1877. https://doi.org/10.21608/EJCHEM.2019.10925.1700.

Al-Madhagy, S.A., Mostafa, N.M., Youssef, F.S., Awad, G.E., Eldahshan, O.A. and Singab, A.N.B. 2019b. Metabolic profiling of a polyphenolic-rich fraction of *Coccinia grandis* leaves using LC-ESI-MS/MS and in vivo validation of its antimicrobial and wound healing activities. *Food and Function* 10:6267–6275. https://doi.org/10.1039/c9fo01532a.

Amalan, V., Vijayakumar, N., Indumathi, D. and Ramakrishnan, A. 2016. Antidiabetic and antihyperlipidemic activity of p-coumaric acid in diabetic rats, role of pancreatic GLUT 2: In vivo approach. *Biomedicine and Pharmacotherapy* 84:230–236. https://doi.org/10.1016/j.biopha.2016.09.039.

Anderson, R.A., Zhan, Z., Luo, R., Guo, X., Guo, Q., Zhou, J., Kong, J., Davis, P.A. and Stoecker, B.J. 2016. Cinnamon extract lowers glucose, insulin and cholesterol in people with elevated serum glucose. *Journal of Traditional and Complementary Medicine* 6:332–336. https://doi.org/10.1016/j.jtcme.2015.03.005.

Anonymous, 1979. *Ayurveda Pharmacopeia*, Department of Ayurveda, Sri Lanka, Part 2.

Attanayake, A.P., Arawwawala, L.D.A.M. and Jayatilaka, K.A.P.W. 2016a. Chemical standardization of leaf extract of *Coccinia grandis* (L.) Voigt (Cucurbitaceae) of Sri Lankan origin. *Journal of Pharmacognosy and Phytochemistry* 5:119–123.

Attanayake, A.P., Jayatilaka, K.A.P.W., Mudduwa, L.K.B. and Pathirana, C. 2016b. In vivo antihyperlipidemic, antioxidative effects of *Coccinia grandis* (l.) Voigt (cucurbitaceae) leaf extract: An approach to scrutinize the therapeutic benefits of traditional Sri Lankan medicines against diabetic complications. *International Journal of Pharmaceutical Sciences and Research* 7:3949–3958.

Attanayake, A.P., Jayatilaka, K.A.P.W., Mudduwa, L.K.B. and Pathirana, C. 2019. β-Cell regenerative potential of selected herbal extracts in alloxan induced diabetic rats. *Current Drug Discovery Technologies* 16:278–284. https://doi.org/10.2174/1570163815666180418153024.

Attanayake, A.P., Jayatilaka, K.A.P.W., Pathirana, C. and Mudduwa, L.K.B. 2013. Efficacy and toxicological evaluation of *Coccinia grandis* (Cucurbitaceae) extract in male Wistar rats. *Asian Pacific Journal of Tropical Disease* 3:460–466. https://doi.org/10.1016/S2222-1808(13)60101-2.

Attanayake, A.P., Jayatilaka, K.A.P.W., Pathirana, C. and Mudduwa, L.K.B. 2015a. Antihyperglycemic activity of *Coccinia grandis* (L.) Voigt in streptozotocin induced diabetic rats. *Indian Journal of Traditional Knowledge* 14:376–381.

Attanayake, A.P., Jayatilaka, K.A.P.W., Pathirana, C. and Mudduwa, L.K.B. 2015b. Phytochemical screening and in vitro antioxidant potentials of extracts of ten medicinal plants used for the treatment of diabetes mellitus in Sri Lanka. *African Journal of Traditional, Complementary and Alternative Medicines* 12:28–33. https://doi.org/10.4314/ajtcam.v12i4.5.

Attari, V.E., Mahluji, S., Jafarabadi, M.A. and Ostadrahimi, A. 2015. Effects of supplementation with ginger (*Zingiber officinale* Roscoe) on serum glucose, lipid profile and oxidative stress in obese women: a randomized, placebo controlled clinical trial. *Pharmaceutical Sciences* 21:184–191. https://doi.org/10.15171/PS.2015.35.

Basavarajappa, G.M., Nanjundan, P.K., Alabdulsalam, A., Asif, A.H., Shekharappa, H.T., Anwer, M. and Nagaraja, S. 2020. Improved renoprotection in diabetes with combination therapy of *Coccinia indica* leaf extract and low-dose pioglitazone. *Separations* 7:58. https://doi.org/10.3390/separations7040058.

Bhutkar, M.A., Bhinge, S.D., Randive, D.S., Wadkar, G.H. and Todkar, S.S. 2018. Screening of in vitro hypoglycaemic activity of *Murraya koenigii* and *Catharanthus roseus*. *Ars Pharmaceutica* 59:145–151.

Bösenberg, L.H. and Van Zyl, D.G. 2008. The mechanism of action of oral antidiabetic drugs: A review of recent literature. *Journal of Endocrinology, Metabolism and Diabetes of South Africa* 13:80–88. https://doi.org/10.1080/22201009.2008.10872177.

Chang, C.L., Lin, Y., Bartolome, A.P., Chen, Y.C., Chiu, S.C. and Yang, W.C. 2013. Herbal therapies for type 2 diabetes mellitus: Chemistry, biology, and potential application of selected plants and compounds. *Evidence-Based Complementary and Alternative Medicine* 2013. https://doi.org/10.1155/2013/378657.

Chaudhury, A., Duvoor, C., Reddy Dendi, V.S., Kraleti, S., Chada, A., Ravilla, R., Marco, A., Shekhawat, N.S., Montales, M.T., Kuriakose, K. and Sasapu, A. 2017. Clinical review of antidiabetic drugs: Implications for type 2 diabetes mellitus management. *Frontiers in Endocrinology* 8:6. https://doi.org/10.3389/fendo.2017.00006.

Choudhury, H., Pandey, M., Hua, C.K., Mun, C.S., Jing, J.K., Kong, L., Ern, L.Y., Ashraf, N.A., Kit, S.W., Yee, T.S. and Pichika, M.R. 2018. An update on natural compounds in the remedy of diabetes mellitus: A systematic review. *Journal of Traditional and Complementary Medicine* 8:361–376. https://doi.org/10.1016/j.jtcme.2017.08.012.

Das, D., Devi, K.P., Asha, S., Asha, S. and Maheswar, T. 2019. Ethnomedicinal review of the plant *Coccinia indiaca* (bimbi) and its utilization in India. *International Ayurvedic Medical Journal* 7:1399–1402.

Deshpande, S.V., Patil, M.J., Daswadkar, S.C., Suralkar, U. and Agarwal, A. 2011. A study on anti-inflammatory activity of the leaf and stem extracts of *Coccinia grandis* Voigt. *International Journal of Applied Biology and Pharmaceutical Technology* 2:247–250.

Doss, A. and Dhanabalan, R. 2008. Antihyperglycemic and insulin release effects of *Coccinia grandis* (L.) Voigt leaves in normal and alloxan diabetic rats. *Ethnobotanical Leaflets* 12:1172–1175.

Dubey, G.P., Agarwal, A., Vyas, N. and Rajamanickam, V.G. 2009. *Herbal formulation for the prevention and management of diabetes mellitus and diabetic micro-vascular complications*. U.S. Patent Application 11/994,362.

Ediriweera, E.R.H.S.S. and Ratnasooriya, W.D. 2009. A review on herbs used in treatment of diabetes mellitus by Sri Lankan ayurvedic and traditional physicians. *AYU* 30:373–391.

Eshrat, M.H. 2003. Effect of *Coccinia indica* (L.) and *Abroma augusta* (L.) on glycemia, lipid profile and on indicators of end-organ damage in streptozotocin induced diabetic rats. *Indian Journal of Clinical Biochemistry* 18:54–63. https://doi.org/10.1007/BF02867368.

Gantait, A., Sahu, A., Venkatesh, P., Dutta, P.K. and Mukherjee, P.K. 2010. Isolation of taraxerol from *Coccinia grandis*, and its standardization. *Journal of Planar Chromatography – Modern TLC* 23:323–325. https://doi.org/10.1556/jpc.23.2010.5.3.

Gupta, R., Sharma, A.K., Dobhal, M.P., Sharma, M.C. and Gupta, R.S. 2011. Antidiabetic and antioxidant potential of β-sitosterol in streptozotocin induced experimental hyperglycemia. *Journal of Diabetes* 3:29–37. https://doi.org/10.1111/j.1753-0407.2010.00107.x.

Hammeso, W.W., Emiru, Y.K., Ayalew Getahun, K. and Kahaliw, W. 2019. Antidiabetic and antihyperlipidaemic activities of the leaf latex extract of *Aloe megalacantha* baker (Aloaceae) in streptozotocin-induced diabetic model. *Evidence-Based Complementary and Alternative Medicine* 2019. https://doi.org/10.1155/2019/8263786.

Howard, M.E. and White, N.D. 2013. Potential benefits of cinnamon in type 2 diabetes. *American Journal of Lifestyle Medicine* 7:23–26. https://doi.org/10.1177/1559827612462960.

IDF. 2019. *International Diabetes Federation Atlas*. 9th edition. https://diabetesatlas.org/upload/resources/material/20200302_133351_IDFATLAS9e-final-web.pdf.

Jayaweera, D.M.A. 1980. *Medicinal Plants (Indigenous and exotic) Used in Ceylon*. National Science Council of Sri Lanka, Sri Lanka.

Jose, E. and Usha, P.T.A. 2011. Interaction of *Coccinia indica* with glibenclamide in alloxan induced diabetic rats. *Indian Journal of Veterinary Research* 20:1–7.

Kamble, S.M., Kamlakar, P.L., Vaidya, S. and Bambole, V.D. 1998. Influence of *Coccinia indica* on certain enzymes in glycolytic and lipolytic pathway in human diabetes. *Indian Journal of Medical Sciences* 52:143–146.

Kasole, R., Martin, H.D. and Kimiywe, J. 2019. Traditional medicine and its role in the management of diabetes mellitus: "Patients' and herbalists' perspectives." *Evidence-Based Complementary and Alternative Medicine* 2019. https://doi.org/10.1155/2019/2835691.

Khan, A.K., Akhtar, S. and Mahtab, H. 1980. Treatment of diabetes mellitus with *Coccinia indica*. *British Medical Journal* 280:1044. https://doi.org/10.1136/bmj.280.6220.1044.

Kohli, S. and Kumar, P.N. 2014. Combined effect of *Coccinia indica* leaf extract with acarbose in type II diabetes induced neuropathy in rats. *Journal of Innovations in Pharmaceutical and Biological Sciences* 1:77–87.

Kumar, G.P., Sudheesh, S. and Vijayalakshmi, N.R. 1993. Hypoglycemic effect of *Coccinia indica*: mechanism of action. *Planta Medica* 59:330–332. https://doi.org/10.1055/s-2006-959693.

Kuriyan, R., Rajendran, R., Bantwal, G. and Kurpad, A.V. 2008. Effect of supplementation of *Coccinia cordifolia* extract on newly detected diabetic patients. *Diabetes Care* 31:216–220.

Lu, W., Xiaole, L., Shufang, Y., Qiwei, W., Zhongtian, O. and Yurou, W. 2018. *A kind of India's Ivy gourd leaf beverage and preparation method thereof with effect of lowering blood sugar*. Patent Application D1CN108967787.

Mallick, C., Chatterjee, K., GuhaBiswas, M. and Ghosh, D. 2007. Antihyperglycemic effects of separate and composite extract of root of *Musa paradisiacal* and leaf of *Coccinia indica* in streptozotocin-induced diabetic male albino rat. *African Journal of Traditional, Complementary and Alternative Medicines* 4:362–371. https://doi.org/10.4314/ajtcam.v4i3.31230.

Mallick, C., De, D. and Ghosh, D. 2009. Correction of protein metabolic disorders by composite extract of *Musa paradisiaca* and *Coccinia indica* in streptozotocin-induced diabetic albino rat: An approach through the pancreas. *Pancreas* 38:322–329. https://doi.org/10.1097/MPA.0b013e318192ebdf.

Medagama, A.B., Bandara, R., Abeysekera, R.A., Imbulpitiya, B. and Pushpakumari, T. 2014. Use of complementary and alternative medicines (CAMs) among type 2 diabetes patients in Sri Lanka: A cross sectional survey. *BMC Complementary and Alternative Medicine* 14:1–5. https://doi.org/10.1186/1472-6882-14-374.

Meenatchi, P., Purushothaman, A. and Maneemegalai, S. 2017. Antioxidant, antiglycation and insulinotrophic properties of *Coccinia grandis* (L.) in vitro: Possible role in prevention of diabetic complications. *Journal of Traditional and Complementary Medicine* 7:54–64. https://doi.org/10.1016/j.jtcme.2016.01.002.

Meenatch, P., Purushothaman, A. and Maneemegalai, S. 2018. Antidiabetic efficacy of two major compounds isolated from *Coccinia grandis* (L.) Voigt and their effect on insulin-producing cell line RINm5F in vitro. *Paper presented at the research symposium on Pure and Applied Sciences, Faculty of Science*, University of Kelaniya, Sri Lanka.

Modak, M., Dixit, P., Londhe, J., Ghaskadbi, S. and Devasagayam, T.P.A. 2007. Indian herbs and herbal drugs used for the treatment of diabetes. *Journal of Clinical Biochemistry and Nutrition* 40:163–173. https://doi.org/10.3164/jcbn.40.163.

Mohammed, S.I., Chopda, M.Z., Patil, R.H., Vishwakarma, K.S. and Maheshwari, V.L. 2016. In vivo antidiabetic and antioxidant activities of *Coccinia grandis* leaf extract against streptozotocin induced diabetes in experimental rats. *Asian Pacific Journal of Tropical Disease* 6:298–304. https://doi.org/10.1016/S2222-1808(15)61034-9.

Momin, Y.H. and Yeligar, V.C. 2021. Synthesis of *Coccinia grandis* (L.) Voigt extract's silver nanoparticles and it's in vitro antidiabetic activity. *Journal of Applied Pharmaceutical Science* 11:108–115. https://doi.org/10.7324/JAPS.2021.110815.

Munasinghe, M.A.A.K., Abeysena, C., Yaddehige, I.S., Vidanapathirana, T. and Piyumal, K.P.B. 2011. Blood sugar lowering effect of *Coccinia grandis* (L.) J. Voigt: path for a new drug for diabetes mellitus. *Experimental Diabetes Research* 2011:978762. https://doi.org/10.1155/2011/978762.

Niture, N.T., Ansari, A.A. and Naik, S.R. 2014. Antihyperglycemic activity of rutin in streptozotocin induced diabetic rats: an effect mediated through cytokines, antioxidants and lipid biomarkers. *Indian Journal of Experimental Biology* 52:720–727.

Ohnishi, M., Matuo, T., Tsuno, T., Hosoda, A., Nomura, E., Taniguchi, H., Sasaki, H. and Morishita, H. 2004. Antioxidant activity and hypoglycemic effect of ferulic acid in STZ-induced diabetic mice and KK-A^y mice. *Biofactors* 21:315–319. https://doi.org/10.1002/biof.552210161.

Okaiyeto, K. and Oguntibeju, O.O. 2021. African herbal medicines: Adverse effects and cytotoxic potentials with different therapeutic applications. *International Journal of Environmental Research and Public Health* 18:5988. https://doi.org/10.3390/ijerph18115988.

Packirisamy, M., Ayyakkannu, P. and Sivaprakasam, M. 2018. Antidiabetic effect of *Coccinia grandis* (L.) Voigt (Cucurbitales: Cucurbitaceae) on streptozotocin induced diabetic rats and its role in regulating carbohydrate metabolizing enzymes. *Brazilian Journal of Biological Sciences* 5:683–698. https://doi. org/10.21472/bjbs.051107.

Patel, A.R. and Ishnava, K.B. 2015. In vitro shoot multiplication from nodal explants of *Coccinia grandis* (L.) Voigt. and it's antidiabetic and antioxidant activity. *Asian Journal of Biological Sciences* 8:57–71. https://doi.org/10.3923/ajbs.2015.57.71.

Pochhi, M. 2019. Evaluation of antidiabetic potential and hypolipidemic activity of *Coccinia indica* (leaves) in diabetic albino rats. *Asian Journal of Medical Sciences* 10:49–54. https://doi.org/10.3126/ajms.v10i4.24180.

Poongunran, J., Perera, H.K.I., Fernando, W.I.T., Jayasinghe, L. and Sivakanesan, R. 2015. α-Glucosidase and α-amylase inhibitory activities of nine Sri Lankan antidiabetic plants. *Journal of Pharmaceutical Research International* 7:365–374. https://doi.org/10.9734/BJPR/2015/18645.

Poongunran, J., Perera, H.K.I., Jayasinghe, L., Fernando, I.T., Sivakanesan, R., Araya, H. and Fujimoto, Y. 2017. Bioassay-guided fractionation and identification of α-amylase inhibitors from *Syzygium cumini* leaves. *Pharmaceutical Biology* 55:206–211. https://doi.org/10.1080/13880209.2016.1257031.

Pulbutr, P., Saweeram, N., Ittisan, T., Intrama, H., Jaruchotikamol, A. and Cushnie, B. 2017. In vitro α-amylase and α-glucosidase inhibitory activities of *Coccinia grandis* aqueous leaf and stem extracts. *Journal of Biological Sciences* 17:61–68. https://doi.org/10.3923/jbs.2017.61.68.

Purintrapiban, J., Keawpradub, N. and Jansakul, C. 2006. Role of the water extract from *Coccinia indica* stem on the stimulation of glucose transport in L8 myotubes. *Songklanakarin Journal of Science and Technology* 28:1199–1208.

Raja, A.M., Sushma, K., Banji, D., Rao, K.N.V. and Selvakumar, D. 2014. Evaluation of standardization parameters, pharmacognostic study, preliminary phytochemical screening and in vitro antidiabetic activity of *Coccinia indica* fruits as per WHO guidelines. *Indian Journal of Pharmaceutical and Biological Research* 2:54. https://doi.org/10.30750/ijpbr.2.3.9.

Rajesh, P., Manish, K., Deepmala, V., Singh, D.K. and Mahesh, C. 2010. Antidiabetic effect of *Morinda citrifolia* and *Coccinia indica* in alloxan induced diabetic rats. *Advances in Bio Research* 1:75–77.

Rashad, H., Metwally, F.M., Ezzat, S.M., Salama, M.M., Hasheesh, A. and Abdel Motaal, A. 2017. Randomized double-blinded pilot clinical study of the antidiabetic activity of *Balanites aegyptiaca* and UPLC-ESI-MS/MS identification of its metabolites. *Pharmaceutical Biology* 55:1954–1961. https://doi.org/ 10.1080/13880209.2017.1354388.

Reddy, G. and Rani, VS. 2020. Antidiabetic effect of methanolic extract of whole plant of *Lindernia ciliata* (Colsm.) Pennell. on streptozotocin induced diabetic rats. *International Journal of Pharmaceutical Sciences and Research* 11:660–668. https://doi.org/10.13040/IJPSR.0975-8232.11(2).660-68.

Saklani, A.K.A.N.K.S.H.A., Parcha, V.E.R.S.H.A., Dhulia, I.S.H.A.N. and Kumar, D.E.E.P.A.K. 2012. Combined effect of *Coccinia indica* (Wight & Arn) and *Salvadora oleoides* (Decne) on blood glucose level and other risk factors associated with type 2 diabetes mellitus in alloxan induced diabetic rats. *International Journal of Pharmacy and Pharmaceutical Sciences* 4:79–84.

Salehi, B., Ata, A., V Anil Kumar, N., Sharopov, F., Ramírez-Alarcón, K., Ruiz-Ortega, A., Abdulmajid Ayatollahi, S., Valere Tsouh Fokou, P., Kobarfard, F., Amiruddin Zakaria, Z. and Iriti, M. 2019. Antidiabetic potential of medicinal plants and their active components. *Biomolecules* 9:551 https://doi.org/10.3390/biom9100551.

Sangeetha, D.N. and Rajamani, S. 2019. In vitro antidiabetic activity of methanolic leaf extract of *Indianthus virgatus* (Roxb.) Suksathan and Borchs by glucose uptake method. *Pharmacognosy Journal* 11:674–677. https://doi.org/10.5530/pj.2019.11.106.

Shibib, B.A., Khan, L.A. and Rahman, R. 1993. Hypoglycemic activity of *Coccinia indica* and *Momordica charantia* in diabetic rats: depression of the hepatic gluconeogenic enzymes glucose-6-phosphatase and fructose-1, 6-bisphosphatase and elevation of both liver and red-cell shunt enzyme glucose-6-phosphate dehydrogenase. *Biochemical Journal* 292:267–270. https://doi.org/10.1042/bj2920267.

Singh, G., Gupta, P., Rawat, P., Puri, A., Bhatia, G. and Maurya, R. 2007. Antidyslipidemic activity of polyprenol from *Coccinia grandis* in high-fat diet-fed hamster model. *Phytomedicine* 14:792–798. https://doi. org/10.1016/j.phymed.2007.06.008.

Soltani, R., Gorji, A., Asgary, S., Sarrafzadegan, N. and Siavash, M. 2015. Evaluation of the effects of *Cornus mas* L. fruit extract on glycaemic control and insulin level in type 2 diabetic adult patients: A randomized double blind placebo controlled clinical trial. *Evidence-Based Complementary and Alternative Medicine* 2015. https://doi.org/10.1155/2015/740954.

Subba, A., Sahu, R.K., Bhardwaj, S. and Mandal, P. 2019. Alpha glucosidase inhibiting activity and in vivo antidiabetic activity of *Fraxinus floribunda* bark in streptozotocin-induced diabetic rats. *Pharmacognosy Research* 11:273–278. https://doi.org/10.4103/pr.pr3219.

Subbiah, V. PhytoMyco Research Corp. 2008. *Method and Composition for Management of Weight and Blood Sugar*. U.S. Patent Application 11/880,701.

Sunny, B., Mathews, M.M., Joseph, D., Mathew, F., George, J. and Varghese, B. 2020. Antihyperglycemic status of *Coccinia grandis*: An extensive overview. *Research Journal of Pharmacy and Technology* 13:1951–1956. https://doi.org/10.5958/0974-360X.2020.00351.0.

Suryawanshi, S.G., Shinde, K.R., Folane, P.N., Khedekar, S.L. and Sagrule, S.D. 2020. Antidiabetic activity of *Coccinia grandis* in alloxan induced diabetic rats. *European Journal of Pharmaceutical and Medical Research* 7:384–388. https://doi.org/10.7324/JAPS.2021.120103.

Tamilselvi, K., Ananad, S.P. and Doss, A. 2018. Evaluation of in vitro antidiabetic activity of *Gardenia Latifolia* Ait. *International Journal of Health Sciences and Research* 8:226–230.

Udayasankar, S. and Santhi, S. 2020. Docking studies on ligand molecules of *Coccinia indica* against human 5′-AMP-activated protein kinase catalytic subunit α-2 a diabetes mellitus. *International Journal of Scientific Research and Engineering Development* 3:617–623.

Umasankar, K. 2020. Studies on antidiabetic activity of *Atylosia Albicans* in streptozotocin-induced diabetic rats. *International Journal of Research in Pharmaceutical Sciences* 11:416–424. https://doi.org/10.26452/ijrps.v11i1.1836.

Venkateswaran, S. and Pari, L. 2002. Effect of *Coccinia indica* on blood glucose, insulin and key hepatic enzymes in experimental diabetes. *Pharmaceutical Biology* 40:165–170. https://doi.org/10.1076/phbi.40.3.165.5836.

Wasana, K.G.P., Attanayake, A.P., Jayatilaka, K.A.P.W. and Weerarathna, T.P. 2021c. Antidiabetic activity of widely used medicinal plants in the Sri Lankan traditional healthcare system: New insight to medicinal flora in Sri Lanka. Evidence-Based Complementary and Alternative Medicine. https://doi.org/10.1155/2021/6644004.

Wasana, K.G.P., Attanayake, A.P., Weerarathna, T.P. and Jayatilaka, K.A.P.W. 2021a. Efficacy and safety of a herbal drug of *Coccinia grandis* (Linn.) Voigt in patients with type 2 diabetes mellitus: A double blind randomized placebo controlled clinical trial. *Phytomedicine* 153431. https://doi.org/10.1016/j.phymed.2020.153431.

Wasana, K.G.P., Attanayake, A.P., Weeraratna, T.P. and Jayatilaka, K.A.P.W. 2021b. Effect of herbal drug *Coccinia grandis* (L.) on antioxidant status and inflammatory markers and their association with glycemic status in newly diagnosed patients with type 2 diabetes mellitus. *Paper presented at the research conference in Health Sciences*, Faculty of Allied Health Sciences University of Sri Jayewardenepura, Sri Lanka.

Yoshikawa, M., Murakami, T., Shimada, H., Matsuda, H., Yamahara, J., Tanabe, G. and Muraoka, O. 1997. Salacinol, potent antidiabetic principle with unique thiosugar sulfonium sulfate structure from the Ayurvedic traditional medicine *Salacia reticulata* in Sri Lanka and India. *Tetrahedron Letters* 38:8367–8370. https://doi.org/10.1016/S0040-4039(97)10270-2.

Section III

Resources

24 Recommended Resources on Diabetes in Relation to Foods, Plants, Herbs and Spices in Human Health

Rajkumar Rajendram, Daniel Gyamfi,
Vinood B. Patel and Victor R. Preedy

CONTENTS

24.1 INTRODUCTION

Diabetes is a chronic disease characterized by insufficient insulin or insensitivity to the activity of insulin. This results in hyperglycemia which is damaging to almost every organ. Diabetes is one of the most common causes of morbidity and mortality worldwide (Guo et al., 2012; World Health Organization, 2022). In the 21st century, the standard treatment of diabetes involves dietary modification and a mixture of medications to control blood glucose. However, some aspects of dietary modifications or restrictions are unpalatable and hypoglycemic medications may have side effects. As the prognosis of uncontrolled diabetes is poor, identifying safer, more effective, and better tolerated alternatives is therefore of paramount importance.

Several cultures use traditional concoctions derived from medicinal plants for the treatment of diabetes (Deutschländer et al., 2009; Grover, Yadav, and Vats, 2002; Li et al., 2004; Abo, Fred-Jaiyesimi, and Jaiyesimi, 2008). However, the scientific basis for the use of these traditional remedies is questioned by many physicians and researchers. Some researchers have extracted individual components from such remedies.

Critical evaluation of the potential benefits of plant-based extracts and nutraceuticals for the treatment of diabetes is required. The knowledge that ancient religious texts have recommended plant-based treatments for a range of ailments has driven the scientific study of these claims (Hossain et al., 2016). For example, the anti-diabetic activity of several metabolites derived from plants including polysaccharides and flavonoids has been investigated (Chen et al., 2015; Putta et al., 2016; Zheng et al., 2019).

Here we have presented resources to assist experienced researchers and clinicians to stay up to date. Those embarking on research into foods, plant-based extracts, or other compounds in human health can also be guided on where to begin their exploration by the tables containing suggested resources in this chapter. The list of acknowledgments below includes all the experts who helped to compile these valuable resources.

DOI: 10.1201/9781003220930-27

24.2   RESOURCES

Tables 24.1–24.5 list the most up-to-date information on the regulatory bodies (Table 24.1), professional societies (Table 24.2), books (Table 24.3), emerging technologies and platforms (Table 24.4), and other resources of interest (Table 24.5). Some organizations are listed in more than one table as they occasional fulfill multiple roles.

TABLE 24.1

Websites, Regulatory Bodies or Organizations Dealing with Foods, Plants, Herbs, Spices and Diabetes or Related Fields and Areas

Regulatory Body or Organization	Web Address
Academy of Cardiovascular Sciences	http://cardiovascularsciences.org/
Indian Section of International Academy of Cardiovascular Sciences	
Academy of Nutrition and Dietetics	www.eatrightpro.org/
Agricultural Biotechnology Research Center, Academia Sinica	https://abrc.sinica.edu.tw/en/
American Congress of Rehabilitation Medicine	https://acrm.org/
Botanical Safety Consortium	https://botanicalsafetyconsortium.org/
Centers for Disease Control and Prevention	www.cdc.gov/
China Academy of Chinese Medical Sciences	www.cacms.ac.cn/zykxyenglish/ zykxy_english_index.html
Chinese Academy of Sciences: Shanghai Institute of Materia Medica	http://english.simm.cas.cn/
Chinese Medicine Council of Hong Kong	www.cmchk.org.hk/index_en.html
Consortium for Globalization of Chinese Medicine (CGCM)	www.tcmedicine.org/
Council of Agriculture	https://eng.coa.gov.tw/
Development Center for Biotechnology	www.dcb.org.tw/
Diabetes Action Research and Education Foundation	https://diabetesaction.org/
Diabetes Australia	www.diabetesaustralia.com.au
Diabetes Malaysia	https://diabetesmalaysia.org.my/
Diabetes New Zealand	www.diabetes.org.nz/
Diabetes South Africa (DSA)	www.diabetessa.org.za/
DiabetesAtWork.org	http://diabetesatwork.org/
Diabetes.co.uk	www.diabetes.co.uk/
Diabetes UK	www.diabetes.org.uk/
European Commission Food Safety	https://ec.europa.eu/food/overview_en/
European Food Safety Authority (EFSA)	www.efsa.europa.eu/en
Food and Agriculture Organization of the United Nations (FAO)	www.fao.org/
Food with Health Claims, Food for Special Dietary Uses, and Nutrition Labeling, Japan	www.mhlw.go.jp/english/topics/ foodsafety/fhc/
HealthPartners Institute	www.healthpartners.com/
International Diabetes Foundation (IDF)	www.idf.org
Juvenile Diabetes Research Foundation	www.jdrf.org/
Linus Pauling Institute: Oregon State University	https://lpi.oregonstate.edu
Micronutrient Forum	https://micronutrientforum.org/
Ministry of Health and Welfare, Taiwan	www.mohw.gov.tw/mp-2.html
National Academy of Medicine	https://nam.edu/
National Agency for Food and Drug Administration and Control	www.nafdac.gov.ng
National Center for Complementary and Integrative Health (NCCIH)	www.nccih.nih.gov/
National Council of Asian Pacific Islander Physicians (AANHPI)	http://ncapip.org/
National Health and Medical Research Council (NHMRC), Australia	www.nhmrc.gov.au/
National Health Research Institutes, Taiwan	www.nhri.edu.tw/eng/

Regulatory Body or Organization	Web Address
National Health Service (NHS)	www.nhs.uk/
National Health Service (NHS) England	www.england.nhs.uk/
National Institute of Diabetes and Digestive and Kidney Diseases (NIDDK)	www.niddk.nih.gov/
National Institute on Aging	www.nia.nih.gov/
National Institutes of Health	www.nih.gov/
National Medical Products Administration, China	http://english.nmpa.gov.cn/
National Research Institute of Chinese Medicine, Taiwan	www.nricm.edu.tw/?Lang=en
Nestlé Nutrition Institute	https://nnia.nestlenutrition-institute.org/
Nutrition.gov: U.S. Department of Agriculture	www.nutrition.gov/
Office of Dietary Supplements: National Institutes of Health	https://ods.od.nih.gov/
Physicians Committee for Responsible Medicine	www.pcrm.org/
Sudan Diabetes Federation	https://sudandiabetes.org/
Swedish Nutrition Foundation	https://snf.ideon.se/
Taiwan Food and Drug Administration	www.fda.gov.tw/ENG/
Texas Health and Human Services	https://dshs.texas.gov/
United Nations System Standing Committee on Nutrition	www.unscn.org/
U.S. Department of Agriculture (USDA)	www.usda.gov/
World Diabetes Foundation	www.worlddiabetesfoundation.org/
World Food Safety Organization (WFSO)	https://worldfoodsafety.org/
World Health Organization (WHO)	www.who.int/

Note: This table lists the regulatory bodies and organizations involved with foods, plants, herbs, spices and diabetes in human health. Some of the links have indirect references to this topic. The links were accurate at the time of going to press but may move or alter. In these cases, the use of the search tabs should be explored at the parent address or site. In some cases, links direct the reader to pages related to biomarkers of trauma within parent sites. Some societies and organizations have a preference for shortened terms, such as acronyms and abbreviations. See also Table 24.2.

TABLE 24.2
Professional Societies Related to Foods, Plants, Herbs, Spices and Diabetes or Related Fields and Areas

Society Name	Web Address
American Diabetes Association	www.diabetes.org/
American Herbal Products Association	www.ahpa.org/
American Nutrition Association	https://theana.org/
American Society for Nutrition	https://nutrition.org
American Society for Parenteral and Enteral Nutrition	www.nutritioncare.org
Arabic Association for the Study of Diabetes and Metabolism	www.aasdonline.com/
Association of Diabetes Care and Education Specialists	www.diabeteseducator.org/
British Herbal Medicine Association	https://bhma.info/
Bulgarian Diabetes Association	https://badiabet.com/
Canadian Diabetes Association	www.diabetes.ca/
Canadian Nutrition Society	www.cns-scn.ca/
Chinese Nutrition Society	www.cnsoc.org/
Czech Society for Nutrition	www.vyzivaspol.cz/
Danish Nutrition Society	www.sfe.dk/dansk1
Diabetes Association of Nigeria	www.diabetesnigeria.org/

(Continued)

TABLE 24.2
(Continued)

Society Name	Web Address
Diabetes Association of the Republic of China (Taiwan)	www.endo-dm.org.tw/dia/english/
European Association for the Study of Diabetes (EASD)	www.easd.org/
European Society for Clinical Nutrition and Metabolism	www.espen.org/
Federation of African Nutrition Societies	http://fanus.org/
Federation of European Nutrition Societies	https://fensnutrition.org/
German Society for Nutritional Medicine	www.dgem.de
Hong Kong Nutrition Association	www.hkna.org.hk/
Humane Society International	www.hsi.org/
Indian Pharmacological Society	www.indianpharmacologicalsociety.org/
International American Association of Clinical Nutritionists	www.iaacn.org
International Association for Plant Taxonomy (IAPT)	www.iaptglobal.org/
International Confederation of Dietetic Associations (ICDA)	www.internationaldietetics.org/
International Union of Nutritional Sciences (IUNS)	https://iuns.org/
National Association of Diabetes Centres, Australia	https://nadc.net.au/
National Association of Nutrition Professionals	https://nanp.org/
Nutrition Society	www.nutritionsociety.org/
Physician Association for Nutrition	https://pan-int.org/
Society for Nutrition Education and Behavior	www.sneb.org/
Swiss Society for Nutrition	www.sfkn.se/
Universal Society of Food and Nutrition	www.usfn.net
World Federation of Chinese Medicine Societies	www.wfcms.org/en/

Note: This table lists the professional societies involved with foods, plants, herbs, spices and diabetes in human health. Some of the links have indirect references to this topic. The links were accurate at the time of going to press but may move or alter. In these cases, the use of the search tabs should be explored at the parent address or site. Some societies and organizations have a preference for shortened terms, such as acronyms and abbreviations.

TABLE 24.3
Books on Foods, Plants, Herbs, Spices and Diabetes or Related Fields and Areas

Book Title	Author(s) or Editor(s)	Publisher	Year of Publication
All-Natural Diabetes Cookbook: The Whole Food Approach to Great Taste and Healthy Eating	Newgent J	American Diabetes Association	2015
American Diabetes Association Vegetarian Cookbook: Satisfying, Bold, and Flavorful Recipes from the Garden	Petusevsky S	American Diabetes Association	2013
Anti-Diabetes and Anti-Obesity Medicinal Plants and Phytochemicals: Safety, Efficacy, and Action Mechanisms	Saad B, Zaid H, Shanak S, Kadan S	Springer	2017
Aromatic Herbs in Food: Bioactive Compounds, Processing, and Applications	Galanakis CM	Academic Press	2021
Benefits of the Mediterranean Diet in the Elderly Patient	Capurso A, Crepaldi G, Capurso C	Springer	2018
Bioactive Food as Dietary Interventions for Diabetes: Bioactive Foods in Chronic Disease States	Watson RR, Preedy VR	Academic Press	2012

Book Title	Author(s) or Editor(s)	Publisher	Year of Publication
Biotechnology of Anti-Diabetic Medicinal Plants	Gantait S, Verma SK, Sharangi AB	Springer Nature	2021
Botanical Medicine and Clinical Practice	Watson RR, Preedy VR	CABI Publishing	2008
Diabetes: Oxidative Stress and Dietary Antioxidants	Preedy VR	Elsevier	2013
Diabetes Comfort Food Diet Cookbook: 200 Delicious Dishes to Help You Lose Weight and Balance Blood Sugar	Cipullo L	Rodale	2015
Diabetes in Clinical Practice: Questions and Answers From Case Studies	Nikolaos K, Evanthia D, Ionnis I, Stavros L, Konstantinos M, Nicholas T, Panagiotis T	Wiley	2006
Diabetes in Clinical Practice	Fonseca V	Springer London Ltd	2009
Diabetes: How Food and Alcohol Affect Diabetes: The Most Important Information You Need to Improve Your Health	Adams Media	Adams Media	2012
Diabetes: Oxidative Stress and Dietary Antioxidants	Preedy VR	Academic Press	2013
Dictionary of Medicinal Plants	Sammbamurty AVSS, Bansal R	CBS Publishers and Distributors	2009
Food Labeling	Codex Alimentarius Commission FAO, WHO	Food and Agriculture Organization of the UN	2008
Functional Foods, Cardiovascular Disease and Diabetes	Arnoldi A	CRC Press	2004
Handbook of Herbal Formulations	Malviya S, Malviya N	CBS Publishers and Distributors	2021
Herbal Biomolecules in Healthcare Applications	Mandal SC, Nayak AK, Dhara AK	Academic Press	2021
Herbal Medicine: Biomolecular and Clinical Aspects, 2nd edition	Benzie IFF, Wachtel-Galor S	CRC Press	2011
Herbal Therapy for Diabetes. Volume 1	Khan IA, Khanum A	Ukaz Publications	2005
Herbs for Diabetes and Neurological Disease Management: Research and Advancements	Kumar V, Veeranjaneyulu A	Apple Academic Press, Inc.	2018
Indian Medicinal Plants, 2nd edition (8 volumes)	Kirtikar KR, Basu BD	Vedic Books	2012
Mastering Diabetes: The Revolutionary Method to Reverse Insulin Resistance Permanently in Type 1, Type 1.5, Type 2, Prediabetes, and Gestational Diabetes	Khambatta C, Barbaro R	Penguin Publishing Group	2020
Medicinal Foods as Potential Therapies for Type-2 Diabetes and Associated Diseases: The Chemical and Pharmacological Basis of Their Action	Habtemariam S	Academic Press	2019
Molecular Nutrition and Diabetes	Mauricio D	Elsevier	2015
New Beginnings: A Discussion Guide for Living Well With Diabetes	National Institutes of Health	National Institutes of Health	2005
New Soul Food Cookbook for People with Diabetes	Gaines FD, Weaver R	American Diabetes Association	2015
Nutraceuticals, Glycaemic Health, and Type 2 Diabetes	Pasupuleti VK, Anderson JW	John Wiley and Sons	2009
Nutrition and Immunology Principles and Practice	Gershwin ME, German JB, Keen CL	Humana Press	2000
Nutritional and Therapeutic Interventions for Diabetes and Metabolic Syndrome	Bagchi D, Nair S	Elsevier	2012

(Continued)

TABLE 24.3
(Continued)

Book Title	Author(s) or Editor(s)	Publisher	Year of Publication
Official Pocket Guide to Diabetic Food Choices	American Diabetes Association	American Diabetes Association	2015
Phytotherapy in the Management of Diabetes and Hypertension. Volume 3	Eddouks M	Bentham Science Publishers	2020
Plant-Based Functional Foods and Phytochemicals: From Traditional Knowledge to Present Innovation	Goyal MR, Nath A, Suleria HAR	Apple Academic Press	2021
Plants With Anti–Diabetes Mellitus Properties	Subramoniam A	CRC Press	2016
Role of Phenolic Phytochemicals in Diabetes Management: Phenolic Phytochemicals and Diabetes	Hoda M, Hemaiswarya S, Doble M	Springer	2019
Structure and Health Effects of Natural Products on Diabetes Mellitus	Chen H, Zhang M	Springer	2021
Treating Endocrine and Metabolic Disorders With Herbal Medicines	Hussain A, Behl S	IGI Global	2021
Understanding Diabetes	Bilous WR	Family Doctor Publications Ltd	2006

Note: This table lists books relevant to foods, plants, herbs, spices and diabetes in human health. Some authors have recommended culinary related text. These effectively allude to traditional and cultural practices related to food proration and the use of herbs and spices, although not necessarily in scientific terms.

TABLE 24.4

Emerging Techniques, Instruments, and Analytical Platforms or Devices for Investigating Foods, Plants, Herbs, Spices and Diabetes or Related Fields and Areas

Organization or Company Name	Web Address
Abbott	www.abbott.com/
Advanced Diabetes Supply (ADS)	www.northcoastmed.com/
Advion Interchim Scientific	www.advion.com/
Agilent Technologies	www.agilent.com/
BeatO Smart Glucometer	www.beatoapp.com/
BectonDickinson	www.bd.com/en-us
Bruker	www.bruker.com/en.html
CAMAG: Chromatography	www.camag.com/
Dexcom	www.dexcom.com/en-ZA
General Electric (GE): Healthcare	www.gehealthcare.com/
Hitachi High Tech	www.hitachi-hightech.com/global/
Jackson Laboratory	www.jax.org/jax-mice-and-services
Leica	https://leica-camera.com/en-int
Medtronic	www.medtronic.com/us-en/index.html
Nestlé Health Science	www.nestlehealthscience.com/
Novo Nordisk Global	www.novonordisk.com/our-products/smart-pens/novopen-6.html
Onedrop	https://onedrop.today/
PerkinElmer	www.perkinelmer.com/
Quality Phytochemicals	www.qualityphytochemicals.com/
Sepiatec: Separation Systems	www.sepiatec.com/

Organization or Company Name	Web Address
Tandem Diabetes Care	www.tandemdiabetes.com/products/t-slim-x2-insulin-pump/control-iq
Thermo Fisher Scientific	www.thermofisher.com
Waters Corporation	www.waters.com/nextgen/us/en.html
ZOE: In-Depth Nutrition	https://joinzoe.com/

Note: This table lists technologies or platforms relevant to foods, plants, herbs, spices and diabetes in human health. Please note, occasionally the location of the websites or web address changes.

TABLE 24.5

Other Resources of Interest or Relevance for Health Care Professionals or Patients Related to Foods, Plants, Herbs, Spices and Diabetes or Related Fields and Areas

Name of Resource or Organization	Web Address
American Type Culture Collection (ATCC)	www.atcc.org/
Australian Regulatory Guidelines for Listed Medicines and Registered Complementary Medicines	www.tga.gov.au/publication/ australian-regulatory-guidelines-listed-medicines-and-registered-complementary-medicines
Ayurvedic Pharmacopoeia of India: Department of Ayush, Government of India	www.ayurveda.hu/api/API-Vol-2.pdf
Center for Advanced Functional Foods Research and Entrepreneurship: Ohio State University	https://u.osu.edu/caffre/
Centers for Disease Control and Prevention: Diabetes Self-Management Education and Support (BSMES)	www.cdc.gov/diabetes/dsmes-toolkit/index.html
ChemFaces	www.chemfaces.com/compound/index.php
Chinese Medicine Development Fund	www.cmresource.hk/main.php
Diabetes Action Research and Education Foundation: Medicinal Plants and Herbs for Diabetes	https://diabetesaction.org/medicinal-plants-and-herbs
Diabetes Diet: Mayo Clinic	www.mayoclinic.org/diseases-conditions/diabetes/ in-depth/diabetes-diet/art-20044295
Diabetes.co.uk: Herbal and Natural Therapies	www.diabetes.co.uk/Diabetes-herbal.html
Diabetes UK: Spice Up Your Seasoning	www.diabetes.org.uk/guide-to-diabetes/enjoy-food/ cooking-for-people-with-diabetes/getting-started/ spice-up-your-seasoning
European Federation of Pharmaceutical Industries and Associations: Working With Patient Groups	www.efpia.eu/relationships-code/patient-organisations/
European Food Safety Authority: Material on Botanicals	www.efsa.europa.eu/en/topics/topic/botanicals
Extrasynthese	www.extrasynthese.com/
FLAVEX Naturextrakte	www.flavex.com/en/
Global Plants Database	https://plants.jstor.org/
HealthPartners Institute: International Diabetes Center	www.healthpartners.com/institute/centers/ international-diabetes-center/
Heart and Stroke Foundation, South Africa	www.heartfoundation.co.za/
Institute of Himalayan Bioresource Technology	www.ihbt.res.in/en/research2/biotechnology
International Plant Name Index	www.ipni.org/
Joslin Diabetes Center	www.joslin.org/
KingNet	www.kingnet.com.tw/tcm/
Micronutrient Information Center: Oregon State University	https://lpi.oregonstate.edu/mic

(Continued)

TABLE 24.5
(Continued)

Name of Resource or Organization	Web Address
National Agricultural Library	www.nal.usda.gov/
National Center for Complementary and Integrative Health: Clinical Practice Guidelines	www.nccih.nih.gov/health/providers/clinicalpractice
National Center for Complementary and Integrative Health: Resources for Health Care Providers	www.nccih.nih.gov/health/providers
National Center for Natural Products Research: The University of Mississippi	https://pharmacy.olemiss.edu/ncnpr/research-programs/medicinal-plant-research/
National Council of Asian Pacific Islander Physicians (AANHPI): Diabetes Coalition	http://ncapip.org/diabetes/AANHPIDC/index.html
National Diabetes Centre	https://national-diabetes-centre.business.site/
National Diabetes Institute: Complementary and Alternative Medicine	www.diabetes.gov/about-diabetes/treatment/cam
National Institute of Diabetes and Digestive and Kidney Diseases: Diabetes	www.niddk.nih.gov/health-information/diabetes
National Institute of Neurological Disorders and Stroke: Patient Organizations	www.ninds.nih.gov/disorders/support-resources/patient-organizations
National Laboratory Animal Center	www.nlac.narl.org.tw/eng/index.asp
Natural and Non-Prescription Health Products Directorate: Government of Canada	www.canada.ca/en/health-canada/corporate/about-health-canada/branches-agencies/health-products-food-branch/natural-non-prescription-health-products-directorate.html
Natural Health Products Regulations: Government of Canada	https://laws-lois.justice.gc.ca/eng/regulations/SOR-2003-196/page-1.html
Oldways: Cultural Food Traditions	https://oldwayspt.org/
Pan American Health Organization (PAHO)	www.paho.org/
Parkinson's UK	www.parkinsons.org.uk/
Physicians Committee for Responsible Medicine: Tackle Diabetes With a Plant-Based Diet	www.pcrm.org/health-topics/diabetes
Plant Identification. University of Massachusetts	https://extension.umass.edu/plant-identification/common/all
Pure Health Dieticians	https://purehealthdieticians.co.za/
Regulatory Frameworks for Nutraceuticals: Australia, Canada, Japan, and the United States	https://pubmed.ncbi.nlm.nih.gov/34345505/
Regulatory Frameworks for Nutraceuticals: Different Countries of the World	https://pubmed.ncbi.nlm.nih.gov/32427089/
Stamford Health: 10 Natural Home Remedies for Type 2 Diabetes	www.stamfordhealth.org/healthflash-blog/integrative-medicine/type-2-diabetes-natural-remedies/
Tang Center for Herbal Medicine Research: University of Chicago	www.uchicago.edu/education-and-research/center/tang_center_for_herbal_medicine_research/
Texas Health and Human Services: Texas Diabetes Council	https://dshs.texas.gov/txdiabetes/tdc/
The Global Biodiversity Information Facility	www.gbif.org/
The Patients Association	www.patients-association.org.uk/
The Plant List	www.theplantlist.org/
Tokiwa Phytochemical	www.tokiwaph.co.jp/en/
UMass Amherst Plant Identification	https://extension.umass.edu/plant-identification/
UniProt Taxonomy	www.uniprot.org/taxonomy/
WebMD	www.webmd.com/
World Flora Online	www.worldfloraonline.org/

Name of Resource or Organization	Web Address
World Health Organization: International Regulatory Cooperation for Herbal Medicines (IRCH)	www.who.int/initiatives/international-regulatory-cooperation-for-herbal-medicines#:~:text=International%20Regulatory%20Cooperation%20for%20Herbal%20Medicines%20(IRCH)%20is%20a%20global,improved%20regulation%20for%20herbal%20medicines
World Health Organization: Healthy Diet	www.who.int/news-room/fact-sheets/detail/healthy-diet
World Health Organization: Nutrition	www.who.int/health-topics/nutrition
WHO Global Report on Traditional and Complementary Medicine 2019	https://apps.who.int/iris/bitstream/handle/10665/312342/9789241515436-eng.pdf?sequence=1&isAllowed=y

Note: This table lists other resources of interest or relevance to foods, plants, herbs, spices and diabetes in human health. Please note, occasionally the location of the websites or web address changes.

24.3 OTHER RESOURCES

The Wellcome Collection (https://wellcomecollection.org/collections) and The British Library (www.bl.uk/) also hold material on topics related to traditional foods, plants-based extracts, and the study of diabetes.

Other chapters on resources relevant to nutrition and cardiovascular disease (recommended by authors and practitioners) have been published previously (Alzaid et al., 2015; Rajendram, Patel, and Preedy, 2014, 2015, 2019a, 2019b, 2020, 2022a, 2022b; Rajendram et al., 2013a, 2013b).

The material in these tables is included to provide general information only. It does not constitute any recommendation or endorsement of the activities of these sites, facilities, or other resources listed in this chapter, by the authors or editors of this book.

24.4 SUMMARY POINTS

Diabetes is one of the most common causes of morbidity and mortality worldwide.

The use and study of traditional remedies for the treatment of diabetes is widespread in many cultures.

The scientific rationale for the use of traditional remedies for the treatment of diabetes must be established.

The study of natural remedies has gained tremendous importance as sources of drugs for the treatment of diabetes.

This chapter lists resources relevant to the foods, plants, herbs, and spices used to treat diabetes.

24.5 ACKNOWLEDGMENTS

We thank the following authors for their contributions to the development of this resource. We apologize if some of the suggested material was not included in this chapter or has been moved to different sections. Names are listed in alphabetical order.

Agatonovic-Kustrin, Snezana
Chan, Sze Wa
Islam, Md. Shahidul
Liu, Hui-Kang
Mahanty, Biswanath
Ray Mohanty, Ipseeta

REFERENCES

Abo, K., Fred-Jaiyesimi, A., Jaiyesimi, A. Ethnobotanical studies of medicinal plants used in the management of diabetes mellitus in South Western Nigeria. *J. Ethnopharmacol.* 2008, 115, 67–71.

Alzaid, F., Rajendram, R., Patel, V.B., Preedy, V.R. Expanding the knowledge base in Diet, Nutrition and critical care. Electronic and published resources. In Rajendram, R., Preedy, V.R., Patel, V.B. (Editors). *Diet and Nutrition in Critical Care.* Springer, Berlin, Germany, 2015.

Chen, J., Mangelinckx, S., Adams, A., Wang, Z.-T., Li, W.-L., De Kimpe, N. Natural flavonoids as potential herbal medication for the treatment of diabetes mellitus and its complications. *Nat. Prod. Commun.* 2015, 10, 187–200.

Deutschländer, M., Lall, N., Van De Venter, M. Plant species used in the treatment of diabetes by South African traditional healers: An inventory. *Pharm. Biol.* 2009, 47, 348–365.

Grover, J., Yadav, S., Vats, V. Medicinal plants of India with anti-diabetic potential. *J. Ethnopharmacol.* 2002, 81, 81–100.

Guo, X., Li, H., Xu, H., Woo, S., Dong, H., Lu, F., Lange, A.J., Wu, C. Glycolysis in the control of blood glucose homeostasis. *Acta Pharm. Sinica B.* 2012, 2, 358–367.

Hossain, M. S., Urbi, Z., Evamoni, F. Z., Zohora, F. T., and Rahman, K.M.H. A secondary research on medicinal plants mentioned in the Holy Qur'an. *J. Med. Plants.* 2016, 3(59), 81–97.

Li, W., Zheng, H., Bukuru, J., De Kimpe, N. Natural medicines used in the traditional Chinese medical system for therapy of diabetes mellitus. *J. Ethnopharmacol.* 2004, 92, 1–21.

Putta, S., Sastry Yarla, N., Kumar Kilari, E., Surekha, C., Aliev, G., Basavaraju Divakara, M., Sridhar Santosh, M., Ramu, R., Zameer, F., Prasad, M. Therapeutic potentials of triterpenes in diabetes and its associated complications. *Curr. Topics Med. Chem.* 2016, 16, 2532–2542.

Rajendram, R., Gyamfi, D., Patel, V.B., Preedy, V.R. Recommended resources for biomarkers of nutrition. In Preedy, V.R. and Patel, V.B. (Editors). *Biomarkers of Nutrition.* Elsevier, New York, 2022a.

Rajendram, R., Gyamfi, D., Patel, V.B., Preedy, V.R. Recommended resources for Biomarkers in diabetes: Methods, discoveries, and applications. In: Patel, V.B., Preedy, V.R. (Editors). *Biomarkers in Diabetes. Biomarkers in Disease: Methods, Discoveries and Applications.* Springer, Cham, 2022b. https://doi.org/10.1007/978-3-030-81303-1_58-2

Rajendram, R., Patel, V.B., Preedy, V.R. Web based resources and suggested reading. In Rajendram, R., Patel, V.B., Preedy, V.R. (Editors). *Glutamine in Health and Disease.* (pp. 527–532). Springer, New York, 2014.

Rajendram, R., Patel, V.B., Preedy, V.R. Web based resources and suggested reading. In Rajendram, R., Patel, V.B., Preedy, V.R. (Editors). *Branched Chain Amino Acids in Health and Disease.* Springer, New York, 2015.

Rajendram, R., Patel, V.B., Preedy, V.R. Recommended resources on maternal nutrition. In Rajendram, R., Patel, V.B., Preedy, V.R. (Editors). *Nutrition and Diet in Maternal Diabetes* (pp. 495–500). Springer, New York, 2017.

Rajendram, R., Patel, V.B., Preedy, V.R. Resources in famine, starvation, and nutrient deprivation. In Patel, V.B., Preedy, V.R. (Editors). *Famine, Starvation, and Nutrient Deprivation* (pp. 2399–2406). Springer, New York, 2019a.

Rajendram, R., Patel, V.B., Preedy, V.R. Resources in diet, nutrition and epigenetics. In Patel, V.B., Preedy, V.R. (Editors). *Nutrition and Epigenetics* (pp. 2309–2314). Springer, New York City, 2019b.

Rajendram, R., Patel, V.B., Preedy, V.R. Recommended resources for nutrition, oxidative stress, and dietary antioxidants. In Martin, C.R., Preedy, V.R. (Editor). *Nutrition, Oxidative Stress, and Dietary Antioxidants* (pp. 393–397). Elsevier, New York, 2020.

Rajendram, R., Rajendram, R., Patel, V.B., Preedy, V.R. Interlinking diet, nutrition, the menopause and recommended resources. In Hollins-Martin, C.J., Watson, R.R., Preedy, V.R. (Editors). *Nutrition and Diet in Menopause.* Springer, Berlin, Germany, 2013a.

Rajendram, R., Rajendram, R., Patel, V.B., Preedy, V.R. Diet quality: What more is there to know? In Preedy, V.R., Hunter, L.-A., Patel, V.B. (Editors). *Diet Quality: An Evidence-Based Approach* (pp. 397–401). Springer, Berlin, Germany, 2013b.

World Health Organization. *Fact Sheet,* 16 September 2022. Available online: www.who.int/news-room/factsheets/detail/diabetes (accessed on 10 October 2022).

Zheng, Y., Bai, L., Zhou, Y., Tong, R., Zeng, M., Shi, J., Lib, X. Polysaccharides from Chinese herbal medicine for anti-diabetes recent advances. *Int. J. Biol. Macromol.* 2019, 121, 1240–1253.

Index

Note: **Boldface** page references indicate tables. *Italic* references indicate figures.

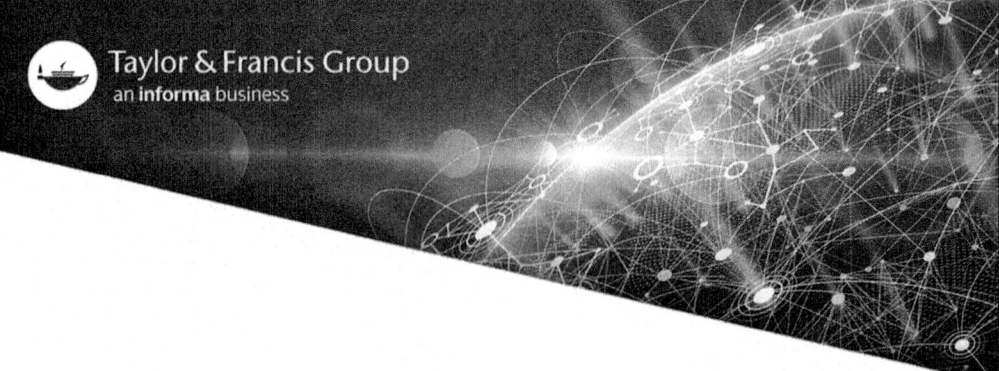
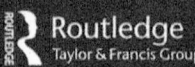
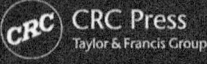